Mental Disorders in the Classical World

Columbia Studies in the Classical Tradition

VOLUME 38

The titles published in this series are listed at brill.com/csct

Mental Disorders in
the Classical World

Edited by

W.V. Harris

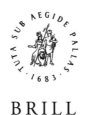

BRILL

LEIDEN · BOSTON
2013

Cover illustration: Detail of Galen from the title-page of 'Herbarius. Kreüterbuch von neüwem mit höstem fleiss durch sucht und gebessert', Strasbourg: Balthasar Beck, 1527. Woodcut and letterpress. © Trustees of the British Museum.

Library of Congress Cataloging-in-Publication Data

Mental disorders in the classical world / edited by W.V. Harris.
    pages cm. – (Columbia studies in the classical tradition, ISSN 0166-1302 ; volume 38)
    Includes bibliographical references and index.
    ISBN 978-90-04-24982-0 (hardback : alk. paper) – ISBN 978-90-04-24987-5 (e-book) 1. Mental illness. 2. Mental illness–History. I. Harris, William V. (William Vernon) editor of compilation.

RC438.M46 2013
    616.89–dc23

2013000782

This publication has been typeset in the multilingual "Brill" typeface. With over 5,100 characters covering Latin, IPA, Greek, and Cyrillic, this typeface is especially suitable for use in the humanities. For more information, please see www.brill.com/brill-typeface.

ISSN 0166-1302
ISBN 978-90-04-24982-0 (hardback)
ISBN 978-90-04-24987-5 (e-book)

This book is printed on acid-free paper.

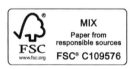

Printed by Printforce, the Netherlands

CONTENTS

PART III

PARTICULAR SYNDROMES

PART IV

SYMPTOMS, CURES AND THERAPY

PART V

FROM HOMER TO ATTIC TRAGEDY

PART VI

MENTAL DISORDERS AND RESPONSIBILITY

PART VII

A ROMAN CODA

ACKNOWLEDGEMENTS

This volume addresses a large problem of cultural, medical, social and intellectual history that is explained in Chapter I. I would not have been able to organize this interdisciplinary response to the problem at hand had it not been for the fortuitous and generous gift of an Andrew W. Mellon Distinguished Achievement Award in 2008. That allowed me to organize two conferences in 2010 under the title "Mental Disorders in the Classical World: Concepts, Diagnosis and Treatment" at Columbia's Center for the Ancient Mediterranean. I believe that others too found those meetings stimulating, and I wish to thank the distinguished scholars who agreed to take part in what was for me one of the most exhilarating intellectual experiences of my professional life.

I wish to thank Bennett Simon, Glenn Most (once again) and Chiara Thumiger for timely advice during the process of editing this collection. And a number of people besides the contributors deserve especial thanks for their roles in bringing this volume to completion. In particular, three Columbia graduate students played important roles, Molly Allen, who was Coordinator of the Center for the Ancient Mediterranean in 2010, Anne Hunnell Chen and Emily Cook. The last two were successively my research assistants in the period in question, and labored hard to help get the manuscript into shape. I also wish to thank Caroline Wazer most warmly for her work on translating Jacques Jouanna's paper. Finally, I should like to express my regret that my former student Alissa Gafford Abrams was prevented by ill health from completing her paper on madness in Athenian law.

W.V. Harris
New York

NOTES ON CONTRIBUTORS

Véronique Boudon-Millot is the Director of Research on Ancient Medicine at the CNRS at the Sorbonne. She has published extensively on ancient medicine, philosophy and science and has written critical essays on six of Galen's works, which have been published in the Collection des Universités de France. She is also the co-editor of *Les Pères de l'Eglise face à la science médicale de leur temps* (Paris, 2005), *La science médicale antique: nouveaux regards* (Paris, 2007), and *René Chartier, éditeur et traducteur d'Hippocrate et Galien* (Paris, 2012), among other works. She has just published a biography of Galen (Paris, 2012).

Christopher Gill is Professor of Ancient Thought at the University of Exeter. His work is centered on psychology and ethics in Greek and Roman thought, especially ideas about personality and self. He is the author of *Personality in Greek Epic, Tragedy, and Philosophy: The Self in Dialogue* (1996), *The Structured Self in Hellenistic and Roman Thought* (2006), and *Naturalistic Psychology in Galen and Stoicism* (2010). He has edited several volumes, including *The Person and the Human Mind: Issues in Ancient and Modern Philosophy* (1996) and *Virtue, Norms, and Objectivity: Issues in Ancient and Modern Ethics* (2005) (all published by Oxford University Press).

W.V. Harris teaches history at Columbia University and directs its Center for the Ancient Mediterranean. He is the author of *Restraining Rage: the Ideology of Anger-Control in Classical Antiquity* (2002), *Dreams and Experience in Classical Antiquity* (2009), and *Rome's Imperial Economy* (2011). He is currently working on a book about Roman power, 400 BC to 650 AD, as well as on mental disorders in the Greek and Roman worlds.

Brooke Holmes is an Associate Professor in the Department of Classics at Princeton University, working at the intersection of literature, the history of medicine and science, and the history of philosophy. Her first book, *The Symptom and the Subject: The Emergence of the Physical Body in Ancient Greece* was published by Princeton in 2010, and a second book, *Gender: Antiquity and Its Legacy* (I.B. Tauris and OUP) appeared in 2012. She has also co-edited two volumes: *Aelius Aristides between Greece, Rome, and the Gods* (Leiden: Brill, 2008), and *Dynamic Reading: Studies in the Reception of Epicureanism* (New York: OUP, 2012).

Julian Hughes is a consultant in old age psychiatry at North Tyneside General Hospital and honorary professor of philosophy of ageing at the Institute for Ageing and Health in Newcastle University, UK. His research is in the fields of ethics and philosophy in connection with dementia and ageing. He previously chaired the Philosophy Special Interest Group of the Royal College of Psychiatrists. He served on the working party of the Nuffield Council on Bioethics which produced *Dementia: Ethical Issues*. His most recent books, both published by Oxford University Press in 2011, were *Thinking Through Dementia* and *Alzheimer's and Other Dementias*.

Jacques Jouanna is a Member of the Institut de France (Académie des Inscriptions et Belles-Lettres) and Professor Emeritus of Greek at the Université de Paris-Sorbonne, where he taught from 1981 to 2004 and where he founded and directed the CNRS 'Groupe Médecine grecque'. His publications include *Hippocrate. Pour une archéologie de l'école de Cnide* (1975), *Hippocrate* (1992, Engl. tr. 1999), *Sophocle* (2007), and numerous critical editions of Hippocratic and Galenic medical texts. See also *Greek Medicine from Hippocrates to Galen. Selected Papers* (Leiden: Brill, 2012).

George Kazantzidis has recently completed a doctoral thesis entitled 'Melancholy in Hellenistic and Latin Poetry: Medical Readings in Menander, Apollonius Rhodius, Lucretius and Horace' (Oxford, 2011). He is currently a Junior Research Associate at the Department of Classics, Oxford University, working for the project 'The Social and Cultural Construction of Emotions: The Greek Paradigm' (funded by the European Research Council). Articles on madness in New Comedy and the Hellenistic poets and on the idea of disease as a closural device in Latin poetry are forthcoming.

Helen King is the Professor of Classical Studies at the Open University, and a Visiting Professor at the Peninsula Medical and Dental School, Truro. Following a first degree in Ancient History and Social Anthropology at UCL, she has specialised in ancient medicine and its reception up to the nineteenth century, focusing in particular on gynaecology and obstetrics in the Renaissance, and has published seven books. A former Fellow of the Netherlands Institute of Advanced Studies, she has also held visiting positions at Sackville, New Brunswick; University of Victoria, British Columbia; and the University of Texas. She is committed to public engagement.

David Konstan is Professor of Classics at New York University, and Emeritus Professor of Classics and Comparative Literature at Brown University.

Among his publications are *Sexual Symmetry: Love in the Ancient Novel and Related Genres* (1994), *Greek Comedy and Ideology* (1995), *Friendship in the Classical World* (1997), *Pity Transformed* (2001), *The Emotions of the Ancient Greeks: Studies in Aristotle and Classical Literature* (2006), *"A Life Worthy of the Gods": The Materialist Psychology of Epicurus* (2008), and *Before Forgiveness: The Origins of a Moral Idea* (2010). He is currently working on a book on the idea of beauty in classical antiquity.

Roberto Lo Presti received his doctorate in Classical Philology in 2008 from the University of Palermo. He subsequently held a Post-doc Research Fellowship at the University of Palermo (2008–2010) and various visiting scholarships from the Fondation Hardt, the Scaliger Institute of Leiden University Library, the Universities of Paris IV-Sorbonne, Newcastle, Leiden and Lausanne and the Descartes Centre for the History and Philosophy of the Sciences of Utrecht University (2010). Since 2010 he has been a lecturer at the Humboldt University in Berlin, within Prof. Philip van der Eijk's research programme "Medicine of the Mind, Philosophy of the Body".

Glenn W. Most has taught at Yale, Princeton, Michigan, Siena, Innsbruck, and Heidelberg. Since 2001 he has been Professor of Greek Philology at the Scuola Normale Superiore di Pisa, and since 1996 he has been a visiting Professor on the Committee on Social Thought at the University of Chicago. He has published numerous books and articles on ancient and modern literature and philosophy, the history and methodology of Classical studies, comparative literature, cultural studies, the history of religion, literary theory, and the history of art. Most recently he has co-edited a one-volume companion to the Classical tradition, and, among current projects, he is co-editing a four-volume Loeb edition of the Presocratic philosophers.

Vivian Nutton is professor emeritus of the history of medicine at University College London, and a fellow of the British Academy and the German Academy of Sciences. He has worked extensively on the classical tradition in medicine from Antiquity to the Renaissance, with a particular interest in Galen. His edition of Galen's *On Problematical Movements* appeared in 2011, and his translation and commentary on his *Avoiding Distress* in 2012. He is at present preparing a study of the renaissance anatomist Vesalius.

Peter E. Pormann is Professor of Classics and Graeco-Arabic Studies at the University of Manchester. After studying Classics, Islamic Studies, and French at Paris (Sorbonne), Hamburg, Tübingen, Leiden, and Oxford (Corpus Christi College), he obtained his D.Phil. with a thesis on Paul of Aegina's *Pragmateía* (or medical handbook); it won the Hellenic Foundation's 2003 Award and was published by Brill as a monograph in 2004. His recent publications include *Islamic Medical and Scientific Tradition, Critical Concepts in Islamic Studies*, 4 vols (London: Routledge 2011), *Epidemics in Context* (Berlin: De Gruyter 2012), and, with Peter Adamson, *The Philosophical Works of al-Kindī* (OUP 2012). He is Principal Investigator on the ERC-funded project 'Arabic Commentaries on the Hippocratic Aphorisms' (2012–2017).

Suzanne Saïd is professor emeritus at Columbia University and at Paris X—Nanterre. Her books include *La faute tragique* (1978), *Sophiste et Tyran ou le Prométhée enchaîné* (1985), *Approches de la mythologie grecque* (1993, new edition 2008)), *Histoire de la littérature grecque* (together with M. Trédé-Boulmer and A. Le Boulluec) (1997), *Homer and the Odyssey* (OUP 2012). She has published extensively on Homer, Greek tragedy, Aristophanes, Herodotus, Thucydides, Isocrates, the Greek novel, Plutarch and Lucian, She is also interested in the reception of ancient texts (especially Homer and Greek tragedy). She is currently working on a book on myth and historiography.

Maria Michela Sassi studied Classics at the Scuola Normale Superiore, Pisa, and is currently Professor at Pisa University, where she teaches the History of Ancient Philosophy. Her publications, ranging from early and classical Greek philosophy and science to anthropology, from history to methodology of classical studies, include such books as *The Science of Man in Ancient Greece* (Chicago University Press, 2001) and *Gli inizi della filosofia: in Grecia* (Turin: Bollati Boringhieri, 2009), and a number of essays in both Italian and international journals.

Bennett Simon, psychiatrist and psychoanalyst, has retired from private practice, and is now working part-time as a general psychiatrist and consultant in an underserved area of Massachusetts. His professional career has always involved inter-disciplinary work, including connecting the study of antiquity with contemporary concerns in psychiatry. He is Clinical Professor of Psychiatry at Harvard Medical School (Cambridge Health Alliance) and Training and Supervising Analyst at the Boston Psychoanalytic Society and Institute. He is the author of *Mind and Madness in Ancient Greece* (1978), and *Tragic Drama and the Family* (1988), and he has co-authored three books, including *Ritual and Its Consequences* (2010).

Chiara Thumiger is a research associate at the Humboldt Universität (Berlin) within the Alexander von Humboldt Professorship Project 'Medicine of the Mind—Philosophy of the Body'. She has previously worked on the representation of self and mental facts in literary sources (especially tragedy) and published variously about tragedy (in particular, a monograph on Euripides' *Bacchae, Hidden paths*, London, 2007). She is now preparing a monograph on insanity in ancient medicine and non-medical literature, with a focus on fifth- and early fourth-century medical texts.

Jerry Toner is a Fellow and Tutor and Director of Studies in Classics at Hughes Hall, University of Cambridge. His books include *Leisure and Ancient Rome* (London: Polity, 1995), *Popular Culture in Ancient Rome* (Polity, 2009), *Roman Disasters* (Polity, forthcoming 2013) and *Homer's Turk: How Classics Shaped Ideas of the East* (Harvard University Press, forthcoming 2013).

Peter Toohey is a Professor of Classics at the University of Calgary. He was educated in Canada and in his native Australia where he taught for many years at the University of New England. His most recent books are *Boredom: A Lively History* (New Haven: Yale University Press, 2012) and *Melancholy, Love, and Time: Boundaries of the Self in Ancient Literature* (Ann Arbor: University of Michigan Press, 2004).

Philip van der Eijk is Alexander von Humboldt Professor of Classics and History of Science at the Humboldt Universität zu Berlin. He has research interests in ancient medicine, philosophy and science, comparative literature and patristics. Among his publications are *Medicine and Philosophy in Classical Antiquity: Doctors and Philosophers on Nature, Soul, Health and Disease* (Cambridge, 2005), *Diocles of Carystus* (Leiden, 2000–2001), *Philoponus: On Aristotle On the Soul I* (London, 2005–2006), *Aristoteles: De insomniis, De divinatione per somnum* (Berlin, 1994) and (with R.W. Sharples) *Nemesius: On the Nature of Man* (Liverpool, 2008).

Katja Maria Vogt is a Professor of Philosophy at Columbia University and Chair of the Classical Studies graduate program. She specializes in ancient philosophy and ethics. Her first book, *Skepsis und Lebenspraxis* (1998), discusses skeptical belief, language, and action. In her second book, *Law, Reason, and the Cosmic City* (2008), Vogt reconstructs Stoic ethics. Her most recent book, *Belief and Truth* (2012), explores the Socratic commitment to an examined life in Plato and Hellenistic epistemology. Her next project, *Desiring the Good*, applies this Socratic-skeptic perspective to questions of motivation and agency.

ABBREVIATIONS

References to ancient authors follow the conventions of the *Oxford Latin Dictionary*, the *Oxford Classical Dictionary*, or LSJ, or the eccentricities of the individual contributors.

AJPsy   *American Journal of Psychiatry*
ANRW *Aufstieg und Niedergang der römischen Welt*, ed. W. Haase and H. Temporini
CMG   *Corpus Medicorum Graecorum*
CQ   *Classical Quarterly*
Dig.   *Digesta*, ed. T. Mommsen, transl. A. Watson et al.
DSM   *Diagnostic and Statistical Manual of Mental Disorders* (American Psychiatric Association)
ICD   *International Statistical Classification of Diseases and Related Health Problems* (World Health Organization)
JRS   *Journal of Roman Studies*
LIMC *Lexicon Iconographicum Mythologiae Classicae*
LSJ   Liddell, Scott, Jones, *Greek-English Lexicon* (ninth edition)
OED   *Oxford English Dictionary*
OSAP *Oxford Studies in Ancient Philosophy*
P.Oxy. *Oxyrhynchus Papyri*
QUCC *Quaderni Urbinati di Cultura Classica*
SVF   *Stoicorum Veterum Fragmenta*, ed. H. von Arnim

THINKING ABOUT MENTAL
DISORDERS IN CLASSICAL ANTIQUITY

W.V. Harris

This book is a work of historical scholarship which also touches on a highly fraught scientific, and also social, mega-problem—the conceptualization, diagnosis and treatment of mental disorders. It attempts to span both history and psychiatry, though not in equal depth. Its authors, whether scholars or scientists, operate with contemporary concepts and knowledge, but they concern themselves with the background and the foundations of those concepts and that knowledge. Starting with the Greeks, they raise far-reaching questions about ways of detecting, classifying and treating mental disorders, and about the nature of mental illness and madness.

No one suggests here that the ancients devised more accurate or more serviceable diagnostic categories than the ones that are used now. It may be salutary, however, for all who are concerned with the history or the practice of psychiatry to consider how some of the best ancient minds perceived mental illness and madness (and the ancients' avoidance of what has been called 'nosologorrhea', the tendency to multiply to excess the number of recognized syndromes, has something to recommend it).[1] All the more so, since modern medicine, though it displaced the medicine of Hippocrates and Galen, also grew out of it. The aim is to speak intelligibly—and indeed persuasively—to mental health professionals concerned about the foundations and current state of modern psychiatry as well as to historians and classicists.

---

[1] Greek has a profusion of words to refer to abnormal mental states and the behaviour that goes with them (Padel 1995, 22; Thumiger this volume), but until at least the second century AD quite a small number of names for actual mental disorders. Some medical writers were aware that their terminology had to cover multiple phenomena: Aretaeus of Cappadocia begins his discussion of *mania* by saying that 'the ways of madness are myriad in form, though they all belong to a single *genos*' (*On Chronic Diseases* 1.6). Aetius also wrote (*Iatrika* 6.8) that 'the forms of *mania* are myriad', but few modern people would agree with his opinion that 'it would be excessive to describe them all'.

Fundamental questions about what constitutes mental illness and mental disorders more generally, and how to treat their victims, have never been more pressing. The whole edifice of modern psychiatric medicine, while not built on sand, stands in a highly seismic zone. Definition and diagnosis are a large part of the problem. The current strife surrounding the not-yet-completed fifth edition of the DSM—the *Diagnostic and Statistical Manual* of the American Psychiatric Association[2]—has gone far beyond the sort of dispute that can commonly be encountered in scientific and scholarly fields. The other standard reference work is the equally problematic *International Statistical Classification of Diseases and Related Health Problems*, commonly known as the ICD, which went into its tenth edition in 1992 (ICD-10), and has not been brought up to date. What most hinders the revision of the DSM, as far as a non-psychiatrist can tell, is disagreement about eminently practical matters, but there are undoubtedly deep theoretical disagreements at work too.

Meanwhile the (U.S.) National Institute of Mental Health has begun to create a rival classification entitled 'Research Domain Criteria' (RDoC).[3] This is a readily intelligible response to the perceived need to correlate the latest developments both in brain-scanning and in genetics with the clinical observation of mental disorders. The exponents of this new project candidly observe that existing categories 'have not been predictive of treatment response'.[4] They also note that their project is 'daunting', and its clinical utility may clearly be a very long time in coming.

The urgency of the classificatory challenge stems, obviously, from the fact that, the world over, psychiatrists and many others are having to deal day-by-day with real-life patients and others who need to be listened to and understood and humanely treated. The number of such people is increasing, at least in developed countries, as their populations age.[5] How to treat people who behave strangely or say strange things is a question that every modern society has to decide, and the ancients had to decide too.

Since the fifth century BCE, and probably before, the western world has been seeking for 'oblivious antidotes' (Macbeth's words) for mental disorders of all kinds. The Greeks made scant progress in this area, as far as the more severe disorders were concerned, though they managed a great

---

[2] Much can be learned about the new edition at www.dsm5.org (now itself in its third edition). DSM-5 is currently scheduled for publication in May 2013.

[3] Insel et al. 2010. See also www.nimh.nih.gov.

[4] Insel et al. 748.

[5] Cf. Petsko 2012.

deal of perceptive and vivid description. The nineteenth century and especially the twentieth century made a much more concerted and systematic
effort in this direction, and now we have the blessings of a complex array of
pharmaceuticals, the use and abuse of which have given rise to enormous
debates.

Yet to draw a stark contrast between ancient ineffectiveness and cruelty
on the one hand and the humanity of modern practice on the one other
would be quite foolish. It is true that one traditional Greek reaction to
mad people was to throw stones at them,[6] and some ancient authorities
recommended forms of physical abuse;[7] Socrates himself is said to have
thought that mad people—whatever he meant by that—should be placed
under physical restraint—whatever he meant by *that* (Xenophon, *Mem.*
1.2.50). The results of medicalizing mental illness, which may already have
begun before the classical Greeks,[8] were in ancient times decidedly mixed.
But a certain modest degree of both rationality and humanity entered in,[9]
and several contributors to this volume, most conspicuously Christopher
Gill, suggest that with respect to some of the less acute mental disorders,
ancient therapies are likely to have had positive effects—and could have
positive effects here and now. The twentieth century, meanwhile, with its
lobotomies and insane asylums, had plenty of its own horror stories. And
what to say of the twenty-first? We in the United States, at least, have things
to be ashamed of when it comes to the responses of the state—or at least of
some states—, above all because of the periodic execution of citizens who
are beyond doubt suffering from severe mental illness;[10] but that is not the
fault of psychiatrists.

---

[6] Aristophanes, *Acharnians* 1166–1169, *Wasps* 1491, *Birds* 524–525; cf. Euripides, *Heracles*
1004.
   [7] This seems to have been a special proclivity of the authoritative medical writer Asclepiades of Bithynia: see the evidence mentioned by Toohey, this volume p. 460, n. 18.
   [8] This is the view taken by the authors of a standard book about Assyrian and Babylonian
medicine: Scurlock and Anderson 2005, chapter 16, but in the texts they cite the treatments
prescribed for mental disorders are by any reasonable definition of the term magical.
   [9] For an explicit reference to humanity as a criterion for dealing with a mentally ill person
see *Digest* 24.3.22.7 (Ulpian).
   [10] For instance: on 18 May 2004 one Kelsey Patterson, a paranoid schizophrenic according
to state-appointed psychiatrists, was executed in Texas, after Governor Rick Perry, a rising star
in the Republican party, had refused him clemency in spite of a very rare recommendation
for clemency by the Texas Board of Pardons and Parole. Patterson had given ample proof of
both mental illness and a propensity for violence for at least eight years before committing an
apparently unmotivated double murder with a firearm in 1992. If he had received clemency,
he would have spent the rest of his active life in institutions. My main source is the *New York
Times*, 31 October 2011; some minor details I learned from other sources. Another kind of

Madness and mental illnesses and disorders of various kinds receive a huge amount of attention in Greek and Roman texts, and some of the writings in question, especially Athenian tragedies and certain philosophical works, have received even huger amounts of learned commentary. But the diversity of the texts in question, given the partly unavoidable compartmentalization of classical scholarship, has made it impossible to get a synoptic view.[11]

It follows from the above that the contributors had to come from diverse fields, and I have been fortunate enough to enroll distinguished psychiatrists as well as historians of medicine, classicists, philosophers and ancient historians (see the List of Contributors for further details).

I will set out in this section the main contentions of the contributing authors, relating them to each other as occasion arises. I must emphasize, however, that I shall not really be summarizing my colleagues' work, for one could not do full justice in a brief essay even to their most essential arguments. And since I shall occasionally express disagreement, it is all the more important for the reader to go to the contributors' own words.

One crucial question here, raised at the outset by Bennett SIMON, is whether mental illnesses do in fact fall into natural categories. The many fuzzy distinctions enshrined in the DSM may make one doubt it, though they can probably be made less fuzzy. The Platonic metaphor 'cutting nature at the joints' may by implication be too optimistic, for what needs to be classified is a good deal more complex than any carcass; and the experience of mental disorder is often a prolonged sequence of events, turning this way or that.

In any case the world needs a classification that is pragmatic, that will in other words form the foundation for a system of effective and humane treatment in so far as that is possible. Simon points out with candour and clarity the obstacles that hinder a satisfactory classification of mental illnesses,[12] which I can epitomize as follows: (1) competition between professions and between professionals, (2) subjective and culturally restricted ideas about normality, (3) 'nosologorrhea', or more exactly the question

---

absurdity is that in 2010 American doctors wrote 51.5 million prescriptions for drugs, 'with a total sales value of $7.42 billion', to treat what is known as Attention-Deficit/Hyperactivity Disorder, drugs that are widely abused (*New York Times*, 1 January 2012).

[11] And no one has really tried to provide one since Heiberg 1927.

[12] Cf. Meehl 1978.

whether a classification should have few or very many categories, (4) the awkwardness of individual cases ('often', writes Simon, who is among other things a practising psychiatrist, 'the more one knows about the patient, the harder it becomes to slot the patient into a category'), (5) the desirability of differentiating between mental disorders and non-pathological traits, (6) 'the aspiration [of mental health professionals] to have a drug or other intervention specific to a disorder', and finally (7) the 'magnetic' quality of diagnoses that are *à la mode*.

Simon's answer is optimistic, but only in the long term. No one is about to provide us with the 'perfect schema', but the increasing awareness of the problems of classification and the fact that they are explicitly debated are positive developments. At least we know that we do not know. He adds a final declaration, which indicates the significance of this volume for mental health professionals: there is a 'tension in the whole study of causes and treatment of mental disorders ... between the need to harken to the personal, narrative voice, the *cri de coeur* of the individual suffering person, and the need to find a slot, or box, for that person's suffering'. And literary texts can have a powerful effect in making professionals more inclined to listen to the voice of the patient.

In Julian HUGHES' view the immediate objective should be a practical classification, since a grand theory of causation is still far beyond us, while there are unwell people who need immediate help. The best we can do is to observe patients carefully and identify 'commonalities'—like the adherents of the Methodist school of medicine under the Roman Empire. There are many obstacles to such an enterprise, including the increasing dominance of a 'technological' attitude among mental health professionals. What might save us from this trend, he contends, is more attention to 'values', that is to say to what constitutes a good human life for the patients and potential patients; he suggests somewhat adventurously that the Methodists shared this view. Hughes also calls in here John Z. Sadler and his book *Values and Psychiatric Diagnosis*,[13] in which Sadler analysed in great detail the values expressed, more or less explicitly, in DSM-IV. Sadler's argument does not reject scientific approaches, but it sets up against values such as 'research utility' and 'administrative utility' quite different values, which he sums up as creativity, tradition, personal discipline, nature, connectedness and engagement, and *eudaimonia* (which is 'happiness', but not in any superficial sense; in Aristotle's famous definition, it is 'activity of the soul in

---

[13] Sadler 2005.

accordance with *aretê* or ... the best and most perfect *aretê*').[14] We have
to work out for ourselves what constitutes *eudaimonia*, and about that, as
many of us will agree, the classical Greeks have much to teach us. But how
many of us would want to be treated by psychiatrists who frankly relied on
intuition, another Hughes theme, I am not sure.

As Vivian Nutton has pointed out, however, the Methodist text available
to us in the work of Soranus' translator Caelius Aurelianus does demonstrate
a more humane attitude to mental patients than some of the Methodists'
rivals in other schools.[15] As to the possible practical utility now of ancient
forms of therapy, the question will arise again later in the paper by Christopher Gill.

A first step towards understanding Greek thinking on this subject is obviously to study the actual language Greek medical writers used to describe
mental disorders. This has never been done in a thorough and systematic
fashion, in spite of a number of useful contributions.[16] Hence the enormous
value of Chiara THUMIGER's account of the language used in the Hippocratic
corpus.[17] She demonstrates that these writers made a vigorous effort to create a more technical and a more precise terminology in this area, using a
wide variety of verbs and adjectives as well as names for symptoms and syndromes; but that later writers, beginning as early as the fourth century BC,
to a great extent 'dismiss[ed] the richer nuances of the Hippocratic vocabulary'. Time, on this view, did not bring progress, in spite of the fact that
there was a continuous medical tradition. Thumiger also shows, and this is
particularly important for a book such as this which is aimed partly at non-
classicists, that existing translations of the Hippocratic texts have very often
missed these nuances.

Greek thinking about mental illnesses combines a prolonged struggle to
systematize the results of observation and an irresistible but futile drive to
find physiological explanations. Some Hippocratics already 'knew'—but it
was merely a conjecture, and others thought otherwise—that mental illness
occurred in the brain. They were in any case able to construct—and it was
a notable achievement—what Jacques JOUANNA calls a binary division of
madness (*mania*): at one extreme was 'a type of madness that, from its

---

[14] *Nicomachean Ethics* 1.6.1098a16–18.
[15] Cf. *On Chronic Diseases* 1.5 (= *Fragments of the Methodists* fr. 57 Tecusan). See further
Nutton 2004, 200.
[16] One might single out the work of Berrettoni 1970 on the Hippocratics.
[17] For an introduction to the problems of Hippocratic authorship see Jouanna 1992.

low-energy nature, we might call a depressive madness', at the other extreme 'what we might qualify as a hyperactive madness'. They did not of course agree in their speculations about the aetiology of these conditions.

Students of antiquity already know, but others may be rather surprised to learn, that in the Graeco-Roman world the line between a lay-person and a doctor was not well-defined,[18] and the right of physicians to decide what mental disorders were, and who was suffering from one, was by no means agreed. Philosophers certainly felt entitled to speak about many aspects of the matter, so it should come as no surprise that Plato receives a great deal of attention here.[19]

Plato, in his principal 'scientific' work, the *Timaeus*, also, in a summary fashion, makes a binary division of mental disorders like the Hippocratics, and introduces for the first time the notion that madness is a condition of the *psuchê* (Jouanna; so too Michela Sassi later in this volume).[20] But Plato's binary division is not between two types of *mania*, it is between two types of *anoia*, namely *mania* and *amathia*.[21] In Jouanna's view this classification corresponds to the Hippocratic division between hyperactive and depressive madness. (In my view, this claim illustrates the great difficulty involved in following the evolution of this phase of Greek thinking about mental illness, for the polarity in the *Timaeus* which corresponds to the Hippocratic one is not the polarity between *mania* and *amathia*—since *amathia* is either 'ignorance' or possibly 'stupidity' but in any case not 'madness'[22]—, but between different forms of *mania*, which as Plato briefly notes (*Timaeus* 86b), are characterized by excessive joy or the opposite. One sees here, in my opinion once again, how Plato sacrifices observation to theory and rhetoric).[23]

It is not entirely clear who first replaced this binary classification of mental illness with a tripartite classification *mania-phrenitis-melancholia*. *Phrenitis* was a concept devised in the fifth century BC, or quite possibly

---

[18] The literature bearing on his topic is large; see esp. Lloyd 1991, Nutton 2004, chapter 17.

[19] Plato ranked medicine among the least exact of the *technai* (*Philebus* 56b).

[20] To my mind this view is already present in [Hippocrates], *On Regimen* 1.35, which is probably though not necessarily pre-Platonic. And see below on Aeschylus, *Persians* 750.

[21] In my view Jouanna is in error to translate *anoia* as 'démence'; see *Tim.* 92c. Other Plato passages that clearly show that *anoia* did not mean madness include *Phaedo* 93b, *Symposium* 210b, *Laches* 197a and b, etc.; there is no counter-evidence.

[22] On the meaning of this term see van der Eijk this volume p. 316 n. 23, Sassi this volume p. 418.

[23] Timaeus insists that *amathia* is a sickness (*Tim.* 86b, 88b). I cannot find a passage in Plato where *amathia* must mean madness, depressive or otherwise. It certainly does not in *Timaeus* 88b or 92b.

somewhat earlier, to signify something like *mania* accompanied by fever.[24] The triple classification, first attested in detail in Celsus (3.18), must have gone back to Hellenistic doctors; to which ones, it is hard to tell, and I will not pursue the question here.[25]

Jouanna maintains, however, that a binary classification persists in the writings of Galen. In *On the Differences of Symptoms* and *On the Causes of Symptoms*, he states, in Jouanna's analysis, that sicknesses of the hegemonic part of the 'soul' are either *anoia* (folly), consisting of a complete loss of energy, foolishness (*môria* and similar expressions), or 'faulty movements of the hegemonic faculty'. Jouanna argues that the first two of these three categories are essentially one. Galen subdivides each category (and ends up with a more specific definition of *mania* than the one the Hippocratics had used). It is in any case a difficulty for Jouanna, as he recognizes, that *melancholia*, by his time a major category of mental illness, cannot be fitted into an essentially binary scheme.

Perhaps, on this subject, we tend to expect something from Galen that he does not want to give us. As Vivian NUTTON remarks, he 'is not interested in nosography, in distinguishing and describing diseases in the manner of Aretaeus [of Cappadocia] .... What concerns him is what might be termed the theoretical and intellectual bases of medical practice, from which his therapeutics flow'.[26] Nonetheless he has much to say about mental illness, and in *On the Causes of Symptoms*, while *phrenitides* and *maniai* are both forms of *paraphrosunê* (mental disorder), they are distinct categories; in addition there is *melancholia*.

In fact Galen's understanding of mental illness is by ancient standards sophisticated; such is Nutton's view. Galen is aware that it takes many forms. He knew, partly from his own experience, that mental disorders might be temporary concomitants of other diseases. He knew from his own observation that attacks of *paraphrosunê* can affect some of a person's brain

---

[24] As pointed out by McDonald 2009, 15–16, [Hippocrates], *Regimen in Acute Diseases* 5, asserts that 'the ancients' (*hoi archaioi*) had identified *phrenitis* as an acute disease.

[25] Stok 1996, 2314–2317, takes the triple classification back to Diocles of Carystus and Praxagoras in the fourth century, without sufficient reason. Asclepiades of Bithynia, one of the leading physicians and medical writers of the first century BC, might have been a plausible candidate, but we know that he did not distinguish *mania* from *melancholia* (Caelius Aurelianus, *On Chronic Diseases*, preface 15), and neither did his influential student Themison of Laodicea (*On Chronic Diseases* 1.6.183).

[26] Aretaeus (cf. n. 1), probably an approximate contemporary of Galen, 'provides the best disease descriptions of any surviving ancient author' (Porter 1997, 71). He inherited the tripartite division of mental disorders but realized that he was up against terrible complexity.

functions without affecting others. And his remedies are more thoughtful than those of most others, which accords well with the acuteness of much of what he has to say about therapy for anger.[27] While he sometimes advocates humoral remedies, he also describes other approaches: in his commentary on the Hippocratic *Epidemics VI*, for instance, he describes a number of cases in which he applied distraction therapy.

Yet,

> compared with mental aberrations and hallucinations, Galen says very, very little about ... *mania*, less even than *melancholia*. Is this because he saw *mania* as something almost incurable, brought about by primarily physical changes? Or is this because, as so often, he never produces a completely systematic account, but follows a trail that leads to a concentration on something slightly different from what may have been his original intention? The latter seems to be at least a possible explanation, and would still allow us to view Galen as a physician the records of whose practice are far more interesting than the traditional theory that underlies them.

Véronique BOUDON-MILLOT also examines Galen, starting from questions of definition and diagnosis. It emerges again that he is not in fact much interested in definitions. Mental illnesses are just conditions that affect the functioning of the brain. The best way of diagnosing a mental illness, Galen paradoxically claims, is to observe the sleep of those who have lost their memories or their intelligence,[28] for whether the sick person sleeps a lot or very little will tell the physician (and this was in line with Hippocratic tradition) whether the patient's brain is cold or warm; other physical signs will help here. Yet Galen is able to distinguish a variety of different mental illnesses, sub-types of *phrenitis* for example.

But Galen makes matters more complicated for himself by including harmful passions among psychological illnesses as well as malfunctions of the brain. Which takes him into the field of ethics, which modern psychology, as Boudon-Millot observes, largely regards as extraneous (or, one might say, brings in disguised as part of 'normality'). Towards the end of her paper, Boudon-Millot argues that Galen 'agrees with the increasing number of people who are beginning to think that the model of mental illness adopted by the neurosciences is far from self-evident, and that other approaches can be equally legitimate'. But I wonder whether it is proper to say that Galen agreed with scientists whose methods he could not possibly

---

[27] Cf. Harris 2001, 385–387.
[28] *On Affected Places* 3.7 (VIII.164 K).

imagine. Admittedly he was not a thoroughgoing materialist, but his approach to mental illnesses, in any strict sense of that expression, was for the most part physiological and analytic.

But what exactly were Galen's opinions about how soul or mind and body interacted? Brooke HOLMES connects this question to another problem, namely the role that Galen assigned to sympathy (*sumpatheia*) between soul/mind and body, a discussion which takes her back to Galen's heroes Hippocrates and Plato but also to Hellenistic philosophers' thinking about the nature of the mind. Galen often uses sympathy as a pathological concept, but seems reluctant to apply it to the soul. Holmes's answer to this problem is that while Galen was able to develop the medical tradition about *sumpatheia* to create a picture of the body, including the brain, as an interconnected unity, he could not work out a clear relationship between the soul/mind and its physical location. Thus 'his understanding of sympathy privileges the one-way movement of affections from the gut to the brain (and, to a lesser degree, the heart), affections that are cast as pathological'.

Non-medical writers often held views of mental disorders that were quite different from those of the doctors. The most influential among them were Plato and the great tragic poets. Katja VOGT expounds Plato's opinions under three headings, (1) 'rational madness', which we may interpret as extreme enthusiasm for the good, (2) god-given madness, in other words inspiration from some superhuman source, and (3) mental illness, which means for Plato the pursuit of harmful pleasures. In fact it is only the last kind of madness that is harmful. What is particularly valuable here, I think, is Vogt's analysis of the real and apparent differences between the views Plato expressed in dialogues written over a considerable period of years.

To my mind *mania* and related terms are in Plato's usage almost always metaphorical or ironical, a fact that is intimately related to the promiscuous use of *mania* words in the non-philosophical Athens of his time (see further below). Even the mental-illness madness which Vogt describes is not about delusions in the sense of delusions recognized by 'normal' people as such; it is about delusions labelled by Plato as such because they do not accord with his opinions about ethics (and politics). As for 'rational madness', Vogt takes the position that 'it counts as madness only in a relatively thin sense'. I will not attempt to lay down the law as to how we should take two key passages in the *Symposium*, but it is reasonably clear that they are not about madness in any clinical sense: in the first (173e), quoted by Vogt, the narrator Apollodorus simply asks his interlocutor ironically whether he, Apollodorus, is mad (*mainomai*) to hold certain opinions; in the second, more striking, passage (218b), Alcibiades, in his wonderful semi-inebriated encomium of Socrates, refers to the philosopher and his companions as all having 'shared philosophical *mania* and *bakcheia* [Bacchic frenzy]'. A powerful metaphor indeed. English also uses madness words in a promiscuous way, though not of course exactly in the same promiscuous way as Greek: 'My friend Mrs. Fraser is mad for such a house' (Jane Austen, *Mansfield Park*). Michela Sassi also points out the similarity between classical and modern usages.

Vogt's paper, I should add, offers a succinct analysis of Plato's theory of god-given madness which is unsurpassed, as far as I know, in its clarity and perceptiveness.

Next we turn to some particular illnesses, epilepsy (Roberto Lo Presti), *melancholia* (Peter Pormann, George Kazantzidis), and a pair of phobias described in the Hippocratic corpus (Helen King). It will be noticed incidentally that the contributors to this book have in general avoided the sort of retrospective diagnosis of individual cases that has plagued the study of mental illness in antiquity (Jerry Toner's paper offers a vigorous counterargument).

Epilepsy is unique among mental disorders (if in fact that is where it belongs) in that it has survived from antiquity as a major nosological category, and, in spite of differences, 'there is ... quite a remarkable continuity between the ancient and the modern *clinical* accounts of the epileptic seizure' (Lo Presti). Lo Presti's approach is to ask how 'Greek scientific discourse drew a distinction, or vice versa accounted for the intertwinement, between the somatic and the cognitive/behavioural manifestations of epilepsy'. Was epilepsy in fact, in Greek thinking, a mental illness in some non-physiological sense? Fifth- and fourth-century Greek medical accounts of epileptic conditions are strictly physiological—that is their great strength. Lo Presti, however, shows that for the Plato of the *Timaeus* matters were considerably more complicated, even though he classifies epilepsy as a disease of the body not the soul. The point is that the Greeks did not posit a strict mind-body opposition such as has been familiar since Descartes. Thus it can be argued that the classical Greek concept of epilepsy should be understood through contemporary 'embodied mind' theories.

Pormann, who recently edited Rufus of Ephesus' fragmentary two-book work on melancholy (which is known to us partly from Arabic sources),[29] here approaches Rufus through the tenth/eleventh-century Baghdadi schol-

---

[29] Tübingen, 2008. For an introduction to Rufus of Ephesus, a physician who wrote in the late first century AD, see the essays by the various contributors to that volume.

ar Ahmad ibn Muhammad Miskawayh, and investigates the latter's understanding of the concept. Rufus gave the name *melancholia* to a type of
madness that he thought occurred in different forms, 'ranging from general despondency and fear to hallucinations, ravings, and aggressive streaks'.
What is specifically at issue here is his claim (fragments 33–36 Pormann)
that too much thinking leads to clinical *melancholia*, a development of
the well-known question in the pseudo-Aristotelian *Problems* (30.1): 'Why
is it that all men who have achieved distinction in philosophy, public life,
poetry or the *technai* seem to have been *melancholikoi*?' Miskawayh could
not believe that an authority such as Rufus can have meant that all intense
thinking can lead to *melancholia*, and preferred to suppose that he was referring only to 'instances of imaginary knowledge, and acts of imagination
in general', by which Miskawayh meant delusional fantasies. He developed
a novel physiological theory as to how such fantasies engendered *melancholia*; and he advocated therapy by means of reasoning with the patient.
Miskawayh did not always understand Rufus correctly but was nonetheless
stimulated by him.

What did the Greeks in fact mean by *melancholia*? For the most part,
an aggressive form of madness, and not 'melancholy', and Cicero reflects
this fact when he translates the term as *furor* (*Tusculan Disputations* 3.11).
But matters are more complicated than that, for occasionally, starting with
pseudo-Hippocrates, *Aphorisms* 6.23, classical authors associate the term
with a pathological state of lasting sadness and fear. Both aspects of *melancholia* are present when it is discussed in the passage of pseudo-Aristotle's
Problems 30.1 that I mentioned just now, though the emphasis is on its manic
manifestations.[30] Kazantzidis' paper argues that Cicero, both in the *Tusculans* and elsewhere, engages critically with this text. According to him, there
is an allusion in *Tusculans* 3.63 to ps.-Aristotle's treatment of Bellerophon as
a *depressive* melancholic and this shows that Cicero was familiar with both
sides of the disease. Both sides are also visible, as mentioned above, in the
fragments of Rufus of Ephesus' treatise.[31] This two-sidedness one might take
to be a victory of humoral theory over actual observation.

The history of modern psychiatry since the sixteenth century features in
several papers in this book, but in particular in Helen KING's, where she
traces the way in which the learned have reacted to two cases of phobia
that are described in the Hippocratic *Epidemics*. One of these concerns a

---

[30] Pormann 2008, 223.
[31] Fragment 11 Pormann.

banal fear of heights, the other a puzzling culture-specific fear of night-time 'flute' music played by 'flute-girls' at symposia (the *aulos* was played rather like an oboe, not like a flute, but somehow such translations as 'oboe-girls' and 'girl pipers' fail to conjure up the right image). So what was so scary about the sexually available 'flute-girls' and their music? 'Whenever [the patient] heard the voice of the flute begin to play at a symposium, masses of terrors rose up'. The music of the *aulos* was known to release inhibitions. What made it potentially frightening, in King's view, is that the symposium, a somewhat ritualized event in classical Athens, was a *competitive* occasion; she hypothesizes that the *aulos* music reminded the patient of 'a past failure, sexual or otherwise, during a symposium'.

It is a small step from specific syndromes to specific symptoms.[32] If we want to gain an idea of how a wide range of Greeks and Romans regarded a particular class of symptoms of mental disorder, hallucinations are eminently worth investigating, all the more since, though they are not altogether easy to define, they were easier to recognize as symptoms than, say, mild delusions or mild behavioural disorders. They are the subject of my main contribution to this volume.

Both medicine and philosophy most definitely led the lay-person towards a secular understanding of hallucinatory experiences—but who was willing to follow? Doctors did not write about the hallucinations of Orestes, but for anyone else who had even a moderate education, he was real enough, and it was easy to think that his 'Furies' were outside him. All the evidence suggests that ordinary people, not surprisingly, tended to attribute hallucinations to supernatural forces. And it is scarcely surprising either, that with the methods at their disposal ancient physicians could make no demonstrable progress in post-Hippocratic times in the understanding of hallucinations. It can be argued on the other hand that while one would not want to prettify the way in which the Greeks and Romans treated the mentally ill, it was safer then than it is now to hallucinate involuntarily, for who would want to be labelled as a schizophrenic?

So we pass on to the vital matter of treatment. Philip van der Eijk, in a paper of outstanding lucidity, surveys the question which mental disorders Greek medical and philosophical writers considered to be curable and by what means, selecting five texts to concentrate on: the Hippocratic *On Regimen*, the *Timaeus*, *Nicomachean Ethics* VII, Galen's *On the Diagnosis and*

---

[32] In this essay I use the word 'symptom' to include also what technically speaking were formerly known as 'signs'.

Treatment of Affections and Errors of the Soul, and, less familiar, Ptolemy's account of affections of the soul and their curability in the *Tetrabiblos.* These texts describe a great variety of mental disorders, 'ranging from what we would call clinical conditions to character flaws, cognitive as well as moral and behavioural failure'. What is perhaps most striking of all is the apparent conviction of these (and, it may be said, many other) ancient writers that such disorders—not indeed all of them, but many of them—could be cured or at least alleviated. They claim that diet and other therapies, and drugs, actually produce positive results, within limits. In some cases Galen advocates surgery.

How could these Greeks be so optimistic? The Hippocratic writers and Galen were certainly not short of practical experience or of opportunities to observe the consequences of their recommendations. Van der Eijk does not speculate about the reasons for this apparent optimism. Perhaps the answer is mostly obvious: it was a professional necessity, just as in any other area of medical practice. Sometimes patients must indeed have got better, and in occasional cases their recovery may have been helped by regimen, which always tended towards exercise and moderation. But that hardly accounts for the attitudes of the philosophers.[33]

Van der Eijk raises several fascinating questions which he does not have space to explore. One is the question of authority. Who in the ancient world was regarded as entitled to say that someone was suffering from a mental disorder and to decide or recommend what to do about it? Since doctors did not distinguish between physical and mental disorders as such, all or many of them certainly felt entitled to judge and recommend what should be done about mental and indeed moral disorders of all kinds. But nothing in Athenian or Roman law would lead us to think that doctors were credited by society at large with the prerogative of deciding whether or not an individual was mentally ill.

It is also intriguing that it is Ptolemy the astronomer and astrologer, of all the ancient authors discussed in this book, who makes the most definite distinction between mental afflictions (*pathê psuchika*) and bodily injuries and afflictions (*sinê kai pathê sômatika*) (as we have seen, the distinction had been made before). Might one infer that ordinary educated persons in the second century AD Alexandria, less concerned than the physicians were with the aetiology of illness, *normally* made the distinction that Ptolemy makes?

---

[33] This optimism about the curability of mental illnesses appears in many other classical texts: see for example Plautus' *Menaechmi* (with my comments, this volume p. 294), and Lucian's *Abdicatus* [*The Disowned*].

Christopher GILL concentrates on one calling in particular and its contribution to the treatment of mental illness—philosophy. 'To what extent', he asks 'can we ... recognize in these essays [those of Greek and Roman writers about philosophical themes] a credible response to mental illness?' He argues that the philosophical essays of the quite numerous classical writers who concerned themselves with the more moderate kind of mental ill-health, such a depression, were meant to function as rough equivalents of such modern phenomena as advice about 'life-style management' and 'preventive medicine'. Differentiating carefully between Platonic-Aristotelian approaches and Stoic approaches, he nevertheless identifies a 'core strategy' which has much in common with modern cognitive therapies.

In one of the most important sections of this book, Gill discusses whether the classical texts in question could be of current use in treating 'long-term states of depression or anxiety or of situational distress', identifying some specific reasons for giving a positive answer. Could we not benefit from preventive psychological therapy, 'designed to enable people to build up emotional resilience against setbacks and disasters before they have actually happened'? In some ancient milieux at least, it was assumed among educated males (a minority of the population of course) that 'one can and should take care of one's psychological health and well-being and manage [one's] life accordingly'. The point being not so much to ward of illness as to pursue positive personal aims.

All this is in accord with the stronger emphasis in contemporary medicine on prevention. 'One might argue that ancient culture provides a paradigm we would do well to adopt, in which people can reasonably be expected to manage their lives in a way that promotes psychological well-being as well as a sound bodily condition'. Gill anticipates of course the objection that the therapeutic texts are not based on scientific inquiry in a modern sense.[34] But they are based on centuries-long experience, and in some cases at least on acute psychological insight.

Michaela SASSI, for her part, concentrates on the *Timaeus*. Like Jouanna, she gives Plato the credit for being the first Greek to conceptualize mental disease as such, whereas the Hippocratics had for the most part—but not invariably, as she points out—treated disturbances of the cognitive and behavioural functions as symptoms. This picture is certainly complicated by the Hippocratic *Diseases of the Virgins (peri partheniôn)* and by *On the*

---

[34] There is scarcely any need to point out how much current psychotherapy, even after the decline of Freudianism, is based on imperfectly scientific knowledge.

Sacred Disease and Book I of *On Regimen*. And more perhaps needs to be said about *phrenitis*, the one technical term for a mental illness that doctors had definitely invented before Plato came on the scene.

Sassi also raises the question how much Plato owed to Socrates in this area. As for Plato himself, she considers him to have shown 'remarkably sensitivity' to some of the pathological manifestations of *mania*. That is a generous judgement. Plato included an absurd number of moral aberrations and psychic conflicts under the heading of madness, as Sassi herself in effect points out. But one could not argue with her conclusion that 'the general theory of human behavior emerging from the *Timaeus* is ... functional ... to his concern for social cohesion and the psychological basis for it'. And she is clearly right to see the *Timaeus* as a sort of preparation for the regimented ideal that Plato created in the *Laws*.

We turn to the enormous role that madness played in non-philosophical Greek literature, though we can only hope to cover selected genres. Athenian tragedy is clearly the central interest, which Suzanne SAID and Glenn MOST approach in very different styles, Said meticulously accumulating evidence to build a nuanced analysis of the tragic vocabulary of madness (but rightly starting with Homer), Most staking all on an ingenious and original solution to a large problem in understanding what we can call the 'madness tragedies'.

The only passage in Homer which describes cognitive impairment is the Theoclymenos story in *Odyssey* 20, but madness words are everywhere. The key terms are ἄτη ('disastrous folly') and μαίνομαι ('I am mad'). Said points out that the poems distinguish fairly clearly between ἄτη words, which always refer to 'some harm experienced by the subject' and not to any one mental condition, and μαίνομαι and λύσσα words (the latter relatively rare), which always refer to 'some harm inflicted by the subject on others' and often involve physical symptoms. μαίνομαι words are often, as later, employed in face-to-face abuse. The strong tendency is of course to see both *ate* and *mania* as the work of the gods.

Aeschylus no longer observes the older distinction between these terms in a regular fashion. It is still the gods who cause madness, in Said's view, but as she observes, Aeschylus now has a concept of 'mental illness' (*nosos phrenôn*, *Persians* 750)—which ought to give pause to those who think that it was Plato who devised the concept (see above). There is still of course in Euripides madness sent by the gods, but in *Orestes* (and not only there in my opinion; see below, p. 293) we are offered a psychological explanation. All three tragic poets put on stage the gods/goddesses who caused attacks of madness, but 'it is only Aeschylus in the *Oresteia*, who makes visible for the audience the true visions of Cassandra and Orestes'.

Vision is at the centre of the paper by Most. He begins, however, with the suggestion that madness in fifth-century tragedy still exercised fascination in Athens a century and more after the plays in question were produced (evidence of Menander). The main figure in question is Orestes, whose madness 'consists essentially in visual hallucinations'. In Most's view, this is at odds with the supposed prevalence of auditory rather than visual hallucinations in modern psychiatry (I take a different view of this matter: below, p. 287). How to explain this visuality of the madness that the tragic dramatists put on the stage? Our author's explanation is that 'the depiction of tragic madness is being influenced by the essential visuality of the tragic medium itself'. 'Other forms of madness cannot easily be staged as effectively as visual hallucinations can'. But not only that: when the tragic poets represent visual hallucination on the stage, they are also bringing home to the members of the audience that they, like the hallucinator, are seeing what is not really there. Most then explores how this principle helps us to understand other plays, especially Euripides' *Heracles* and *Bacchae*.

Are people who are suffering from mental illnesses responsible for their actions? And what follows from the various possible answers that we may give? The already-mentioned papers by Boudon-Millot, van der Eijk, Gill and Sassi show some of the various ways that the ancients answered these questions. It was all the harder for them to answer the basic question about responsibility because they lacked clear lines between mental and physical illness and between mental illness and a proclivity towards bad behaviour— though the same might be said about us. How Roman law dealt with these matters we shall see in the chapter by Toohey. The most plausible view is that both philosophers and lawyers tended to think that mental illness meant that a person was not responsible for his/her actions and should not be held responsible for them, while public opinion was a great deal less forgiving.

David KONSTAN's paper deals briefly with the rhetorical aspects of this problem, in other words the types of excuses that the ancients habitually offered or were recommended to offer. Agamemnon blamed his *atê* for his having confiscated Briseis (*Iliad* 19.78–144).[35] This strategy of shifting the blame was known later to rhetorical theorists as *metastasis*.

---

[35] It is significantly more complicated than that: what Agamemnon says is that 'Zeus and Fate (*moira*) and an air-walking Fury (*erinus*)' inflicted *ate* on him (19.87), and then he tells a long tale to show that *ate* could afflict even Zeus.

A historian who desires to know how people came to be classified as mentally ill in antiquity, and how they were really treated in consequence, can learn a good deal from the medical sources, but also, in certain periods, from what we can loosely called the legal sources. The classical Athenian sources are admittedly frustrating (I planned to include a paper on this topic, but as explained in the preface the author's ill health prevented this). We know that there was an old law that invalidated a will made by a person suffering from *mania*,[36] but we really have no idea at all what an orator might have put forward as a minimum proof of *mania*, or what would have convinced a jury. The argumentation involved is likely to have varied hugely from case to case, since the Athenians, while being proud of their adherence to the rule of law, judged not so much the cases they heard as the litigants themselves, and 'the congruence of the interests of the litigants with those of the *demos*'.[37] The same applies to the other statutory provision we know about, which authorized the *graphê paranoias*,[38] the 'charge of madness', which apparently allowed one citizen to dispossess another if he could prove that the other was 'wasting' his property. What counted as waste in Athenian eyes? What sort of defence did the mentally ill have against ruthless relatives?

The Roman evidence is more instructive. Peter TOOHEY provides an in- valuable summary of what Justinian's *Digest* has to tell us in this area, and analyses it from several different angles, concluding that the humane aspects of Roman ways of treating the mentally ill deserve more emphasis than the frankly brutal ones.[39]

I cannot, I have to admit, agree with Toohey's view that all the terms for mental illness that he sets out on p. 444 are indistinguishable from each other. There is no doubt a fair amount of synonymity in practice, but *animi vitia* ('mental defects') and *mentis alienatio* ('insanity'), for instance, seem not to be interchangeable, as witness *Dig.* 21.1.1.9 (Ulpian).[40] As to who counted as mentally ill in varying degrees, the *Digest* offers no systematic guidance, unsurprisingly. It is plain, however, that just as the Romans in general used at least some of their terms for madness in a fast and loose

---

[36] [Aristotle], *Constitution of Athens* 35.2.

[37] Cohen 1995, 115. Not everyone would agree with this formulation.

[38] [Aristotle], *Constitution of Athens* 56.6.

[39] The classic study of madness in Roman law is Nardi 1983, but it was narrowly conceived.

[40] 'The question is raised ... whether a slave who ... associates with religious fanatics and joins in their utterances is nonetheless to be regarded as healthy. Vivianus says that he is, for he says that we should still regard as sane those who have *animi vitia* ...'.

way—like the Greeks—, so the jurists occasionally applied them to what we may call deviance from social norms. A will that required the *heres* to cast the testator's remains into the sea could be suspected of being the work of someone not *compos mentis* (*Dig.* 28.7.27 pr., Modestinus); on balance, however, one would have to say that there is little evidence in the *Digest* that insanity claims were used to regulate the social behaviour *of free people*. Slaves on the other hand were considered to show a mental defect (*animi vitium*) if they 'wandered' or ran away (*Dig.* 21.1.4.3, Ulpian). Venuleius had already categorized other behaviour on the part of slaves as proof of mental defects, such as a constant desire to watch the 'games', studying paintings (!), or lying (*Dig.* 21.1.65 pr.).

Two kinds of treatment can be distinguished, the treatment that a mentally ill person received from society at large and the treatment that he or she received from the law. Family care was of course central, and heaven help the individual who had no family that was willing to provide care;[41] Ulpian assumes that it is the responsibility of the *necessarii* (a term which includes friends as well as relatives) to keep the *furiosus* under control if that is possible (*Dig.* 1.18.13.1). We can hardly be shocked if *furiosi* were locked up, put in prison or subjected to physical restraints, since we do that to some people too; the unanswerable question is whether such methods were also applied to people who offered no physical threat. And it was doctors not jurists who recommended the most brutal methods.[42]

As to how the law and its human agents treated the mentally ill, Toohey rightly points to Ulpian's assurance (*Dig.* 1.5.20) that 'a person who has become insane ('qui furere coepit')' retained his or her previous status, such a Roman citizenship, rank and property'. Nonetheless the state could intervene, once it had decided that a person was *furiosus*. It recognized, and if necessary appointed, one or more *curatores* for any *furiosus* over the age of twenty-five.[43] 'The curator's concern and care should extend over the health and well-being of the *furiosus* as well as his property' (*Dig.* 27.10.7 pr., Julian). There is some reason to think that a conscientious provincial governor in the second century might actually take notice of whether the *curator* was doing his job properly.[44]

---

[41] Cf. Dover 1974, 127; M. Smith 1978, 9.

[42] See Toohey this volume, p. 460 n. 18.

[43] This was a very old institution, mentioned in the Twelve Tables: *Dig.* 27.10.13 (Gaius).

[44] See *Dig.* 27.10.7.2, Julian. A whole chapter (26.10) deals with what could be done about untrustworthy *tutores* and *curatores* (but not all *curatores* were responsible for the mentally ill).

Roman criminal law may at first glance seem to be rather kind and reasonable towards the mentally ill, but as much depended on who was considered to be *furiosus* as now depends on what courts decide, under the McNaughton rules or otherwise, about whether a defendant is of sound mind. Certain hints suggest that Roman courts set the bar quite high: Marcus Aurelius and Commodus stated that it had to be 'clearly ascertained that [a certain defendant] is in such a state of insanity that he lacks all understanding through the continuous alienation of his mental faculties' (reported by Macer, *Dig.* 1.18.14). Then there was the problem of the so-called 'lucid interval', during which, if a *furiosus* committed a crime, he was held to be fully liable to pay the penalty.[45] But the Roman law of homicide seems more humane with respect to mentally ill defendants than that of a several American states in the twenty-first century. An insane parricide (in the wide Roman sense of the term) was to be imprisoned not put to death, an insane matricide 'is being punished enough by his own madness (*furore ipso*)', and insane murderers were not held liable under the standard homicide law.[46]

Jerry TONER concludes our book with a refreshing consideration of a precise historical situation. We are in Amida, on the extreme eastern fringe of the Roman Empire, late in the reign of Justinian, in the year 560. The population, deeply disturbed by events of the preceding two generations, is now terrified of another Persian invasion, and much of it shows symptoms of derangement, at least according to the chronicler John of Ephesus (c. 507–c. 588). Toner describes the modern concept of Post-traumatic Stress Disorder. How much of this (I think we may say) typically late-twentieth century narrative-type is applicable to antiquity in general and sixth-century Amida in particular? Appropriate caveats immediately come to the fore, especially with regard to the specific religious characteristics of the Romans, always somewhat inclined to attribute disasters to the gods, and of sixth-century Christians, who were inclined, at least officially, to see disasters as the result of the victims' supposed 'sins' and an occasion for repentance. Deeper social tensions were also at work. When the crisis had passed, so John of Ephesus claimed, many repented.

---

[45] Apparently: *Dig.* 1.18.14 (Macer), 14.4.4 (Paul).

[46] See respectively *Dig.* 1.18.13.1 (Ulpian); 1.18.14 (Macer) and 48.9.9.1 (Modestinus) (evidently the same case); 48.8.12 (Modestinus). 21.1.23.2 is an intriguing passage because it suggests that at one time intent was considered less important, with the effect that *furiosi* may have been held liable (but Ammianus Marcellinus 15.12.4 implies that the Cato the Censor considered *furor* madness to be involuntary). If an insane person damages property, he is not to be punished (6.1.60, Pomponius).

This paper opens an entirely new problematic, quite apart from the unavoidable question of the reliability of John of Ephesus as a source. Even with much better sources, should be willing to indulge in retrospective diagnosis? And a society which adhered to a soteriological religion, which its leaders defined in such as way as to exclude fiercely those devotees who defined it differently (in this case, Monophysites, who made up most of the population of Amida), a religion that stimulated repentance and extreme asceticism, clearly had ideas about normality very different from those that prevail now.[47]

This book thus represents a concerted effort to understand how the Greeks and to a lesser extent the Romans saw mental disorders. But a grand systematic synthesis lies in the future, and it will not be difficult for reviewers to identify aspects of the problem that are not covered here. Some of them concern very wide problems, such as how the ancients regarded stupidity, senile dementia, senile forgetfulness and a number of other conditions. Others concern specifically ancient or at least non-modern phenomena: I should have found someone to write about demoniac possession in ancient Israel and Christianity, for example, and someone to write about the origins and effects of using hellebore to treat mental illnesses (though such treatment is mentioned in this volume by both Nutton and van der Eijk),[48] and about the treatment of mental disorders by seeking divine intervention, by means of Corybantic rites or visits to shrines of the healing god Asclepius.[49] Work for the future.

The point of this book, though it is built on the work of earlier scholars like any work of scholarship, is to lay some new interdisciplinary foundations for further work and a hoped-for synthesis. The field is so large, and some of the authors concerned are so little studied (I particularly regret the absence of a chapter on Aretaeus of Cappadocia), that any single book of reasonable dimensions, put together in a reasonable amount of time, has unavoidable gaps.

In the concluding part of this introduction I should like to advocate a particular approach to the history of the way mental illness was understood

---

[47] Religiosity does not make it into the DSM, which is after all an American production. The psychology of religion seems to be progressing (see esp. Burkert 1996, Boyer 2001, brilliant books that have attracted much criticism), but there is a great deal more to do.

[48] On this topic see Diliberto 1984, 35 n. 101, Padel 1995, 48–49.

[49] Cf. Aristophanes, *Wasps* 118–123, with commentators.

in antiquity, an approach that is also relevant to the history of modern
psychiatry. I am concerned here with vocabulary. We should, I suggest,
give more space to the possibility (to put it no more strongly) that the
ancient writers whom we regard as experts on mental disorders—mostly
medical writers and philosophers—operated within and were imprisoned
by ordinary language. We may of course envy them their freedom from
jargon, acronyms and 'nosologorrhea', but some specialized terminology
such as the Greeks created in many other areas, would have helped to clarify
distinctions.

From Hippocratic times onwards, if not earlier, physicians devised a rich
vocabulary for physical illnesses,[50] and ancient thought about mental disorders is not entirely lacking in technical terminology. φρενῖτις (*phrenitis*)—a condition, sometimes fatal, mainly characterized by fever and delirium[51]—is a clear example: it is used very often in the Hippocratic corpus
but never by a non-medical writer until it appears twice, very interestingly, in Menander's *Shield*. The first philosopher to use it was Chrysippus,
and though it is sometimes used by other non-medical writers it clearly
remained a term of art; so much so that the learned layman Celsus got it
slightly wrong and wrote it as *phrenesis*.[52] λήθαργος (*lêthargos*) was another
such technical term for a mental illness, but whatever it meant exactly it
attracted relative little attention from the doctors. Now it may be that *phrenitis* was a misconceived entity, and we can certainly say that about *melancholia*, but at least it allowed medical writers to discuss a perceived condition
without the continuous osmosis from ordinary language that affected Gk.
mania, Lat. *furor*, and many other ordinary-language terms that are mentioned in this book.

Asclepiades of Bithynia regarded *furor* as a satisfactory technical term,
whereas *insania*, he said, was merely part of ordinary language (the words he
actually discussed were respectively, I suppose, μελαγχολία and μανία).[53] He
was unduly optimistic, because μελαγχολία words were part of the ordinary
language too, and the confusion about what they meant (see Kazanztidis'
paper in this volume) may well have derived in part from their having being
in general use (so that they appeared in Aristophanes, for example). Plato's
manipulation of *mania* words shows how the wide meaning of a term in
ordinary language could be exploited and how such a meaning then passed

---

[50] See Schironi 2010.
[51] See especially McDonald 2009, 28–45, for the Hippocratic understanding of this term.
[52] 2.1.15, 3.18.2–3; but a copyist may have been responsible.
[53] Caelius Aurelianus, *On Acute Diseases* 1 *praefatio* 15.

into the canon. Someone might object here that the physicians at least kept their nosological terms reasonably clear even if laymen muddled them up. No doubt there is some truth in that, but even Galen could get things wrong. When he analyses the terminology for delirium employed in the Hippocratean *Epidemics* III, he asserts quite reasonably that Hippocrates uses different terms for delirious states according to their intensity (XVIIA.481 K). But this happens not to be true.[54] More work for the future.

---

[54] Thumiger forthcoming.

PART I

CURRENT PROBLEMS IN THE
CLASSIFICATION OF MENTAL ILLNESS

'CARVING NATURE AT THE JOINTS':
THE DREAM OF A PERFECT CLASSIFICATION
OF MENTAL ILLNESS

Bennett Simon

> It is indisputable today that, despite hon-
> est efforts, we are still unable to catego-
> rize quite a vast number of cases within
> the frame of the known forms in the sys-
> tem.
>
> (Emil Kraepelin, 1910)[1]

This is a paper on the ancient and ongoing effort to define and classify mental illness. 'Carving Nature at the Joints', is a modern paraphrase of Plato's image for the dialectical mode of making classifications, 'To have the power, conversely, to cut up a composition, form by form according to its natural joints and not to try to hack through any part as a bad butcher might.'[2] Sometime in the 1960's, the distinguished psychologist Paul Meehl began to use this phrase to characterize the quest for the ideal classification of mental illnesses.[3] The centuries before and the decades since have seen many schemas arise, many disappear, and many remain as geological agglomerates with still newer schemas. All observers agree that we have not achieved anything approaching an ideal, let alone perfect way of classifying. The current ongoing revision of the fourth *Diagnostic and Statistical Manual* (DSM IV) of the American Psychiatric Association, supposed to culminate in the fifth edition, has been beset by considerable controversy, as has each previous revision.[4]

---

[1] Cited in Trede et al. 2005, a paper that is a major contribution to the history of psychiatric classification.

[2] *Phaedrus* 265B–266C; see also Plato's *Sophist* 298D. Translations are from the translation and edition of Steven Scully (2003).

[3] Waller 2006; Meehl 1995.

[4] For a philosophically based critique, see, among others, R. Cooper 2004. For a good overview of the current debate, see Frances 2010 and the entire issue in which this is published, especially the replies to Allen Frances by Hannah Decker (23–25); S. Nasser Ghaemi

It has been even difficult to get agreement on whether or not to use the term 'mental illness' or the term 'mental disorder.' There is fierce disagreement on the question of whether or not some or most of current major diagnostic entities actually exist, are found 'in nature', or are jerry-rigged constructions.

I first take up literary texts that have been cited in discussions of psychiatric and psychological classification. I examine in detail Plato's *Phaedrus* to exemplify some spoken and unspoken assumptions in any attempt at classifying 'madness.' I then list and detail seven factors that persistently constrain psychiatric classifications.

Next I list and detail a number of the perennial and persistent problems besetting the enterprise of classification, from antiquity onwards. I draw brief examples and illustrations from classical antiquity, Revolutionary France, late nineteenth-century and early twentieth-century German psychiatry, and contemporary disputes within American psychiatry and between psychiatry and the 'allied' (often at odds with each other) mental health professions.

While there are important differences between contemporary psychiatric methods of classification and those developed in Greek and Roman antiquity, there has been an amazing degree of continuity and similarity from late antiquity (e.g beginning in the Byzantine era) until roughly the late eighteenth and early twentieth century. This continuity can be seen qualitatively in the way each schema developed relied heavily on one or two striking symptoms that the patient exhibited. There was also astonishing continuity in the vocabulary of mental illness, though there was over the centuries considerable fluctuation in exactly what was designated by the same word, e.g, mania. Each era had its own plethora of classificatory schemas, and theoretical framework in which the classification was embedded. Frameworks could be amalgamated in interesting ways, such as a theological framework combining with a medical humoral framework to yield the aphorism: *gaudet Diabolus in melancholico humore* ('the Devil revels to find a person with a melancholic humoral predominance'). What began to

---

(33–35) and Joseph Pierre (9–11). Frances takes a kind of 'agnostic position' on the question of the actual existence of our currently defined classes of mental disorder, while Ghaemi (in part using Hippocratic texts) argues for the veracity of some of our major diagnostic categories. The National Institute of Mental Health group is arguing for discarding the entire DSM enterprise and is developing a totally different schema, now called 'Research Domain Criteria'. See Insel et al. 2010. This NIMH schema has aroused considerable controversy, scientific and political.

change, and gradually to become an aspiration of systems during the late eighteenth and nineteenth century was the realization that careful observation of numbers of patients, and—especially in the latter half of the nineteenth century—long-term follow-up of course and outcome was necessary. In the twentieth century, the notion of a life-history of the patient as an integral part of diagnosis and classification gradually became important to the mental health professions. Simultaneously, from several different quarters, the need to have clear, replicable, criteria for diagnosis and classification came to dominate, sometimes tending to displace the need to have a full life-history of the patient, but sometimes in concert with such a history.

I suggest that, while the quest for the perfect schema is unlikely to succeed in our lifetime, our increasing awareness of these problems, our ability to articulate them, and the realization of the imperfectability of this quest, are important and favorable developments.

1. Three Literary Texts on Classification: Shakespeare, Borges and Plato

In *Macbeth*, 3.1.92–108, Macbeth interviews the murderers he has hired to kill Banquo and Fleance. Famously, he compares breeds of dogs to breeds of humans, with the main point of the comparison being which breeds have the necessary qualities to be a murderer. Here the method of classification of the human race is shaped by a very particular motive and need. From the point of view of the structure of the play, this speech further instantiates Shakespeare's examination throughout the play of what it takes to engender and breed murder and a murderer (e.g, 'Bring forth male children only.')

Jorge Luis Borges, in his 1942 story, 'The Analytical Language of John Wilkens', has the narrator describe his experience of laughing at his first reading a classification of animals in an ancient Chinese encyclopedia.[5]

---

[5] Translated in Simms 1993. This piece most famously was used by Michel Foucault as his introduction to *The Order of Things: An Archaeology of Human Sciences* [1964] (1996). 'This book first arose out of a passage in Borges, out of the laughter that shattered, as I read the passage, all the familiar landmarks of thought—*our* thought, the thought that bears the stamp of our age and our geography—breaking up all the ordered surfaces and all the planes with which we are accustomed to tame the wild profusion of existing things and continuing long afterwards to disturb and threaten with collapse our age-old definitions between the Same and the Other.'

Those that belong to the Emperor, embalmed ones, those that are trained, suckling pigs, mermaids, fabulous ones, stray dogs, those included in the present classification, those that tremble as if they were mad, innumerable ones, those drawn with a very fine camelhair brush, others, those that have just broken a flower vase, those that from a long way off look like flies.

Borges' caricature of classification, along with being a statement on the absurdity of striving for an absolute classification of life and the universe, is also a caricature of literary-genre classification. The master of 'meta-fiction' prepares his attack on those who might try and categorize, crib and confine, his own writing.

For a more detailed examination of the need to examine the context and accompanying motives of any method of classification of mental disorder, let us now turn to the passage in Plato's *Phaedrus* where we encounter the image of 'carving at the joints' (265b–266c). For students of classics of my generation, this and preceding passages (244a–245c) on 'The Blessings of Madness' have been made famous by E.R. Dodds' discussion in his germinal work, *The Greeks and the Irrational*. For mental health professionals, it has rarely been examined in detail, apart from it providing a certain model of how to classify things—cutting at the 'natural joints'. For Paul Meehl, the passage provided the armature for his belief that there were genuine entities of disease in nature and that he was developing a method for a taxonomy, whose units he called 'taxons.' Ironically, in my reading of the passage, I find rather a somewhat playful set of reminders of several reasons why the quest for 'natural' divisions is so fraught.

The dialogue is a complex, multi-layered discourse on *eros*, on the possibility of describing its nature, its effects, and its sub-divisions. The relationship between *eros*, especially homoerotic *eros*, and the process of philosophical inquiry, of dialogue and dialectic, is critical to the dialogue.[6] Important too is the Socratic effort to distinguish his method of inquiry and persuasion, namely dialogue and dialectic, from that of the practitioners of rhetoric, with their methods of charm and seduction. In the course of the examination of *eros*, Socrates has just been considering the forms of madness, *mania*, invoking a number of terms that appear in contemporary Greek medical writings. His diagnostic schema divides first into 'two forms of madness, one caused by human illness, the other from a divine upheaval of normal customs. [265a].' The second category divides into four kinds of divinely sent

---

[6] The word 'philosophy' was a recent coinage, probably by Plato.

madness (see below).[7] This is an ambitious project—the classification of both love and madness!

> SOCRATES: And that there were two forms of madness, one caused by human illness, the other by a divine upheaval of customary beliefs.
>
> PHAEDRUS: Yes, exactly.
>
> SOCRATES: Of the divine type, we separated out four parts assigned to four gods: a seer's inspiration coming from Apollo, mystical initiation ascribed to Dionysos, a poetic madness coming from the Muses, and fourth madness coming from Aphrodite and Eros (Love) which we called an erotic madness and the best. In some way, though I can't say exactly how, we offered an image of erotic experience and perhaps touched upon a truth in some instances and in others were wide of the mark blending together a not totally unpersuasive account in playful way—but also in a measured way and with due reverence—a mythic hymn to your master and mine, Phaedrus, to Eros, the guardian of beautiful boys.
>
> PHAEDRUS: And, for me, certainly not unpleasant to the ear.
>
> SOCRATES: Then, let's take up what follows from this point: how was the speech able to pass from censure to praise.
>
> PHAEDRUS: What do you have in mind?
>
> SOCRATES: I'd say that everything else was in fact done in play for sport, but that some things were mentioned by chance and two of these hit upon forms or aspects of speech which would not be unpleasant to seize upon if someone had the power to capture their power by means of a systematic art.
>
> PHAEDRUS: What things?
>
> SOCRATES: The first involves someone whose sight can bring into a single form things which have previously been scattered in all directions so that by defining each thing he makes clear any subject he ever wants to teach about. So just now speaking about Eros, we defined what it is, whether well or poorly. The definition, at least, allowed the speech to progress with clarity and internal consistency.
>
> PHAEDRUS: And what do you say the second form is, Socrates?
>
> SOCRATES: To have the power, conversely, to cut up a composition, form by form, according to its natural joints and not to try to hack through any part as a bad butcher might. Rather take the example of the two recent speeches which seize upon one common form to explain the loss of coherent thought; just as the body, which is one thing, is naturally divided into pairs of things with both parts having the same name (called, for example, left arm and right arm), so also the two speeches assumed that madness is by its nature one form in us, though capable of being divided into two parts. One of the speeches cut the

---

[7] Earlier in the dialogue there is a three fold classification of divinely (and beneficently) sent madness (244A–245A): prophetic madness, such as at the oracular sites; a form of madness in conjunction with a gift for healing prophecy and rituals that arises in some individuals from certain families where this an ancient blood guilt leading to severe illnesses and troubles; poetic madness, Dionysiac and from the Muses.

part on the left and did not cease cutting until it found among these parts
something called 'left love' and the, with absolute justice, abused; the other
speech, however, led us to the madness on the right side and discovered there
a love with the same name as the other but of some divine nature. Setting this
before us, the speech praised it as the greatest cause of good for us.

PHAEDRUS: This is very true.

SOCRATES: I myself am certainly a lover [*erastes*], Phaedrus, of these processes
of division [*diairesis*] and collection [*sunagoge*], so that I may have the ability
to speak and think. If I believe that someone else has the capacity to see into
a single thing and to see the natural outgrowth from a single thing toward
many things, I pursue him, following 'right behind in his tracks as if he were a
god.'[8] And furthermore—god knows whether I've been speaking correctly or
not—up to now I have been calling those who can do this, dialecticians.

Classification, then, is a two-step procedure: first we gather together 'the
scattered particulars', the seemingly disparate pieces or entities. Second,
having collected these in one place, we then proceed to make divisions
according to 'natural joints', making meaningful and 'natural' subdivisions.
The first step clearly involves a bold intellectual or even intuitive leap—to
claim many diverse particulars as actually forms of love—however weird
or even slightly counter-intuitive. The particulars that Plato in effect brings
together include: love/attraction/lust between man and man, man and
woman, between deities and mortals, intellectual *eros*, and passionate and
painful yearning of the psyche for return to the realm of the Form of the
Beautiful. In modern terms, influenced by a century of psychoanalysis, not
only do we call certain relations between man and woman, man and man,
woman and woman, child and parent, children with each other, 'love', but
even relations that seem to be painful, full of more anguish than pleasure,
as, for example, a dominatrix whipping the subjected male. Second, there
are reasons for wanting to subdivide this entity of love (or madness) into
divisions, classes, not just particulars. The divisions of madness are part of
Plato's philosophic (and rhetorical) purposes.

These purposes include demonstrating the superiority of dialectic over
rhetoric.[9] But, above all, he is concerned how the philosophic/dialectical
enterprise must draw upon some form of *eros*, some form of 'enthusiasm',

---

[8] Paraphrase of *Odyssey* 2.406 and 5.193.

[9] A few sections later (270) Plato considers how the craft, the *techne*, of medicine makes
classifications, implicitly comparing it to his own, but perhaps also critiquing medicine as
it usually practiced. See the elegant discussion by Wesley Smith, demonstrating that the
Hippocratic text to which Plato refers is in fact *On Regimen*. Smith adds, 'But we cannot tell
what Plato really thought of Hippocrates' (1979, 50).

as in a Dionysiac frenzy, a dialectical Bacchanalia, as it were. And, Socrates is definitely erotic in his classifying activity. Plato does not need here to make distinctions among the disturbances that might bring someone to a physician,[10] but rather a kind of classification of what might bring a person to a philosopher, and keep him coming to the philosopher.

But the two stages of classifying that Plato delineates—collecting the particulars under one heading, and then making 'natural' divisions—are not neatly separable. The process captures something recurrent in the history of psychiatric classification. Eugen Bleuler, for example, in his 1910 monograph, *Dementia Praecox, or the Group of Schizophrenias*, first collected a number of illnesses variously described and labeled in the nineteenth century, and pronounced them as being one. More precisely, at the moment of carving out the category schizophrenia from the mélange of numerous other disorders, he speaks of 'the group of schizophrenias': catatonic, hebephrenic, paranoid, and simple. To this day, both stages of Bleuler's operation remain quite problematic, and redefinition and drawing of new borders continue apace.[11]

But what Plato's discourse here illustrates is the need to carefully examine any proposal for classification of mental disturbance for its spoken and unspoken assumptions. The designation of a classification as 'natural' is especially in need of close scrutiny, for so much of what has been, and is, called 'natural', is often largely a culturally constructed version of the natural. One can envision the construction of categories of mental illness as overlapping with the process of colonial powers drawing boundaries of their African possessions in the nineteenth and early twentieth centuries. These boundaries satisfied certain needs of the powers, and often disregarded tribal, ethnic divisions. But those ethnic and tribal divisions were not necessarily entirely 'natural' either, having their own complex origins and histories.

I do not believe that categorization per se is an evil to be avoided, but rather it is both inevitable and necessary. A schema may be provisional,

---

[10] See in this volume, M.M. Sassi's paper, 'Mental Illness, Moral Error, and Responsibility in Late Plato'; Plato's discussion and classifying in the *Timaeus* is driven by a different set of considerations than his discussion in the *Phaedrus*.

[11] In the mélange of terms around schizophrenia, there have variously appeared: schizophreniform psychoses, pseudo-neurotic schizophrenia, borderline schizophrenia, schizophrenic spectrum disorders, schizoid and schizoid personality. 'Schizoid' underwent many changes of meaning from Bleuler's use of the term, describing features of first degree relatives of schizophrenic patients or schizophrenic patients that had recovered from their severe psychosis, but had some residual peculiarities.

and regarded as such, but nevertheless pragmatic and useful.[12] The human impulse to classify, perhaps starting with classifications such as pain and pleasure, mother and father, baby and grown-up, good girl/bad girl, is universal, though the contents of categories can vary historically and cross-culturally. And all such early classifications universally appear to the 'classifiers' as 'natural.' Further, the professional need to communicate, to understand, to find commonalities—all demand some schema of classification. But 'nature' and its 'joints' turn out to be quite complex, even when as today there are sophisticated ways of studying the genetics of mental disorders. Modern genetics is no simple matter, and at this stage it is definitely 'complexifying' the picture of how molecular and environmental factors interact in a variety of ways at virtually every stage of human development, from gamete formation to mature brain functioning.[13]

2. Seven Constraints on a Perfect System of Classification

Let us now turn to a detailed examination of some perennial and persistent issues that are part and parcel of the process of classifying mental illness, mental disturbance. The reader may notice that my own schema of classifying these constraints is a bit haphazard, and certainly has its own context, motives, and history.

1. The dream of a theory-free method of classification and that such a method will uncover and discover 'natural' entities, without theoretical presupposition. In fact, historically and contemporaneously, any schema has, at the least, a shaping and defining perspective, a set of motives for what is selected to be classified, and/or a theory with a small 't', if not a theory with a capital 'T.' This inevitability makes the 'dream' unrealistic. My own notion (borrowed from others) of 'models of mind and mental illness'—poetic, philosophical, and medical—is one attempt to identify particular perspectives

---

[12] In the current debates on revision of DSM, there has even been debate on the meaning of the word 'pragmatic',—with one author, Ghaemi 2010, arguing the real pragmatism, such as defined by Pierce, requires recognizing that the category of bipolar illness is a robust category and a true entity.

[13] A major impetus for reexamining the role of environmental and family-interaction factors in shaping mental illness came from studies of the genetics of certain behaviors, indicating that the genetics seemed to account for only half of the statistical variance in the findings. See Reiss et al. 1991. For a recent example of the complexity of researching gene/environment interactions, see Arseneault et al. 2011.

that shape classification and provide theories of etiology and treatment.[14] Doctors in antiquity, as do doctors today, had vested interests in classifications and diagnoses that enhanced their professional importance, as well as their income. Competition among doctors as well as between doctors and other 'practitioners' was probably as intense then as now. The Hippocratic doctor was advised not to quote the poets or playwrights, lest he not be taken seriously as a professional. Philosophers of various persuasions and schools in antiquity spawned characterizations of psychic disturbances that fitted their philosophical predilections and devised methods of healing, perhaps gratis, perhaps for a fee. Anecdotes from later antiquity have a certain Sophist named Antiphon (5th–4th century, BCE), setting up a shop in the Agora at Corinth, with a 'shingle' proclaiming that he had a therapy for pains of the soul, a *techne alupias*.[15] In the last decades of the twentieth century, some professional philosophers began to do 'philosophical counseling' of clients whom they saw as having problems of living amenable to philosophical discourse. Their theory revived an ancient category of psychic distress, along with a specific treatment. Thus, there is an element of competition for who has, or who should have, the power to classify.

2. *Cultural, political and economic biases and perspectives inevitably shadow and shape the diagnosis and classification of the 'others', whether other cultures and groups, or of sub-groups within the same culture (e.g. women, children, slaves).* Ancient medicine and philosophy had suppositions about women and slaves, as well as about foreign groups.[16] Modern medicine, psychiatry and psychology, have often overlooked the specific characteristics and needs of various different groups, *and* entertained fantasies about their uniqueness that have tended to exclude them from normative human beings, i.e., 'us.' The fields of 'cross-cultural psychiatry' and 'cross-cultural psychology' are in continuous flux, constantly wrestling with how to deal

---

[14] Simon 1978, and an amendment to the presentation of models ('folk medicine') in Simon 2008.

[15] See Nussbaum 1994 and Pigeaud 1981. On Antiphon, see Lain Entralgo 1970, 103–104. Four late testimonia have slightly different versions of the story. He gave up the effort after a while—in one version because he thought it beneath him, and in another because he was greedy and it was not profitable enough, so he moved to rhetoric. See Pendrick 2002, 94–97.

[16] Sassi 2001. Herodotus was extraordinary both for registering such beliefs and the accompanying pseudo-observations (e.g. in Book 2, he records that Egyptian men urinate squatting, and the women urinate standing up; Egypt is the country where everything is reversed because the Nile runs from South to North), and at the same time he was able to exercise some skepticism and caution about some such reports.

with the 'etic'– how the outside observer sees phenomena in a culture versus the 'emic'–how those within the culture view the same phenomena. A
perennial question in psychiatry has been whether or not 'primitive cultures' have less major mental illness than does 'ours', a question in part
motivated by a romanticizing of the 'primitive.' A small tribe in Ethiopia
had been reported to have no cases of schizophrenia or bipolar psychosis,
but it took a major conceptual and investigative effort to cross the emic/etic
polarity and establish that indeed such cases exist.[17] Considerable controversy exists around whether or not certain entities are cultural constructions or are naturally occurring mental disorders, most recently around
Post-Traumatic Stress Disorder.[18] Closer to home, we have debates around
sexuality, sexual orientation, and various sexual practices—are they abnormal, and why? Homosexuality moved from a 'sexual deviation' in earlier
DSM editions (Diagnostic and Statistic Manual) to being removed as a disorder from DSM III. 'Perversions' got renamed 'paraphilias' and there is much
controversy about their inclusion in DSM revisions.

3. How many entities do you want to posit? Four or four hundred? It seems
difficult to find some number in between. Pinel's first (1798) classification
of mental illness, found in his larger classification of all illnesses, distinguished several hundred, while only a few years later, (1801), his second classification relied on four basic divisions: Mania, ou Délire Général, Mélancolie, ou Délire Exclusif, Démence, ou Abolition de la Pensée, Idiotisme,
ou Obliteration des Facultés Intellectuelles et Affectives.[19] Karl Menninger
(1963) had assembled a chronological listing of classificatory schemes from
antiquity to his time, neatly illustrating this problem. Sometime in the nineteenth century, I believe, the derisive term, 'nosologorrhea',—a disease of
uncontrollable flow of classifications—came into discussions of classifica-

---

[17] Shibre et al. 2010.

[18] See the issue of the journal *Culture, Medicine, Psychiatry* 28: June 2004, dedicated to this
controversy, with the lead article by Joshua Breslau as well as the follow-up debate between
de Jong and Breslau in volume 29: Sept. 2005.

[19] Karl Menninger's *The Vital Balance: The Life Process in Mental Health and Illness* (1963),
11 and 20, endnote 1, originally called my attention to the Pinel material, which I then had
to check out. In Pinel's 1798 work, *Nosographie philosophique, ou, La méthode de l'analyse
appliquée à la médecine,* the last section is 'nervous disorders', and even with the large number
of entities he has a 'classe non determinée'. He is aware there of the classificatory zeal of
'les nosologistes', and the difficulties of neat definition and classification. The 1801 work,
Traité médico-philosophique sur l'aliénation mentale, is specifically about mental disorders.
Pinel himself was a gifted naturalist, and like many in his day, was profoundly influenced by
Linnaeus' method of botanical classification.

tion. Menninger himself argued for a unitary disorder, characterized by different degrees of disorganization or disequilibrium, Today, there is some push to create a basic dichotomy between 'internalizing' and 'externalizing' mental disorders, which, for some researchers, helps make sense out of an otherwise bewildering array of disorders.[20] A further problem, absent clear understanding of etiology and pathogenesis, is that it is difficult to construct a valid 'family, genus, species' schema, such as biological classification traditionally does.

4. There is a tension between the specifics of an individual patient and the generalities of the diagnostic category. It takes both skill and patience to gather the right amount of detail and depth of knowledge of the patient to find the appropriate category. Often, the more one knows about the patient, the harder it becomes to slot the patient into a category. Those who are uneasy with the larger enterprise of classifying mental illness can evoke the overlap of the Greek word for category with the word for accuser, or prosecuting attorney (*kategoros*): the prosecuting attorney's job is to make a given situation fit into a known category of crime. The degree to which it does indeed fit is of course the subject matter of the trial and the jury deliberations.[21] Some historians of medicine have lined up the Greek 'schools' of Cos and Cnidos as a dichotomy between valorizing the diagnostic category or valorizing the specifics of each patient. Emil Kraepelin the great categorizer (and observer) of the late nineteenth and twentieth century, knew not only that many cases did not fit even his own categories, but argued that the study of just such cases was vital to advancing our understanding. From the perspective of the patient, one patient may find comfort in being placed into a known category of illness, and yet another may resent being categorized, as a diminution of her or his individuality.

5. What is the boundary between a trait, a temperament, a constitution, and a disorder or a disease? Is there a continuum from a trait (obsessiveness) to a disease (obsessive-compulsive disorder), or, does the disease actually have no real connection with the trait? Ancient medicine posited varying humoral constitutions which could shade off or predispose to humorally generated diseases. The famous section XXX of the pseudo-Aristotelian

---

[20] See for example Kendler et al. 2011.
[21] I believe this overlap of category and prosecution was pointed out by Kelsen 1946, though I cannot locate that passage in my current reading of the book. See OED entries, 'categorical' and 'category', as well as LSJ, the standard Greek dictionary.

Problemata, 'Why are so many men of genius melancholic?' reflects the position of continuum. Modern classification continues to struggle, for example,
with the boundary between a personality trait and a personality disorder, or
with the definition of normal grief versus 'pathological mourning.' Or, consider a highly traumatized collectivity—what is 'normal mourning' for the
group of survivors of the Cambodian killing-fields, and what is 'pathological mourning'? Ancient philosophy, especially Stoicism, tried to deal with
normal human states of unhappiness, metaphorically, as a disease, and prescribed philosophy as a treatment.[22] A modern development would extend
the spectrum beyond normal to 'supernormal.' Should not we regard, and
treat the 'normal' as a problem, as an artificially defined limit, and have the
medical and psychiatric professions work at 'enhancement?'[23]

6. *Does the classification scheme and the specific diagnosis lead to specificity
in treatment? When they do not, do we call into question the classification
scheme?* Looking just at Hippocratic texts, let alone the larger corpus of
Hellenistic and Graeco-Roman works, one would be hard pressed to find
consistently that phrenitis is treated totally differently from melancholia. In
modern clinical practice, there is the aspiration to have a drug or other intervention specific to a disorder, but this is far from the actual state of affairs.
If the treatment specific to the disorder does not cure the patient, the clin-
ician 'mixes and matches', hoping for a better outcome. At best, there can
be a fruitful feedback from observations about the non-specificity of particular drugs for particular illnesses, a feedback that pushes us to reconsider
our original categories. At worst, there can ensue a chaos of indiscriminate
'polypharmacy',—adding epicycles, as it were, of categories to an individual
case, each of which requires a specific drug. Prompted in part by the problem
of non-specificity of treatment for specific mental disorders, the National
Institute of Mental Health Group is developing a schema that would treat
specific traits, identified as having a genetic contribution, with (often as yet
to be developed) drugs or psychotherapies specific to them. Thereby, they
discard all present diagnostic categories.[24]

---

[22] See Nussbaum 1994 and Pigeaud 1981.

[23] See, for example, Kass 2003, esp. the section 'Happy Souls' (205–273) for a thoughtful
critique of 'enhancement'. The vision decried in this volume stands in stark contrast to
one early statement by Freud about the goal of psychoanalysis: '... much will be gained if
we succeed in transforming your hysterical misery into common unhappiness' (Freud 1957
[1895], 305).

[24] See Insel et al. 2010.

7. There is often a magnetic attraction of a really catchy diagnostic category.
This problem is caricatured in George Bernard Shaw's *Doctor's Dilemma*,
with the surgeon who cheerfully discovers how virtually everyone he encounters suffers from some form or other of a diseased 'nuciform sac.' Once
a clinically plausible *and/or* culturally meaningful category is established,
there is a tendency to draw more and more patients into that category.[25]
This process makes for increasing heterogeneity (and confusion) of who and
what is included in the category. The diagnoses over the centuries of entities
such as melancholia, neurasthenia, chlorosis, attention deficit disorder, bipolar disorder, and post-traumatic stress disorder have all had this magnetic
field pulling in a multitude of patients.

I have attempted to catalog some persistent and probably ineluctable problems in defining and classifying mental illness. I began with a discussion of
Plato's *Phaedrus*, 'carving nature at the joints' and how that model has been
invoked by Paul Meehl, a most serious and influential psychological investigator. Passages from Shakespeare and more recently, Borges, have also been
frequently invoked. I would like to suggest that the recurrent use of literary
passages to help frame, or to caricature, discussions of diagnostic schemas,
hints at a basic tension in the whole study of causes and treatment of mental
disorders, of 'madness' in its various incarnations. That tension is between
the need to harken to the personal, narrative voice, the *cri de coeur* of the
individual suffering person, and the need to find a slot, or box, for that person's suffering. The recourse to literary passages, then, represents that press
to attend to the voice of the patient. The presence of such passages in serious
systematic discourse on diagnosis is a kind of ghost in the wings, or perhaps
an uninvited guest, that demands some attention. Insistently, it is this very
tension that characterizes the mental health professions, for better and for
worse. For better—when the tension is recognized and owned; for worse,
when one or the other pole is granted absolute hegemony. In addition, the
playful nature of the *Phaedrus* dialogue, and the comedy in Borges' caricature, are useful reminders of the tentativeness of even our best efforts at
classification.

These two recognitions—of the need to heed the patient's voice and
the need for our own humility—are necessary in order to avoid despair

---

[25] See, for example, Draaisma 2009 for examples of how a crystallized eponymous disease
entity takes on a life and centrality of its own, becoming a reference point for, e.g., 'Parkinson-
like diseases' (I thank M.M. Sassi for this reference). On neurasthenia and chlorosis, see the
excellent monograph of Helen King (2004).

in facing all of the above difficulties, in persisting to clarify our thinking about classification, and to improve the products of that thinking. Over the long haul, we need an ongoing acknowledgment of the subjectivity of both patients and the treating professionals, of motives latent and blatant, as a *starting point*. We then need to continually 'parse' and clarify these factors in order to see what kinds of more durable perspectives and truths emerge.

IF ONLY THE ANCIENTS HAD HAD DSM, ALL WOULD HAVE BEEN CRYSTAL CLEAR: REFLECTIONS ON DIAGNOSIS

Julian C. Hughes

Introduction

Ludwig Wittgenstein wrote that 'the truly apocalyptic view of the world is that things do *not* repeat themselves'.[1] He went on to make a typically acerbic comment, suggesting that the age of science and technology might be 'the beginning of the end for humanity'. Exactly how this should be interpreted is controversial; but, more simply, I want to use Wittgenstein's remark to justify my discussion, namely that things do repeat themselves, that we face the same intellectual problems today with respect to diagnosis in connection with psychiatry that the Ancients faced before us in relation to diagnosis generally. I am going to draw some parallels—no more than that—to shed light on continuing debates. But that it is possible for such parallels to be drawn might be a source of surprise, perhaps, to anyone inclined to believe that if the ancients had had the *Diagnostic and Statistical Manual* (DSM), all would have been crystal clear. In the passage cited above, Wittgenstein went on to suggest that the idea of great progress is a delusion. There is something striking about the way in which, to some extent at least, so little progress has been made despite scientific and technological advances.

In this chapter, therefore, I shall draw some parallels between discussions that have underpinned (and continue to tax) those involved in the nosology of DSM and the divisions between some of the different schools of ancient medicine. I shall focus on the Methodic School in order to draw some lessons that still seem pertinent. I shall then draw from current thinking in the philosophy of psychiatry to suggest why, seemingly, there has been so little progress in terms of the debates around diagnosis in the field of mental

---

[1] Wittgenstein 1980 [1947], 56.

health. Finally, I shall suggest that, rather than the Ancients learning from DSM, the framers of current psychiatric nosologies, including DSM, should learn from the Ancients. Moreover, these lessons, derived from psychiatry, are none the less pertinent to the whole of medical practice.

Whilst I shall draw on parallels in connection with Methodism in particular, comparisons with the other main schools or sects of ancient medicine also encourage clearer thoughts about current nosological problems. The Dogmatic School, said to follow Hippocrates, regarded the hidden causes of diseases as important. According to Nutton, they were linked by 'their belief in the use of reason to establish a chain of causation'.[2] The Empiric School derived their knowledge from experience. They were interested in evident causes of disease, but not in hidden causes, the search for which they regarded as dogmatic and unhelpful. Effective treatments might emerge on the basis of inspiration, but mostly it was a matter of experience—the more experience the better.[3] The Methodist School will be discussed in more detail below, but their emphasis was on generalities or commonalities. Having observed the general symptoms of an illness, the treatment followed in response to these generalities, without then the need for too much theory concerning underlying causes. The differences between these sects is not, however, completely clear. In particular, part of the attraction of Methodism is precisely that it

> ... may be said to have steered a kind of middle course between two extremes by reacting critically to both the Empiricists and the Dogmatists, while at the same time combining accurate observation of a patient's symptoms with a moderately strong theoretical apparatus.[4]

At least in outline, then, we can sense a division between those who believe illnesses should be classified according to their underlying causes, those who feel that the purpose is simply to arrive at empirical treatments, and those who emphasize observation as a means of picking out the generalities that encapsulate the condition.[5]

---

[2] Nutton 2004, 124.
[3] Nutton 148.
[4] Van der Eijk 2005a, 321–322.
[5] Perennial problems around classification are nicely discussed in this volume by Bennett Simon (see the previous chapter).

New York 1959

In 1959, the World Health Organization (WHO) and the American Psychopathological Association held a meeting in New York.[6] One of the most significant events at the meeting was an address by Carl Hempel (1905–1997), a logical empiricist philosopher of science. Hempel was born and studied in Germany, gained his doctoral degree from Berlin in 1934, and ended up in the USA, having previously met Rudolf Carnap (1891–1970) and having established connections with the logical positivists of both the Berlin and Vienna Circles. In the USA he held positions at various universities and finally at Princeton, where he remained until he retired in 1973.

Hempel was invited to give a paper to the 1959 conference on psychiatric classification. The aim of the conference was to establish a classification of mental disorders that might gain international currency. The WHO had achieved this in other branches of medicine in 1948 in its *Manual of the International Statistical Classification of Diseases, Injuries and Causes of Death*. But, 11 years later, only four countries had adopted the mental disorders section of the Manual. In order to try to rectify this state of affairs, the WHO commissioned the Austrian-born psychiatrist, Erwin Stengel (1902–1973), who was professor at Sheffield, to make recommendations for a classification that might be more widely accepted.

The 1959 conference led to the Eighth Revision of the *International Classification of Diseases* (ICD-8) in 1967. The ICD-8 nomenclature was subsequently adopted by the American Psychiatric Association in the second version of its *Diagnostic and Statistical Manual* (DSM-II). The WHO then published a glossary in 1974, which was 'the first predominantly symptom-based modern classification of mental disorders'.[7] The DSMs and the ICDs have continued to evolve. We are now up to ICD-10, which appeared in 1992,[8] and DSM-IV, which appeared in 1994, with text revisions made in 2000.[9] And recommendations from the working groups of the DSM-5 are now on the web,[10] with the aim that this should appear at about the same time as this chapter. We shall then see ICD-11 following in the next few years.

---

[6] I shall draw throughout on the accounts and commentaries offered by Fulford et al. 2006.

[7] Fulford et al. 2006, 325.

[8] World Health Organization 1992.

[9] American Psychiatric Association 2000.

[10] The change from Roman to Arabic numerals seems to be part of the process of modernizing the DSM. Details can be found on the website of the American Psychiatric Association (DSM-5 Development).

The 1959 conference in New York was very significant in setting the pattern and underpinning logic of the classification of mental disorders that has ensued. In his paper, Hempel set out two requirements for a classification to be scientific.

> Broadly speaking, the vocabulary of science has two basic functions: first, to permit an adequate *description* of the things and events that are the objects of scientific investigation; second, to permit the establishment of general laws or theories by means of which particular events may be *explained* and *predicted* and thus *scientifically understood* ....[11]

The requirements are for *description* (or 'descriptive adequacy') and systematic *explanation*, where, in the development of a science, description comes first and explanation increasingly follows. Hempel continued:

> The vocabulary required in the early stages of this development will be largely observational; it will be chosen so as to permit the description of those aspects of the subject matter which are ascertainable fairly directly by observation. The shift toward theoretical systematization is marked by the introduction of new, 'theoretical' terms, which refer to various theoretically postulated entities, their characteristics, and the processes in which they are involved; all these are more or less removed from the level of directly observable things and events.[12]

Despite his logical empiricist background, Hempel, in talking about psychiatric classification, allowed his natural inclination to insist on knowledge that is objective to slip from view in favour of the more speculative views of psychodynamic theory that dominated at the time. It did not seem to be a pressing issue for Hempel whether the theoretical basis of psychiatry turned out to be psychodynamic or biophysiological. The other historical feature is that, in the event, although Hempel's first requirement, for descriptive adequacy, was picked up, the emphasis on systematic explanation—which Hempel clearly felt was more important for the development of psychiatric classification if it were to acquire the standing of a scientific enterprise—was not pursued.[13]

Why did the framers of ICD and DSM move so strongly in the direction of a descriptive basis for their nosologies? According to Fulford et al., it was because of an intervention during the discussion that followed Hempel's paper by Professor Sir Aubrey Julian Lewis (1900–1975),[14] and because of

---

[11] Hempel 1994.
[12] Hempel.
[13] These issues are brought out well in the discussion by Fulford et al. 2006.
[14] Lewis 1961.

his subsequent influence on how things developed.[15] Lewis was the first Professor of Psychiatry at the Institute of Psychiatry in London and a driving force in British psychiatry after the Second World War. The important point to note is that Lewis's view was based on the need to reach a *practical* conclusion, which was that an international system of classification was required. Awaiting a unified, systematic, theoretical, agreed underpinning to the classification seemed senseless.

From this discussion of the New York conference we can derive three things in connection with psychiatric diagnosis. First, there is the need for close observation or description (Hempel's 'descriptive adequacy'). Secondly, there is Hempel's further requirement for systematic explanation; a requirement which, however, was rejected in the event as not being achievable. Thirdly, there is the need to arrive at a workable, practical, classificatory diagnostic system.

Links to Methodism

Turning now to Methodism, which Nutton describes as 'arguably the dominant medical theory throughout the Roman world for at least three centuries',[16] it is possible to start drawing some parallels between the discussions in New York in 1959 and the concerns of the Methodic School of ancient medicine. It is relevant to recall Hempel's requirement—for descriptive adequacy—that a psychiatric classification should meet if it is to be scientific:

> The vocabulary ... will be largely observational; it will be chosen so as to permit the description of those aspects of the subject matter which are ascertainable fairly directly by observation.[17]

The emphasis on the observable can also be found in the work of Caelius Aurelianus:

> Like other Methodist authors, Caelius challenges the more traditional, humoural theories of disease in favour of a form of medicine that focuses on the practical treatment of illness. The Methodists' motivation in creating this new approach is the belief that if entities such as humours and *pneuma* are not physically observable, their very existence cannot be proven, and should not be used as the basis of a theory of medicine.[18]

---

[15] Again, see Fulford et al. 2006.
[16] Nutton 2004, 188.
[17] Hempel 1994.
[18] McDonald 2009, 154.

My aim here is not to suggest that the Methodists would or would not be happy with current psychiatric classifications. Such an argument would have to be enormously complex, probably impossible and ultimately pointless. But there is something important to be derived from a comparison of contemporary arguments and those that occurred almost 2000 years ago. In this vein, therefore, it is instructive to note that Stengel had himself produced a review in 1959,[19] which included the recommendation that:

> ... since the widespread use of diagnostic terms with aetiological implications impeded agreement on a common nomenclature, there should be a set of neutral, operational definitions which were primarily descriptive ....[20]

There is, therefore, a clear parallel between Hempel's first requirement, for good description based on observation, and an important plank in the Methodist approach, which emphasized close observation too.

The other pressing issue for those involved in the New York conference in 1959 was that any diagnostic system had to be practical. Again there is a parallel to be drawn with Methodism, which is said to have originated in the approach of Themison in the first century BC. According to Nutton,

> Themison declared that good medicine was effective practice, no more, no less: there was no need for complex nosological classifications (though nosology and close observation of symptoms were essential), still less for any investigation into the hidden causes of disease.[21]

Aubrey Lewis was obviously *not* against nosology, but he did want the system of classification to be practical. Hence, in the discussion after Hempel's paper in New York in 1959, we find Lewis attempting to steer matters in the following way:

> I would suggest that for the purpose of public classification we should eschew categories based on theoretical concepts and restrict ourselves to the operational, descriptive type of classification.[22]

Once again, the emphasis is on description, which is based on careful observation, but this is for practical purposes, because the underlying mechanisms are not known. This emphasis is based on a long tradition of empirical observation, without commitments to underlying theory, which had characterized British psychiatry. Thus Henry Maudsley's (1835–1918) comment:

---

[19] Stengel 1959.
[20] Shepherd 1994.
[21] Nutton 2004, 190.
[22] Lewis 1961.

classifications which pretend to go to the root of the matter go beyond what knowledge warrants and are radically faulty.[23]

This does not, however, mean that there are no grounds for positing some theoretical background. Themison, according to Nutton, held that

> empirical observation by itself was not enough. What was required was the understanding that all diseases shared some general and plainly visible characteristics, 'commonalities', and that once these were recognized the choice of treatment followed easily. An examination of the patient would provide a good indication of the appropriate commonality.[24]

According to the critics of Methodism, even the less hostile ones such as Celsus, the practitioners of Methodism ignored the needs and characteristics of individual patients. They,

> ... lacked the subtlety of diagnostic and prescriptive reasoning to be able to view each patient as an individual requiring individual care and individual treatment.[25]

And yet,

> ... to the Methodists their ability to see beyond the individual and to grasp the commonalities was something to be proud of.[26]

Nutton links the emergence of Methodist theories to the realities of providing medical care in a city the size of Rome, where the ability to offer a swift diagnosis and treatment was valued.[27] There is something similar to be said in favour of the approach of Aubrey Lewis to international classification. Despite uncertainties, the requirement was for a public system that could be applied with facility in many different countries. The critical thing would be good observation, which would have to lead to common diagnoses, rather than private, idiosyncratic determinations of what might be wrong at the level of aetiology. The two situations, the need for quick and effective treatment in a city the size of Rome and the requirement for an international system of psychiatric classification, are dissimilar; but the underlying concern, that similar things should be picked up similarly, is the same. As Aubrey Lewis was to write in his Foreword to the WHO's 1974 *Glossary*,

---

[23] Maudsley 1879.
[24] Nutton 2004, 190–191. For the Methodist texts outside Soranus that refer to "commonalities" see Tecusan 2004, 88.
[25] Nutton 201.
[26] Nutton 201.
[27] Nutton 187–188.

It would seem … that accurate observation is still the gate that needs the clos-est guard. A.R. Feinstein put it bluntly: 'the current psychiatric debates about systems of classification, the many hypothetical and unconfirmed schemas of 'psychodynamic mechanisms', and the concern with etiological inference rather than observational evidence are nosologic activities sometimes remi-niscent of those conducted by the mediaeval taxonomists.' Since the disorders listed in this glossary are identified by criteria that are predominantly descrip-tive, its use should encourage an emphasis on careful observation.[28]

Remember that at about this time the roots of the US-UK Diagnostic Project, which ran from 1966 to 1971 and brought together London and New York, were being formed, where the aim was to establish whether similar diagnos-tic categories were being used in the two countries.[29] Establishing a common diagnostic language, based on close observation, was obviously key to these developments and it could be argued that the process was similar to that of seeing the commonalities. This may be to stretch the point a little, because what seeing the commonalities amounted to throughout the Methodist tra-dition is not altogether certain—it seems to have included a degree of intu-ition as well as observation. This raises a question concerning the extent to which intuition might be involved in the process of diagnosis using DSM or ICD, to which I shall return.

But first I shall consider a little more closely the contentious doctrines that were thought to mark out Methodism. Van der Eijk usefully summarizes these in his chapter on the Methodism of Caelius.[30] The details of his argu-ment concern the extent to which Caelius presents a consistent Methodist account. Van der Eijk argues convincingly, to my eyes, that Caelius can accommodate apparent aberrations. But the cogency of the argument is not my concern. I am only going to comment on one aspect of the argu-ment, which is to do with definitions. Recall that it was said that Methodists refused to give definitions. But, first, we should consider a more general comment. Van der Eijk points out that recent scholarship suggests, 'Method-ism is not a philosophy but a way of doing medicine'.[31] And he contin-ues:

> The point is that doctrinal and methodological tensions may, in the case of Methodism, find their origin in the fact that the primary concern of Method-ism is the successful diagnosis and treatment of diseases, and in the Method-

---

[28] Lewis 1974.
[29] See Cooper et al. 1969; And for a brief discussion see Shepherd 1994.
[30] Van der Eijk 2005a, 299–327.
[31] Van der Eijk 305.

ists' belief that all issues that are not necessarily related to this ... are considered to be irrelevant or inappropriate.[32]

When he turns to consider definitions, van der Eijk cites Caelius, who lists some antecedent causes of cholera, but states:

> ... quorum sane intellectus aptus rationi est ob causarum scientiam, inutilis uero ac ⟨non⟩ necessarius curationi uel naturae.

> Yet while the understanding of these is certainly appropriate to the theoretical knowledge of the causes, it is useless and not necessary for the treatment or for the nature of the disease.[33]

Commenting on this passage, van der Eijk says that it shows,

> ... first, that Caelius (and Soranus) have no difficulty with giving a definition, provided that it is a proper definition—in this case, a concise statement of the generality (*coenotes*), of the affected parts, and of the acuteness of the disease—where properness is determined not only by factual correctness but also by the relevance of the components of the definition to diagnosis and treatment.[34]

Later, he summarizes thus:

> ... as far as definitions as such are concerned, it seems that when Caelius ... says that he, or Soranus, refuses to give definitions, he means that he and Soranus object to the uncritical, automatic procedure of trying to catch the essence of a disease in a definition.[35]

Now, I want to draw a parallel between this and Hempel's first requirement for objective description (in the absence of his second requirement for the explanation that leads to scientific understanding). It is also relevant to notice a related parallel, which is still relevant, namely the fight against the tendency to what Scadding has termed Essentialism, where this implies that the name of a disease stands for a discrete entity with an essence.[36] Scadding contrasted this view with Nominalism:

> Avoiding essences—inasmuch as these Nominalists recognise that diseases have no existence apart from that of patients with them, and that the causal implications of a diagnosis in current disease terminology are widely varied.[37]

---

[32] Van der Eijk 305.
[33] *Acute Affections* 3.19.190; cited in Van der Eijk 318.
[34] Van der Eijk 319.
[35] Van der Eijk 320.
[36] Scadding 1996.
[37] Scadding 1996.

Avoiding essences—inasmuch as these tie us to a particular causal account of the disease—sits happily with the approach of Methodism.

One of the other extremely important elements of Hempel's paper to the 1959 conference was his advocacy of 'operational definitions'. These were meant to provide the objectivity that was required for *scientific* psychiatric classification. Hempel described such definitions as follows:

> Schematically, an operational definition of a scientific term S is a stipulation to the effect that S is to apply to all and only those cases for which performance of test operation T yields the specified outcome O.[38]

This would seem to suggest that the descriptive part of Hempel's classification requires precise definitions. But this is not the case:

> Hempel was aware of the considerable difficulties in providing *complete* operational definitions for all things in science, and was willing to settle for, for instance, *observations alone* as qualifying for the test operation ...

> Hempel also emphasized that the criteria of application must be relevant to the scientific question and practical in use.[39]

Without wishing to push the similarity too far, this sounds familiar. Methodism, remember, 'is not a philosophy but a way of doing medicine'.[40] It has to be practical. It was also for this reason, remember too, that Aubrey Lewis felt the second requirement of Hempel was not practicable:

> In psychiatry to make a classification based on theory is what we all would like, and what we believe we cannot at the moment attain—because, as Dr. Hempel clearly stated, the requirements are not met by any of the theories prevailing in psychiatry at the present time.

> Therefore I would suggest that for the purpose of public classification we should eschew categories based on theoretical concepts and restrict ourselves to the operational, descriptive type of classification ....[41]

In summary, therefore, emerging from the New York conference and evident in the work of the Methodists is an emphasis on careful observation and description, the need for a practical approach and the importance of operationalization, which I have suggested can be compared to the idea of looking for generalities or commonalities.

---

[38] Hempel 1994.
[39] Sadler 2005, 76.
[40] Van der Eijk 2005a, 305.
[41] Lewis 1974.

I want to move on to look at why there is a problem—one that *was* implicit in ancient medicine and *is* implicit in persisting problems to do with psychiatric classification. At which point we need to remind ourselves of the continuing tensions. In several publications, Allen Frances, Emeritus Professor in the Department of Psychiatry at Duke University and previous chair of the DSM-IV Task Force, has been overtly critical of the process now underway to establish DSM-5. There has been talk of the need for a 'paradigm shift' amongst those involved in DSM-5. Frances asserts:

> Simply stated, descriptive psychiatric diagnosis does not need and cannot support a paradigm shift. There can be no dramatic improvements in psychiatric diagnosis until we make a fundamental leap in our understanding of what causes mental disorders.[42]

In other words, we still cannot move on to pursue Hempel's second requirement of systematic explanation. Frances goes on to say:

> Undoubtedly, the most reckless suggestion for *DSM-5* is that it include many new categories to capture the subthreshhold (e.g. minor depression, mild cognitive disorder) or premorbid (e.g. prepsychotic) versions of the existing official disorders. ...
>
> The result would be a wholesale imperial medicalization of normality that will trivialize mental disorder and lead to a deluge of unneeded medication treatments—a bonanza for the pharmaceutical industry but at huge cost to the new false-positive patients caught in the excessively wide *DSM-5* net.[43]

Highlighted here, therefore, are two connected issues: first, that the developments in the neurosciences and in genetics have not yet led to clinically useful advances for patients in terms of explaining diseases; and, secondly, that 'early' diagnosis is not at a point at which it differentiates between normal and abnormal, so attempts at early diagnosis will only serve to label many normal people as abnormal.

Values in Practice

To cut to the chase, the common issue is to do with values. In the case of the distinction between normal and abnormal—think, for instance, of what might distinguish between normal and abnormal ageing—that an evaluative judgement is required is obvious. People might doubt that this is true

---

[42] Frances 2009.
[43] Frances.

in dementia, because no one wants to consider dementia a normal part of ageing. Biologically, however, there is a continuum from the 'normal' to the 'abnormal' ageing brain. Pathologists have marked out boundaries that have a good deal of utility, so that on the whole it can be said that if you have this degree of pathology you will have dementia. The point is, however, that this cannot be said with complete certainty and at the margins there is no certainty whatsoever: normal people have the pathology of dementia and people with marked dementia can be remarkably free of pathology. There are many other reasons to be critical of the notion of 'dementia' and one safe tactic, it might be supposed, would be to avoid this syndromal (umbrella) diagnosis and instead stick to specific diagnoses such as Alzheimer's disease.[44] But the same evaluative questions arise in connection with 'Alzheimer's', which some have said should itself be regarded as a syndrome, rather than as a discrete disease entity (it is the problem of Essentialism again).[45]

The problem to do with the advance of science and the lack of advance in connection with psychiatric diagnosis is also, however, to do with values. This line of thought has been convincingly argued for many years by Fulford.[46] The point is that, more than perhaps in any other specialisms in medical practice (a competitor would be general practice), values are central to psychiatry. Even in diagnosis, even in conditions as diverse as schizophrenia and Alzheimer's disease, let alone Attention Deficit Hyperactivity Disorder and Post Traumatic Stress Disorder, evaluative judgements are required. The further point is that non-psychiatric diagnoses *also* involve value judgements; they are just not to the fore. But they *are* there. This is, actually, the first principle of what Fulford has called Values-Based Medicine (VBM) namely the 'two-feet' principle, that decisions in medicine, including to do with diagnosis, depend on values as well as on facts.[47] Fulford sees VBM as a necessary complement to Evidence-Based Medicine (EBM): values must balance facts in medical practice. The third ('science-driven') principle of VBM is apposite to our discussion:

> Scientific progress, in opening up choices, is increasingly bringing the full diversity of human values into play in all areas of health care ....[48]

---

44 Hughes 2011.
45 Richards and Brayne 2010.
46 Fulford 1989.
47 Fulford 2004, 208–209.
48 Fulford 212.

This principle, in other words, closes down the argument that the problem with psychiatry (not *for* it) is that it is not scientific enough. Rather, the difficulty with psychiatry is that values, which are trickier to handle than facts, are prominent and will become more prevalent as the discipline becomes more scientific. But I have jumped over the second principle of VBM, the 'squeaky wheel' principle, which states,

> We tend to notice values only when they are diverse or conflicting and hence are likely to be problematic.[49]

And with these principles in mind we can return to think about ancient medicine. At the start of his chapter on Methodism, Nutton notes that, 'the expanding population of the capital allowed a ready market for any and all medical theories and practices'.[50] There were Pneumatists, Dogmatists, Methodists, Hippocratics, and so forth, with 'learning and showmanship, practical expertise and eloquence on all sides ...'.[51] This is values diversity and values diversity often seems problematic, but it is at least important to see that the problem is precisely to do with values. Nutton goes on to argue that Methodism was able to combine flexibility with manageable treatment options. Here, then, is an approach that manifests certain values and combines these background values with the practical ability to negotiate between the values of others. So, too, in van der Eijk's discussion of the Methodist attitude to 'unobservable entities or processes', he states that the Methodists,

> ... prefer not to build their therapy on such speculations or commitments; but this is a matter of *preference*, based on the criterion of relevance ....[52]

In other words, it is an *evaluative* decision. Remember, too, van der Eijk's earlier talk of the Methodists' rejection of definition *only* if definition were not *proper*,

> ... where properness is determined not only by *factual* correctness but also by the relevance of the components of the definition to diagnosis and treatment (emphasis now added).[53]

Factual correctness is not the be-all and end-all; there are values at work, to do with practicality and prudence. My aim in this chapter has not been to

---

[49] Fulford 209.
[50] Nutton 2004, 187.
[51] Nutton 201.
[52] Van der Eijk 2005a, 326.
[53] Van der Eijk 319.

champion Methodism; but, in its tendency to eschew some sorts of scientific background theories and to focus on observation and practicalities, it forms a nice parallel to the moves that have underpinned approaches to psychiatric classification. And it does seem to me that one of the comparisons we can make across the ages—given that comparing factual knowledge, whilst interesting, is facile if all we wish to do is point out that their facts were more or less sophisticated than ours, from our own temporally blinkered perspective—is in terms of the values that surround and are embedded in and drive medical practice.

Ancient Horizons

The most detailed work on values in conjunction with DSM has been undertaken by Professor John Sadler. His analysis of DSM in *Values and Psychiatric Diagnosis* has allowed him to elucidate what he calls the 'value-structural elements' of DSM-IV, as shown in Table 1.[54] The idea here is that diagnosis reflects certain values, but the way in which these values are embedded in our diagnostic categories can actually shape or structure our attitudes towards diagnosis. Sadler discusses both how values have guided action in past DSMs and how they should do so in the future.[55]

Table 1. Selected value-structural elements in DSM-IV[56]

Administrative utility	Advocacy	Aiding the ill	Atheoreticism
Clinical utility	Comprehensive coverage	Democratic values	Educational utility
Empiricism	Essentialism	Eudaimonia	Guild interests
Hyponarrativity	Individualism	Naturalism	Pragmatism
Professionalism	Profitability	Research utility	Scientific rigor
Technological values	Traditionalism	Universalism	User-friendliness

The inclusion of 'Eudaimonia' as a value-structural element is striking. According to Sadler, this currently operates only in the background. Elements such as 'Research utility' and 'Administrative utility' are in the foreground. In this connection it should be recalled that in the USA a DSM diagnosis is required for remuneration by the medical insurance companies. So one of

---

[54] Sadler 2005.
[55] Sadler 444–469.
[56] From Sadler, Tables 11.1 and 11.2 (440–444).

the drivers in constructing a new DSM is that it should continue to have this administrative utility. But for Sadler much of this is the wrong way round. He states:

> ... many of the controversies associated with psychiatric diagnosis and the DSMs have to do with an incomplete appreciation of the dual meaning of diagnosis: as denotation and as practice.[57]

Once again we see the two themes of observation and practicality emerging: diagnosis is about seeing and conceptually picking out diseases, but it does this with practical intent (e.g. to cure or to palliate). The spirit of practice means, for Sadler, engagement and relationships. It means a scientific approach as well, but one tempered by what Sadler calls, following Heidegger, the 'poietic' mode of existence, which is contrasted with the technological way of relating, as shown in Table 2. Technological values encourage the diagnostic classification in the direction of structural elements such as administrative utility. But the poietic values of Table 2 turn the structure towards elements in Table 1 such as individualism or even *eudaimonia*.

Table 2. Values demonstrated in our interactions with the world[58]

Technological values	Poietic values
Convenience	Creativity
Economy	Tradition
Efficiency	Personal discipline
Productivity	Nature
Utility	Connectedness and engagement

The quintessential evaluative judgement that is required in clinical practice concerns 'how we should live'.[59] The important framing questions (all of which are redolent of ancient concerns) should typically, according to Sadler, be of this sort: 'What characterizes the good life?', 'How should I relate to others?', 'What is worth doing?'. Hence, for Sadler, it seems important that DSM should articulate its view of the good life, so that, as a structural value, *eudaimonia* moves from the background to the foreground:

> Only then will the public and our patients know what psychiatry stands for and, more specifically, what norms and 'normalities' are involved in a DSM.[60]

---

[57] Sadler 429.
[58] Sadler 328–330.
[59] Sadler 345.
[60] Sadler 452.

I left hanging the notion of intuition, which arose in connection with the commonalities of Methodism. The notion of intuitionism needs a good deal of thought. Here I can only point to one aspect relevant to my discussion, which I shall state quite baldly. Intuition has little part to play where facts dominate the picture. But as soon as values come into play and are regarded as essential to the perspective, then there is room for intuition. Seeing the *right* thing to do under these circumstances based on one's observations is partly a matter of intuition. It is also a matter of practical wisdom (*phronesis*) or prudence. It is knowing what to aim at under the particular circumstances. The Empiricist sect could claim that intuition played a role in their approach, because intuition might also depend on experience and might have guided the sort of 'empirical' treatment which they might offer. In a sense too, but of course the details of this must be vague, we could argue that the intuitive knowledge of what to aim at is also something to do with the commonalities of Methodism. But then the Dogmatists might similarly accept that intuition helps in the discernment of the underlying causes of any particular disease. So here we start to see why the discussion in connection with psychiatric diagnoses is none the less relevant to all the other branches of medicine. For, as soon as we see that at the heart of diagnosis there are evaluative decisions—judgements about what is relevant, about which observation to give priority to—we can start to see that intuitions and value judgements have a role to play throughout clinical practice.

What might the DSM have offered to the ancients? Well, the need for careful observation of an objective nature is in DSM, but is also apparent in the practice of Methodists such as Caelius and his predecessor Soranus. There is the tendency to want to seek a better scientific basis for the classification of mental diseases, but we have seen that this might be a mistake on both practical and conceptual grounds: because (practically) we still do not have an adequate science and (conceptually) the advance of science does not lessen the need to negotiate values—if anything the reverse. The Methodists, at least, saw that theories had to be used in a way that contributed to the treatment of the patient and not used for their own sake.

In short, it is not clear what DSM might have contributed to the practice of ancient medicine, except perhaps an increased unity of approach. But here, again, we come back to the problem of shared and disputed values. DSM holds because of the shared values that underpin modern practice. But not *everyone* wishes to see a psychiatrist or even a physician; and not all practitioners wish to practise in accordance with DSM.

We might, after all, learn more from the Ancients. But I think if we do, it will be at the level of values, where we can pick up some of the humanity of Soranus (as portrayed by Caelius), of whom Nutton comments:

> His treatment of mental diseases combines a similar pragmatism with humane concern. It is better to agree at first with the delusions of a madman and then gradually bring him round to accept the true situation than to attempt to convince him immediately of his folly and to deny any reality to his perceptions.[61]

And, in addition, as well as the humanity (the 'poietic' bringing-forth), we might also learn more from the Ancients about the values that should inspire clinical practice. For there is a problem with our talk of values, which emerges precisely when there is values diversity. If there cannot be consensus concerning the value judgements—about where clinical depression ends and normal unhappiness begins, or where normal forgetfulness becomes pathological, or even over what sort of wheezing constitutes asthma—where do we turn? One possibility, with an ancient pedigree, is that we should turn to the virtues. It might be that the virtues could be conceived as supplying the horizon against which we should judge disputed values. If the virtue words provide a sketch of what constitutes flourishing for human beings, if they outline the ways we should live and what we should be aiming at, they might well provide the sort of horizon which we are looking for. There may be other possibilities, but this discussion has established two things: first, that our diagnostic frameworks are replete with evaluative judgements; secondly, that it is, therefore, relevant to raise questions in connection with diagnosis concerning what might constitute the good life for human beings qua human beings.

Conclusion

There are parallels to be drawn between the concerns of the Ancients and modern psychiatric nosologists. In psychiatry we are still in the business, as were the Methodists, of engaging in careful observation and description in order to achieve a practical approach to the diagnosis and treatment of psychiatric diseases. What constitutes a disease is not to be found in terms of some specific essence. Rather we engage with disease in the world of human beings where there are conflicting values and intuitions. These

---

[61] Nutton 2004, 200.

need to be judged against the backdrop of the virtues inasmuch as they set out what it is to live well humanly. And the reason why history must repeat itself is that our notions of what constitutes *eudaimonia* must be worked out afresh by each of us and by each new generation. One reason why the age of science and technology could spell the end of humanity would be, as Wittgenstein suggested, if the scientific and technological approach to the world suggested that evaluative judgements were no longer a concern; whereas, in fact, science and technology simply increase the problems in terms of what is best for human beings as creatures in the world. For similar reasons there are grounds for arguing that psychiatric nosology will remain problematic. Diagnosis in the field of mental health will always be defeasible, because there will always be the possibility of values diversity. Given this, there will always be broader questions to be asked about our aims. Perhaps we should do well to look backwards to achieve a better perspective on what it is to flourish humanly, on what it is that should form the horizon against which the *values* of medicine must be realized.

PART II

GREEK CLASSIFICATIONS

THE EARLY GREEK MEDICAL VOCABULARY OF INSANITY

Chiara Thumiger

The aim of this study is to offer a review of Greek general terminology of insanity as it is used in fifth- and early fourth-century medical texts.[1] By 'general' I indicate here terminology which signifies insanity without strong specifications of features, or circumstances that distinguish it from other phenomena. These terms are usually translated into English with interchangeable and overlapping terms such as 'derangement', 'delirium', etc.

This is a list of the relevant terms found in our corpus:

παράνοος, παρανοέω, παράνοια, (οὐ) κατανοέω, ἀγνοέω, ἄγνοια; ὑπομαίνομαι, μανιώδης, μανικός, ἐκμαίνω, μανίη, μαίνομαι; παραφρόνησις, ὑποκαταφρονέω, σωφρονέω, ἀλλοφρονέω, ἀφρονέω, ἀφροσύνη, ἔκφρων, φρόνιμος, ἄφρων, ἔμφρων, φρονέω, παραφροσύνη, παραφρονέω; ἔκστασις, ἐξίσταμαι; παράφορος, παραφέρομαι; ἐπιληρέω, ὑποπαραληρέω, λήρησις, ὑποληρέω, ληρέω, παραληρέω, παραλήρησις, λῆρος, παράληρος; ὑποπαρακρούω, παράκρουσις, παρακρουστικόν, παρακρούω; παρακοπή, παρακόπτω; συνίημι, σύνεσις and συνετός/ἀσύνετος.

First of all, our category of 'general terms' calls for discussion. I have excluded from the review the two groups of vocabulary based around *phrenitis* (φρεν-) and *melancholia* (μελαγχ-, while I have included the *mania* (μαν-) group).[2] One of the reasons behind this choice is practical: *melancholia* and *phrenitis* have already received a great deal of scholarly attention, as opposed to the terms and concepts I wish to discuss here.[3] In addition, the

---

[1] This includes most of the text of the so called 'Corpus Hippocraticum'. I exclude the texts of the Corpus generally considered as belonging to the Hellenistic or to a later period, with limited exceptions (see list on pp. 93–94). I include in this statistic only instances relevant to mental insanity of patients (excluding, e.g., hyperbolic instances where 'mad' should mean 'incompetent' or 'misjudged', with reference to physicians or to the ways of man, etc.). The complete list of occurrences for these terms is found at the end, pp. 83–95.

[2] I adopt the latinized version of the names when referring to a general concept of *phrenitis, melancholia,* or *mania* as object of scholarly attention; I use the Greek to highlight the individual historical instance in respect for the linguistic distinction between substantives, adjectives and verbs.

[3] For a review of the tradition on the three entities see Di Benedetto 1986, 52–63; van der Eijk 2000–2001, II, 144–145, 214–215, 153, with bibliography.

different statuses of these three concepts in fifth- and early fourth-century medical texts, where the first two appear to have a more evidently specified and construed meaning (and the first considerably more than the second) supports my choice. μανίη (and cognates), although more specified than the other terms in our list above, remains in the early medical texts a general term, also by virtue of its traditional use to identify 'madness' in other genres and linguistic contexts. In our corpus of reference, only *phrenitis* is a disease recognized and discussed as such,[4] while *melancholia* and *mania* are harder to qualify in the same way, as I will discuss shortly. Rather, the two appear intermittently as inbuilt dispositions of character[5] or constitution,[6] ways of being,[7] what seem to be momentary affections[8] or degenerations of other pathologies.[9] There is then a further distinction between the status of *melancholia* and that of *mania*, which ultimately justifies my choice of excluding also the first from a list of 'general terms'. The *melancholia* group displays in fact greater characteristics of specification in contrast to *mania*.

To illustrate this I must engage briefly with the discussion and problems posed by Hippocratic *melancholia*. We will see that the status of *melancholia* remains obviously much more opaque than that of *phrenitis*; but it is also in turn more construed and composite than that of *mania*.[10] We scrutinise now

---

[4] See e.g. the dedicated discussion in *Aff.* 6.216–218, *Morb.* I 6.200; 204 (= Wittern 30; 34), where the word φρενῖτις is used as a header.

[5] E.g., in *Vict.* I 6.518.4 (= Joly-Byl 35.1.7) μανίη can be of different types, and characterize different blends of the soul: ἔστι δ' ἡ μανίη τοιούτων ἐπὶ τὸ βραδύτερον, or be of a lesser 'degree', ὑπομαίνεσθαι (*Vict.* I. 6.520.19 = Joly-Byl 35.9.20).

[6] See *Epid.* III 3.98.1–2 (= Kühlewein 14.15.16), τὸ μελαγχολικόν καὶ ὕφαιμον· οἱ καῦσοι καὶ τὰ φρενιτικὰ καὶ τὰ δυσεντεριώδεα τούτων ἥπτετο, where the melancholic constitution is prone to fever, phrenitis and dysenteric troubles.

[7] E.g. in *Aph.* 6.23, 4.568.11 (= Magdelaine 6.23.2), ἢν φόβος ἢ δυσθυμίη πολὺν χρόνον ἔχουσα διατελῇ, μελαγχολικὸν τὸ τοιοῦτον, 'fear or depression that is prolonged means/generates a melancholic affection'; *Coan Pren.* 5.602.11, τῶν ἐξισταμένων μελαγχολικῶς, 'those who are out of themselves *in a melancholic way*'; *Epid.* VII 5.374.18 (= Jouanna 5.6.7), 'on the eighteenth, nineteenth and twentieth [they behave?] μανικῶς'.

[8] In *Morb.* III, 7.134.1 (= Potter 3.13.22), about *opisthotonus*: 'sometimes [during an attack] they become somehow manic or melancholics', μανικοί τι ἢ μελαγχολικοί; in *Epid.* III, 3.112.11–12 (= Kühlewein 17, case 2, 6): at the end of a list of temporary aspects of the illness (κῶμα, aversion to food, irritability *et similia*) we find τὰ περὶ τὴν γνώμην μελαγχολικά; in *Epid.* VI, 5.272.2 (= Manetti-Roselli 1.11), 'in autumn ... τὸ μελαγχολικόν'.

[9] For example, in the second constitution in *Epid.* I, 2.638.6 (= Kühlewein 12.19), τὰ μανικά is one of the complications in those 'whose natural heat is failing'; in *Epid.* VI, 5.354.19–356.1–3 (= Manetti-Roselli 6.31) 'melancholics tend to become epileptics, and epileptics melancholics', οἱ μελαγχολικοὶ καὶ ἐπιληπτικοὶ εἰώθασι γίνεσθαι ὡς ἐπὶ τὸ πουλύ, καὶ οἱ ἐπίληπτοι μελαγχολικοί.

[10] Kazantzidis 2011, 31 n. 18 (I thank him for his remarks in conversation about this

the concept in two respects, both 1) as a 'disease' proper and 2) as a psychological disorder in particular. To the second point first: in the Hippocratic texts *melancholia* is not exclusively or primarily psychological, but does display psychological implications from early on;[11] there is however limited trace of the 'depressive' quality melancholic disturbances will acquire in subsequent literature. Explicitly, we find such quality only in *Aph.* 6.23, 4.568.11 = Magdelaine 6.23.2, ἢν φόβος ἢ δυσθυμίη πολὺν χρόνον ἔχουσα διατελῇ, μελαγχολικὸν τὸ τοιοῦτον, 'fear or depression that is prolonged means/generates melancholia'. One might add a possible instance in *Mul.* 8.364.12–17[12] for a connection between psychologically 'depressive' traits (φοβῆται καὶ στυγνὴ ᾖ; ... καὶ ἄση ἔχῃ καὶ δυσθυμίη), black discharges (καὶ οὖρα μέλανα καὶ δι' ὑστέρης ὅμοια) and black bile (μέλαινα χολὴ ἐν τῇσι μήτρῃσιν ἔνι), but without mention of μελαγχολίη/μελαγχολικός (we should of course use caution, as the reference is to black bile, not to *melancholia*).[13] More often, however, psychologically μελαγχολίη/μελαγχολικός seem to signify a degree of insanity:[14] in *Morb.* I, 6.200.18–21 (= Wittern 30.7–11) 'patients with φρενῖτις (οἱ ὑπὸ τῆς φρενίτιδος ἐχόμενοι) are said to resemble 'melancholics' κατὰ τὴν παράνοιαν.[15] Like phrenetics, melancholics also 'become παράνοοι' (γίνονται), and some (ἔνιοι δὲ καί) even μαίνονται: the disease of the melancholics is in this

---

passage) comments on the distinction between παραφρονεῖν and μελαγχολᾶν at Aristophanes' *Eccl.* 250–252, where a woman inquires from Praxagora her line of defense against Cephalus ([Πραξαγόρα] φήσω παραφρονεῖν αὐτόν. [Γυ. α'] ἀλλὰ τοῦτό γε ἴσασι πάντες. [Πραξαγόρα] ἀλλὰ καὶ μελαγχολᾶν. [Γυ. α'] καὶ τοῦτ' ἴσασιν, Praxagoras: 'I say, that he is mad'. First woman: 'This much, everyone knows'. Praxagoras: 'Mad, and also *affected with melancholia*/ μελαγχολᾶν'), proposing that this could be read, to some degree, as a linguistic comment on a distinction between the two not based on degree, or not primarily on degree, but as a difference between a colloquial and a more specialized term, a 'general term' and 'a more construed and composite category of insanity'.

[11] Cf. e.g. *Epid.* III, 3.112.11 = Kühlewein 17, case 2.6, τὰ περὶ τὴν γνώμην μελαγχολικά.

[12] I thank Georgios Kazantzidis for pointing this passage to me.

[13] The connection between *melancholia* and μέλαινα χολή is one of the most difficult points of this inquiry, with many areas of shadow. See Flashar 1966, 21–49 and Müri 1953, 174–186, and 186–191 on the non-medical tradition for a discussion of the independent trajectories of popular traditional beliefs about bile and psychic affection, black bile as humour, and melancholic pathology, and Klibansky, Panofsky and Saxl 1990, 39–54 for an historical summary. Langholf 1990, 47–48, observes that 'the derivation [of *melagkholiē* from *melaina kholē*] ... is extremely unlikely', and that the noun must rather derive from the adjective *melagkholos* found in Soph. *Trachiniae* 573, akin to other adjectives ending in -*kholos* that 'signify functions of the soul such as wrath or anger' (47); see Jouanna 2007b.

[14] As described in *Morb.* III 7.134.1 = Potter 13.22, where in cases of opisthotonus the patients ἐνίοτε δὲ καὶ ἄφωνοι γίνονται ἅμα ἁλισκόμενοι ἢ μανικοί τι ἢ μελαγχολικοί.

[15] τοῖσι μελαγχολώδεσι Wittern, Potter; Littré chooses τοῖσι μελαγχολῶσι; see below n. 24 on the text.

instance more severe than that of the phrenitics from the point of view of psychological disturbance, as the first reach more extreme levels of insanity (expressed by the use of μαίνομαι). Finally, in the same direction goes the testimony of *Epid.* V 5.204.7 = Jouanna 2.1.8, where a patient is μαινόμενος δὲ ὑπὸ χολῆς μελαίνης, 'raving with/because of the black bile'.[16] These passages offer a good illustration of *mania* as resting at a less construed level: μαίνομαι emerges as a more general term, indicating a phenomenon that can occur *also* in connection with black bile, and befall phrenitics as well as melancholics.[17]

This takes us to the first, more general question, whether or not we can speak of a disease 'melancholia' with a notional status comparable to that of 'phrenitis' (or other diseases). We must notice that the noun μελαγχολίη appears only three times in our sources of choice: for the first time in *Aer.* 2.50.12 (= Jouanna 10.12.9–10) ἐνίοισι δὲ καὶ μελαγχολίαι; in the list of affections in *Morb.* I 6.144.12 (= Wittern 3.13); and in *Aph.* 3.14, 4.492.6 (= Magdelaine 3.14.7). Jouanna considers the passage of *Aer.* 'capital', as it is the first attestation of the noun in Western history; and he argues additionally that the substantive μελαγχολίη designates beyond doubt 'une maladie', even though the text does not offer depiction of a 'syndrome'; this is the proof that it was perfectly known at the time.[18] Even if not with the same degree of specificity and definition as *phrenitis*, in conclusion, an accepted concept of *melancholia* must have been there and taken for granted 'in Greek medicine at a stage before Hippocrates'.[19]

---

[16] On which, again, see the caveats of n. 13.

[17] This characteristic appears to persist in later technical usage: in Aretaeus μαινέσθαι is again a possible σημεῖον and 'part' of μελαγχολία (at *Caus.Chr.* 5, Hude III, 5.3.18–21), but μανίη indicates at the same time an independent disease (*Caus.Chr.* 6, Hude III, 6); this is also reflected in *Therap.Chr.* 5 (Hude VII, 5) and the topic for the lost chapter 6 (Hude VII, 6).

[18] Jouanna 2007b, 17 (my translation). Other scholars have also documented beyond discussion the rich tradition about (black) bile as psychopathogenic and the history of a melancholic disorder prior to the Hippocratic testimony. See Klibansky, Panofsky and Saxl 1990, 53: '[die schwarze Galle] ... zeigte ein so bekanntes und charakteristisches Krankheitsbild (das möglicherweise sogar aus vorhippokratischer Zeit stammte)'; Müri 1953 'die Wortbildung με-λαγχολ- -und die damit verbundene Vorstellung einer geistigen oder seelischen Störung oder einer Erkrankung im letzten Drittel des 5. Jahrhunderts schon Überlieferung ist' (187); Flashar 1966 is more cautious, and comments about the *Aer.* passage that 'die Melancholie wird angesehen als eine Krankheit, die unter bestimmten Bedingungen einen bestimmten Typ befallen kann, aber *nicht muß*', 22; und 'der Text verrät nichts über das Krankheitsbild der μελαγχολίη', 23. On the pre-Aristotelic stage in the history of the concept see also van der Eijk 2005, 140–141. On the Aristotelic testimony about *melancholia*/the *melancholic* and the place occupied by *Problemata* 30.1 see also van der Eijk 2005a, Centrone (2011).

[19] Jouanna 2007, 17 (my translation).

Phrenitis, melancholia, and *mania* are thus in no way three diseases that it is appropriate to take as categorically homogeneous,[20] even if they will be more than once classified as competing types of insanity by the later medical tradition.[21] On the contrary, they enjoy three fundamentally different statuses. Different grammars of vocabulary (nouns, verbs, adjectives ...) are a significant reflection of this difference, and offer us a piece of information that is mostly lost in translation (where 'melancholy', for example, is generously used for many Hippocratic instances in English translations) but would reinforce our understanding of the three psychiatric distinguishable 'syndromes' known in our medical texts. Let us review how grammatical forms are distributed in the corpus we are considering in the case of *phrenitis, mania* and *melancholia*:

- In the μανίη group[22] verbal forms are most frequent (53% of occurrences in this group are forms of ἐκμαίνω and μαίνομαι, 52 in total) and followed by the noun μανίη (28% of occurrences, 27 in total). The adjectives μανιώδης and μανικός recur the 18% of times, 18 times in total (of which 5 times to replace a substantive).
- The μελαγχολίη group, instead, is very rarely present with the actual noun (μελαγχολίη: 3 times[23]) or verb (μελαγχολάω, only two

---

[20] As for instance does Ciani 1983, 28: 'Hippocrates is credited with having isolated the two types of endogen psychosis without fever, mania and melancholia', or Enge 1991, who surveys a selection of items (*epilepsy, phrenitis, melancholy, manie* and *rabies*) under the common heading of 'Psychische Erkrankungen' in the Hippocratic Texts, Celsus and Aretaeus alike, seeking to define for each a 'Symptomatologie', 'Ätiologie', and 'Therapie'. See Matentzoglu 2011 instead for an approach mindful of the risks and problems of leveling the ancient terminology to fit contemporary classifications (esp. discussion at 13–23). I have excluded *epilepsy* in its various forms from discussion for the same reasons for which I have excluded *phrenitis*, as well as for the stronger physiological quality that is ascribed to this disease.

[21] Celsus in *De Medicina*, III.18 divides *insania* into φρένησιν (18.1), acute with fever; *tristitia, quam videtur bilis atra contrahere*, of longer duration (18.17); and the *longissimum* type (such as that of Ajax and Orestes, 18.19). Aretaeus, in his treatments of acute and chronic diseases (*On the Causes and Symptoms of Acute Diseases; On the Causes and Symptoms of Chronic Diseases; Therapeutics of Acute Diseases; Therapeutics of Chronic Diseases*) classifies φρενῖτις as an ὀξὺν πάθος and μανία and μελαγχολία as cases of χρονίον πάθος; Caelius Aurelianus' elaboration of Soranus in *On Acute Diseases* and *On Chronic Diseases* maintains the distinction between *passio phrenitica* (with fever, acute), *furor/insania* (μανία) and *melancholia*, the last two both chronic diseases.

[22] See below pp. 84–86 at the end for the complete listing.

[23] *Aer.* 2.50.12 (= Jouanna 10.12.9–10) ἐνίοισι δὲ καὶ μελαγχολίαι; *Aph.* 3.14, 4.492.6 (= Magdelaine 3.14.7) ἢν δὲ βόρειον ᾖ καὶ ἄνυδρον ... ἐνίοισι δὲ καὶ μελαγχολίαι; *Morb.* I 6.144.12 (= Wittern 3.13), κέδματα, μελαγχολίη, ποδάγρη, ἰσχιάς, τεινεσμός ...

dubious occurrences[24]. It is mostly evoked through the adjectives μελαγχολικός (32 occurrences)[25] and μελαγχολώδης (2 occur-

---

[24] The first instance is the already mentioned passage at *Morb.* I 6.200.19 οἱ ὑπὸ τῆς φρενίτιδος ἐχόμενοι τοῖσι μελαγχολῶσι κατὰ τὴν παράνοιαν, where the verb μελαγχολῶσι found in M is Littré's choice, while Wittern 30.8 and Potter follow Θ, μελαγχολώδεσι); the second is at *Aff.* 6.246.10, ὅσοι δὲ μελαγχολῶσι, τὰ ὑφ' ὧν μέλαινα χολή, on which Potter 1988, 58–59, n. 1 writes: 'W. Artelt (*Studien zur Geschichte der Begriffe Heilmittel und Gift*, Leipzig, 1937, 87) deletes these two clauses because they contain the sole reference in the treatise to the humours "black bile" and "water", in contradiction to the two-humour theory expounded in Ch. 1 and 37, and otherwise followed'; cf. also Jouanna 2007b, 16 n. 2, on these verbal occurrences, which are ultimately 'not certain'. Kazantzidis (2011, 28) notes that an absence of the verb from the Hippocratic texts is made even more puzzling by the fact that the verb is used five times already in Aristophanes (*Aves* 14: μελαγχολῶν; *Ecclesiazusae* 251: μελαγχολᾶν; *Plutus* 12: μελαγχολῶντ'; *Plutus* 366: μελαγχολᾷς and *Plutus* 903: μελαγχολᾶν).

[25] *Aph.* 4.9, 4.504.6 (= Magdelaine 4.9.6) τοὺς δὲ μελαγχολικοὺς ἁδροτέρως τὰς κάτω, τῷ αὐτῷ λογισμῷ τὰ ἐναντία προστιθείς; 6.11, 4.566.5 (= Magdelaine 6.11.11) τοῖσι μελαγχολικοῖσι καὶ τοῖσι νεφριτικοῖσιν αἱμορροΐδες ἐπιγενόμεναι, ἀγαθόν; 3.20, 4.494.16 (= Magdelaine 3.20.8) τοῦ μὲν γὰρ ἦρος, τὰ μελαγχολικὰ καὶ τὰ μανικά, καὶ τὰ ἐπιληπτικά ...; 3.22, 4.496.8 (= Magdelaine 3.22.8) τοῦ δὲ φθινοπώρου ... καὶ εἰλεοί, καὶ ἐπιληψίαι, καὶ τὰ μανικά, καὶ τὰ μελαγχολικά; 6.23, 4.568.11 (= Magdelaine 6.23.2) ἢν φόβος ἢ δυσθυμίη πολὺν χρόνον ἔχουσα διατελῇ, μελαγχολικὸν τὸ τοιοῦτον; 6.56, 4.576.19 (= Magdelaine 6.56.4) τοῖσι μελαγχολικοῖσι νουσήμασιν ἐς τάδε ἐπικίνδυνοι αἱ ἀποσκήψιες; 7.40, 4.588.9 (= Magdelaine 7.40.1) ἢν ἡ γλῶσσα ἐξαίφνης ἀκρατὴς γένηται ἢ ἀπόπληκτόν τι τοῦ σώματος, μελαγχολικὸν τὸ τοιοῦτο; *Acut.* 2.358.2 (= Joly 61.1.11), ἐν κεφαλαίῳ δε εἴρησθαι, αἱ ἀπὸ ὄξεος ὀξύτητες πικροχόλοισι μάλλον ἢ μελαγχολικοῖσι συμφέρουσι; *Acut.* (*sp.*) 2.426.4 (= Joly 16.1.1) δοκεῖ οὖν μοι τὰ τοιάδε μελαγχολικὰ εἶναι (with reference to such beahviours as crocydism and lack of initiative to speak); 2.450.8 (= Joly 29.1.9–10) καὶ ἢν ἀκμάζῃ τῇ ἡλικίῃ καὶ τὸ σῶμα ἐκ γυμνασίων [ἢ] εὐσάρκως ἔχῃ, ἢ μελαγχολικὸς ᾖ, ἢ ἐκ πόσιος χεῖρες τρομεραί, καλῶς ἔχει παραφροσύνην προειπεῖν ἢ σπασμόν; 2.468.10 (= Joly 37.1.20–21), ἀπὸ μελαγχολικῶν διὰ φλεβῶν πνευμάτων ἀπολήψιες ὅταν ἔωσι, φλεβοτομίη ῥύεται; 2.488.3 (= Joly 68.1.3) τὰ μὲν γὰρ μελαγχολικὰ παροξυνθείη ἂν παθήματα ὑπὸ βοείων κρεῶν; *Epid.* II 5.128.9, νοσήματα δὲ ἔχουσι τραυλὸς ἢ φαλακρὸς ἢ ἰσχνόφωνος ἢ δασὺς ἰσχυρῶς μελαγχολικά; 5.132.17, οἱ τραυλοί, ταχύγλωσσοι, μελαγχολικοί, κατακορέες, ἀσκαρδαμύκται, ὀξύθυμοι; *Epid.* III, 3.98.1 (= Kühlewein 14.15) τὸ μελαγχολικὸν καὶ ὕφαιμον· οἱ καῦσοι καὶ τὰ φρενιτικά, καὶ τὰ δυσεντεριώδεα τούτων ἥπτετο; 3.112.11 (= Kühlewein 17, case 2.6) τὰ περὶ τὴν γνώμην μελαγχολικά; *Epid.* V, 5.252.16 (= Jouanna 87.2) καὶ ὁ τοῦ Τιμοχάριος θεράπων ἐκ μελαγχολικῶν δοκεόντων εἶναι καὶ τοιούτων καὶ τοσούτων ἔθανεν; *Epid.* VI 5.272.2 (= Manetti-Roselli 11.2) τὸ θηριῶδες φθινοπώρου, καὶ αἱ καρδιαλγίαι καὶ τὸ φρικῶδες καὶ τὸ μελαγχολικόν; 5.330.7 (= Manetti-Roselli 14.7) τὸ ἐπίχολον καὶ ἔναιμον σῶμα μελαγχολικόν, μὴ ἔχον ἐξεράσιας; 5.352.1 (= Manetti-Roselli 20.7) ὁ μελαγχολικὸς ὁ Ἀδάμαντος ἀπὸ πεπλίων πλειόνων ἤμεσέ ποτε μέλανα, ἄλλοτε ἀπὸ κρομύων; 5.354.19 (= Manetti-Roselli 31.10) and 5.356.1 (= Manetti-Roselli 31.1), οἱ μελαγχολικοὶ καὶ ἐπιλημπτικοὶ εἰώθασι γίνεσθαι ὡς ἐπὶ τὸ πουλύ, καὶ οἱ ἐπίληπτοι μελαγχολικοί; 5.356.3 (= Manetti-Roselli 31.5) τουτέων (i.e., the disease of the melancholics and that of the epileptics) δ' ἑκάτερον μάλλον γίνεται, ἐφ' ὁπότερα ἂν ῥέψῃ τὸ ἀρρώστημα, ἢν μὲν ἐς τὸ σῶμα, ἐπίληπτοι, ἢν δὲ ἐπὶ τὴν διάνοιαν, μελαγχολικοί; *Epid.* VII 5.448.1 (= Jouanna 91.5) καὶ ὁ τοῦ Τιμοχάριος θεράπων ἐκ μελαγχολικῶν δοκεύντων εἶναι καὶ τοιούτων ἐτελεύτησεν; *Morb.* III 7.134.1 (= Potter 13.22) ἐνίοτε δὲ καὶ ἄφωνοι γίνονται ἅμα ἁλισκόμενοι ἢ μανικοί τι ἢ μελαγχολικοί (in cases of opisthotonus); *Nat. Hom.* 6.68.9 (= Jouanna 15.15) οἱ τεταρταῖοι πυρετοὶ μετέχουσι τοῦ μελαγχολικοῦ (in a discussion of quartan fevers caused by black bile; *Prorrh.* I 5.552.6 (= Polack 123.16), τὰ ἐπ' ὀλίγον θρασέως παρακρούοντα μελαγχολικά; *Prorrh.* II 9.26.5–6 (about internal suppuration) μάλιστα δὲ περιγίνονται ἐκ τῶν τοῦ αἵματος ἀναρρήξεων οἷσιν ἂν ἀλγήματα ὑπάρχῃ μελαγχολικὰ ἔν τε τῷ νώτῳ καὶ ἐν τῷ στήθει, καὶ μετὰ τὴν

rences);[26] these two are the 80% of all occurrences, of which 7 times used in a substantive way.

- As expected, φρενῖτις is much present in noun form, 35% of occurrences (29 times in total).[27] There is no verb that expresses the action or state of being subject to the disease; the adjective (or noun for the

---

ἀνάρρηξιν ἀνωδυνώτεροι γένωνται; 9.28.20, αἱ μὲν γὰρ μελαγχολικαὶ αὗται ἐκστάσιες οὐ λυσιτελέες; 9.64.7, αἱ κνιδώσιες δὲ καὶ τὰ μελαγχολικὰ ταύτησιν ἧσσον ἢ τοῖσιν ἀνδράσιν; 9.74.14, αἱ δὲ λέπραι καὶ οἱ λειχῆνες ἐκ τῶν μελαγχολικῶν; Judic. 9.290.3, τοῖς μελαγχολικοῖς μετὰ φρενιτικῶν ἐχομένοις αἱμορροΐδες ἐγγενόμεναι ἀγαθόν; adverb, μελαγχολικῶς: Coac. 5.602.11–12, τῶν ἐξισταμένων μελαγχολικῶς, οἱ τρομώδεες γενόμενοι, κακοήθεες; 5.602.18, τῶν ἐξισταμένων μελαγχολικῶς, οἷς τρόμοι ἐπιγίνονται, κακόν; 5.602.19, οἱ ἐξιστάμενοι μελαγχολικῶς, τρομώδεες γινόμενοι καὶ πτυαλίζοντες, ἠρά γε φρενιτικοί; 5.610.2–3, ἐν τοῖσι καυσώδεσιν, ἤχων προσγενομένων μετὰ ἀμβλυωγμοῦ καὶ κατὰ ῥῖνας βάρους, ἐξίστανται μελαγχολικῶς; Prorrh. I 5.514.7 (= Polack 13.12), τοῖσιν ἐξισταμένοισι μελαγχολικῶς, οἷσι τρόμοι ἐπιγίνονται καὶ κακόηθες; 5.514.14 (= Polack 18.6), ... ἐξίστανται μελαγχολικῶς.

26 Twice at Morb. I 6.200.19, (= Wittern 30.8), προσεοίκασι δὲ μάλιστα οἱ ὑπὸ τῆς φρενίτιδος ἐχόμενοι τοῖσι μελαγχολώδεσι κατὰ τὴν παράνοιαν, and (= Wittern 30. 8–9) οἵ τε γὰρ μελαγχολώδεις, ὅταν φθαρῇ τὸ αἷμα ὑπὸ χολῆς καὶ φλέγματος, τὴν νοῦσον ἴσχουσι καὶ παράνοοι γίνονται.

27 Acut. 2.232.7 (= Joly 5.1.22) ἔστι δὲ ταῦτα ὀξέα, ὁκοῖα ὠνόμασαν οἱ ἀρχαῖοι πλευρῖτιν, καὶ περιπλευμονίην, καὶ φρενῖτιν; Aff. 6.214.7, πλευρῖτις, περιπλευμονίη, καῦσος, φρενῖτις, αὗται καλέονται ὀξεῖαι; 6.216.21, φρενῖτις ὅταν λάβῃ, πυρετὸς ἴσχει βληχρὸς τὸ πρῶτον, καὶ ὀδύνη πρὸς τὰ ὑποχόνδρια, μᾶλλον δὲ πρὸς τὰ δεξιὰ ἐς τὸ ἧπαρ; 6.220.11, ὅταν, τῶν δύο κεκινημένων τοῦ φλέγματός τε καὶ τῆς χολῆς, μὴ τὰ ξυμφέροντα προσφέρηται τῷ σώματι, συστρεφόμενα αὐτὰ πρὸς ἑωυτὰ τό τε φλέγμα καὶ ἡ χολὴ προσπίπτει τοῦ σώματος ᾗ ἂν τύχῃ, καὶ γίνεται ἢ πλευρῖτις, ἢ φρενῖτις, ἢ περιπλευμονίη; Aph. 3.30, 4.500.13 (= Magdelaine 3.30.12) τοῖσι δὲ ὑπὲρ τὴν ἡλικίην ταύτην, ἄσθματα, πλευρίτιδες, περιπλευμονίαι, λήθαργοι, φρενίτιδες ...; 7.12, 4.580.8 (= Magdelaine 7.12.3) ἐπὶ περιπλευμονίῃ φρενῖτις, κακόν; Coac. 5.602.14, ἐνύπνια τὰ ἐν φρενίτιδι, ἐναργῆ; 5.602.15, ἐν φρενίτιδι διαχωρήσιες λευκαί, καὶ νωθρότης, κακόν; Epid. I, 2.654.6 (= Kühlewein 18.11) ἔστι δ' οἶσι καὶ εἰκοσταίοισι, οἶσιν οὐκ εὐθὺς ἐξ ἀρχῆς ἡ φρενῖτις ἤρξατο ⟨ἢ⟩ περὶ τρίτην ἢ τετάρτην ἡμέρην; Epid. III 3.62.10 (= Kühlewein 1, case 11.2) [φρενιτιαία]; Galen φρενῖτις (this is one of the labels at the end case descriptions in Epid. III); 3.142.4 (= Kühlewein 17, case 14.25) [φρενῖτις], again the label; 3.146.6 (= Kühlewein 17, case 15.16), [φρενῖτις], again the label; 3.148.5 (= Kühlewein 17, case 16.8) [φρενῖτις], again the label; Epid. V, 5.236.24 (= Jouanna 52.1.7), τῷ μαγείρῳ ἐν Ἀκάνθῳ τὸ κύφωμα ἐκ φρενίτιδος ἐγένετο; Epid. VII, 5.432.12 (= Jouanna 71.1.14), τῷ μαγείρῳ ἐν Ἀκάνθῳ τὸ κύφωμα ἐκ φρενίτιδος ἐγένετο; Judic. 9.290.3, τοῖς μελαγχολικοῖς μετὰ φρενιτίδων ἐχομένοις αἱμορροΐδες ἐγγενόμεναι ἀγαθόν (Littré prints Linden's correction μετὰ φρενιτικῶν); Morb. I 6.144.7 (= Wittern 3.6) περιπλευμονίη ἢ καῦσος λάβῃ ἢ πλευρῖτις ἢ φρενῖτις, ἢ ἐρυσίπελας ...; 6.144.9 (= Wittern 3.9) περιπλευμονίη, καῦσος, πλευρῖτις, φρενῖτις ... 6.144.20 (= Wittern 3.5) καῦσος δέ, φρενῖτις ...; 6.146.1 (= Wittern 3.7) μεταπίπτει δὲ τάδε· ... καὶ ἐκ φρενίτιδος ἐς περιπλευμονίην; 6.200.11 (= Wittern 30.19), φρενῖτις δ' οὕτως ἔχει; 6.200.18 (= Wittern 30.7), προσεοίκασι δὲ μάλιστα οἱ ὑπὸ τῆς φρενίτιδος ἐχόμενοι τοῖσι μελαγχολώδεσι κατὰ τὴν παράνοιαν; 6.200.22 (= Wittern 30.11), καὶ ἐν τῇ φρενίτιδι ὡσαύτως; 6.204.5 (= Wittern 34.7) ὑπὸ τῆς φρενίτιδος ἀπόλλυνται οὕτως; Morb. III 7.128.5 (= Potter 9.20) φρενῖτις δὲ γίνεται καὶ ἐξ ἑτέρης νόσου; 7.140.3 (= Potter 15.7.27) οὐ μέντοι ἐξαμαρτήσῃ καὶ πλεῦριτιν καὶ φρενῖτιν οὕτω μεταχειριζόμενος; 7.146.14 (= Potter 16.11.9) θεραπεύειν δὲ χρὴ τὰς πλευρίτιδας ὧδε· τὰ μὲν πολλὰ ὡς τὴν φρενῖτιν καὶ τὴν περιπλευμονίην; Prog. 2.122.6 (= Alexanderson 4.2) ὁκόσοισιν ἐν πυρετοῖσιν ὀξέσιν ... καὶ ἐν φρενίτισι καὶ ... πρὸ τοῦ προσώπου φερομένας καὶ θηρευούσας καὶ καρφολογεούσας, καὶ κροκύδας ἀπὸ τῶν ἱματίων ἀποτιλλούσας καὶ ἀπὸ τοῦ τοίχου ἄχυρα σπώσας, πάσας εἶναι κακὰς καὶ θανατώδεας; 2.188.1 (= Alexanderson 24.124.7) οἷά περ ἐπὶ τῇσι φρενίτισι γίνεται.

ill) φρενιτικός[28] appears in the 65% of occurrences (55 times in total, in 8 of which cases it is used as a substantive).[29]

---

[28] *Aph.* 4.72, 4.528.2 (= Magdelaine 4.72.8) ὁκόσοισιν οὖρα διαφανέα λευκά, πονηρά· μάλιστα δὲ ἐν τοῖσι φρενιτικοῖσιν ἐπιφαίνεται; 7.82, 4.606.3 (= Magdelaine 7.82.11) ὁκόσοι ὑπὲρ τὰ τεσσαράκοντα ἔτεα φρενιτικοὶ γίνονται, οὐ πάνυ τι ὑγιάζονται; *Coac.* 5.598.18, οἱ μετὰ καταψυξίων οὐκ ἀπύρων ἐφιδρῶντες ἄνω, δύσφοροι, φρενιτικοί τε καὶ ὀλέθριοι; 5.600.8, αἱ τρομώδεες, ψηλαφώδεες παρακρούσιες, φρενιτικαί; 5.600.14, ἠρά γε καὶ φρενιτικοὶ οἱ τοιοῦτοι παροξυσμοί; 5.602.16, ἐν τοῖσι φρενιτικοῖσιν ἐν ἀρχῆσι τὰ ἐπιεικῶς ἔχοντα, πυκνά τε μεταπίπτοντα, κακόν; 5.602.20, οἱ ἐξιστάμενοι μελαγχολικῶς, τρομώδεες γινόμενοι καὶ πτυαλίζοντες, ἠρά γε φρενιτικοί; 5.602.20, οἱ ἐκστάντες ὀξέως ἐπιπυρέξαντες, φρενιτικοὶ γίνονται; 5.602.21, οἱ φρενιτικοὶ βραχυπόται, ψόφου καθαπτόμενοι, τρομώδεες ἢ σπασμώδεες; 5.604.1, τὰ ἐν φρενιτικοῖσι νεανικῶς τρομώδεα, θανάσιμα; 5.604.7, τὰ ἐν φρενιτικοῖσι πυκνὰ μεταπίπτοντα, σπασμώδεα, πονηρά; 5.604.8, οἱ ἐν φρενιτικοῖσι μετὰ καταψύξιος πτυαλίζοντες, μέλανα ἔμετον δηλοῦσιν; 5.608.1–2, κεφαλαλγίη ἐν ὀξεῖ, ὑποχόνδριον ἀνεσπασμένον, μὴ ῥυέντος αἵματος ἐκ ῥινέων, ἐς φρενιτικὸν περιίσταται; 5.622.2, οἱ κωματώδεες ἐν ἀρχῆσι γενόμενοι μετὰ κεφαλῆς, ὀσφύος, τραχήλου, ὑποχονδρίου ὀδύνης, ἀγρυπνέοντες, ἠρά γε φρενιτικοί; 5.630.6, μετώπου ξυναγωγὴ ἐπὶ τουτέοισι, φρενιτικόν; 5.632.21, πρὸς τὴν ἁφὴν μὴ περικαέες, φρενιτικοὶ γίνονται, καὶ μᾶλλον ἢν αἷμα ῥυῇ; 5.634.17, αἱ δασεῖαι γλῶσσαι καὶ κατάξηροι, φρενιτικαί; 5.636.12, ἀνάχρεμψις πυκνή, ἢν δή τι καὶ ἄλλο σημεῖον προσῇ, φρενιτικόν; 5.642.12, τὰ ἐν ὀξέσι κατὰ φάρυγγα μικρὰ ὀδυνώδεα, ὅτε χάνοι, μὴ ῥηϊδίως συνάγοντι, ἰσχνῷ, παρακρουστικά· ἐκ τουτέων φρενιτικοί, ὀλέθριον; 5.676.7–8, μετὰ πλευρέων ἀλγήματος, μὴ πλευριτικοῦ δέ, καὶ ταραχωδέων λεπτῶν ἐπιεικῶν, οὗτοι φρενιτικοὶ ἀποβαίνουσιν; 5.714.11, λευκὸν δὲ καὶ καταχεόμενον διαφανὲς οὖρον, πονηρόν· μάλιστα ἐν φρενιτικοῖσιν ἐπιφαίνεται; 5.716.16, τὰ δ' ἄχροα μέλασιν ἐναιωρεύμενα μετὰ ἀγρυπνίης καὶ ταραχῆς, φρενιτικά; *Epid.* I 2.636.6 (= Kühlewein 12.9) φρενιτικοῖσι μὲν σπασμοί; 2.650.10 (= Kühlewein 18.14–15) ἀτὰρ καὶ οἱ φρενιτικοὶ τηνικαῦτα πλεῖστοι ἐγένοντο δὲ καὶ κατὰ θέρος ὀλίγοι; 2.654.3 (= Kühlewein 18.8) τοῖσι δὲ φρενιτικοῖσι συνέπιπτε μὲν καὶ τὰ ὑπογεγραμμένα πάντα; 2.620.6 (= Kühlewein 6.1) οὐδένα οἶδα τότε καύσῳ οὐδὲ φρενιτικὰ τότε γενόμενα; 2.666.11 (= Kühlewein 22.16) ὑπὸ δὲ χειμῶνα ... παρέμενον μὲν καὶ οἱ καῦσοι καὶ τὰ φρενιτικά; *Epid.* III 3.70.6 (= Kühlewein 3.1–2) καῦσοι φρενιτικοί; 3.80.2 (= Kühlewein 5.25) φωναί τε πολλοῖσιν ἐπεσήμαινον κακούμεναι καὶ κατίλλουσαι ... καὶ τοῖσι καυσώδεσι καὶ τοῖσι φρενιτικοῖσιν; 3.80.3 (= Kühlewein 5.26) ἤρξαντο μὲν οὖν οἱ καῦσοι καὶ τὰ φρενιτικὰ πρωῒ τοῦ ἦρος; 3.82.15 (= Kühlewein 6.21), παραπλήσια δὲ καὶ τοῖσι φρενιτικοῖσιν; 3.82.16 (= Kühlewein 6.22–23), οὐδ' ἐξεμάνη τῶν φρενιτικῶν οὐδείς; 3.90.14 (= Kühlewein 11.14), κωματώδεες δὲ μάλιστα οἱ φρενιτικοὶ καὶ οἱ καυσώδεες ἦσαν; 3.98.2 (= Kühlewein 14.15–16) οἱ καῦσοι καὶ τὰ φρενιτικὰ καὶ τὰ δυσεντεριώδεα τούτων ἥπτετο; 3.116.15 (= Kühlewein 17, case 4.11), ὁ φρενιτικὸς τῇ πρώτῃ κατακλινεὶς ἤμεσεν ἰώδεα πολλά, λεπτά ...; 3.140.13 (= Kühlewein 17, case 13.12) [φρενιτικός]; *Epid.* IV, 5.186.19, οἷσι κατὰ τὰ δεξιὰ ὑπολάπαρος ἔντασις, φρενιτικοί; *Epid.* VII 5.422.4 (= Jouanna 53.1.21) ἡ Ἵππιος ἀδελφὴ χειμῶνος φρενιτικός; 5.434.20 (= Jouanna 78.1.8) ὁ γραφεὺς ὁ ἐν Σύρῳ ὁ φρενιτικός; 5.460.11 (= Jouanna 112 1.9) παρέκρουσε τρόπον φρενιτικόν; 5.460.13 (= Jouanna 112.1.12), φρενιτικὴ γενομένη ἀπέθανε; 5.460.19 (= Jouanna 112.3.21) φρενιτικὸς ἐγένετο; *Judic.* 9.290.3, τοῖς μελαγχολικοῖς μετὰ φρενιτικῶν ἐχομένοις αἱμορρόιδες ἐγγενόμεναι ἀγαθόν; *Prorrh.* I 5.510.3 (= Polack 1.3), τραχήλου ὀδύνης ἀγρυπνέοντες ἠρά γε φρενιτικοί εἰσιν; 5.510.8 (= Polack 3.8), αἱ δασεῖαι γλῶσσαι κατάξεροι φρενιτικαί; 5.512.1 (= Polack 4.10), τὰ ἐπὶ ταραχώδεσιν ἀγρύπνοισιν οὖρα ἄχροα, μέλασιν ἐνηωρημένα παρακρουστικά. ἐφιδρῶντι φρενιτικά; 5.512.1 (= Polack 5.11), ἐνύπνια τὰ ἐν φρενιτικοῖς ἐναργέα; 5.514.2 (= Polack 11.6) φρενιτικοί. ὀλέθριοι; 5.514.3 (= Polack 13.9), ἐν τοῖσι φρενιτικοῖσιν ἐν ἀρχῆσι τὸ ἐπιεικές, πυκνὰ δὲ μεταπίπτειν, κακὸν τὸ τοιοῦτον; 5.514.4 (= Polack 13.9), ἐν φρενιτικοῖσι λευκὴ διαχώρησις κακόν; 5.514.8 (= Polack 15.14), οἱ ἐκστάντες ὀξέως ἐπιπυρέξαντες σὺν ἱδρῶτι φρενιτικοί; 5.516.11 (= Polack 27.2–3), αἱ μετὰ καταψύξεως οὐκ ἀπύρῳ, ἐφιδρῶοντι τὰ ἄνω δυσφορίαι φρενιτικά; 5.516.12 (= Polack 28.4), τὰ ἐν φρενιτικοῖσι πυκνὰ μεταπίπτοντα σπασμώδεα (Littré φρενίτισι); 5.518.2 (= Polack 31.8), τὰ ἐν φρενιτικοῖσι μετὰ καταψύξιος πτυελίζοντα μέλανα ἐμεῖται; 5.518.10 (= Polack 34.15–11), αἱ τρομώδεες, ἀσαφέες, ψηλαφώδεες παρακρούσιες πάνυ φρενιτικαί.

[29] We may also notice that the adverb μανικῶς occurs twice and μελαγχολικῶς six times in

We can then propose the following observations: the use of nouns implies a concept that has already reached some reasonable degree of definition; this applies less to the case of *melancholia,* whose occurrence in the noun με-λαγχολίη are very few; while it is more so for *mania* (a familiar non-medical concept) and definitely so for *phrenitis,* which is acknowledged as a well-defined concept. Conversely, verbs express a shared and recognized set of relevant actions and behaviours in absence of the abstract concept; they are the first, more direct level of observed reality.

Partly pertinent to this discussion are Halliday's theories on the formation of scientific language, in which he observes that verbs and nouns carry different degrees of scientific authoritativeness.[30] In terms of functional linguistics he establishes verbal forms as 'historically prior'[31] to nominalized forms. The latter are taken as *metaphorically* connected to verb forms (if via a 'grammatical', not a 'lexical' metaphor).[32] The use of nouns contributes in this way to the creation of a more abstract and authoritative ('scientific') language opposed to everyday communication.[33]

In the case of *phrenitis,* we have a disease 'proper', characterised by various organic ailments and phenomena; the verb here would be redundant (it would mean simply 'to have the described-as-such-and-such φρενῖτις') or fall under the very general meaning suggested by the root φρεν- (the denominal verb φρονέω, significantly, just means 'to think' or 'to be of sound mind').[34]

---

the Hippocratic texts, while indeed no adverb φρενιτικῶς is found in extant Greek literature (see end of nn. 25, 81). These are small numbers across the Hippocratic Corpus; however, with some caution, so we can see the datum as in line with a status of φρενῖτις as more clearly defined composite entity, which cannot be inflected as adverb. Adverbs describe a way of being, of existing 'in certain way', with an implication of chronicity: φρενῖτις is an acute disease, episodic by definition, not a way of being or a physiological trait; this 'aoristic' quality of phrenitic insanity, as opposed to the 'imperfect' quality of *melancholia* and *mania* is well revealed by the grammar of its terminology.

[30] Halliday 2004, 102, to clarify this point, contrasts the sentence 'prolonged exposure will result in rapid deterioration of the item' (nominal) with 'if the item is exposed for two long it will rapidly deteriorate' (verbal).

[31] In Halliday's sense 2004, 107: 'in the grammar's construction of reality, the mapping of process into verb and of entity into noun preceded the mapping of process into noun'.

[32] Halliday 2004, 102–134.

[33] Halliday 2004, 103; 132–133 calls the metaphorical/nominal form that comes second 'Attic' (sophisticated, scientific) as opposed to the 'Doric' ('naïve, everyday') which uses verbs. They are different ways of 're-construing', recapitulating reality; the choice of noun or verb is thus non-neutral.

[34] The verbs φρενιτίζω and φρενιτιάω are a later coinage, found in Plutarch, Galen and later authors. One might object that the nature of the noun φρενῖτις, with the -τις suffix and its alleged etymological formation from the locus of the disease (the φρένες) or from

For μαινέσθαι and ἐκμαίνω the level of observable action is instead the most important: as we have noticed, expressions of *mania* appear often as general 'raving' within illnesses otherwise defined. *Melancholia* tends to escape formulation as external output formed by a set of fixed elements ('verb') and as abstract conceptualisation ('noun'). It rather fluctuates, in the Hippocratic texts, between affect, behavioural traits and episode, best expressed by the multifarious figure of the μελαγχολικός, the individual 'melancholic', or the substantival τὰ μελαγχολικά.

On the whole, we may conclude that it would be more appropriate to speak of φρενῖτις ('phrenitis'), οἱ μελαγχολικοί/τὸ μελαγχολικόν ('the melancholic(s)') and μαίνεσθαι/μανίη ('being insane'/'insanity') in the sources we are discussing rather than simply φρενῖτις, μελαγχολίη and μανίη. This confirms μαίνεσθαι as an activity that can characterize different ailments, while φρενῖτις ('phrenitis') and to a lesser extent οἱ μελαγχολικοί/τὸ μελαγχολικόν indicate on the contrary entities that contain other affections and call for a descriptive definition—they are, so to say, like ingredients in a recipe; a recipe that in the case of *phrenitis* appears to be already reasonably fixed and clear, while in the case of *melancholia* competing versions are co-present.

General Terms of Insanity: Semantics[35]

We should now offer a review of the most important of these terms, broadly divided by etymological families:

παρακρούω, one of the key terms in *Epid.* I–III literally means 'I strike', 'I hit' on the side, 'I lead astray' (παρα + κρούω).[36] The domains in which the verb κρούω is used in its concrete sense are fighting (wrestling, military) and music (with the meaning 'to play the guitar', 'to play the flute', generating the first meaning of the noun παράκρουσις as 'a strike of the wrong note', which might provide a bridge to the meaning 'to be insane'). For παρακρούω

---

the damaged faculty, the φρόνησις, τὸ φρονεῖν (on these see van der Eijk 2000–2001, II, 144–146) makes the creation of a denominative verb more difficult than, say, μανίη. Our linguistic analysis, however, is aimed at asking the significance of the fact that an affection (*phrenitis*) is conceptualised primarily around a technical noun in -τις, rather than, say, around a verb, like *mania* is; and what informations about the concept this difference might offer to us.

[35] Matentzoglu 2011 is partly organised around a review of Greek terms of psychiatric disorder divided by Hippocratic text, or group of texts; as such it is informative and useful. See Byl 2006 for a discussion of the Hippocratic terminology of insanity, focussing on compounds with παρα-.

[36] On versions of 'strike'/'striking' in association with insanity see also Mattes 1970, 104–105.

Chantraine gives the more neutral 'tromper, se tromper' ('to deceive', 'to mislead') as first meaning. Use in the psychological sense, 'to be mad' is not common in Greek literature outside the medical corpus, and it is used with the meaning 'to be deranged' in the active form in the Hippocratic texts only.[37] παράκρουσις is not a very common term (in Ps.-Aristotle it occurs perhaps for checking temperature, παράκρουσις τοῦ θερμοῦ in *Pr.* 872b29–30[38]); apart from the musical sense ('note out of tune', e.g. Plut. *Mor.* 826), it is used with the meaning 'fraud', 'deceit' (e.g. in Demosthenes). The recurrent adjective παρακρουστικός is used exclusively with reference to conditions and causes, not to patients ('leading to derangement', 'relative to derangement'). Surprisingly, Liddell-Scott-Jones gives a circular entry, 'παρακρουστικός = παρακοπτικός (*Prorrh.*1.11 [...]); deceitful, Poll.4.21', not even attempting a translation of one of the key terms for mental affection in the Hippocratic texts.

The use of παρακόπτω (mostly found in *Coac.* and *Epid.* V, and absent from *Epid* I–III) with reference to mental health also appears to be specific to the Hippocratic texts. As with παρακρούω, the term implies the idea of striking and hitting as well as deceit, but with specific concrete reference to 'false coinage' ('I adulterate', 'I falsify'): 'to be deranged', therefore, in the sense of 'to be misled/deceived' in judgment. Money and coinage and the purity of precious metals are increasingly present as metaphors for soundness and value in the fifth century.[39] In this way, the term appears indeed as a neologism and a technical term established exclusively in the medical context. Accordingly, the idea of 'hitting', 'striking' deserves a more precise qualification than is usually offered,[40] as the term is only at first sight homologous to the popular, wider metaphor of being hit by a disease as externalized entity, an affection that possesses the individual. παρακόπτω (like

---

[37] See Berrettoni 1970, 222.

[38] Dubious passage: Bonitz prefers κατάκρουσις in analogy with 3.25 a (= 874b12).

[39] The adjective κίβδηλος is important in this sense: see Euripides' *Medea* 516–519:

ὦ Ζεῦ, τί δὴ χρυσοῦ μὲν ὃς κίβδηλος ἦι
τεκμήρι' ἀνθρώποισιν ὤπασας σαφῆ,
ἀνδρῶν δ' ὅτωι χρὴ τὸν κακὸν διειδέναι
οὐδεὶς χαρακτὴρ ἐμπέφυκε σώματι;

Again, *Hipp.* 616, where women are a κίβδηλον κακόν planted among men by the gods. See Seaford 2004, 153–156, and *passim* about money and Greek imagination in the fifth century. The image is not absent from the Hippocratic texts: κίβδηλος occurs at *Epid.* II 5.120.5 with reference to a deceitful sign for the doctor to interpret (τὰ οἰδήματα τὰ παραλόγως ῥηΐζοντα, κίβδηλον ...).

[40] E.g. Pigeaud 1995, 21: 'παρακρούω means to have the mind hit'.

παρακρούω above) seem to refer to 'striking' in a different sense: '"frapper d' un coup sec, tailler, frapper une monnaie, trancher, hacher", d' où au figuré "fatiguer"' (κόπτω in Chantraine), with the added sense of deviation, applied to the example of production of false money. The cognate noun παρακοπή appears to have as a first meaning the psychological, 'metaphorical' one (it is used thus also in Aeschylus *Ag.* 223 and *Eu.* 329/342[41]). In summary, the ideas of deceit, falsity, and leading astray, not 'possession' appear to dominate. This is of importance, as the chief image for mental derangement in non-medical literature is precisely that of possession, seizing, 'taking hold of': by a Fury, by an emotion coming upon the subject, by Lyssa, by Dionysus, with verbs of seizing such as λαμβάνομαι.[42] In this way, the etymological meaning of the characteristic terms adopted by the Hippocratic writers appears to differ interestingly from the most loaded representation in previous and contemporary tradition, that of possession.

μαίνομαι/ἐκμαίνω (and the cognate noun, μανίη, and adjectives, μανικός and μανιώδης). The two verbs appear to be synonymous in the Hippocratic texts; the second has the primary meaning of 'getting someone to become furious'; therefore a stronger ingressive/intensive quality might be present when used in the active with a reflexive meaning, 'to burst out with the most violent derangement'. This semantic group is obviously very familiar to modern readers and contemporary audiences from other sources (tragedy, lyric poetry) and contexts (religion) than the medical. They have the widest range of implications, and are loaded with traditional and every-day associations. The verbs are not modified by adverbs of degree, duration or quality (unlike παρακρούω, which receives adverbs such as σμικρά, πάντα, πολλά, κοσμίως, κατόχως, θρασέως with regularity), which suggests that it has a superlative quality and represents a higher degree of insanity.[43]

---

[41] See Berrettoni 1970, 221.

[42] Onians 1954, 147–149 and 159–160, discusses some of these wide spread representations. Traces of those are indeed present in the Hippocratic ἐμβρόντητος, 'thunder-struck' (*Vict.* 1 6.518.3 = Joly-Byl I, 35.7.8), an obviously poetic term, as well as βλητός, 'hit' (*Morb.* II 7.16.5 = Jouanna 8.1.1, 7.38.19 = Jouanna 25.1.10, *Morb.* III 7.120.17 = Potter 3.10). Cf. also ἄκανθα, κεντέειν at *Morb.*II 7.110.1 (Jouanna 72.16 maintains φροντίς ΘΜ, Littré; Potter corrects with φρενῖτις): 'goad/sting', 'to prick' ('something like a thorn seems to be in the inward parts and to prick them'), evocative of οἶστρος imagery (materialized as 'gadfly' in the myth of Io, and used variously in poetic imagery of frenzy: see Mattes 1970, 110 on 'die Bremse' as imagery of madness in Greek literature). These are however a minority in the Hippocratic texts, which appear to suggest, if not a totally different view, a shift away from the straightforwardly exogenous representation of insanity traditional elsewhere.

[43] On μαίνομαι, λύσσα and βαγχεύω see Perdicoyanni-Paleologou (2009) for a wide ranging, if unqualified terminological survey.

(οὐ) κατανοέω, ('I reason', 'I understand', with the idea of 'grasping with the mind'), παραφρονέω and (οὐ) φρονέω ('I am of (un)sound mind', 'I do (not) reason well') are examples of denominal verbs common in Hippocratic language (in -έω, often compounded with prepositions).[44] They appear to have a strong cognitive connotation and to refer to reasoning capacities, habilities, as opposed to signposting the visible behaviour of the mad.

κατανοέω is first attested in Herodotus and only in the Hippocratic texts is it used in the sense of 'to be of sound mind', 'to recover from insanity' (in particular, only in the *Epidemics*, and predominantly in *Epid.* I–III). This use remains exclusive to the Hippocratics, while it is generally employed elsewhere with the meaning 'to understand', 'to grasp with the mind'.[45]

παραφρονέω and (οὐ) φρονέω appear to have a more general connotation not characterised by the alternating states of soundness and derangement. παραφρονέω is found in Herodotus, and will have a history to denote general, unqualified impaired cognitive abilities in subsequent medical literature. In the Hippocratic testimony it occurs in *Epidemics*, but not as characteristically as κατανοέω, and in fact in numerous other texts. The indication of cognitive soundness is also reinforced by the interesting compound ἀλλο-φρονέω, which indicates literally 'to think something else', 'to change one's mind', but also 'to be senseless', 'to deviate in one's thought', therefore 'to be taken by derangement'.[46]

---

[44] Use of negative expressions or litotes to assess one's state of mental sanity appears only with this group of denominal verbs, and to express insanity, not its reverse: (οὐ) παρακρούω, for instance, or similar negative phrases with terms expressing insanity are not found to convey mental soundness or recovery. We find instead οὐ/σμικρὰ κατανοέω, e.g. in *Epid.* I, 2.686.9 (= Kühlewein 26, case 2.3), 2.692.9 (= Kühlewein 26, case 4.1), 2.692.16 (= Kühlewein 26, case 4.14), 2.710.7 (= Kühlewein 26, case 11.9–10), or *Epid.* III 3.140.6 (= Kühlewein 17, case 13.5), 3.142.3 (= Kühlewein 17, case 14.24), *Epid.* V, 5.230.22 (= Jouanna 39.2) and οὐ φρονέω, e.g. in *Epid.* V, 5.240.10 (= Jouanna 60.2); *Epid.* VII 5.402.4 (= Jouanna 32.2); *Morb.Sacr.* 6.372.8 (= Jouanna 7.1); *Mul.* II, 8.390.1. This suggests a greater technicalism of denominal verbs: their meaning is more neatly determined, and can be 'polarized' into sanity and its opposite through the use of privative suffixes (ἀ-φρονέω and the like) and of litotes (with οὐ, σμικρά and so on). These terms will have greater fortune in later medical and philosophical literature. Also, the implication is that 'insanity' appears to be more straightforward and uncomplicated than 'sanity', so that while an aspect of 'madness' can be defined as a failure in 'sound reasoning' the reverse is not the case.

[45] See Berrettoni 1970, 81, who notes that Galen seems to feel he needs to offer an interpretation to its meaning (*Comm. in Hipp. Epid. III*, 17.538.9 K).

[46] See *Il.* 23.698, the description of Euryalus' head trauma after the boxing match against Epaeus, where the concussed champion swoons, dragging his feet (696) and shaking his head from one side to the other (697) and is led away ἀλλοφρονέοντα. Aristotle returns to the use of the verb with reference to the Homeric passage twice, in *De Anima* 404a30 and in *Metaph.*

A clear distinction between νόησις and φρόνησις (and their verbs) is impossible to make, even though the usage of the verbs we have seen suggests a more circumscribed, episodic significance of the first as 'cognitive performance' as opposed to the second, which comprises potentiality and capacity. The two are differentiated rather cryptically with reference to Erasistratus in Anonymus Parisinus (1), where the text speaks of the meninx as οὗ γὰρ τόπου κατ' αὐτὸν ἡ νόησις φρόνησις, ἐπὶ τούτου ἡ παρανόησις παραφρόνησις ἂν εἴη. Fuchs' translation has 'intelligence' and 'mental sanity' for νόησις and φρόνησις respectively, a distinction possibly functioning in the instance but not seen elsewhere—as φρόνησις can also refer to intellectual abilities.[47] These are not clearly established as two different types of reasoning, or of being mentally (in)sane.

ἄφρων, ἔμφρων, ἔκφρων, φρόνιμος. The denominal compound ἄφρων (from φρήν) is very common in Greek literature from Homer onwards. The other two, ἔμφρων and ἔκφρων appear mostly in prose (philosophical, medical, historiography, oratory ...) and post-classical poetry, and when present in tragedy have arguably medical or technical overtones. The adjective φρόνιμος occurs outside medicine, and is also used in the ethical sense of 'intelligent, prudent, and appropriate'.

The abstract noun παραφροσύνη is derived from the common adjective παράφρων (almost absent from the Hippocratic texts). Galen makes large use of the term, and he considers παραφροσύνη to be a broad category of insanity,[48] with reference to which more precise degrees can be specified.[49] This is not confirmed by the Hippocratic evidence,[50] although the term is

---

1009b30, φασὶ δὲ καὶ τὸν Ὅμηρον ταύτην ἔχοντα φαίνεσθαι τὴν δόξαν, ὅτι ἐποίησε τὸν Ἕκτορα, ὡς ἐξέστη ὑπὸ τῆς πληγῆς, κεῖσθαι ἀλλοφρονέοντα, ὡς φρονοῦντας μὲν καὶ τοὺς παραφρονοῦντας ἀλλ' οὐ ταὐτά, 'Homer ... had Hector stand up again after the blow he has received and then 'lie down *allophroneonta*', as if those who do not reason (*paraphronountas*) actually did reason (*phronountas*), but just not with the same objects as content' (my translation; the philosopher quotes approximatively and mistakes the character, referring the episode to Hector: on the passage in *De Anima* see Hicks 1907, 219; Ross ad loc., and Polansky 2007, 70 n. 21; Ross 1924, vol. 1 275 on the *Metaphysics* occurrence).

[47] For instance at *Morb.Sacr.* 6.390.14–15 (16.2.10–11 Jouanna), γίνεται γὰρ ἐν ἅπαντι τῷ σώματι τῆς φρονήσιος, τέως ἂν μετέχῃ τοῦ ἠέρος (if we accept φρονήσιος, which Jouanna prints *inter cruces*) 'in fact the whole body participates in intelligence in proportion to its participation in air', where 'φρόνησις' would be conceptualized as faculty as much as externalized substance.

[48] I shall discuss this matter on another occasion.

[49] Galen, *Comm. in Hipp. Epid. III*, 17.481.17–482.1 K.

[50] Compare, to give just one example, the use of παραφρονέω in *Morb.Sacr.* 6.354.4–5 (= 1.3 Jouanna), μαινομένους ἀνθρώπους καὶ παραφρονέοντας, where the verb is used, it appears, in

frequent in the Hippocratic texts and does not have a strong connotation, so perhaps it expresses a broader category. First attested in Hippocratic texts, παραφροσύνη arguably maintains a technical sense, used extensively by Plutarch and Galen, and in a variety of late philosophical and medical sources. The verb παραφρονέω (and (οὐ) φρονέω) has wide use and it occurs in drama (tragedy but especially Aristophanes), oratory, Herodotus and other prose sources (apart of course from medical and philosophical texts) after the fifth century. παραφρόνησις appears only once in the Hippocratic writings and rarely otherwise, only in medical contexts and late authors.

The nouns παραλήρησις and λῆρος/λήρησις, the denominal verbs παραληρέω and ληρέω, and the adjective παράληρος are used to describe the behavior of the insane as perceived by the observer, rather than the cognitive process or psychological state. This explains why the vast majority of occurrences appear in the cases of the *Epidemics* books, and in this respect they are symmetrical to the φρονέω/νοέω group. λῆρος (which is related to λάλος, 'chatty', 'loquacious' and λάσκω, 'I echo, resound', 'I shout, I scream') may refer in particular to inarticulate or inappropriate sounds and as a consequence to the nonsensical muttering of the insane. Unlike παραλέγω or ἀλλοφάσσω, however, the verbal aspect is not so clearly established (it should be more generally translated with 'to act foolishly'; the etymology is uncertain). As Berrettoni points out, the term λῆρος is attested starting from the second half of the fifth century, with the meaning 'thing of little value', while ληρέω is found in Archilochus with a more general meaning of 'talking nonsense', suggesting therefore that it was a term used in a general, non-technical sense.[51] παράληρος is however first attested in the Hippocratic texts, and παραληρέω the verb is typically medical, but also found in Aristophanic characterization and in the orators, among others, perhaps with medical overtones. Therefore, although this group is not exclusive to the Hippocratic context it seems to acquire a technical medical quality.[52]

συνίημι, σύνεσις and συνετός/ἀσύνετος appear in the Hippocratic texts only in a handful of cases with a pathological meaning, or with explicit reference to cognitive capacities; more often they are used to qualify the competence

---

hendiadys with μαίνομαι. On the other hand, Theophrastus is also known to have composed a treaty περὶ παραφροσύνης (fr. 328 FHS&G), which suggest that the term might have reached a more precise acceptation by his time.

[51] Berrettoni 1970, 95.

[52] λήρησις is also the nonsensical chattering connected to old age: in Aretaeus' *De causis et signis acutorum et diuturnorum morborum* (Hude III 6.2.19) *mania* is compared with senile λήρησις (see Godderis 1989, 90–91).

and prudence of the good physician and the intelligent man more generally (we also find παρασύνεσις in *De Articulis*, for practical mistake and misjudgement). These terms play a greater role in philosophical prose, and seem to have a technical weight when used in the Hippocratic texts. The term σύνεσις, first of all, occurs only rarely in classical authors (Herodotus, Pindar) and is more common in prose, used by philosophical authors (Democritus, Aristotle and Plato) and by the orators. It is more important in later writings, notably those of Galen and Plutarch. The term is used however by Euripides,[53] where it is employed at least once in a loaded way, at *Or.* 396. It is worth exploring the passage: σύνεσις is used in fact to qualify the bad conscience of Orestes, his awareness of what he has done which becomes the cause of his derangement, in opposition to some alleged physiological νόσος. Menelaus asks the hero, who is lying in bed, τί χρῆμα πάσχεις; τίς σ' ἀπόλλυσιν νόσος, to which he replies ἡ σύνεσις, ὅτι σύνοιδα δείν' εἰργασμένος. The term is used self-consciously to indicate some sort of deep awareness, deeper understanding of the situation and of one's actions, which can accommodate guilt and remorse. This σύνεσις is symmetrical to the external possession by a wave of emotions or by a daemonic entity that seems to befall Orestes in his Aeschylean counterpart. The other uses in Euripides do not share in this moral and personal sense but maintain the idea of correct, lucid understanding.[54]

In the Hippocratic testimony both verb and related adjectives are used few times in the pathological sense, to indicate disorientation and general mental disturbance, like in *Epid.* II 5.136.4, στρεβλοί, ἀσύνετοι, ἢ λιθιῶντες, ἢ μαινόμενοι. Interesting and more technical is the passage in *Vict.* I 6.488.11 (= Joly-Byl 12.13), where the stomach *in itself* is said to be 'unaware', while it is precisely *through* it that *we* become *aware* of thirst or hunger: ἀσύνετον γαστήρ· ταύτῃ συνίεμεν ὅτι διψῇ ἢ πεινῇ. The author opposes the stomach and 'its' needs or drives to the governing reason of the individual—it is perhaps useful to compare what in terms of modern neurology is called 'interoception', the subject's awareness of one's organs at work.

The abstract noun σύνεσις indicates the mental faculty located in the blood (*Morb.* I, 6.200.12), and on a different theoretical frame, in *De Morbo Sacro*, that 'intelligence' to which the brain is ἑρμηνεύς, 'interpreter' (6.390.12 = Jouanna 16.1.6) or ὁ διαγγέλλων, 'messenger' (6.390.16= Jouanna 16.1.12);

---

[53] The only tragedian to use the term—see Assael 1996.

[54] *Or.* 1524 (meaning intelligence, common sense, prudence) and *Suppl.* 203 (to signify the gift of 'reason' given to men by a Promethean figure).

in addition, it is used in a variety of cases to signify the competence and knowledge of the physician.

On the whole, medical and non medical examples seem to associate this group to awareness that comes out of comprehension and learning, in a moral-spiritual sense (in the Euripidean *Orestes*, perhaps with medical overtones, in line with the idiom of the whole scene); but also competence or skill, as the passage in *Airs Waters Places* 2.92.9 (= Jouanna 24.9.6) seems to suggest: ἔς τε τὰς τέχνας ὀξυτέρους τε καὶ συνετωτέρους καὶ τὰ πολέμια ἀμείνους εὑρήσεις (the reference is to men inhabiting bare and waterless lands with harsh winters and burning summers).[55] Finally, we find the expression 'a part in/of σύνεσις' both in *Morb.* I, 6.200.12 (= Wittern 30.20), τὸ αἷμα ἐν τῷ ἀνθρώπῳ πλεῖστον συμβάλλεται μέρος συνέσιος, 'blood has a part/share in intelligence', and *Epid.* II (5.136.12), φλὲψ ἔχει παχείη ἐν ἑκατέρῳ τιτθῷ· ταῦτα μέγιστον ἔχει μόριον συνέσιος,[56] 'the veins in the breast have a part/share in intelligence'. These expressions also suggest a more abstract, potential quality to σύνεσις, the idea of a 'faculty' that can be possessed in degrees.

ἐξίσταμαι and other compound verbs (and phrases) with *ἐκ/ἐξ* (alongside *παρά, ἐν, ἐντός* and *ἐξ, ἐκτός*) are expressions familiar from poetic sources to qualify mental soundness and its opposite.[57] The imagery of reference here is that of possession from an external force that belongs to tragic representations of *mania* in particular, and more generally Homeric (and traditional) portrayal of emotions and mental processes. This group of terms is the least exclusive to the medical field, and the least 'technical' of all. The same representation is active in medical contexts outside the Hippocratic texts in the symmetrical concept of ἐνθεαστικά, which is found as a disease in Praxagoras (*An. Par.* 20). This 'fanaticism' (in Garofalo's translation) is connected with inflammation around the heart, and may sometimes cause shaking of the hands and head, the familiar phenomenology of religious possession (well portrayed, for example, in Euripides' *Bacchae*). Likewise, ἐνθουσιασμός is also a religious concept that comes to the attention of medicine: to be 'in-god' is a counterpart of being 'out of oneself'.[58] The

---

[55] The noun σύνεσις is also used in the same sense at *Aer.* 2.24.2 (= Jouanna 5.4.4).

[56] Further on this, see below at *Epid.* II, 5.138.19–20, τῷ μέλλοντι μαίνεσθαι τόδε προσημαίνει τὸ σημεῖον· αἷμα συλλέγεται αὐτῷ ἐπὶ τοὺς τιτθούς.

[57] On tragedy, but with many general points about the Greek conceptualization of 'inside' and 'outside' the mind see Padel 1992.

[58] A medical treaty περὶ ἐνθουσιασμοῦ (-ῶν) is ascribed to Theophrastus (fr. 328 FHS&G); Aretaeus will devote a paragraph in his treatment of chronic diseases to 'another kind of

pseudo-Aristotelian *Problemata* 30.1 systematically uses ἐκστῆναι and ἐκστα-τικός to indicate generic insanity.

General Terms of Insanity:
Morphological Variations and Distribution

As far as morphology is concerned, verbs dominate as a whole, with 56% of occurrences, followed by nouns (23%) and adjectives (20%).[59] The most common verbs used are παρακρούω (25%) and μαίνομαι/ἐκμαίνω (11% + 7%), followed by (οὐ) κατανοέω (15%) and παραφρονέω (13%). ἐξίστημι and (οὐ) φρονέω follow (7% and 4%), then ληρέω and cognates (5%) and παρακό-πτω (3%). All the other verbs listed are rarer. Among nouns παραφροσύνη has the 28%, followed by μανίη (23%); then λῆρος and cognates (13%), πα-ράκρουσις (9%) and παρακοπή (7%) follow; other terms are rarer. Finally, among adjectives three terms stand out: μανικός/μανιώδης (18%, and with several substantival uses, τὸ μανικόν, τὰ μανικά), παρακρουστικός (17%, and often used as a substantive, in τὸ παρακρουστικόν, τὰ παρακρουστικά) and ἔμ-φρων (17%) followed by φρόνιμος (11%), ἄφρων (6%) and παράληρος (11%) παράφορος (8%).

Distribution, secondly, is not even among the Hippocratic texts. While there are terms, like παραφρονέω, which occur across all texts, some others are specific to one text or group of texts: ἐξίστημι, ἔκστασις, παρακρουστικός and ἐκμαίνω characterise *Prorrheticon I/Coa Presagia* (ἐκμαίνω also *Epid.* 1 and 3); μαίνομαι, παραφρονέω and φρον-/φρεν- terms (φρόνιμος, ἄφρων, ἔμ-φρων) stand out in *De Morbo Sacro*. The *Epidemics* are generally the main texts of reference for our topic, containing around the 40% of all instances of the terms we are analyzing. One notices that παραφροσύνη and φρόνιμος, common overall, are absent from these texts,[60] and the otherwise very fre-quent παρακρουστικός appears only 3 times (all found in *Epid.* VI). On the other hand, the *Epidemics* are characterized by an abundant use of the com-pounded diminutive: ὑποπαρακρούω, ὑποπαραληρέω, ὑποκαταφρονέω; and

---

mania', described as ἔνθεος (Hude III, 6.11). See Delatte 1934 for a history of the concept in the pre-Socratics.

[59] This in itself might well reflect a more general linguistic mode, and not be specific to our terminology; but it is a useful measure against which to evaluate the variations observed in the case of *mania*, *melancholia* and *phrenitis*, discussed above.

[60] It is interesting to notice that Galen, in the passage I refer to above, n. 48, quotes precisely παραφροσύνη as a Hippocratic general term commenting on *Epid.* III, in which it does not feature.

also ὑποδυσφορέω, ὑποκαρούμαι, ὑπονοέω are exclusive to them. In addition, *Epid.* I and III stand out in a number of ways. They seem to display a simplifying tendency: the vast majority of hapaxes (or rarer terms and expressions that recur only a few times) appear elsewhere; in *Epid.* I and III fewer terms are used, and a fixed vocabulary seems to be favoured. They also appear to be less free and 'poetic', avoiding more complex expressions that we find in *Epid.* II, IV, VI and V, VII. And so, in *Epid.* I and III the verb παρακρούω, the adjective παράληρος, the expression κατανοέω and οὐ κατανοέω visibly dominate; we then find sporadically παραφρονέω (*Epid* I) and παρακοπή (*Epid.* III); but the overall common μανίη or μαίνομαι are never used here, and ἐκμαίνω is systematically preferred. *Epid* II, IV, VI and the later V and VII, instead, show much greater variety and freedom in their terminology for insanity: παράφορος, μαίνομαι, μανίη, παραφρονέω, μανιώδης, παραφέρω, ἐκμαίνω, παρακόπτω, παρανοέω, οὐ φρονέω, λήρησις, ἔκτοθεν γίνεσθαι, παρακρουστικόν; παρακρούω is used too, but it is not so dominant as in *Epid.* I–III. There are also more imaginative expressions used here to qualify the mental state of the subject, e.g. ἡ γνώμη ταράσσεται (*Epid.* VI, 5.344.6 = Manetti-Roselli 8.5) or the more metaphorical and general opposition between θόρυβος and ἡσυχίη (*Epid.* VII, 5.384.13= Jouanna 11.5.6–7), or in *Epid.* IV, 5.156.20, πυρετοί ... πλανώδεες, 'fever that induce wandering'. The image of being 'in-out of oneself' (familiar from tragedy) is typical of these latter texts: ἐν-ἔκφρων are recurrent,[61] we find phrases like οὐκ ἐντὸς ἑωυτοῦ ἐγένετο (*Epid.* VII 5.366.5 = Jouanna I, 7.20) and analogous expressions using ἐκ, παρά, ἐντός, ἐκτός with the reflexive pronoun to denote (loss of) control over oneself.

Concluding Remarks

On the whole, we do not have a common and evenly shared Hippocratic vocabulary of insanity, but specific preferences, and even 'key-words' in different texts (or groups of texts). In particular, *Epid.* I and III show an attempt towards a more specific and precise use of fewer terms, avoiding loans from the more loaded tragic (and generally poetic) imagery or lexicon that the other books of the *Epidemics* allow, and choosing specific forms as 'technical terms' (for instance, ἐκμαίνω over μανία or μαίνομαι).

We can also briefly compare other medical sources that are broadly relevant to our period. These are handed down through a scarse and largely

---

[61] In *Epid.* 5.378.15 (= Jouanna 7.4) we find even the *hapax* ἐμφρονώδεες for the patient's lucidity (on which see Jouanna 2003 lxiv).

indirect tradition, which makes a lexical analysis especially problematic. It is simply impossible to reckon the extent to which terminology found in these sources reflects the original.[62] In the testimony for Diocles and Praxagoras, for example, much in the vocabulary of the psychological sphere is clearly post-Aristotelian; it is exclusively nominal (not surprisingly, given the indirect and doxographic nature of the fragments); finally, it shows a strong technical-philosophical quality and a tendency to abstraction. Thus, the thought of Diocles in fr. 77 van der Eijk is reported in terms of διάνοια and τὸ ψυχικόν in opposition to τὸ σωματικόν (grouped together with the views of other interpreters of 'Hippocrates' such as Asclepiades, while discussing the affected 'mental' function in cases of *errhipsis*).[63] The adjective ψυχικός, absent from the Hippocratic texts, recurs more than once. In the Anonymus Parisinus 18 Praxagoras and Diocles are credited with the view that black bile 'changes the psychic faculty', ψυχικὴ δύναμις, causing melancholia; there is also one direct fragment for the use of ψυχή in Diocles, the (dubious) 183a, 44 van der Eijk: ἀηδῶς ἔχειν τὴν ψυχήν, 'to be distressed in one's psyche', is used to describe psychological discomfort.[64] In the surviving fragments of Praxagoras of Cos one finds remarks on φρενῖτις (fr. 62) as an affection of the heart, where the last is qualified as the source of φρόνησις.[65]

With all the caution necessary in dealing with this kind of material and its accidents of transmission, and bearing in mind that there is gap in the medical material available to us that extends to the 1st century AD, the general impression we can register is that the richness in semantic variation found in the Hippocratic texts we have considered is a remarkable 'linguistic experiment' towards establishing a vocabulary of technical definitions, part

---

[62] See van der Eijk 2000–2001, I, xv–xvi on the difference between a 'fragment' (in the strict sense of literal quotation) vs. 'testimonium', and the necessary reservations in taking the first as a faithful quotation of a Dioclean text (and, conversely, in ranking the second as substantially less reliable).

[63] Reported by Ps. Galen, *Comm. on De Humoribus*.

[64] We should notice that ψυχή never features, somehow paradoxically, in the psychological contexts in which insanity is treated in the Hippocratic texts. Partial exceptions are *Reg.* 1.35–36, where we have the only (and extensive) theoretical discussion of types of ψυχή in man, where forms of insanity are ascribed to some of the blends, and *Hum.* 9, 5.488.90 where a number of ethical traits, emotional states and inclinations (some of which relevant to insanity) are listed under the heading ψυχῆς. The use of the term in the Hippocratic texts is otherwise 'non-psychological' in our sense of the expression, i.e. not linked to personal identity (cognitive, emotional or ethical), but belonging to the general physiological account of man.

[65] See also fr. 72 for a discussion of Praxagoras' physiological interpretation of μανία as inflammation of the heart without fever, with the heart again as organ of τὸ φρονεῖν.

of an inquiry into terminology. The richness and variety in the semantic range offered here goes through a curbing in the later authors. The very fact that Galen, on two different occasions,[66] praises explicitly Hippocrates for his precision in describing insanity with the (for Galen) diligent use of a rich terminology to express nuances of the disorder can be taken in support of this view. Non-fragmentary texts confirm the impression. In the description of the 'disease of the soul', νόσον ψυχῆς, in the famous passage *Timaeus* 86b, Plato posits the affection as dependent on two types of ἄνοια: μανία and ἀμαθία. Regardless of the details in his distinction, there is no clear engagement with the Hippocratic technicalities here, but rather the use of common, familiar terminology of insanity to establish an extemporaneous distinction between diseases caused by an excess of pleasure or pain in the body (μανία), and by those dependent on a failure in the institutions (where ἀμαθία evokes precisely the issue of education, rather than mental soundness and lack thereof).

The pseudo-Aristotelian *Problemata* 30.1, its stated topic being 'φρόνη-σις, νοῦς and σοφία', should also be considered for comparison in our lexical inquiry; the general terms for insanity used here are however also very restricted by comparison with the Hippocratic sources. We find fundamentally two groups, the ἔκστασις/ἐκστῆναι/ἐκστατικός family, and the adjective μανικός. There are then specifications of different nuances of mood and emotional distress characterizing the melancholics (such as δυσθυμία, ἀθυμία, φόβος ...); the general indication of insanity is however played around the two items mentioned.

In conclusion, the Hippocratic texts we have reviewed display an impressive linguistic effort to develop a range of terms to describe insanity: out of these, however, only some will persist in medical usage (such as ληρέω), while some others will be abandoned (such as παρακρούω). Conversely, the peculiar terminological multiplication of the Hippocratic texts is accompanied by a narrower use of more traditional, 'colloquial' psychological (and other medical) terms. Langholf explores this aspect with reference to Homeric and Aristophanic examples for χολή, φρήν and κραδίη,[67] describing a process of 'narrowing down in the meaning of "medical words"' in the Hippocratic texts.[68] In summary, the Hippocratic writers seek to create a technical

---

[66] See n. 49 and *De comate secundum Hippocratem* 3 (7.657–658 K).
[67] Langholf 1990, 40–51.
[68] Langholf 1990, 51.

terminology that might confer more precise (and restricted) meaning to traditional, 'folk' terms, while including new ones to afford greater precision and range. As we have seen above,[69] later tradition will generally prefer the 'polarized' families of terms (in-out, or insane-sane couplets, with negatives or privatives, mostly denominal) and retain some traditional terms, like μανία, but dismiss the richer nuances of the Hippocratic vocabulary.

It is perhaps the fact that only a selection from this vocabulary continues to be used in later medical texts that invited translators to ignore the hugely wide range in the Hippocratic passages. Thus, notwithstanding the variety of semantics and unevenness in use we have observed, these terms are almost completely interchangeable in modern translations, which makes all the observations just made about frequency, technicality, semantics and register entirely inaccessible to readers. 'Delirium', 'to be delirious', accordingly, are the first-choice for individual items in Jones's Loeb translation into English, with or without qualifying adverbs; in longer and richer narratives, when differentiation is needed, we find also 'derangement' as the staple translation for παρακρούω and παρακόπτω; 'wandering' for παραλέγω or παραληρέω, 'to be beside oneself' or 'not to be oneself' for the metaphorical 'being carried away' (παραφέρομαι, etc), while for μανίη/μαίνομαι the qualifier 'wildly' may be added (but not always) to the more general 'delirium'. When degrees and differentiations are applied, these are rather arbitrarily and variably assigned to the modern version. The problem is widespread: in Lichtenthaeler's German commentary on the first twelve cases of the *Epidemics* variants are sometimes employed for the same Greek term, leaving unclear what differentiation is introduced and why (for instance, in the third case in *Epid.* III instances of παρέκρουσε are translated with 'verwirrt', then 'phantasierte', then 'Verstörtheit', and 'verstört').[70] The same is true when the same German term is used for different Greek words (e.g., 'phantasierte' is in turn used to translate λῆρος in the first case in *Epid.* III).[71]

This review, therefore, must conclude with the suggestion of retaining as much as possible the variety of vocabulary when commenting and translating Hippocratic texts on insanity (for instance, by including a transliteration, and remaining, as much as possible, faithful to the grammar of the

---

[69] See above p. 73 n. 44.

[70] Lichtenthaeler 1994, 60–63.

[71] Lichtenthaeler 1994, 22. Lichtenthaeler states more clearly his approach to these terms later (46), discussing παρέκρουσεν: 'deliriert der Patient, er phantasiert wortreich (vgl. παραληρέω, παρανοέω, παραφρονέω)'—the three appear to be equated. See Matentzoglu (2011) 103 for a discussion of translations for παρακρούω and other similar concerns.

original). In addition, the narrative and pragmatic functions played by terminological variety in the individual text have to be highlighted, in the belief that history of medical ideas and of linguistic usage cannot be told but in dialogue with one another.[72]

General Terms for Insanity:
A Review of the Occurrences in Fifth- and
Early Fourth-Century Medical Texts

παράνοος (1)[73]
παρανοέω (5)[74]
παράνοια (5)[75]
(οὐ) κατανοέω (42)[76]

---

[72] See Thumiger, 'Mental insanity in the Hippocratic texts: a pragmatic perspective', forthcoming.

[73] *Morb.* I, 6.200.21 (= Wittern 30.8–9) (describing patients with phrenitis and οἱ μελαγχολώδεις).

[74] *Epid.* III, 3.140.7 (= Kühlewein 17.13.5–6), πάλιν δὲ ταχὺ παρενόει; 3.140.22 (= Kühlewein 17, case 13.6) πάλιν δὲ ταχὺ παρενόει; *Epid.* V, 5.232.2, (40.1.6 Jouanna) καὶ πρῶτον μὲν παρενόησε, τῆς δὲ νυκτὸς ἐπαύσατο; *Morb.* I, 6.200.16 (Wittern 30.3), καὶ παρανοεῖ τε ὤνθρωπος καὶ οὐκ ἐν ἑωυτῷ ἐστιν; *Mul.* I, 8.128.2 ... καὶ δάκνεται, καὶ κεφαλὴν ἀλγέει σφοδρῶς, καὶ παρανοεῖ.

[75] *Morb.* I, 6.200.19 (= Wittern 30.8), προσεοίκασι δὲ μάλιστα οἱ ὑπὸ τῆς φρενίτιδος ἐχόμενοι τοῖσι μελαγχολώδεσι κατὰ τὴν παράνοιαν; *Prog.* 2.178.7–8 (= Kühlewein 23.2–3) ἢν δὲ ἐς τὸν πνεύμονα τρέπηται, παράνοιάν τε ποιεῖ); *Morb.Sacr.* 6.362.4 (= Jouanna 1.11.11), οἷσι δὲ νυκτὸς δείματα παρίσταται καὶ φόβοι καὶ παράνοιαι; *Mul.* I, 8.100.9, καὶ καρδιώξει, καὶ ἐρεύξεται, καὶ ἀλλοφάσσει, καὶ παράνοιαι γίνονται μανιώδεες *Virg.* 8.466.19–20 (= Lami 2.4.17), εἶτ᾽ ἐκ τῆς νάρκης παράνοια ἔλαβεν.

[76] *Epid.* I 2.686.9 (= Kühlewein 26, case 2.3), σμιχρὰ κατενόει; 2.690.1 (= Kühlewein 26, case 3.4) νύχτα κατενόει; 2.690.2 (= Kühlewein 26, case 3.5) κατενόει πάντα; 2.692.4 (= Kühlewein 26, case 4.1) πάλιν κατενόει; 2.692.9 (= Kühlewein 26, case 4.6) σμιχρὰ κατενόει; 2.692.16–17 (Kühlewein 26, case 4.14) σμιχρὰ κατενόει; 2.702.6–7 (= Kühlewein 26, case 7.14) κατενόει; 2.702.17 (= Kühlewein 26, case 8.23) κατενόει πάντα; 2.706.10 (= Kühlewein 26, case 10.4) κατενόει μᾶλλον; 2.706.13 (= Kühlewein 26, case 10.7–8) πάντα κατενόει; 2.710.7 (Kühlewein 26, case 11.9–10) πάλιν ταχὺ σμιχρὰ κατενόει; 2.714.10 (= Kühlewein 26, case 13.20) ἕχτῃ κατενόει; 2.714.14 (= Kühlewein 26, case 13.2) πάντα κατενόει; *Epid.* II 5.100.12, κατενόουν πάντα; *Epid.* III, 3.34.6 (= Kühlewein 1, case 2.4) οὐ κατενόει; 3.36.1 (= Kühlewein 1, case 2.8) ἡσυχῇ κατενόει; 3.36.2 (= Kühlewein 1, case 2.9) κατενόει πάντα; 3.36.6 (= Kühlewein 1, case 2.13) κατενόει πάντα; 3.40.15 (= Kühlewein 1, case 3.17) κατενόει μᾶλλον; 3.40.18 (= Kühlewein 1, case 3.20); κατενόει; 3.42.11 (= Kühlewein 1, case 3.8) κατενόει μᾶλλον; 3.42.14 (= Kühlewein 1, case 3.12) οὐ κατενόει; 3.42.15 (= Kühlewein 1, case 3.13), κατενόει πάντα; 3.44.3 (Kühlewein 1, case 3.17) κατενόει πάντα; 3.48.12 (= Kühlewein 1, case 5.21) κατενόει; 3.50.11 (= Kühlewein 1, case 6.15) πάλιν ταχὺ κατενόει; 3.62.7 (= Kühlewein 1, case 11.22) πάλιν ταχὺ κατενόει; 3.64.12 (= Kühlewein 1, case 12.16–17) πάλιν ταχὺ κατενόει; 3.82.5 (= Kühlewein 6.10) καὶ πάλιν κατενόεον καὶ διελέγοντο, 3.110.6 (= Kühlewein 17, case 2.9) ταχὺ πάλιν κατενόει; 3.110.7 (= Kühlewein 17, case 2.11) ἑνδεκάτῃ κατενόει; 3.112.5 (= Kühlewein 17, case 2.26) καὶ ταχὺ πάλιν κατενόει (κατενόει at 3.112.8 deleted by Kuhlewein); 3.122.8 (= Kühlewein 17, case 7.23) κατενόει; 3.128.10 (= Kühlewein

ἀγνοέω (1)⁷⁷
ἄγνοια (3)⁷⁸
ὑπομαίνομαι (1)⁷⁹
μανιώδης (5)⁸⁰
μανικός (13)⁸¹

17, case 9.16) κατενόει μᾶλλον; 3.134.12 (= Kühlewein 17, case 11.16) πάντα κατενόει; 3.140.6 (Kühlewein 17, case 13.5) σμικρὰ δὲ κατενόησεν; 3.142.3 (= Kühlewein17, case 14.24), οὐδὲν ἔτι κατενόει. *Epid.*V, 5.204.18 (= Jouanna 3.1.8), κατανόεων; 5.206.8 (= Jouanna 5.1.4–5) ἰητρευόμενος κατενόησε; 5.230.22 (= Jouanna 39.2.3) τὸ δὲ πνεῦμα πυκινὸν εἶχε καὶ οὐ κατενόει; *Epid.* VII, 5.396.15 (= Jouanna 25.6.16–17) ἀτρεμίζουσα τὸ σῶμα καὶ κατανοέουσα; 5.462.9 (= Jouanna 114.3.13) ὑπεκαθάρθη δὲ πρότερον· καὶ κατανόει.

⁷⁷ *Hebd.* 8.671.4 (= Roescher 106), in a context of psychopathology: ... ὑπολυσσέων ἄτρεμα καὶ ἀγνοέων καὶ μὴ ἀκούων μηδὲ ξυνιεὶς θανατώδες.

⁷⁸ *Epid.*VII, 5.444.1 (= Jouanna 85.1.17), ἀνδροθαλεῖ ἀφωνίη, ἄγνοια, παραλήρησις; *Coac.* 5.588.6, μετὰ ῥίγεος ἄγνοια κακόν· κακὸν δὲ καὶ λήθη; *Prorrh.* I, 5.526.6 (= Polack 64.6), μετὰ ῥίγεος ἄγνοια κακόν· κακὸν δὲ καὶ λήθη.

⁷⁹ *Vict.* I. 6.520.19 (= Joly-Byl 35.11.4), describing one of the intermediate blends of fire and water in the soul, εἰ δ᾽ ἔτι πλέον ἐπικρατηθείη τὸ ὕδωρ ὑπὸ τοῦ πυρός, ὀξέα ἡ τοιαύτη ψυχὴ ἄγαν, καὶ τούτους ὀνειρώσσειν καλέουσιν, οἱ δὲ ὑπομαίνεσθαι.

⁸⁰ *Aer.* 2.28.10 (= Jouanna 7.5.1) μανιώδεα νοσεύματα; *Coac.* 5.690.11, ἐν τοῖσι μανιώδεσι σπασμὸς προσγινόμενος ἀμαύρωσιν ἴσχει; *Epid.* II 5.132.8–9, μανιώδεις; *Epid.* IV 5.136.3, μανιώδεες, both times in connection with the φαλακροί, bold people; *Mul.* I, 8.100.9, καρδιώξει, καὶ ἐρεύξεται, καὶ ἀλλοφάσσει, καὶ παράνοιαι γίνονται μανιώδεες.

⁸¹ *Aph.* 3.20, 4.494.16 (= Magdaleine 3.20.8) τοῦ μὲν γὰρ ἦρος, τὰ μελαγχολικὰ καὶ τὰ μανικὰ καὶ τὰ ἐπιληπτικά; 3.22, 4.496.8 (= Magdaleine 3.22.8) τοῦ δὲ φθινοπώρου ... καὶ τὰ μανικὰ καὶ τὰ μελαγχολικά; *Coac.* 5.626.4 (ἐν ὀξεῖ πυρετῷ ὦτα κωφοῦσθαι, μανικόν), 5.634.19 (ὀδόντας συνερίζειν ἢ πρίειν, ᾧ μὴ σύνηθες ἐκ παιδίου, μανικὸν καὶ θανάσιμον); 5.710.1 (τὰ ἐξ ἐμέτων ἀσώδεα, κλαγγώδεα, ὄμματα ἐπίχνουν ἴσχοντα, μανικά); 5.706.19 (τὰ μανικὰ πυρετοὺς ὀξεῖς ταραχώδεας ἀχόλῳ καρδιαλγικῷ λύουσιν); *Epid.* I 2.638.6 (= Kühlewein 12.19) μανικά; *Epid.* II 5.130.19, οὗ ἂν ἡ φλὲψ ἡ ἐν τῷ ἀγκῶνι σφύζῃ, μανικὸς καὶ ὀξύθυμος; *Morb.* III 7.134.1 (= Potter 13.22), ἐνίοτε δὲ καὶ ἄφωνοι γίνονται ἅμα ἁλισκόμενοι ἢ μανικοί τι ἢ μελαγχολικοί (where τι is Potter's correction for the ms. τε ἢ); *Epid.* IV 5.194.8 (= Langholf 294), ἅμα ἠσθένει τῇ ἑωυτοῦ, τῇ κεκρυμμένον μανικόν τι ἐνῆν (Littré has ἅμα ἠσθένει τῇ ἑωυτοῦ γυναικί, τῇ κεκριμένη, μανικόν τι ἐνῆν, 'he was ill at the same time as his wife *who reached a crisis, there was some mania* (*in her*) ...', while Langholf's text would translate 'he was ill at the same time as his wife, there was some *hidden* mania (in her) ... (Langholf ad loc.: 'welche latent manisch war ...'). This passage, with Langholf's reading, is remarkable for the notion of a κεκρυμμένον μανικόν that is only to an extent comparable to the examples Langholf quotes (κρυπτοὶ καρκίνοι in *Aph.* 6.38, 4.572.5 (= Magdelaine 6.38.6), as well as *Mul.* II, 8.282.12, *Prorrh.* II, 9.32.5 and 9.32.8), where the reference is to tubercles and cysts, while the concept of a hidden insanity deserves a further, and differently framed discussion; *Progn.* 2.120.10 (= Alexanderson 3.6) ὀδόντας δὲ πρίειν ἐν πυρετῷ, ὁκόσοισι μὴ ξύνηθές ἐστιν ἀπὸ παίδων, μανικὸν καὶ θανατῶδες; *Prorrh.* I 5.514.11 (= Polack 17.2), τὰ ἐξ ἐμέτου ἀσώδεος, φωνὴ κλαγγώδης, ὄμματα ἐπίχνουν ἴσχοντα, μανικά; *Prorrh.* II 9.64.1 (ὁκόσους δὲ ξὺν τῇσιν ὀδύνῃσιν σκοτόδινοι λαμβάνουσι, δυσαπάλλακτον καὶ μανικόν); cf. also the adverbial form at *Epid.* VII 5.374.18 (= Jouanna 5.7.7) ὀκτωκαιδεκάτῃ· ἐννεακαιδεκάτῃ καὶ εἰκοστῇ, μανικῶς; 5.386.10 (= Jouanna 11.7.10), λάβρως καὶ μανικῶς κατέπιε καὶ ἐρρύμφανε).

ἐκμαίνω (21)[82]
μανίη (27)[83]

---

[82] *Coac.* 5.620.4, τὰ ἐν κεφαλαλγίῃσιν ἰώδεα ἐμέσματα μετὰ κωφώσιος, ἀγρύπνοισι, ταχὺ ἐκμαίνει; 5.642.8, τραχήλου πόνος, κακὸν μὲν ἐν πυρετῷ παντί, κάκιστον δὲ ἐν οἶσι καὶ ἐκμανῆναι ἐλπίς; 5.686.12, τὰ δυσεντεριώδεα, ὑπέρυθρα, ἰλυώδεα, λάβρα διαχρωρήματα, ἐπὶ φλογώδεσιν ἐξερύθροισι χρώμασι λυόμενα, ἐλπὶς ἐκμανῆναι; 5.690.14, ἀτὰρ καὶ ἐκμαίνονται οὗτοι; 5.726.18, οἶσιν ἐπὶ φλογώδεσι καὶ ἐξερύθροις λυομένοις δυσῶδες, λάβρον, ὑπέρυθρον, ἐλπὶς ἐκμανῆναι; 5.730.13, ἐπὶ κοιλίῃ ὑγρῇ, κοπιώδει, κεφαλαλγικῷ, διψώδει, ἀγρύπνῳ, ἐξερύθρῳ χρώματι λυομένους ἐλπὶς ἐκμανῆναι; *Epid.* I 2.702.18 (= Kühlewein 26, case 8.24), πολὺ δὲ πρὸ μέσου ἡμέρης ἐξέμανῃ; 2.704.12 (= Kühlewein 26, case 9.12–13), πυρετὸς ὀξύς, ἐξέμανῃ; *Epid.* III 3.46.6 (= Kühlewein 1, case 4.6) ἐξέμανῃ περὶ μέσον ἡμέρης; 3.82.16 (= Kühlewein 6.22) ἄδιψοι δὲ πάνυ οὗτοι ἦσαν οὐδ' ἐξέμανῃ τῶν φρενιτικῶν οὐδείς, ὥσπερ ἐπ' ἄλλοισιν ...; 3.138.13 (= Kühlewein 17, case 13.23), ῥιγώσας ἐπεθερμάνθη· ἐξέμανῃ; 3.140.22 (= Kühlewein 17, case 14.21) περὶ δὲ ἑνδεκάτην ἐοῦσα, ἐξέμανῃ, καὶ πάλιν κατενόει; 3.148.4 (= Kühlewein 17, case 16.6) εἰκοστῇ, ἐξέμανῃ; *Epid.* IV 5.154.3 ἔπειτα ἐξέμανῃ τε αὖθις, καὶ ἀπέθανε ταχέως; 5.154.4 προφάσιος, οἶμαι, πιεῖν ἄκρητον συχνόν, πρὶν ἐκμανῆναι; 5.186.9, κωματώδης, παραφερόμενος ἐξ ὕπνου, οὐκ ἐξέμανῃ; *Prorrh.* I 5.512.8 (= Polack 10.4), τὰ ἐν κεφαλαλγίῃσιν ἰώδεα ἐμέσματα μετὰ κωφώσιος ἀγρύπνῳ ταχὺ ἐκμαίνει; 5.514.11 (= Polack 17.3), ἡ τοῦ Ἑρμοζύγου ἐκμανεῖσα ὀξέως ἄφωνος ἀπέθανεν; 5.528.10 (= Polack 73.1), τραχήλου πόνος κακὸν μὲν ἐν παντὶ πυρετῷ· κάκιστον δὲ καὶ οἶσιν ἐκμανῆναι ἐλπίς.

[83] *Aph.* 5.40, 4.544.16–17 (= Magdaleine 5.40.7), γυναιξὶν ὁκόσῃσιν ἐς τοὺς τιτθοὺς αἷμα συστρέφεται, μανίην σημαίνει; 5.65, 4.558.8 (= Magdaleine 5.65.3), τούτων δὲ ἀφανισθέντων ἐξαίφνης, τοῖσι μὲν ὄπισθεν σπασμοί, τέτανοι, τοῖσι δὲ ἔμπροσθεν μανίη, ὀδύνη πλευροῦ ὀξεία ...; 6.21, 4.568.8 (= Magdaleine 6.21.8), τοῖσι μαινομένοισι κιρσῶν ἢ αἱμορροΐδων ἐπιγενομένων, τῆς μανίης λύσις; 6.56, 4.576.20 (= Magdaleine 6.56.5) ἀποπληξίην τοῦ σώματος ἢ σπασμὸν ἢ μανίην ἢ τυφλώσιν [σημαίνει]; 7.5, 4.578.14 (= Magdaleine 7.5.5), ἐπὶ μανίῃ δυσεντερίη ἢ ὕδρωψ ἢ ἔκστασις, ἀγαθόν; *Coac.* 5.690.10, ἐκ μανίης ἐς βράγχον μετὰ βηχὸς ἀπόστασις; *Epid.* II, 5.120.4, τούτων δὲ ἀφανισθέντων ἐξαίφνης, οἶσι μὲν ἐς τὸ ὄπισθεν, σπασμοὶ μετὰ πόνων, οἶσι δὲ ἐς τοὔμπροσθεν, ἢ μανίαι, ἢ ὀδύναι πλευροῦ ὀξέαι, ἢ δυσεντερίη ἐρυθρή; 5.128.13, ὅσοι τῇ γλώσσῃ παφλάζουσι, χειλῶν μὴ ἐγκρατέες ἐόντες, ἀνάγκη, ... λύει ... μανίη; *Epid.* IV, 5.144.15 (= Langholf 72), ἐκρίθη ὡς εἰκὸς περὶ πληϊάδων δύσιν τὸ πρῶτον, μετὰ δὲ πληϊάδων δύσιν χολώδης ἐς μανίην; *Epid.* VII 5.384.20 (= Jouanna 11.6.15) ἡ δὲ μανίη καὶ τὸ παρὰ καιρὸν καὶ ἡ βοὴ καὶ ἡ μεταβολὴ ἡ εἰρημένη παρηκολούθει ἐς τὸ κῶμα; 5.396.11 (= Jouanna 25.5.12), περὶ δὲ τὸν πρῶτον ὕπνον, δίψα πολλή· μανίη· καὶ ἀνεκάθιζε καὶ τοῖσι παρεοῦσιν ἐλοιδορεῖτο καὶ πάλιν ἀπεσιώπησε καὶ ἐν ἡσυχίῃ ἦν; *Gland.* 8.570.12 (= Joly 15.17) καὶ πάθεα ἐγκεφάλου καὶ ἄλλαι νοῦσοι, παραφροσύναι καὶ μανίαι, καὶ πάντα ἐπικίνδυνα, καὶ πονεῖ ὁ ἐγκέφαλος καὶ αἱ ἄλλαι ἀδένες; *Judic.* 9.290.6, ὅσοι μαίνονται, αὐτόματοι ἢ ἀπαλλασσόμενοι ἐκ τῶν νούσων, τουτέοις τὴν μανίην ὀδύνη ἐς τοὺς πόδας εἰσελθοῦσα ἢ ἐς [τὸ] στῆθος, ἢ βὴξ ἰσχυρὴ γενομένη λύει; 9.290.8, ἐὰν τουτέων μηδὲν γένηται, λυομένης τῆς μανίης, στέρησις τοῦ ὀφθαλμοῦ γίνεται; 9.290.11, ὁκόσοι τῇ γλώσσῃ παφλάζουσι τῶν χειλέων μὴ κρατέοντες, ἐὰν ταῦτα παύσηται, ἔμπυοι γίνονται, ἢ ὀδύνη ἰσχυρὴ ἐν τοῖς κάτω χωρίοις λύει, ἢ κυφότης, ἢ αἷμα πολὺ ἐκ τῶν ῥινῶν ῥυὲν, ἢ μανίη; 9.294.11, ὁπόταν ξυντεταμένος τὰς χεῖρας καὶ τοὺς πόδας [ᾖ], μανίην ἐμποιεῖ; *Loc. Hom.* 6.324.16 (= Joly 33.1.17) πρὸς δὴ τὸ ἀπὸ τοῦ πυρετοῦ θερμὸν τὸ ἀπὸ τοῦ φαρμάκου προσελθὸν μανίην ποιεῖ; 6.330.4 (= Joly 39.2.13), ὁπόταν ἄνθρωπος συντεταμένος ᾖ τοὺς πόδας καὶ τὰς χεῖρας, μανίην ἑωυτῷ ποιεῖ; *Morb* I 6.200.22 (= Wittern 30.11), οὕτω δὲ ἧσσον ἡ μανίη τε καὶ ἡ παραφρόνησις γίνεται, ὅσωπερ ἡ χολὴ τῆς χολῆς ἀσθενεστέρη ἐστίν; *Prorrh.* II 9.6.14, ἕτερος δὲ τρόπος προρρήσιος, ὠνεομένοισί τε καὶ διαπρησσομένοισι προειπεῖν τοῖσι μὲν θανάτους, τοῖσι δὲ μανίας, ...; 9.8.13, ἐλπίζω δὲ καὶ τἆλλα προρρηθῆναι ἀνθρωπινωτέρως ἢ ὅσα περ τοῖσιν ὠνεομένοισί τε καὶ περναμένοισι λέγεται προρρηθῆναι, θανάτους τε καὶ νοσήματα καὶ μανίας; 9.10.7, γὰρ ἐκ τῶν γεγραμμένων προειπεῖν καὶ θάνατον καὶ μανίην καὶ εὐεξίην; *Vict.* I 6.518.4 (= Joly-Byl I, 35.7.9) ἔστι δ' ἡ μανίη τοιούτων ἐπὶ τὸ βραδύτερον; 6.520.13 (Joly-Byl I, 35.10.32) ὅταν δὲ τοῦτο πάθῃ ἡ τοιαύτη ψυχή, ἐς μανίην

μαίνομαι (31)[84]
παραφρόνησις (1)[85]
ὑποκαταφρονέω (1)[86]
σωφρονέω (2)[87]
ἀλλοφρονέω (2)[88]
ἀφρονέω (3)[89]

καθίσταται κρατηθέντος τοῦ ὕδατος, ἐπισπασθέντος τοῦ πυρός; 6.520.19 (= Joly-Byl I, 35.11.5) οἱ δὲ ὑπομαίνεσθαι· ἔστι δὲ ἔγγιστα μανίης τὸ τοιοῦτο; *Vict.* IV 6.662.4 (= Joly-Byl IV, 93.5.8) ποταμῶν διαβάσιες καὶ ὁπλῖται πολέμιοι καὶ τέρατα ἀλλόμορφα νοῦσον σημαίνει ἢ μανίην; *Virg.* 8.468.7 (= Lami 2.8.24) ἐπικάρσιαι γὰρ αἱ φλέβες καὶ ὁ τόπος ἐπίκαιρος ἔς τε παραφροσύνην καὶ μανίην.

[84] *Aph.* 5.65, 4.558.7 (= Magdaleine 5.65.2), ὁκόσοισιν οἰδήματα ἐφ᾽ ἕλκεσι φαίνεται, οὐ μάλα σπῶνται, οὐδὲ μαίνονται; 6.21, 4.568.7 (= Magdaleine 6.21.7), τοῖσι μαινομένοισι κιρσῶν ἢ αἱμορροΐδων ἐπιγενομένων, τῆς μανίης λύσις; *Coac.* 5.710.1, ὀξέως μανέντες θνήσκουσιν ἄφωνοι; *Epid.* II 5.120.2, οἷσιν οἰδήματα ἐφ᾽ ἕλκεσιν, οὐ μάλα σπῶνται, οὐδὲ μαίνονται; 5.136.4, τουτέων ὅσοι ἐκ γενεῆς καὶ στρεβλοὶ, ἀσύνετοι, ἢ λιθιῶντες, ἢ μαινόμενοι; 5.138.19, τῷ μέλλοντι μαίνεσθαι τόδε προσημαίνει τὸ σημεῖον; *Epid.* IV 5.196.11 (= Langholf 306), θεραπευθεὶς ἐμάνη; *Epid.* V 5.204.7 (= Jouanna 2.1.8) μαινόμενος δὲ ὑπὸ χολῆς μελαίνης; *Epid.* VII 5.396.23 (= Jouanna 25.6.6) ἐμαίνετο; *Int.* 7.242.26, ἡ δὲ χροιὴ μέλαινα· τοῦ δὲ ἥπατος ἡ χολὴ φλέγματος καὶ αἵματος πλησθεῖσα, ὡς λογιζόμεθα, διαρρήγνυται, καὶ ὁκόταν διαρρηχθῇ, τάχιστα μαίνεται; *Judic.* 9.290.5, ὅσοι μαίνονται, αὐτόματοι ἢ ἀπαλλασσόμενοι ἐκ τῶν νούσων, τουτέοις τὴν μανίην ὀδύνη ἐς τοὺς πόδας εἰσελθοῦσα ἢ ἐς [τὸ] στῆθος, ἢ βὴξ ἰσχυρὴ γενομένη λύει; 9.290.20, ὅσοις ἂν ἐν τοῖσι πυρετοῖσι τὰ ὦτα κωφωθῇ, τουτέοισι μὴ λυθέντος τοῦ πυρετοῦ μανῆναι ἀνάγκη; *Loc. Hom.* 6.324.10 (= Joly 32.1.10), (ἰχώρ) λυπεῖ καὶ μαίνεσθαι ποιεῖ τὸν ἄνθρωπον; 6.324.14 (= Joly 33.1.15), πυρεταίνοντι κεφαλὴν μὴ κάθαιρε, ὡς μὴ μαίνηται; 6.328.17 (= Joly 39.1.3) μανδραγόρου ῥίζαν πρωὶ πιπίσκειν ἔλασσον ἢ ὡς μαίνεσθαι; 6.328.19 (= Joly 39.1.5), καὶ μανδραγόρου ῥίζαν πιπίσκειν ἔλασσον ἢ ὡς μαίνεσθαι); *Morb.* I 6.200.21 (= Wittern 30.10–11), οἵ τε γὰρ μελαγχολώδεις ... παράνοοι γίνονται, ἔνιοι δὲ καὶ μαίνονται; *Morb.* II 7.36.22 (= Jouanna 22.3.19), ἢν δ᾽ ἀνιστάμενος χολὴν ἐμῇ μαίνεται; *Morb. Sacr.* 6.354.4 (= Jouanna 1.3.8) τοῦτο δὲ ὁρῶ μαινομένους ἀνθρώπους καὶ παραφρονέοντας ἀπὸ οὐδεμιῆς προφάσιος ἐμφανεῖς; 6.386.22–23 (= Jouanna 14.3.5), τῷ δ᾽ αὐτῷ τούτῳ (the brain) καὶ μαινόμεθα καὶ παραφρονέομεν; 6.388.6 (= Jouanna 14.5.13) καὶ μαινόμεθα μὲν ὑπὸ ὑγρότητος; 6.388.13–14 (= Jouanna 15.1.7) οἱ μὲν ὑπὸ φλέγματος μαινόμενοι ἥσυχοί ... εἰσι; 6.388.16 (= Jouanna 15.1.10–11) ἢν μὲν οὖν συνεχέως μαίνωνται, αὗται αὐτοῖς αἱ προφάσιές εἰσιν. ...; *Prog.* 2.126.6 (= Alexanderson 7.4) ἢν γὰρ αἱ ὄψιες πυκνὰ κινέωνται, μανῆναι τούτους ἐλπίς; *Prorrh.* II 9.8.18, εἴ τις εἰδείη οἷσι τὸ νόσημα τοῦτο ἢ ξυγγενές ἐστιν, ἢ πρόσθεν ποτ᾽ ἐμάνησαν; 9.10.12, ἁμαρτοίη δ᾽ ἄν τις πρὸς τῷ μισεῖσθαι τάχ᾽ ἂν καὶ μεμηνέναι δόξειεν; *Superf.* 8.504.22 (= Lienau 34.16) ... καὶ ἐξεμεῖ καὶ μαίνεται καὶ πάλιν σωφρονέει; *Vict.* I 6.496.12 (= Joly-Byl I, 24.2.30) πίνοντες καὶ μαινόμενοι ταὐτὰ διαπρήσσονται); 6.520.20 (= Joly-Byl I, 35.11.5) καὶ γὰρ ἀπὸ βραχέης φλεγμονῆς καὶ ἀσυμφόρου μαίνονται; *Vict.* IV 6.648.8 (= Joly-Byl IV, 89.7.19) εἰ δὲ τρεφθῆναι δοκέοι ἐς φυγὴν τὸ ὑπάρχον, φεύγειν δὲ ταχέως, τοὺς δὲ διώκειν, κίνδυνος μανῆναι τὸν ἄνθρωπον, ἢν μὴ θεραπευθῇ; *Virg.* 8.468.10 (= Lami 3.1.1), ὑπὸ μὲν τῆς ὀξυφλεγμασίης μαίνεται.

[85] *Morb.* I, 6.200.22–23 (= Wittern 30.12), οὕτω δὲ ἧσσον ἡ μανίη τε καὶ ἡ παραφρόνησις γίνεται.

[86] *Epid.* IV, 5.176.1, καὶ ἴσως ἄλλως ὑποκατεφρόνει, ἐρρίπταζετο, καί τι ἐσπᾶτο.

[87] *Artic.* 4.220.4 (= Kühlewein 50.7), ἀτὰρ καὶ ἰησίος σκεθροτέρης οἱ τοιοῦτοι δέονται, εἰ σωφρονοῖεν; *Superf.* 8.504.22 (= Lienau 34.16–17) ... ἐξεμεῖ, καὶ μαίνεται καὶ πάλιν σωφρονέει.

[88] *Morb.* II, 7.30.3 (= Jouanna 16.1.15–16), ἀλύει καὶ ἀλλοφρονεῖ ὑπὸ τῆς ὀδύνης; *Mul.* I, 8.100.8, καὶ καρδιώξει, καὶ ἐρεύξεται, καὶ ἀλλοφρονήσει, καὶ παράνοιαι γίνονται μανιώδεες (Littré prints θ ἀλλοφάσσει).

[89] *Gland.* 8.566.12 (= Joly 12.2.20), ὁ νοῦς ἀφρονεῖ (Littré prints ἀφραίνει); *Morb.* II 7.82.15–16 (= Jouanna 54.1.10 writes instead ἀφρὸν ἱεῖ) ἀφρονέει καὶ πυρετὸς ἴσχει.

ἀφροσύνη (1)[90]
ἔκφρων (5)[91]
φρόνιμος (11)[92]
ἄφρων (6)[93]
ἔμφρων (17)[94]
φρονέω (12)[95]

[90] *Vict.* I, 6.512.20 (= Joly-Byl I, 35.29) περὶ δὲ φρονήσιος ψυχῆς ὀνομαζομένης καὶ ἀφροσύνης ὧδε ἔχει.

[91] *Epid.* V, 5.258.19 (= Jouanna 106.7), ἔκφρων νύκτα καὶ ἡμέρην· ἔθανεν; *Epid.* VII 5.392.11 (= Jouanna 21.2.5), ἔκφρων νύκτα καὶ ἡμέρην, ἐτελεύτησεν; *Morb.* III, 7.128.7 (= Potter 9.21), τὰς φρένας ἀλγέουσιν, ὥστε μὴ ἐᾶσαι ἂν ἅψασθαι, καὶ πῦρ ἔχει, καὶ ἔκφρονές εἰσι, 7.128.9 (= Potter 9.23), ὅταν [οἱ ἐν τῇ περιπλευμονίῃ] ἔκφρονες ἔωσι; *Mul.* III 8.252.20, καὶ θέρμη πολλή, δίψα, ἀγρυπνίη, καὶ ἔκφρονες γίνονται.

[92] *Morb. Sacr.* 6.390.19 (= Jouanna 16.3.16), καταλελοιπὼς ἐν τῷ ἐγκεφάλῳ ἑωυτοῦ τὴν ἀκμὴν καὶ ὅ τι ἂν ᾖ φρόνιμόν τε καὶ γνώμην ἔχον (on the brain); *Vict.* I 6.512.22 (= Joly-Byl I, 35.1.30) πυρὸς τὸ ὑγρότατον καὶ ὕδατος τὸ ξηρότατον κρῆσιν λαβόντα ἐν τῷ σώματι φρονιμώτατον; 6.514.11 (= Joly-Byl I, 35.2.9), φρόνιμοι μὲν καὶ οὗτοι, ἐνδεέστεροι δὲ τῆς προτέρης; 6.514.15 (= Joly-Byl I, 35.2.13), εἰ δὲ ὀρθῶς διαιτῷντο, καὶ φρονιμώτερος καὶ ὀξύτερος ⟨ἂν⟩ γένοιτο παρὰ τὴν φύσιν; 6.518.1–2 (= Joly-Byl I, 35.6.7), ταῦτα ποιέων ὑγιεινότερος ἂν καὶ φρονιμώτερος εἴη; 6.518.12 (= Joly-Byl I, 35.8.14), ἐν ὑγιαίνουσι σώμασι φρόνιμος ἡ τοιαύτη ψυχή; 6.518.20 (= Joly-Byl I, 35.8.21), τῆς ψυχῆς φρόνιμος ⟨ἡ⟩ σύγκρησις; 6.520.11 (= Joly-Byl I, 35.10.30) συμφέρει δὲ καὶ ἀσαρκεῖν τοῖσι τοιούτοισι πρὸς τὸ φρονίμους εἶναι; 6.522.15 (= Joly-Byl I, 35.12.17–18), ἐκ ταύτης τῆς ἐπιμελείης ἡ τοιαύτη ψυχὴ φρονιμωτάτη ἂν εἴη; 6.522.17 (= Joly-Byl I, 36.1.19) περὶ μὲν οὖν φρονίμου καὶ ἄφρονος ψυχῆς ἡ σύγκρησις αὕτη αἰτίη ἐστίν; 6.522.21–22 (= Joly-Byl I, 36.1–2.22–23) ἐκ τούτων δὲ φρονιμώτεραι καὶ ἀφρονέστεραι γίνονται (all these discussing the different blends of the soul).

[93] *Morb.* III 7.120.20 (= Potter III, 3.1.13), καὶ κῶμά μιν ἔχει, καὶ ἄφρονές εἰσι (Littré ἔκφρονες); *Morb. Sacr.* 6.374.1 (= Jouanna 7.5.22) αἱ φλέβες τοῦ ἠέρος ὑπὸ τοῦ φλέγματος καὶ μὴ παραδέχωνται, ἄφωνον καθιστᾶσι καὶ ἄφρονα τὸν ἄνθρωπον; *Vict.* I 6.514.8–9 (= Joly-Byl I, 35.1.7), εἰ δέ τινι ἐπαγωγῇ χρεώμενον τούτων ὁποτερονοῦν αὐξηθείη ⟨ἢ⟩ μαραίνοι, ἀφρονέστατον ἂν γένοιτο; 6.518.3 (= Joly-Byl I, 35.7.8) τούτους ἤδη οἱ μὲν ἄφρονας ὀνομάζουσιν, οἱ δὲ ἐμβροντήτους; 6.522.17 (= Joly-Byl I, 36.1.19), περὶ μὲν οὖν φρονίμου καὶ ἄφρονος ψυχῆς ἡ σύγκρησις αὕτη αἰτίη ἐστίν; 6.522.22 (= Joly-Byl I, 36.1.23) ἐκ τούτων δὲ φρονιμώτεραι καὶ ἀφρονέστεραι γίνονται.

[94] *Coac.* 5.610.18, ἔμφρονες δὲ γενόμενοι (about patients with lethargy); *Epid.* V, 5.214.4 (= Jouanna 14.4.11) τὰς δὲ πέντε ἡμέρας, τοτὲ μὲν ἔμφρων ἦν, τοτὲ δὲ οὔ; 5.258.18 (= Jouanna 105.2.4) ἔμφρων ἔθανε; *Epid.* VII, 5.378.23–24 (= Jouanna 8.1.25) ἥ τε φωνὴ ψελλὴ διὰ τὸ παραλελυμένον καὶ ἀκίνητον καὶ ἀσθενὲς εἶναι τὸ σῶμα· ἔμφρων δέ), 5.380.24 (= Jouanna 10.2.6) καὶ ἔμφρων τὸ πρῶτον; 5.388.6 (= Jouanna 12.3.8) ῥυφήμασιν ἐχρῆτο, ἔμφρων ἅπαντα τὸν χρόνον; 5.388.21 (= Jouanna 14.4.24), ἔμφρων δὲ πάντα τὸν χρόνον ἐών, ἐτελεύτησεν; 5.390.2 (= Jouanna 15.2.22) ἔμφρων, ἐτελεύτησε; 5.390.7 (= Jouanna 16.4.9) ἔμφρων δὲ σφόδρα ἐὼν τεταρταῖος ἐτελεύτησεν, 5.390.13 (= Jouanna 17.2.17) οὐκ ἔμφρων; 5.412.9 (= Jouanna 44.3.6) ἐτελεύτησεν ἔμφρων; 5.418.17 (= Jouanna 50.3.12) ἐτελεύτησε μετὰ τὴν ἄφεσιν ἑβδόμη ἔμφρων; 5.420.9 (= Jouanna 51.4.27) ἔμφρων διετέλει; 5.448.15 (= Jouanna 92.5.5) διψώδης, ἄγρυπνος, ἔμφρων; 5.458.12 (= Jouanna 107.5.8) ἔμφρων ἐτελεύτησε τριταῖος ἀπὸ τῆς ὑποστροφῆς; *Morb.* II 7.36.9 (= Jouanna 21.3.3) ἦν δ᾽ ἔμφρων γένηται καὶ ἐκφεύγῃ τὴν νοῦσον; *Morb.* III 7.120.2 (= Potter 2.1.23) οὕτω δὲ ἡ ὀδύνη παύεται, καὶ ἔμφρων γίνεται; see also *Epid.* VII, 5.396.6 (= Jouanna 25.5.6). ἐμφρόνως διετίθετο τὰ ἑωυτῆς.

[95] *Epid.* V 5.240.10 (= Jouanna 60.2.5) ἤκουεν οὐδὲν οὐδὲ ἐφρόνει· οὐκ ἀτρεμέως; 5.254.9 (= Jouanna 91.2.7), ἤκουε δὲ καὶ ἐφρόνει· καὶ ἐσήμαινε τῇ χειρὶ περὶ τὸ ἰσχίον εἶναι τὸ ἄλγημα; *Epid.* VII

παραφροσύνη (33)[96]
παραφρονέω (37)[97]

5.402.4 (= Jouanna 32.2.8) ἤκουεν οὐδὲν οὐδ' ἐφρόνει· οὐδ' ἠτρέμιζεν; 5.454.2 (= Jouanna 100.2.7) ἤκουε δὲ καὶ ἐφρόνει· καὶ τῇ χειρὶ ἐσήμαινεν ἀμφὶ τὸ ἰσχίον εἶναι τὸ ἄλγημα; 5.458.16 (= Jouanna 108.2.14) ἐγχεόμενος χυλὸν πτισάνης κατείχετο, ἐφρόνει, εὔπνοος ἦν; *Morb.* I, 6.174.13 (= Wittern 19.2) λεσχηνευομένου δὲ αὐτοῦ καὶ φρονέοντος πάντα χρήματα; *Morb. Sacr.* 6.354.9 (= Jouanna 1.3.14) ἔπειτα δὲ ὑγιέας ἐόντας καὶ φρονέοντας ὥσπερ καὶ πρότερον; 6.372.8 (= Jouanna 7.1.2) καὶ οὐδὲν φρονέουσιν; 6.374.20 (= Jouanna 7.11.23) ἐδέξαντο τὸν ἠέρα αἱ φλέβες καὶ ἐφρόνησαν; 6.388.11 (= Jouanna 14.5.4) φρονεῖ ὥνθρωπος; *Mul.* II 8.390.1, καὶ οὐδὲν φρονέει; *Virg.* 8.468.17 φρονεούσης δὲ τῆς ἀνθρώπου (Lami 3.3.7–8 corrects in ⟨ἀ⟩φρονεούσης).

[96] *Acut.* 2.314.8–9 (= Joly 42.3.14) ταῦτα δ᾽ ἐν ἀρχῇσιν ἐπιφαινόμενα παραφροσύνης δηλωτικά ἐστι σφοδρῆς; *Acut.* (*Sp.*) 2.440.11 (= Joly 23.1.13) παραφροσύνην ἐσομένην προσδέχου; 2.446.11 (= Joly 26.2.3–4), σπασμός ... ἐπιλαμβάνει καὶ παραφροσύνη; 2.448.2 (= Joly 26.3.7) καὶ ἡ παραφροσύνη μέγα τι ἐπιδιδοῖ; 2.448.3 (= Joly 26.3.9) αἱ δὲ νύκτες μᾶλλον σημαίνουσιν ἢ αἱ ἡμέραι τὰ περὶ τὴν παραφροσύνην (however ἀφροσύνην A); 2.450.9 (= Joly 29.1.10–11), καλῶς ἔχει παραφροσύνην προειπεῖν ἢ σπασμόν; *Aph.* 2.2, 4.470.11 (= Magdelaine 2.2.3), ὅκου παραφροσύνην ὕπνος παύει, ἀγαθόν; 4.50, 4.520.10 (= Magdelaine 4.50.9), ὅκου ἐν πυρετῷ μὴ διαλείποντι δύσπνοια γίνεται καὶ παραφροσύνη, θανάσιμον; 6.53, 4.576.13 (= Magdelaine 6.53.10), αἱ παραφροσύναι αἱ μὲν μετὰ γέλωτος γινόμεναι, ἀσφαλέστεραι; 7.7, 4.580.1 (= Magdelaine 7.7.8), ἐκ πολυποσίης ῥῖγος καὶ παραφροσύνη, κακόν; 7.9, 4.580.4 (= Magdelaine 7.9.11), ἐπὶ αἵματος ῥύσει παραφροσύνη ἢ σπασμός, κακόν; 7.10, 4.580.5 (= Magdelaine 7.10.1), ἐπὶ εἰλεῷ ἔμετος ἢ λὺγξ ἢ σπασμὸς ἢ παραφροσύνη, κακόν; 7.14, 4.580.10 (= Magdelaine 7.14.5), ἐπὶ πληγῇ ἐς τὴν κεφαλὴν ἔκπληξις ἢ παραφροσύνη, κακόν; 7.18, 4.582.2 (= Magdelaine 7.18.1), ἐπὶ ἀγρυπνίῃ σπασμὸς καὶ παραφροσύνη; 7.24, 4.582.9 (= Magdelaine 7.24.8), ἐπὶ ὀστέου διακοπῇ, παραφροσύνη, ἢν κενεὸν λάβῃ; *Coac.* 5.602.12, παραφροσύνη ἐν πνεύματι καὶ ἱδρῶτι, θανατώδης; 5.604.2, αἱ περὶ ἀναγκαῖα παραφροσύναι, κάκισται, οἱ ἐκ τούτων παροξυνόμενοι, ὀλέθριοι; 5.604.6; αἱ προεξαδυνατησάντων παραφροσύναι, κάκισται; 5.634.22, ἐπὶ ὀδόντος σφακελισμῷ πυρετὸς ἐπιγενόμενος σφοδρὸς, καὶ παραφροσύνη, θανάσιμον; 5.638.17, πνεῦμα ... μέγα δὲ καὶ διὰ πολλοῦ, παραφροσύνην ἢ σπασμόν; 5.694.6, καίτοι τὸν τοιοῦτον τρόπον διελθοῦσα σημαίνει πονηρὸν καὶ παραφροσύνην; 5.694.13, τὸ δ᾽ ἐπὶ γαστέρα κεῖσθαι οἶσι μὴ σύνηθες, παραφροσύνην σημαίνει; *Gland.* 8.570.11 (= Joly 15.1.7), καὶ πάθεα ἐγκεφάλου καὶ ἄλλαι νοῦσοι, παραφροσύναι καὶ μανίαι, καὶ πάντα ἐπικίνδυνα, καὶ πονεῖ ὁ ἐγκέφαλος καὶ αἱ ἄλλαι ἀδένες; *Judic.* 9.306.3, βάρος ἐν τοῖσι στήθεσι καὶ παραφροσύναι; *Morb.* III, 7.136.15 (= Potter III, 15.25), βάρος ἐν τοῖσι στήθεσι καὶ παραφροσύνη (in pneumonia); *Prog.* 2.120.5 (= Alexanderson 3.2), παραφροσύνην τινὰ σημαίνει; 2.122.13 (= Alexanderson 5.8), διὰ πολλοῦ χρόνου παραφροσύνην δηλοῖ; 2.126.4 (= Alexanderson 7.3) θόρυβον σημαίνει ἢ παραφροσύνην; 2.174.7 (= Alexanderson 22.12) οἱ γὰρ πυρετοὶ καὶ αἱ παραφροσύναι; *Prorrh.* I, 5.512.5 (= Polack 8.1), αἱ προαπαυδησάντων παραφροσύναι κάκισται; 5.516.5 (= Polack 22.12), τὰ ἀραιὰ κατὰ πλευρὸν ἐν τουτέοισιν ἀλγήματα παραφροσύνην σημαίνει; *Prorrh.* II 9.40.4, τῇσι δ᾽ ἀρχῇσι τῶν πυρετῶν ἤν τε παραφροσύνη ἐπιγένηται; *Virg.* 8.468.7 (= Lami 2.8.24), ἐπικάρσιαι γὰρ αἱ φλέβες καὶ ὁ τόπος ἐπίκαιρος ἔς τε παραφροσύνην καὶ μανίην.

[97] *Acut.* 2.312.6–7 (= Joly 42.1.4–5), περίλυποι δε καὶ πικροὶ γίνονται καὶ παραφρονέουσι; *Acut.* (*Sp.*) 2.426.11–12 (= Joly 17.1.8–9), οὐ θαυμάσαιμι δ᾽ ἂν οὐδ᾽ εἰ παραφρονήσειαν; *Coac.* 5.624.10, ὠτὸς πόνος σύντονος, μετὰ πυρετοῦ ὀξέος, καὶ ἄλλου του σημείου τῶν ὑποδυσκόλων, τοὺς μὲν νέους ἑβδομαίους κτείνει καὶ συντομώτερον, παραφρονήσαντας; 5.624.13, τά τε γὰρ ὦτα φθάνει ἐκπυέειν, καὶ παραφρονέουσιν ἧσσον; 5.634.19, ἤδη δὲ παραφρονέως ἦν ποιῇ τοῦτο, παντελῶς ὀλέθριον; 5.670.12, κίνδυνος θανεῖν καὶ παραφρονῆσαι; 5.694.22, ἢ παραφρονήσει ἀπὸ τούτου τοῦ σημείου; *Dieb.Judic.* 9.300.17–18, καὶ ὁκόταν τὸ ἧπαρ μᾶλλον ἀναπτυχθῇ πρὸς τὰς φρένας, παραφρονέει; 9.300.28–29, ὅταν δὲ παύσηται παραφρονέων, εὐθὺς ἔννοος γίνεται; *Epid.* I 2.688.15 (= Kühlewein 26, case 3.2) ἀπὸ κοιλίης ὀλίγα διῆλθε μέλανα, παρεφρόνησεν; 2.704.10 (= Kühlewein 26, case

ἔκστασις (6)[98]
ἐξίσταμαι (21)[99]
παράφορος (8)[100]
παραφέρομαι (8)[101]

9.10), ἐς νύκτα παρεφρόνησεν; 2.706.2 (= Kühlewein 10.20), τετάρτῃ ἐς νύκτα παρεφρόνει; *Epid.*
II 5.128.17, ἢν δὲ παραφρονέῃ, τὴν κεφαλὴν καταβρέχειν, ἢν μὴ τὰ ὑποχόνδρια ἐπηρμένα ᾖ; *Epid.*
VII 5.422.9 (= Jouanna 54.1.2) φαγὼν παρεφρόνει, ἐτελεύτησε ταχέως; *Int.* 7.284.22 παραφρονέει;
7.286.11 ὁκόταν δὲ παύσηται παραφρονέων; *Morb.* I 6.204.5 (= Wittern 34.7–8), ὑπὸ δὲ τῆς φρενίτιδος ἀπόλλυνται οὕτως· παραφρονέουσιν ἐν τῇ νούσῳ διὰ παντός; 6.204.7 (= Wittern 34.9–10)
ἅτε παραφρονέοντες οὔτε τι τῶν προσφερομένων δέχονται; *Morb.* II 7.10.5 (= Jouanna 3.1.1) παραφρονεῖ; 7.10.6 (= Jouanna 3.2.2–3) παραφρονεῖ; 7.24.22 (= Jouanna 14.1.10) παραφρονεῖ; *Morb.* III
(= Potter 2.22) 7.118.22, καὶ παραφρονέει καὶ ἀποθνήσκει; *Morb.Sacr.* 6.354.4–5 (= Jouanna 1.3.9)
τοῦτο δὲ ὁρῶ μαινομένους ἀνθρώπους καὶ παραφρονέοντας; 6.354.8 (= Jouanna 1.3.13) … φεύγοντας
ἔξω καὶ παραφρονέοντας μέχρι ἐπέγρωνται; 6.386.23 (= Jouanna 14.3.5) τῷ δ' αὐτῷ τούτῳ καὶ μαινόμεθα καὶ παραφρονέομεν καὶ δείματα καὶ φόβοι …; *Prog.* 2.120.11 (= Alexanderson 3.7), ἢν δὲ καὶ
παραφρονέων τοῦτο ποιῇ, ὀλέθριον κάρτα ἤδη γίνεται; 2.134.11 (= Alexanderson 10.1) ἢ παραφρονήσει ἀπὸ τούτου τοῦ σημείου; 2.138.8 (= Alexanderson 11.9) καὶ οὕτω διεξελθοῦσα σημαίνει πονεῖν
τι τὸν ἄνθρωπον, ἢ παραφρονεῖν; 2.162.3 (= Alexanderson 18.2), κίνδυνος γάρ, μὴ παραφρονήσῃ καὶ
ἀποθάνῃ; 2.174.2 (= Alexanderson 22.7), παραφρονῆσαι γὰρ κίνδυνος τὸν ἄνθρωπον καὶ ἀπολέσθαι;
Prorrh. II 9.8.16, ἔπειτα τοὺς παραφρονήσοντας ἐστὶ μὴ πολὺ λανθάνειν; 9.8.20, πολλαὶ ἐλπίδες ἐκ
τουτέων τῶν διαιτημάτων παραφρονῆσαι αὐτούς; 9.34.2, ἀλλ' ὅτε ἕλκος ἔχων μὴ παραφρονέει εὐ-
πετέως τε φέρει τὸ τρῶμα; 9.34.11, τὸ μὲν πνεῦμα ἀνήνεγκαν, παρεφρόνησαν δὲ καὶ πυρετήναντες
ἀπέθανον; *Superf.* 8.504.23 (= Lienau 34.1.18), ἐξεμεῖ καὶ πυρέσσει καὶ παραφρονεῖ; *VC* 3.254.4 (=
Hanson 19.3.10), ὅταν δ' ἤδη ὑπόπτυον ᾖ, ἐπὶ τῇ γλώσσῃ φλύκταιναι γίνονται καὶ παραφρονέων τε-
λευτᾷ; *Virg.* 8.466.7 (= Lami 1.2.5) περὶ τῶν δειμάτων, ὁκόσα φοβεῦνται ἰσχυρῶς ἄνθρωποι, ὥστε
παραφρονέειν.
   [98] *Aph.* 7.5, 4.578.14 (= Magdelaine 7.5.5), ἐπὶ μανίῃ δυσεντερίη ἢ ὕδρωψ ἢ ἔκστασις, ἀγαθόν;
Coac. 5.598.10, αἱ ἐν πυρετοῖσιν ἐκστάσιες σιγῶσαι μὴ ἀφώνῳ, ὀλέθριαι; 5.638.4, αἱ μετὰ ἀφωνίης
ἐκστάσιες, ὀλέθριοι; 5.648.16, οἱ κατὰ κοιλίην ἐν πυρετῷ παλμοὶ ἐκστάσιας ποιέουσιν; 5.690.12, αἱ
σιγῶσαι ἐκστάσιες; *Prorrh.* II 9.28.20, αἱ μὲν γὰρ μελαγχολικαὶ αὗται ἐκστάσιες οὐ λυσιτελέες.
   [99] *Coac.* 5.602.11, τῶν ἐξισταμένων μελαγχολικῶς; 5.602.17, τῶν ἐξισταμένων μελαγχολικῶς;
5.602.18–19, οἱ ἐξιστάμενοι μελαγχολικῶς; 5.602.20 οἱ ἐκστάντες ὀξέως; 5.604.5, ἐξίστανται;
5.610.2, ἐξίστανται μελαγχολικῶς; 5.620.16, ἠρά γε ἐξίστανται; 5.636.16, ἐκστάσαι σιγῇ; 5.676.17–
18, ἀλόγως ἀφανισθὲν, ἐξίστανται; 5.690.9, ὅσοι ἐκ φόβου μετὰ καταψύξιος ἐξίστανται, 5.702.21, ἐξίστανται ὀλέθριοι; *Prorrh.* I, 5.514.7 (= Polack 14.12), τοῖσιν ἐξισταμένοισι μελαγχολικῶς; 5.514.8 (=
Polack 15.13), οἱ ἐκστάντες ὀξέως; 5.514.14 (= Polack 18.5–6), ἐξίστανται μελαγχολικῶς; 5.516.1 (=
Polack 19.7–8), ἐξίστανται; 5.520.5 (= Polack 38.12), ἐλπὶς ἐκστῆναι; 5.524.4 (= Polack 54.8), αἱ ἐν
πυρετοῖσιν ἀφωνίαι σπασμώδεα τρόπον ἐξίστανται; 5.536.5 (= Polack 96.9–10), ἐξίσταται; 5.550.1
(= Polack 117.7), ἐξίσταται καύματι πολλῷ.
   [100] *Coac.* 5.592.11, γνώμης παράφοροι; 5.600.9, γνώμης παράφοροι; 5.602.1, αἱ ταραχώδεες θρα-
σύτητι ἐγέρσιες παράφοροι, 5.648.21, γνώμης παράφορον; *Epid.* II, 5.100.11, κωματώδεες ἦσαν καὶ
παράφοροι, οἱ δὲ ἐξ ὕπνων τοιοῦτοι ἐγίνοντο; *Mul.* II 8.282.15, παράφοροι δὲ τῇ γνώμῃ; *Prorrh.* I
5.518.12 (= Polack 36.3), γνώμης παράφορον; 5.528.2 (= Polack 71.5) οἱ ἐπανεμεῦντες μέλανα ἀπό-
σιτοι, παράφοροι.
   [101] *Coac.* 5.652.6, παρενεχθέντες ἄφωνοι; 5.722.9, ὀσφὺν πεπονηκότι, καὶ παρενεχθέντι; *Epid.*
II 5.94.6 (= Langholf 36), πνεῦμα ἐνεδιπλασιάζετο, οὐ μὴν μέγα. παρεφέρετο; *Epid.* IV, 5.152.16,
ὁ πρῶτος παρενεχθείς; 5.188.5–6, ἐν τοῖσιν ὕπνοισι παραφερόμενοι; 5.194.12, παρηνέχθη κοσμίως;
Mul. I 8.196.14, παραφέρεται δὲ ὁ πίνων; *Prorrh.* I, 5.532.1 (= Polack 83.5), παρενεχθεῖσαι ἄφωνοι.

ἐπιληρέω (1?)[102]
ὑποπαραληρέω (1)[103]
λήρησις (2)[104]
ὑποληρέω (2)[105]
ληρέω (2)[106]
παραληρέω (6)[107]
παραλήρησις (7)[108]
λῆρος (6)[109]
παράληρος (11)[110]
ὑποπαρακρούω (1)[111]
παράκρουσις (10)[112]

---

[102] At *Epid.* VII, 5.458.20–21, καὶ ἐπελήρει καὶ πυρετὸς ὀξύς (however Jouanna 109.2.20–21 has ὑπελήρει καὶ πυρετὸς ὀξύς).

[103] *Epid.* VII, 5.372.21 (= Jouanna 5.2.9) πέμπτῃ ὑποπαρελήρει.

[104] *Epid.* V 5.248.23 (= Jouanna 80.1.7), ἀφωνίη, λήρησις; *Epid.* VII 5.398.19 (= Jouanna 26.5.6), ληρήσιος.

[105] *Epid.* VII 5.394.20 (= Jouanna 25.3.19) ὑπελήρει ἄλλοτε καὶ ἄλλοτε, καὶ πάντ᾽ ἐπὶ τὸ χεῖρον; 5.458.20–21 (= Jouanna 109.2.20–21), κῶμα ὀλίγον χρόνον ἐπεῖχε καὶ ὑπελήρει (ἐπελήρει Littré).

[106] *Epid.* I 2.688.15 (= Kühlewein 26, case 3.2) ἕκτῃ ἐλήρει; *Epid.* VII 5.396.7 (= Jouanna 25.5.7) ἐλήρει.

[107] *Acut.* (*Sp*) 2.450.2 (= Joly 28.2.2), φιλεῖ παραληρεῖν; *Epid.* I 2.706.12 (= Kühlewein 26, case 10.6) παρελήρει; 2.712.11 (Kühlewein 26, case 12.5), παρελήρει πολλά (Kühlewein); 2.712.12, παρεληρει (= Kühlewein 26, case 12.6–7); 2.714.2 (Kühlewein 26, case 13.13), παρελήρει πάντα; *Epid.* III 3.50.12 (= Kühlewein 1, case 6.17), πάλιν πολλὰ παρελήρει.

[108] *Epid.* VII 5.366.17 (= Jouanna 2.4.16) παραλήρησις ... ἅμα τῷ ὕπνῳ; 5.366.20 (= Jouanna 2.4.20) παραλήρησις ἐν τῷ ὕπνῳ; 5.374.16 (= Jouanna 5.7.6) παραλήρησις; 5.382.20 (= Jouanna 11.2.6) παραλήρησις; 5.410.6 (= Jouanna 43.1.22), παραλήρησις ἐς νύκτα; 5.440.9 (= Jouanna 83.6.18) παραλήρησις; 5.444.1 (= Jouanna 85.1.17) παραλήρησις.

[109] *Epid.* I 2.684.3 (= Kühlewein 26, case 1.3), ὕπνοι σμικροί, λόγοι, λῆρος; *Epid.* III 3.24.5 (= Kühlewein 1, case 1.2), λῆρος; 3.48.6 (= Kühlewein 1, case 5.15), λῆρος; *Epid.* VII 5.394.15 (= Jouanna 25.2.13) λῆρος βραχύς; 5.396.4 (= Jouanna 25.5.3) χαλεπῶς καὶ λῆρος; 5.422.19 (= Jouanna 56.2.15) λῆρος τις.

[110] *Epid.* I 2.610.1 (= Kühlewein 2.18), παράληροι πολλοί; 2.620.2 (= Kühlewein 6.20), οὔτε οἱ παράληροι; 2.688.16 (= Kühlewein 26, case 3.3), παράληρος παρέμενεν (λῆρος V), *Epid.* III 3.82.1 (= Kühlewein 6.4), οὐ παράληροι; 3.96.2–3 (= Kühlewein 13.11), παράληροι περὶ θάνατον; 3.122.12 (Kühlewein 17, case 7.1–2), ἐνὴν καὶ παράληρος; 3.122.13 (Kühlewein 17, case 7.2–3), παράληρος ἀπέλιπεν; 3.124.5 (= Kühlewein 17, case 8.13), ἕκτῃ παράληρος; 3.128.19–20 (= Kühlewein 17, case 9.3), οἱ παράληροί τε μείους ἦσαν; 3.140.9 (= Kühlewein 17, case 13.8), παράληρος; 3.140.12 (= Kühlewein 17, case 13.11–12), παράληρος διὰ τέλεος.

[111] *Epid.* VII 5.440.4 (= Jouanna 85.5.13) ἤδη τι ὑποπαρέκρουε.

[112] *Coac.* 5.600.8, αἱ τρομώδεες, ψηλαφώδεες παρακρούσιες, φρενιτικαί; 5.602.4, αἱ ἐν καύμασι παρακρούσιες, σπασμώδεες; 5.602.5, αἱ ἐπ᾽ ὀλίγον θρασέες παρακρούσιες, θηριώδεες, καὶ σπασμοὺς δὲ προσημαίνουσιν; 5.604.4, αἱ παρακρούσιες, φωνὴ κλαγγώδεες, γλώσσῃ σπασμώδεες, καὶ αὐτοὶ τρομώδεες γινόμενοι, ἐξίστανται; 5.616.6, αἱ ἐπ᾽ ὀλίγον θρασέες παρακρούσιες, καὶ θηριώδη καὶ σπασμὸν σημαίνουσιν; 5.636.14, αἱ ἐπ᾽ ὀλίγον θρασέες παρακρούσιες, πονηρὸν καὶ θηριῶδες; *Epid.* VI 5.328.10 (= Manetti-Roselli 6.10.1–2), οὖρον πολλὴν ὑπόστασιν ἔχον ῥύεται τὰς παρακρούσιας; *Prorrh.* I 5.514.14 (= Polack 19.6), αἱ παρακρούσιες σὺν φωνῇ κλαγγώδει; 5.516.9 (= Polack 26.1), αἱ ἐπ᾽ ὀλίγον θρασέως παρακρούσιες θηριώδεες; 5.518.9 (= Polack 34.15), αἱ τρομώδεες, ἀσαφέες, ψηλαφώδεες παρακρούσιες πάνυ φρενιτικαί.

παρακρουστικόν (17)[113]
παρακρούω (71)[114]

---

[113] *Coac.* 5.626.1, ἤχοι μετὰ ἀμβλυωσμοῦ, καὶ κατὰ ῥῖνας βάρεος, παρακρουστικόν; 5.626.7, κώφωσις, καὶ οὖρον ὑπέρυθρον, ἀκατάστατον, ἐναιωρεύμενον, παρακρουστικόν; 5.638.1, ἠρά γε καὶ παρακρουστικόν; 5.642.11, τὰ ἐν ὀξέσι κατὰ φάρυγγα μικρὰ ὀδυνώδεα, ὅτε χάνοι, μὴ ῥηϊδίως συνάγοντι, ἰσχνῷ, παρακρουστικά; 5.646.4, σφυγμὸς ἐν ὑποχονδρίῳ μετὰ θορύβου, παρακρουστικόν; 5.650.21, τὰ ἐξ ὀσφύος ἐς τράχηλον καὶ κεφαλὴν ἀναδιδόντα ... παρακρουστικά; 5.706.12, αἱ ναρκώδεες ἐκλύσιες, δύσκολοι μὲν ἐκ τῶν τόκων ἀποβαίνουσι καὶ παρακρουστικαί, οὐ μέντοι ὀλέθριοι; *Epid.* VI 5.276.1 (= Manetti-Roselli 1.15.4), ὄμματος θράσος, παρακρουστικόν; 5.304.1 (= Manetti-Roselli 3.22.1), τὰ στρογγυλούμενα πτύαλα παρακρουστικά; 5.328.7 (= Manetti-Roselli 6.9.7), τὰ στρογγυλούμενα πτύαλα, παρακρουστικά; *Prorrh.* I, 5.510.8 (= Polack 4.9–10), τὰ ἐπὶ ταραχώδεσιν ἀγρύπνοισιν οὖρα ἄχροα, μέλασιν ἐνηωρημένα παρακρουστικά; 5.514.1 (= Polack 11.6), τὰ ἐν ὀξέσι κατὰ φάρυγγα ὀδυνώδεα σμικρά, πνιγώδεα ... παρακρουστικόν; 5.516.8 (= Polack 25.16), ἀρά γε καὶ παρακρουστικὸν τὸ τοιοῦτον; 5.518.4 (= Polack 32.10), κώφωσις καὶ οὖρα ἐξέρυθρα, ἀκατάστατα, ἐναιωρήματα, παρακρουστικόν; 5.520.1 (= Polack 37.7), τὰ κατὰ μηρὸν ἐν πυρετῷ ἀλγήματα ἔχει τι παρακρουστικόν; 5.550.5 (= Polack 118.2–3), τὰ ἐξ ὀσφύος ἐς τράχηλον καὶ κεφαλὴν ἀναδιδόντα παραλύσαντα παραπληκτικὸν τρόπον σπασμώδεα παρακρουστικά; 5.550.11 (= Polack 120.9), ἠρά γε καὶ παρακρουστικὸν τὸ τοιοῦτον.

[114] *Coac.* 5.602.9, παρακρούσαντα; 5.604.9–10, τοῖσι ποικίλως διανοσέουσι καὶ παρακρούουσι ...; 5.618.7, κατόχως παρακρούοντες; 5.618.9, παρακρούοντα σαφῶς; 5.622.12, παρακρούσαντα ἀλυσμῷ; 5.652.12, ὀλίγα θρασέως παρακρούσασιν; 5.652.19, παρακρούειν τι; 5.718.16, ἀρά τι καὶ παρακρούουσιν *Epid.* I, 2.682.12 (= Kühlewein 26, case 1.19), πάντα παρέκρουσε; 2.686.3 (= Kühlewein 26, case 2.20), σμικρὰ παρέκρουσε; 2.690.1 (= Kühlewein 26, case 3.4), παρέκρουσε; 2.690.9 (= Kühlewein 26, case 3.13), οὐδὲ παρέκρουσεν ἐπὶ τῇ ὑποστροφῇ; 2.692.3–4 (= Kühlewein 26, case 4.23), ἑκταίη ἐς νύκτα παρέκρουσε πολλά; 2.692.10 (= Kühlewein 26, case 4.7), ταχὺ δὲ πάλιν παρέκρουσε; 2.692.17 (= Kühlewein 26, case 4.14), διὰ ταχέων δὲ πάλιν παρέκρουσεν; 2.694.13 (= Kühlewein 26, case 5.1), ἐς νύκτα ἑκταίη παρέκρουσεν; 2.694.14 (= Kühlewein 26, case 5.2), παρέκρουσεν; 2.694.17 (= Kühlewein 26, case 5.6), οὐ παρέκρουεν; 2.696.7 (= Kühlewein 26, case 5.13), παρέκρουσεν; 2.696.8 (= Kühlewein 26, case 5.14), παρέκρουσε; 2.702.13 (= Kühlewein 26, case 8.19), ἐς νύκτα παρέκρουσε; 2.702.14 (= Kühlewein 26, case 8.20), πολλὰ παρέκρουσε; 2.710.6 (= Kühlewein 26, case 11.9), περὶ δὲ μέσον ἡμέρης, πολλὰ παρέκρουσε; 2.710.8 (= Kühlewein 26, case 11.11), παρέκρουσεν; 2.712.4 (= Kühlewein 26, case 12.22), ἕκτη δείλης πολλὰ παρέκρουσεν; 2.712.9–10 (= Kühlewein 26, case 12.4), δείλης πολλὰ παρέκρουσε; 2.714.7 (= Kühlewein 26, case 13.17), παρέκρουσε πάντα; 2.714.9 (= Kühlewein 26, case 13.19), παρέκρουε πάντα; 2.714.13 (= Kühlewein 26, case 13.23), σμικρὰ παρέκρουσεν; 2.716.9–10 (= Kühlewein 26, case 14.11), σμικρὰ παρέκρουσεν; *Epid.* III 3.34.5 (= Kühlewein 1, case 2.3), ἐς νύκτα παρέκρουσεν; 3.36.4 (= Kühlewein 1, case 2.11), παρέκρουσεν; 3.40.12 (= Kühlewein 1, case 3.13–14), παρέκρουσε σμικρά; 3.40.14 (= Kühlewein 1, case 3.16), παρέκρουσεν; 3.40.16 (= Kühlewein 1, case 3.18–19), παρέκρουσε; 3.40.19 (= Kühlewein 1, case 3.22), παρέκρουσε; 3.42.4 (= Kühlewein 1, case 3.26), πάντα παρέκρουσεν; 3.42.6 (= Kühlewein 1, case 3.3), πάντα παρέκρουσεν; 3.42.9 (= Kühlewein 1, case 3.6), παρέκρουσεν; 3.42.16–44.1 (= Kühlewein 1, case 3.15), παρέκρουσεν; 3.48.4 (= Kühlewein 1, case 5.13), πάντα παρέκρουσεν; 3.48.16–17 (= Kühlewein 1, case 5.1), οὐδὲ παρέκρουσε; 3.48.19 (= Kühlewein 1, case 5.3), σμικρὰ παρέκρουσεν; 3.50.10 (= Kühlewein 1, case 6.15), μετὰ τὸν ἱδρῶτα τὸν γενόμενον, παρέκρουσε; 3.52.2 (= Kühlewein 1, case 6.19), ἀφ' ἧς δὲ παρέκρουσε τὸ ὕστερον; 3.56.8–9 (= Kühlewein 1, case 8.18), παρέκρουσεν; 3.60.6 (= Kühlewein 1, case 10–11), τετάρτη, παρέκρουσεν; 3.62.4 (= Kühlewein 1, case 11.19), τετάρτη παρέκρουσε; 3.64.12 (= Kühlewein 1, case 12.16), σμικρὰ παρέκρουσε; 3.104.2–3 (= Kühlewein 17, case 1.25), παρέκρουσε; 3.104.10 (= Kühlewein 17, case 1.8–9), παρέκρουσεν; 3.106.8 (= Kühlewein 17, case 1.19), περὶ τὰς ὑποστροφὰς παρέκρουσεν; 3.110.5 (= Kühlewein 17, case 2.8–9), πολλὰ παρέκρουσε; 3.116.8 (= Kühlewein 17, case 3.5),

παρακοπή (7)[115]
παρακόπτω (9)[116]
συνίημι (3)[117]
συνετός (1)[118]
ἀσύνετος (2)[119]
σύνεσις (5)[120]

Isolated terms:

μωρόομαι (3)[121]
μώρωσις (4)[122]

παρέκρουσεν; 3.118.2 (= Kühlewein 17, case 4.16), παρέκρουσεν; 3.128.9 (= Kühlewein 17, case 9.15), πολλὰ παρέκρουσε; 3.132.2 (= Kühlewein 17, case 10.20), παρέκρουσε πολλά; 3.132.8 (= Kühlewein 17, case 10.1), σμικρὰ παρέκρουσεν; 3.136.7 (= Kühlewein 17, case 11.1), παρέκρουσεν ἐς νύκτα; 3.146.15 (= Kühlewein 17, case 16.2), παρέκρουσεν ἀτρεμέως; 3.148.3 (= Kühlewein 17, case 16.6), παρέκρουσεν; *Epid.* IV, 5.152.19, παρέκρουσεν; 5.154.15, κοσμίως παρέκρουσεν; 5.184.16, παρέκρουσε; *Epid.* VI, 5.326.2 (= Manetti-Roselli 6.5.2–3), ὅτι τοῖσι παρακρούουσι λήγουσιν ὀδύναι πλευρέων; 5.354.16 (= Manetti-Roselli 8.30.11 = Langholf 334), παρέκρουσεν; *Epid.* VII 5.460.10 (= Jouanna 112.1.8–9), παρέκρουσε τρόπον φρενιτικόν; *Prorrh.* I 5.532.3 (= Polack 85.8), ἣν ὀλίγα θρασέως παρακρούσωσιν; 5.532.8 (= Polack 88.13), κατόχως παρακρούοντες; 5.552.6 (= Polack 123.15–16), τὰ ἐπ' ὀλίγον θρασέως παρακρούοντα μελαγχολικά; 5.558.2 (= Polack 132.5), παρακρούσαντα.

[115] *Aph.* 6.26, 4.570.1–2 (= Magdelaine 6.26.6), ὁκόσοισιν ἐν τοῖσι καύσοισι τρόμοι γίνονται, παρακοπὴ λύει; *Epid.* III 3.118.13 (= Kühlewein 17, case 5.2–3), παρακοπὴ δὲ τῆς γνώμης; 3.122.15–16 (= Kühlewein 17, case 7.5), παρακοπή; *Coac.* 5.596.6, πονηρὸν καὶ πλησίον παρακοπῆς; 5.600.18, θαῦμα δὲ οὐδέν, εἰ καὶ παρακοπὴ καὶ ἀγρυπνίη γένοιτο; 5.610.4, τοὺς ἐν καύσοισι τρόμους παρακοπὴ λύει; 5.724.14, τὸ δὲ ἐξέρυθρον ἐν πυρετῷ, παρακοπήν.

[116] *Aff.* 6.216.25 καὶ τοῦ νοῦ παρακόπτει (Potter, Θ); παρακοπῇ (Littré); 6.218.4 τοῦ νοῦ παρακόπτοντος; *Coac.* 5.670.14, ὅσοι δὲ τῶν περιπλευμονικῶν μὴ ἀνεκαθάρθησαν ἐν τῇσι κυρίῃσιν ἡμέρῃσιν, ἀλλὰ παρακόψαντες διέφυγον τὰς τεσσαρεσκαίδεκα; *Epid.* V 5.204.17 (= Jouanna 3.1.7), ἀπέθανεν ἑβδομαῖος παρακόπτων; 5.204.19 (= Jouanna 3.1.9) καθαιρόμενος δὲ παρέκοψεν; 5.206.8 (= Jouanna 5.1.4) δεκαταῖος ἤρχετο παρακόπτειν; 5.212.25 (= Jouanna 14.2.5) παρακόπτειν ἤρχετο; 5.228.20 (= Jouanna 31.2.18) καὶ παρέκοψε καὶ ἔθανεν; *Morb.* II 7.96.21 (= Jouanna 63.1.8) παρακόπτει.

[117] *Hebd.* 8.671.5 (= Roscher 77.107), ὑπολυσσέων ἄτρεμα καὶ ἀγνοέων καὶ μὴ ἀκούων μηδὲ ξυνιεὶς θανατῶδες; *Morb.* II 7.36.3 (= Jouanna 21.2.13), ξυνιεῖ δ' οὐδὲν ...; *Vict.* I 6.488.11 (= Joly-Byl 12.13) ἀσύνετον γαστήρ· ταύτῃ συνίεμεν ὅτι διψῇ ἢ πεινῇ.

[118] *Aer.* 2.92.9 (= Jouanna 24.9.6) ἔς τε τὰς τέχνας ὀξυτέρους τε καὶ συνετωτέρους καὶ τὰ πολέμια ἀμείνους εὑρήσεις.

[119] *Epid.* II 5.136.4, τουτέων ὅσοι ἐκ γενεῆς καὶ στρεβλοί, ἀσύνετοι, ἢ λιθιῶντες, ἢ μαινόμενοι, *Vict.* I 6.488.10 (= Joly-Byl 12.13) ἀσύνετον γαστήρ.

[120] *Aer.* 2.24.2 (= Jouanna 5.4.4) λαμπρόφωνοί τε οἱ ἄνθρωποι ὀργήν τε καὶ ξύνεσιν βελτίους εἰσὶ τῶν πρὸς βορέην, εἴπερ καὶ τὰ ἄλλα τὰ ἐμφυόμενα ἀμείνω ἐστίν; *Epid.* II 5.136.12, φλὲψ ἔχει παχείη ἐν ἑκατέρῳ τιτθῷ· ταῦτα μέγιστον ἔχει μόριον συνέσιος; *Morb.* I, 6.200.12 (= Wittern 30.20) φρενῖτις δ' οὕτως ἔχει· τὸ αἷμα ἐν τῷ ἀνθρώπῳ πλεῖστον συμβάλλεται μέρος συνέσιος; *Morb.Sacr.* 6.390.16 (= Jouanna 16.3.12) ἐς δὲ τὴν σύνεσιν ὁ ἐγκέφαλός ἐστιν ὁ διαγγέλλων; 6.392.4 (= Jouanna 17.1.4) διότι φημὶ τὸν ἐγκέφαλον εἶναι τὸν ἑρμηνεύοντα τὴν ξύνεσιν.

[121] *Coac.* 5.622.15, μεμωρωμένα; *Prorrh.* I 5.534.2 (= Polack 92.10), μεμωρωμένα; *Virg.* 8.466.18 (= Lami 2.4.16), ἐμωρώθη ἡ καρδίη.

[122] *Coac.* 5.626.8, ἐπὶ ἰκτέρῳ μώρωσις; *Prorrh.* I 5.518.5 (= Polack 32.11), κακὸν δὲ καὶ ἐπὶ ἰκτέρῳ

παραλλάξις (1)[123]
ἐμβρόντητος (1)[124]
βλητός (4)[125]

Texts Used (Unless Otherwise Stated) and Abbreviations

Hippocratic Texts

Airs Waters Places (Aer.) J. Jouanna (ed. and transl.) *Airs-Eaux-Lieux.* Paris (1996)
Aphorismi (Aph.) C. Magdelaine (ed.) Diss. Universite de Paris-Sorbonne. Paris IV
   Paris (1994)
Articulations (Artic.) H. Kühlewein (ed.) *Hipp. Opera Omnia* II. Leipzig (1902)111–244.
Humours (Hum.) O. Overwien (ed. and transl.) *Hippokrates, De humoribus* (CMG I
   3,1) Berlin (forthcoming)
Diseases I (Morb. I) R. Wittern (ed. and transl.) *Die hippokratische Schrift De Mor-
   bis I. Ausgabe, Übersetzung und Erläuterungen.* Hildesheim, New York (1974).
Diseases II (Morb. II). J. Jouanna (ed. and transl.) *Hippocrate. Maladies II.* Paris (1983)
Diseases III (Morb. III). P. Potter (ed. and transl.) *Hippokrates: Über die Krankheiten
   III.* Berlin (1980 CMG I 2, 3).
Diseases of Women I (Mul. I) H. Grensemann (ed.) *Hippokratische Gynäkologie. Die
   gynäkologischen Texte des Autors C nach den pseudohippokratischen Schriften "De
   Mulieribus" I, II und "De Sterilibus".* Wiesbaden (1982)
Epidemics I, (Epid. I) H. Kühlewein (ed.) *Hipp. Opera Omnia* I. Leipzig (1894) 180–245.
Epidemics III, (Epid. III) H. Kühlewein (ed.) *Hipp. Opera Omnia* I Leipzig (1894)
   180–245.
Epidemics (Epid. V, VII) V, VII. J. Jouanna (ed. and transl.) *Epidémies V et VII.* Paris
   (2000).
Epidemics II, IV, VI (Epid. II, IV, VI) (Partial edition) V. Langholf (ed.) *Syntaktis-
   che Untersuchungen zu Hippokrates-Texten. Brakylogische Syntagmen in den Indi-
   viduellen Krankheits-Fallbeschreibungen der hippokratischen Schriftensammlung.*
   Wiesbaden (1977).
Epidemics VI (Epid. VI) D. Manetti, A. Roselli (ed. and transl.) Ippocrate. *Epidemie.
   Libro sesto. Firenze* (1982).
Girls (Virg.) A. Lami (ed. and transl.) 'Lo scritto ippocratico sui disturbi virginali'.
   Galenos 1 (2007) 15–59.

μώρωσις (Potter 32, κώφωσις); 5.572.4 (= Polack 168.8), φωνῆς μώρωσις (μώρωσις/μώρωσιν mss.;
φωνῆς μώρωσις Potter 168; Littré κώφωσις); *Virg.* 8.466.19 (= Lami 2.4.16) ἐκ τῆς μωρώσιος νάρκη.
   [123] *Acut. (sp.)* 2.396.1 (Joly 1.2.11), παραλλάξιες φρενῶν.
   [124] *Vict.* I 6.518.3–4 (Joly-Byl 35.7.8), οἱ δὲ ἐμβρόντητους.
   [125] *Acut.* 2.260.8 (= Joly 17.1.2–5), τὴν γνώμην βλάβεντες ... μάλα δὲ τοὺς τοιούτους οἱ ἀρχαῖοι
βλητοὺς ἐνόμιζον εἶναι (see also *Coac.* 5.672.8, ἐκάλεον οἱ ἀρχαῖοι βλητούς for the idea of 'blow',
'stroke'). These instances seem to refer to being stricken in the brain, with consequent mental
impairment: *Morb.* II 7.16.5, ἢν βλητὸς γένηται; 7.38.19, ἢν βλητὸς γένηται; *Morb.* III 7.120. 17 (=
Potter 3.10), οἱ δὲ βλητοὶ λεγόμενοι.

Glands (Gland.) R. Joly (ed. and transl.) *Des Lieux dans l'Homme. Du Système des glandes. Des Fistules. Des Hémorroïdes. De la vision. Des Chairs. De la Dentition.* Paris (1978)

Nature of man (Nat.Hom.) J. Jouanna (ed. and transl.) *De Natura Hominis.* Berlin, CMG I 1.3 (1975; revised edition 2002).

On Wounds on the Head (CV) M. Hanson (ed. and transl.) *Hippocratis De capitis vulneribus* (CMG I 4,1) Berlin 1999.

Places in Man (Loc.Hom.) R. Joly (ed. and transl.) *Des Lieux dans l'Homme. Du Système des glandes. Des Fistules. Des Hémorroïdes. De la vision. Des Chairs. De la Dentition.* Paris (1978).

Prognostikon (Prog.) B. Alexanderson (ed.) *Die Hippokratische Schrift 'Prognostikon'.* Stockhols (1968).

Prorrhetikon I (Prorrh. I) H. Polack (ed.) *Textkritische Untersuchungen zu der Hippokratischen Schrift Prorrhetikos I.* Diss. Hamburg 1954. Hamburg (1976).

Regime in Acute Diseases (Acut.). R. Joly (ed. and transl.) *Du Régime des maladies aiguës, Appendice. De l'aliment. De l'usage des liquids.* Paris (1972)

Regime in Acute Diseases, Appendix (Acut. Sp.) R. Joly (ed. and transl.) *Du Régime des maladies aiguës, Appendice. De l'aliment. De l'usage des liquids.* Paris (1972)

Regimen I–IV (Vict. I–IV) R. Joly and S. Byl (ed. and transl.) *Hippocratis De Diaeta.* Berlin (1984, CMG I, 2,4)

Sacred Disease (Morb.Sacr.) J. Jouanna (ed. and transl.) *La maladie sacrée.* Paris (2003).

Sevens (Hebd.) W.H. Roscher (ed.) *Die Hippokratische Schrift von der Siebzahl in ihrer vierfachen Überlieferung zum erstenmal hrsg. U. erläutert.* (1913)

Superfetations (Superf.). C. Lienau (ed. and trans.) *Hipp.De Superfetatione.* Berlin (1973, CMG I, 2,2).

For the others Hippocratic texts, I have used Littré's edition (*Œuvres completes d'Hippocrate.* Ed. and trans. Paris 1839–1861).

Affections (Aff.) Littré VI. 208–271.

Internal Affections (Aff. Int.) Littré VII. 166–303.

Diseases of Women (Mul. II–III) Littré VIII. 1–463.

Prorrhetikon II (Prorrh. II) Littré IX. 1–75.

Crises (Judic.) Littré IX. 274–295.

Coan Prenotions (Coac.) Littré V. 588–733.

Critical Days (Dieb. Judic.) Littré IX. 276–307.

Epidemics II (Epid. II) Littré V. 43–139.

Epidemics IV (Epid. IV) Littré V. 140–177.

Other Texts

Anonymi Medici. *De Morbis Acutis et Chroniis.* Ed. by I. Garofalo, transl. by B. Fuchs. Leiden (1997).

Galen, *On the affected parts (De Loc. Aff.).* In *Claudii Galeni Opera Omnia,* ed. by K.G. Kühn (Leipzig, 1821–1833: Volume 8, 1824). Cambridge (2012).

Aretaeus, *De causis et signis acutorum morborum (Caus.Ac.); De causis et signis diuturnorum morborum (Caus.Chr.); De curatione acutorum morborum (Therap.Ac.); De curatione diuturnorum morborum (Therap. Chr.)* Ed. by C. Hude. Berlin (1958 CMG II).

Caelius Aurelianus. *Caelii Aureliani Celerum passionum libri III, Tardarum passio-num libri V.* Ed. by G. Bendz and transl. by I. Pape. CML VI 1, Berlin (1990/1993; editio altera Berlin 2002).

Celsus. *De Medicina.* Ed. by F. Marx, *A.Cornelii Celsi quae supersunt.* Leipzig and Berlin (1915, CML I).

Diocles of Carystus. *A collection of the fragments with translation and commentary.* Ed. and transl. by P. van der Eijk. Leiden (2000–2001).

Aristotle. *Problems.* Ed. and transl. by R. Mayhew and D.C. Mirhady. London (2011).

Praxagoras. *The Fragments of Praxagoras of Cos and his school.* Ed. and Trans. by F. Steckerl. Leiden (1958)

Theophrastus of Eresus. *Theophrastus of Eresus. Sources for his life, writings, thought and influence.* Volume 5: *Sources on biology: human physiology, living creatures, botany—texts 328–435.* Ed. and transl. by R.W. Sharples. Leiden (1995).

THE TYPOLOGY AND AETIOLOGY OF MADNESS IN ANCIENT GREEK MEDICAL AND PHILOSOPHICAL WRITING[*]

Jacques Jouanna

In order to approach the vast problem of understanding how different types of insanity were classified and explained by physicians and philosophers in ancient Greece, it seems appropriate to begin with an explanation of my method. This study does not take as its basis the abundant secondary literature, but rather engages directly with a selection of fundamental texts in the chronological order of their composition to bring out as far as possible what was constant and what changed in the classification and explanation of manifestations of insanity.

The examination of two texts from the Hippocratic corpus (one from *On the Sacred Disease*, the other from *On Regimen*) according to this method will show that the typology of insanity was binary: two opposite excesses are defined relative to a median equilibrium. At one extreme is a type of madness that, from its low-energy nature, we might call a depressive madness. At the other is what we might qualify as a hyperactive madness. But while the semiotics of these two types of madness are comparable in the two treatises, the aetiology differs from one treatise to the other

What became of this binary typology and aetiology in the later history of medicine and philosophy? To answer this question, I chose from the realm of philosophy Plato's *Timaeus*, the fundamental text regarding illnesses of the soul. This text will be the focus of the second section. From the medical world, it seemed logical to select a writer who was a close reader of both Hippocrates and Plato, namely Galen, and he will be the focus of the third section.

Two deeper questions are related to our principal question about the typology and aetiology of insanity. The first pertains to origin, and the second to form. Origin, or the entry of madness into the roster of illnesses of the soul, is one of the central questions of our discussion: when and how did the soul begin to play an important role in the history of insanity? Form, on the other hand, concerns the problem of the denomination of the two types

---

[*] Translated by Caroline Wazer.

of insanity: by what terms were the two types of insanity originally designated, and how did the vocabulary evolve? These questions will be implicitly present throughout. But some preliminary linguistic considerations are
necessary in order to clear away some of the thicket of madness terminology. These considerations will serve as Ariadne's thread in the semantic
labyrinth. The vocabulary of insanity, like its aetiology, is characterized by
a bipolarity. The first type includes terms positively designating madness,
particularly words of the μανία family, which, at least initially, could signify
all sorts of insanity. In the course of this paper, we will also meet μωρία and,
more importantly, μώρωσις, which are used to designate a particular type
of insanity.[1] The other type consists of compound words. These compounds
are themselves divided into two classes: the negative compounds (ἀ-priva-
tive) refer to loss of thought, while the 'distancing' compounds (παρα- or,
less frequently, ἐκ-) mark distance by comparison with normality and refer
to derangement of thought. Thought is, in this case, expressed by words
from both the φρήν family (negative compounds: ἄφρων, ἀφρονέω, ἀφροσύνη; 'distancing' compounds: παράφρων, παραφρονέω, παραφροσύνη, and more
rarely ἔκφρων, ἐκφρονέω and ἐκφροσύνη) and the νοῦς family (ἄνους, ἄνοια,
more rarely παράνους and ἔκνους). We must also take diachronic change into
account. For example, the νοῦς family compounds appear later than those in
the φρήν family.[2] These facts about the formation of the vocabulary of insanity will allow us to assess better the choices made by the Hippocratic writers,
Plato, and Galen, and the overall evolution of the relevant vocabulary.

1. Binary Insanity in the Hippocratic Corpus: Typology and Aetiology

1.1. On the Sacred Disease

In his monograph on epilepsy, the Hippocratic author of *On the Sacred
Disease* includes an important excursus on the physiological explanation of
thought (ch. 14–17 Jouanna = ch. 17–20 Jones):[3] he demonstrates, for the first
time in the surviving texts, the role of the brain in perception, feeling, and

---

[1] The term μώρωσις, an action noun formed from the denominative verb μωρόομαι,
though well attested by Galen, is not mentioned in Pierre Chantraine's *DELG* (2009), where
one would expect it s.v. μωρός.

[2] In the Hippocratic Corpus, negative compounds from the νοῦς family (ἄνους, ἄνοια) are
not used; they do appear, however, in Plato's *Timaeus*.

[3] The text cited is that of Jouanna 2003. I refer to the introduction and to the notes of this
edition for a general presentation of the treatise and for commentary.

thought. As long as the brain is healthy, all its faculties are intact, but when it is unhealthy, it creates disruptions within itself. It is because of the brain, he claims, that 'we are mad and we are delirious' (c. 14, 36, 4 sq. Jouanna = c. 17 Jones τῷ δ' αὐτῷ τούτῳ μαινόμεθα καὶ παραφρονέομεν).[4] The author explains insanity as a modification of the elemental qualities of the brain, namely an excess of wetness (c. 14, 26, 13 Jouanna = c. 17 Jones Καὶ μαινόμεθα ὑπὸ ὑγρότητος), which leads to movement in the brain and a disruption in sensation and thought, whereas the stability of the brain is necessary for normal thought. The humor that provokes the deterioration of the brain can manifest itself in two opposing forms, bile and phlegm, the former hot and the latter cold. Opposing symptoms correspond to each of these opposing humors. The following excerpt states both the typology and the aetiology of these two opposing insanities (c. 15, 27, 7–10 = c. 18 Jones):

> οἱ μὲν ὑπὸ φλέγματος μαινόμενοι ἥσυχοί τέ εἰσι καὶ οὐ βοηταὶ οὐδὲ θορυβώδεις, οἱ δὲ ὑπὸ χολῆς κεκράκταί τε καὶ κακοῦργοι καὶ οὐκ ἀτρεμαῖοι, ἀλλ' ἀεί τι ἄκαιρον δρῶντες

> Those who are mad because of the effect of phlegm are calm and neither scream nor are violent, whereas those who are mad because of the effect of bile are raucous, maleficent, and will not remain in one place, but rather always set themselves to doing something inappropriate.

The wording is very precise.[5] The author opposes a calm insanity to an agitated one. He specifies that he is speaking of states of ongoing madness (c. 15, 27, 10 sq. Jouanna = c. 18 Jones, ἢν μὲν οὖν συνεχέως μαίνωνται, αὗται αἱ προφάσιές εἰσιν, 'But if the madness is ongoing, here are the causes').

This binary typology is also applicable to temporary aberrations, even if the symptoms are different: the onset of agitation manifests itself in fears and frights (c. 15, 27, 11 sq. = c. 18 Jones δείματα καὶ φόβοι), and they are caused by bile, which ascends to the brain and heats it.[6] Conversely, the onset of depression is characterized by sorrow and disgust at inappropriate moments, and eventually by loss of memory (c. 15, 28, 4 sqq. Jouanna = c. 18 Jones: ἀνιᾶται δὲ καὶ ἀσᾶται παρὰ καιρόν ... καὶ ἐπιλήθεται, 'one displays sorrow

---

[4] The two possibilities that the Greek language offers for referring to insanity are accumulated here to designate insanity in general: the term referring to insanity positively (μαίνομαι) and the 'distancing' compound (παραφρονέω).

[5] Three adjectives serve to describe the symptoms on each side. They are paired, although there is a variation in the order of the adjectives that oppose each other. The first pair refers to general comportment, the second describes vocalizations, and the third designates action.

[6] The sole aetiological element that is added in relation to continuous madness is that a rush of blood to the head can also provoke the heating of the brain.

and revulsion at inappropriate times … and memory losses.'). The cause is also opposite: this onset of depressive insanity is a result of the cooling and contraction (?) of the brain caused by the action of phlegm.

Within the surviving literature, this text is the foundation of two themes in the history of insanity: first, it associates madness with the state of the brain, which Alcmaeon of Croton seems to have already suggested in the sixth century BCE,[7] and, secondly, it distinguishes two opposing types of insanity, a calm madness and an agitated one, which are explained by the opposing effects of two elemental qualities, heat and cold, in the framework of a humoral theory that opposes hot bile with cold phlegm. Still absent is an important agent in the history of madness—the 'soul' (ψυχή).[8] Insanity was not yet an illness of the ψυχή, strictly speaking, in the second half of the fifth century BCE.

1.2. *The Treatise from* On Regimen

This duality of madness appears again in a second Hippocratic treatise probably dating to the first half of the fourth century BCE, *On Regimen*, chapter 35, which treats the intelligence of the spirit and madness as follows (150, 28 Joly = I, 35 Jones):

Περὶ δὲ φρονήσιος ψυχῆς ὀνομαζομένης καὶ ἀφροσύνης ὧδε ἔχει

Regarding that which we call intelligence of the spirit and dementia, it is thus.[9]

A long and important discussion follows, important not least because it is one of the rare pre-Platonic theories about intelligence and madness that is not fragmentary or in the form of a watered-down doxography. In this discussion appears the agent whose absence we noted above, the ψυχή. The presence of the ψυχή is made clear in the conclusion of the discussion:

Περὶ μὲν οὖν φρονίμου καὶ ἄφρονος ψυχῆς ἡ σύγκρησις αὕτη αἰτίη ἐστίν, ὥσπερ μοι καὶ γέγραπται

Regarding intelligence and dementia of the soul, the mixture is the cause, as I have written.

---

[7] For Alcmaeon of Croton, a possible source of *On the Sacred Disease*, see Jouanna 2003, LXII–LXV.

[8] The word ψυχή is absent from *On the Sacred Disease*. As Pigeaud rightly points out (1981, 41), it is the Hippocratic letter 19 on madness that attributes to the brain the 'works of the soul' (ψυχῆς ἔργα).

[9] The text cited is that of the edition of Joly 1984 in the series *CMG*. For the dating of the treatise, see 44–49 in the same.

I have written about the assembly of this theory in detail in a recently published article,[10] although the question at hand here, that of the bipolarity of insanity, was not central.

The author of the treatise in *On Regimen* systematically expounds both a typology and an explication of the degrees of intelligence and madness in terms of the variable mixture of the two primary elements that compose man's body and spirit, namely fire and water. Whereas optimal intelligence occurs when the equilibrium of the two elements of the spirit is balanced, one reaches the state of insanity when the discrepancy between the two elements is greatest, after passing through two intermediary stages. This author distinguishes two opposing types of madness, according to whether the predominant element is water or fire. If fire is dominated by water, the result is a calm insanity (154, 7–11 Joly = I, 35, 76–83 Jones):

Εἰ δὲ κρατηθείη ἐπὶ πλέον τὸ πῦρ ὑπὸ τοῦ ἐόντος ὕδατος, τούτους ἤδη οἱ μὲν ἄφρονας ὀνομάζουσιν, οἱ δὲ ἐμβροντήτους· ἔστι δ' ἡ μανίη τοιούτων ἐπὶ τὸ βραδύτερον· οὗτοι κλαίουσί τε οὐδενὸς ἕνεκα δεδίασί τε τὰ μὴ φοβερὰ λυπέονταί τε ἐπὶ τοῖσι μὴ προσήκουσιν αἰσθάνονταί τε ἢ τι ἢ οὐδέν, ὡς προσήκει τοὺς φρονέοντας

If the fire is further dominated by existing water (in the soul), those so afflicted are said to be devoid of reason (ἄφρονας) by some, and by others struck by lightning (ἐμβροντήτους); their madness (μανίη) tends more toward slowness (ἐπὶ τὸ βραδύτερον); these people cry for no reason, fear what is not frightening, grieve for reasons that are not appropriate, do not feel, either in part or entirely, as is appropriate for sane people.

In contrast to this depressive madness caused by a deceleration of the soul's movements is an agitated madness caused by an inverse disequilibrium, with water dominated by fire (156: 3–6 Joly = I, 35, 125–130 Jones):

Εἰ δ' ἐπὶ (Jouanna cf. 154: 7: δ' ἔτι Ermerins Joly δέ τι M δέ τινι θ) πλέον ἐπικρατηθείη τὸ ὕδωρ ὑπὸ τοῦ πυρός, ὀξέα ἡ τοιαύτη ψυχὴ ἄγαν, καὶ τούτους ⟨οἱ μὲν⟩ (add. Jouanna cf. 154, 8) ὀνειρώσσειν καλέουσιν, οἱ δὲ ὑπομαίνεσθαι· ἔστι δὲ ἔγγιστα μανίης τὸ τοιοῦτο· καὶ γὰρ ἀπὸ βραχέης φλεγμονῆς (M: πλησμονῆς Ermerins Joly) ⟨καὶ⟩ ἀσυμφόρου μαίνονται,

If water is even further dominated by the fire, the afflicted spirit is too alive (ὀξέα ... ἄγαν), and this sort of person is said by some to dream (ὀνειρώσσειν), by others to be half-mad (ὑπομαίνεσθαι). For such a state is very close to insanity. In fact, following a short and untimely inflammation (*vel* plethora), they become entirely mad (μαίνονται).

---

[10] Jouanna 2007. A rather long summary of that study had already been published much earlier, in Jouanna 1966. See now Jouanna 2012, 195–227.

These two passages, though situated at a certain distance from one another in the text, are remarkably parallel and contrasting. Their juxtaposition
allows us to propose here two new improvements to the tradition of the
text.[11] There is no doubt that the author was conscious of the parallelism
and opposition between the two types of insanity.

This theory has some elements in common with the one we encountered
in *On the Sacred Disease*. The opposition between the two types of insanity
is similar, with one characterized by agitation and the other by sluggishness.
One notes in particular a significant parallel regarding depressive insanity—
the mention of grief without reason (*On Regimen* 154, 10 Joly = I, 35, 81–82
Jones: λυπέονταί τε ἐπὶ τοῖσι μὴ προσήκουσιν, 'they mourn for inappropriate
reasons'; cf. *On the Sacred Disease* c. 15, 28, 4 Jouanna = c. 18 Jones, quoted
above). Concerning aetiology, however, the elemental explanation given in
On Regimen is a remarkable exception in the Hippocratic Corpus, in which
humoral theory is predominant. But it is possible to establish a connection
even with respect to aetiology, by means of the elements. Fire, in the *On
Regimen* treatise, incites movement (κίνησις), as does the heat of bile in *On
the Sacred Disease*. Accordingly, water brings about the deceleration of the
spirit in the *On Regimen* treatise, just as phlegm, the cold humor, does in *On
the Sacred Disease*.[12]

The great innovation of *On Regimen* when compared with *On the Sacred
Disease*, however, is that the ψυχή or 'soul' has now become an agent in the
explanation of perceptions, feelings, and intelligence. The author's notion is
very concrete:[13] the soul, formed from a mixture of fire and water, occupies a

---

[11] The two proposed corrections here result from the comparison of the two passages. The
compound ὑπομαίνεσθαι is rare (with a single other attestation: Menander, *Epitrepontes* 457,
where there are, like here, two degrees of insanity: ὑπομαίνεσθαι and μαίνεσθαι).

[12] However, the two elemental qualities dry/wet are primordial in the *On Regimen* aetiology, and not the qualities hot/dry, which do not come into it. This is, however, no more than
an appearance; since fire is hot by nature, water, even though it is not said explicitly, is cold
by nature (cf. 32, 148, 20–22 Joly). In detail, these things are more complex, since there are
many types of water and fire, which produce different combinations; see in c. 32, discussing
the body, the mixtures of varieties of water and fire which give a cold and wet nature (148, 22
Joly), a wet and hot nature (148, 29 Joly), a dry and hot nature (148, 35), and finally a cold and
dry nature (150, 5 Joly). Another particularity that must be mentioned regarding the author
of *On Regimen* is the conviction that it is possible to treat insanity by means of a regimen.
In *On the Sacred Disease*, the therapy for disorders of the spirit is certainly possible, since
the disease called 'sacred' that affects the spirit is curable (cf. c. 18 Jouanna 31–33); but the
author of this text is not devoted, as is that of *Regimen*, to a particular therapy for each type
of insanity. Regarding the question of the treatment of madness in *On Regimen* and *On the
Sacred Disease*, see Pigeaud 2010 and van der Eijk 2011 and this volume.

[13] See above, note 10, and Jouanna 2007.

central circuit in the body (around the stomach), which corresponds to the orbit of the sun in the universe.[14] It moves more or less quickly according to the proportions of water and fire: it moves too slowly in 'calm' madness and too quickly in the 'agitated' kind. It is remarkable that the author gives concrete support to an abstract psychological vocabulary. The vivacity or sluggishness of the mind corresponds to the speed or slowness of the soul, a mixture of fire and water that circulates in a closed circuit in the body, in contact with the exterior through the senses.

This conception of a soul in constant circular motion heralds the conception of the soul in Plato's *Timaeus*. Plato employs a sort of synthesis of the representation in *On the Sacred Disease*, which places thought in the brain, and the one in *On Regimen*, which depicts the soul as a circuit around the stomach. The philosopher situates the revolutions of the thinking soul within the head.

2. *The Typology of the Two Forms of Dementia in Plato's* Timaeus

Before we discuss dementia in the *Timaeus*, we should recall that Plato, discussing madness or delirium (μανία) in the *Phaedrus*, has already made the distinction between two types (265a):

Μανίας δέ γε εἴδη δύο, τὴν μὲν ὑπὸ νοσημάτων ἀνθρωπίνων, τὴν δὲ ὑπὸ θείας ἐξαλλαγῆς τῶν εἰωθότων νομίμων γιγνομένην.

There are two types of madness, one caused by human illnesses and one by a divine impulse that does away with habitual rules.

Divine madness is divided into four types (265b): prophetic (μαντική), ritual (τελεστική), poetic (ποιητική), and erotic (ἐρωτική).[15] This clarification serves to show that the typology of madness that interests us, human madness, is, in Plato's works, integrated into a broader ensemble. This ensemble is binary, encompassing both human madness and delirium inspired by the gods.

In his *Timaeus*, Plato only envisages one of these two types of madness— human madness—in the context of the medical tradition. After explaining the illnesses of the body, he distinguishes two types of dementia (86b):

---

[14] See also Jouanna 1998.
[15] For these species of madness, see the classic chapter by E.R. Dodds, 'The Blessings of Madness' (Dodds 1951).

Καὶ τὰ μὲν περὶ τὸ σῶμα νοσήματα ταύτῃ συμβαίνει γιγνόμενα, τὰ δὲ περὶ ψυχὴν διὰ σώματος ἕξιν τῇδε. Νόσον μὲν δὴ ψυχῆς ἄνοιαν συγχωρητέον, δύο δ᾽ ἀνοίας γένη, τὸ μὲν μανίαν, τὸ δὲ ἀμαθίαν

The illnesses of the body come about in this way, while the illnesses of the soul due to the state of the body are produced in the following way. We must acknowledge that the illness of the soul is dementia, and that there are two types of dementia: madness and ignorance.[16]

In this transitional, introductory formula, one notices the continuities with and the differences from the texts written by the Hippocratic physicians. The essential continuity is found in the bipolarity of dementia, which Plato expresses even more systematically than do the Hippocratic physicians, since he plainly states that there are two types of dementia.

At the same time, a lag in the vocabulary is apparent. Madness in general is designated by the negative composite ἄνοια, which takes the function that ἀφροσύνη occupies in *On Regimen*.[17] The more significant difference lies in the use of the words positively designating madness, namely the μαίνεσθαι/μανία family. In the Hippocratic corpus, the word μανία designates the general concept of insanity and applies to two categories: here, however, this word is used to designate only one of the two types of insanity, with the other designated by a negative compound, ἀμαθία, 'ignorance,' which is never used in this particular sense by the Hippocratic physicians.

Plato's principle innovation seems to me to be that he articulates for the first time (in the surviving literature) a vitally important notion, the illness of the soul (νόσον ... ψυχῆς).[18] The expression does not, in any case, appear in the Hippocratic corpus, even in *On Regimen*, although the latter does make mention of the ψυχή. The new idea had a great future before it.

So begins Plato's discussion regarding the illnesses of the soul.[19] What does he mean by these two species of madness and how does he explain them? The bipolarity consists of two opposing excessive sentiments, pleasure (ἡδονή) and sorrow (λύπη), which are the two most serious illnesses

---

[16] On the justification of this translation and of this interpretation of the end of the phrase, see below, n. 24.

[17] *On Regimen*, c. 35 cited above; cf. also the distancing composite παραφρονέομεν in *On the Sacred Disease*, c. 14 cited above.

[18] Plato, *Timaeus* 86b. The expression is used just after the transition where Plato concludes his discussion of illnesses of the body (τὰ μὲν περὶ τὸ σῶμα νοσήματα) in order to come to illnesses of the soul (τὰ δὲ περὶ ψυχὴν sc. νοσήματα).

[19] The article by Miller 1962 treats solely the illnesses of the body (82a–86a), and does not approach the sicknesses of the soul (86b sq.).

of the soul leading to dementia (ἄνοια) by an analogous process, which is well analysed by Plato.[20] This corresponds in large part to the binary model of hyperactive and depressive madness that held sway with the physicians. Particularly evident are the correspondences in the semiotics of depressive madness between Plato's *Timaeus* and *On the Sacred Disease*. Plato, in 87a, speaks of δυσθυμίας ... ἔτι δὲ λήθης ἅμα καὶ δυσμαθίας, 'of discouragement ... and even of forgetfulness and difficulty learning', which corresponds to *On the Sacred Disease*, c. 15: ἀνιᾶται δὲ καὶ ἀσᾶται παρὰ καιρόν ... καὶ ἐπιλήθεται, 'one displays sorrow and repulsion at inappropriate times ... and lapses of memory'.[21]

If we compare the aetiologies of these two analogous types of insanity described by the philosopher and by the author of *On the Sacred Disease*, we will notice both similarities and differences. Most similar is that the two types of madness are caused by humoral fluctuations. The great difference is that the two humors, bile and phlegm, which provoke the two opposing types of insanity in *On the Sacred Disease*, are reunited by Plato in order to explain one of the two types of madness, 'depressive' madness (86e ἢ τῶν ὀξέων καὶ τῶν ἁλυκῶν φλεγμάτων καὶ ὅσοι πικροὶ καὶ χολώδεις χυμοὶ κατὰ τὸ σῶμα πλανηθέντες, 'acidic and salty phlegm and all bitter and bilious humors wander throughout the body'). It is not, however, an opposition between the heat of bile and the coldness of phlegm that accounts for the opposition between the two types of madness. In this regard, there was no continuity between the psychology of the *Timaeus* and that of the medical writer who wrote *On the Sacred Disease*.

On the other hand, if we compare the *Timaeus* to the psychology of the other Hippocratic physician who presents a binary theory of madness, the author of *On Regimen*, we will note an analogy in the representation of the soul, similar to the one discussed in the paper cited above.[22] According to

---

[20] People under the effect of excessive joy or sorrow rush into inappropriate ethical choices (86c σπεύδων τὸ μὲν ἐλεῖν ἀκαίρως, τὸ δὲ φυγεῖν) as a result of the incapacity to hold correct perceptions (86c οὔθ' ὁρᾶν οὔτε ἀκούειν ὀρθὸν οὐδὲν δύναται) and to participate in reasoning (86c λογισμοῦ μετασχεῖν ἥκιστα τότε δὴ δυνατός); this is how a passionate person falls into madness (86c λύττα). The analytic process of passion leading to madness is behind the thought of the Hellenistic and Roman philosophy of madness resulting from excessive passion, as opposed to the self-restraint of the wise. For passion in the *Timaeus*, see Tetamo 1993.

[21] See also *On Regimen*, c. 35 (154, 10 Joly): λυπέονταί τε ἐπὶ τοῖσι μὴ προσήκουσιν αἰσθάνονταί τε ἢ τι ἢ οὐδέν, ὡς προσήκει τοὺς φρονέοντας 'They mourn for inappropriate reasons, and do not feel, either in part or in whole, as is appropriate for sensible people.'

[22] See n. 10.

the physician, as to the philosopher, the elements exuded by the body can
be mixed in the revolutions of the soul and upset the soul's balance. In
order to explain 'depressive' madness, Plato says that phlegmatic or bilious
humors, confined to the interior of the body even in a state of plethora, mix
together in the revolutions of the soul (87a τῇ τῆς ψυχῆς φορᾷ συμμείξαντες)
and eventually move to three locations in the soul. We have already seen
in *On Regimen* the idea that excessive humors can mix with the soul, which
already was understood to revolve, and can upset intellectual faculties. Thus
a runner must take a leisurely walk after a race, 'so that the excretions
issued during the race do not remain in the body and do not mix with
the soul' (152, 22 sq. Joly = I, 35, 42–44 Jones: ὅπως μὴ ἐγκαταλείπηται ἐν τῷ
σώματι τὸ ἀποκριθὲν ἀπὸ τοῦ δρόμου μηδὲ συμμίσγηται τῇ ψυχῇ). So one meets
an analogous physiology of psychic illnesses in both *On Regimen* and the
Timaeus, which is certainly remarkable.[23]

In his *Timaeus*, however, Plato adds a supplementary vision to the bipolarity of insanity and its aetiology. In his discussion of the illnesses of the
spirit, he has considered up to this point only the illnesses of the soul that
are caused by a bad state of the body.[24] In a discussion that he calls an
antistrophe to the preceding (87c τὸ δὲ τούτων ἀντίστροφον αὖ), Plato starts
from human health to demonstrate that this health arises from equilibrium
between the body and the soul. Furthermore, he enumerates the disorders
that spring from a disequilibrium. This disequilibrium is twofold: the soul
can impose it on the body or, inversely, the body can impose it on the soul.
The opposition between hyperactive and depressive madness reappears in
this double disequilibrium. Man is defined by two contradictory desires:
first, to care for the body, namely the desire for food (88b τροφῆς), and second, to provide for the soul, the desire for intelligence (88b φρονήσεως).
When the body is naturally stronger than the soul, it dominates and 'renders the realm of the soul voiceless, difficult to instruct, and forgetful' (88b
τὸ δὲ τῆς ψυχῆς κωφὸν καὶ δυσμαθὲς ἀμνήμόν τε ποιοῦσαι); it also produces the

---

[23] Another analogy could be underlined between *On Regimen* and the *Timaeus*. It is the
conviction that one can treat the illnesses of the soul by a regimen to reestablish equilibrium,
in one case, *On Regimen*, by the equilibrium between the two constitutive elements of the
body and the soul, namely water and fire (see above, n. 12), and in the other, the *Timaeus*, by
equilibrium between the body and the soul (*Timaeus* 88b sqq.)

[24] This is the sense of the introductory phrase regarding the sicknesses of the soul in 86b:
Καὶ τὰ μὲν περὶ τὸ σῶμα νοσήματα ταύτῃ συμβαίνει γιγνόμενα, τὰ δὲ περὶ ψυχὴν διὰ σώματος ἕξιν
τῇδε (*sc.* συμβαίνει γιγνόμενα), 'The sicknesses that affect the body arise in that way, while the
sicknesses of the soul caused by the state of the body arise in this way'.

greatest of sicknesses, ignorance (88b ἀμαθία).[25] On the other hand, when the soul is stronger than the body, it embarks 'headlong', one might say, into excessive study and intellectual research (*Timaeus* 88a; cf. 88c excessive exercise of διάνοια). The soul upsets the balance of the entire interior of the body, filling it with sicknesses (88a ψυχὴ ... διασείουσα πᾶν αὐτὸ ἔνδοθεν νόσων ἐμπίμπλησι), sicknesses that physicians are generally unable to diagnose.[26]

Therefore, binary madness appears once again in Plato's exposé. This binary madness apparently always corresponds to μανία and ἀμαθία, as mentioned at the beginning (86b). In this case, ἀμαθία surely refers to depressive madness. We can deduce, then, that hyperactive madness corresponds to μανία. The aetiology is no longer the same, though, because hyperactive insanity is no longer caused by a humoral effusion of the body into the soul, but rather by a domination of the soul over the body. Therefore, it is appropriate to ask how Plato reconciled these two different aetiologies into one apparently analogous binary madness. Is Plato's binary madness truly analogous? A finer analysis makes apparent a difference in the symptoms of 'madness by excess', depending on whether the madness is due to a poor condition of the body or to the predominance of the soul over the body. In fact, when madness by excess is caused by a poor condition of the body and manifests itself in the form of excessive pleasure, it is characterized by a blindness regarding ethical choices, an incapacity to reason, whereas when it results from a domination of the body by the soul, it is characterized by an excessive activity of διάνοια in study, teaching, or debate. 'Madness by excess' was apparently distinct not only in its aetiology, but also in its terminology. Therefore, Plato's discussion of the illnesses of the soul offers a 'strophe' to the 'antistrophe' mentioned above, despite the continuity of a bipolarity of madness. In this complexity, we find differences of perspective regarding the first species of dementia, μανία, according to whether it is caused by a bodily illness or by the domination of the soul over the body. The second species, ignorance (ἀμαθία), remains fundamentally the same, however, because it is always due to a negative influence of the body over the soul. Plato certainly does not explicitly insist on this difference in μανία after the reorientation of his discussion on illnesses of the soul in the 'antistrophe.' But is this a sufficient reason to ignore it?

---

[25] The word ἀμαθία had disappeared after the articulation of binary dementia at the beginning of the discussion of sicknesses of the soul (86b).

[26] This is the beginning of the theme of intellectual sicknesses; cf. Jouanna 2009.

We will end this section by concluding that the philosopher adds an ethical reflection regarding the responsibility of illness to the purely medical Hippocratic analyses of the duality of madness.[27]

3. Galenic Developments

First, we must acknowledge that Galen cites many of the longer passages in Plato's *Timaeus* that we discussed above in his treatise *Quod animi mores corporis temperamenta sequantur*, but Galen's purpose in reading that treatise was different from ours.[28] His intent was not to study the different illnesses of the soul or their typology, but rather to find in the writings of his predecessor, from whom he borrowed the concept of the tripartite division of the soul, a confirmation of his own theory, according to which the different faculties of the soul stem from the different temperaments of the body. Accordingly, an unfavorable mix of humors can injure the soul.[29] Galen does not seem interested in Plato except as a guarantee of his own theory's veracity.

Galen offers a synthetic discussion regarding the illnesses of the soul primarily in other treatises, three of which will be mentioned here in the

---

[27] Plato adds this ethical reflection on the problem of responsibility to respond to those who condemn the madman and hold him responsible for his faults; cf. *Timaeus* 86d sqq. The person afflicted with madness, considered an illness of the soul, cannot be judged any more responsible than an invalid can for the illness of his body. The soul is the victim of a faulty disposition of the body (86d–87b), without mention of a faulty education (87b). The adage 'No one does wrong willingly' holds in regard to a physician's relationship to a patient. Plato extends the physician's opinion regarding an ill body to include an ill soul.

[28] For Galen's treatment of illnesses of the soul, see, for example, García-Ballester 1988 and Pigeaud 1988b. The central question of this study, however, is not discussed in García-Ballester's study, and is marginal in that of Pigeaud.

[29] In chapter 6, Galen cites two long passages from the *Timaeus* concerning the illnesses of the soul (86b–87b), but he does so in inverse order, and he does not contextualize them in the problematic Platonism of the bipolarity of madness. He first cites the section on the illness of the soul that manifests itself by excessive sorrow (86e ὅπου γὰρ-δυσμαθίας). He adds the following commentary: 'in this passage, Plato clearly recognized that the soul is in poor condition as a result of the poor condition of the humors in the body' (ἐν κακίᾳ τινί … διὰ τὴν ἐν σώματι κακοχυμίαν). Next, he cites a passage from earlier in the text (86c–d τὸ δὲ σπέρμα-νόσος ψυχῆς γέγονεν), and he comments: 'In this passage as well, he sufficiently shows that the soul is ill because of the poor condition of the body.' And he cites the following section (86d–e Καὶ σχέδον-προσγίνεται), ending with: 'That Plato himself recognized that which I explained above is apparent in these quotations themselves, as well as in other sections of the *Timaeus* and in other works.' The treatise contains other citations from the *Timaeus*, but they do not enter directly into the discussion, even if they are important regarding perturbations in the revolutions of the soul.

chronological order of their composition: *De symptomatum differentiis* (= *De diff.*), *De symptomatum causis* (= *De caus.*), and *De locis affectis* III 6 (= *De loc. affect.*)[30] In light of the immense array of illnesses of the soul discussed by Galen, the objective of this last section will be, first of all, to examine what becomes of the familiar binary typology of madness and its aetiology in Galen's work by means of a comparison of parallel discussions in the first two treatises (*De diff.* and *De caus.*). To be even more precise, we will confine ourselves to the illnesses affecting the hegemonic part of the soul, located in the brain. Galen calls these conditions αἱ τῶν ἡγεμονικῶν ἐνεργειῶν βλάβαι (*De diff.*; *De caus.*) or τὰ τοῦ λογιστικοῦ πάθη (*De loc. affect*). Concluding this section, we will consider some complementary texts from the third treatise, *De locis affectis*.

Galen discusses conditions of the hegemonic part of the soul both in *De diff.* III, 9, and in *De caus.* II, 7. The perspective of each discussion is different (in *De diff.*, Galen's object is to distinguish the different illnesses of the soul, while in *De caus.* he primarily examines the causes), but the elements of the typology are fundamentally the same and allow for a close reading of two parallel passages, presented below side-by-side.

De diff. 3, 9 (224, 13 sqq. Gundert)	*De caus.* II, 7 (7, 200, 11 sqq. K)
Ἐφεξῆς δ' ἂν εἴη τὰς τῶν ἡγεμο-	Καὶ περὶ τῶν κατὰ τὰς ἡγεμο-
νικῶν ἐνεργειῶν βλάβας διελθεῖν ...	νικὰς ἐνεργείας ἐροῦμεν. Ἔστι
καὶ μέν γε καὶ αὐτῆς τῆς διανοη-	μὲν οὖν κἂν ταύταις τρία τὰ
τικῆς ἐνεργείας	πρῶτα γένη τῶν συμπτωμάτων
1 a ἡ μὲν οἷον παράλυσις	1 a ἓν μὲν ἀπώλεια τῆς ἐνεργείας,
1 b ἄνοια,	2 a ἕτερον δὲ ⟨μετρία⟩ (add.
2 a ἡ δὲ οἷον ἐλλιπὴς κίνησις	Jouanna) βλάβη,
2 b μωρία τε καὶ μώρωσις,	3 a τὸ δὲ τρίτον εἰς ἑτέραν
3 a ἡ δὲ οἷον πλημμελὴς (s.c. κίνη-	ἰδέαν ἐκτροπή (*Jouanna* :
σις)	εἰς ἑτέραν ἰδέας ἐκτροπὴν *Kühn*).
3 b παραφροσύνη καλεῖται	1 b ἀπώλεια μὲν ἐν ταῖς καλου-
	μέναις μωρώσεσί τε καὶ λήθαις ...
	2 b αἱ δὲ μέτριαι βλάβαι καὶ
	οἷον νάρκαι τοῦ λογισμοῦ καὶ
	τῆς μνήμης ...
	3 b καὶ παραφροσύναι δὲ πᾶσαι,
	πλημμελεῖς ὑπάρχουσαι κινήσεις
	τῆς ἡγεμονικῆς δυνάμεως

---

[30] B. Gundert's 2009 edition of *De symptomatum differentiis* in the *CMG* V 5, 1, with commentary, adds greatly to our understanding of this treatise (see also the bibliography, pp. 9–18). The *De diff.* and the *De caus.* were written one after the other (cf. *De diff.* 3, 8, 224,

These two discussions in *De diff.* and *De caus.* are parallel because they treat the same subject, the disorders of the hegemonic faculties of the soul.[31] Now to classify these disorders he uses in both treatises a tripartite division of the kind he was familiar with.[32] This is an innovation with respect to Hippocrates and Plato. The difference is all the more obvious because the same term γένη is used by both Galen and Plato. There were two kinds of sicknesses of the soul in the *Timaeus* (86b: δύο … γένη), but there are three kinds of disturbance of the hegemonic faculty in Galen (*De caus.* II 7 τρία γένη). The first is the complete loss of the 'energies' of the soul; the second is a slowing-down of these 'energies'; and the third is an erroneous movement of these 'energies'. To each of these categories there correspond sicknesses of the soul.

The three types of deterioration in the faculties of the soul are referred to here as 1a, 2a, 3a,[33] and the names of the sicknesses that correspond to them are designated 1b, 2b, 3b. A slight difference in the mode of exposition distinguishes the two treatises, but it need not greatly concern us here;[34] for clarity's sake, I will here follow the order in *De Diff.*, where the various kinds of disturbance (the a-series) and the illnesses that correspond to them (the b-series) are discussed together.[35]

7–8 Gundert), whereas the *De loc. affect.* is a later text (cf. *De loc. affect.* I 6, 8, 63, 11–13 K). See Ilberg 1896. It seems necessary to take account of the chronological order of composition, which has not always been done in studies of Galen's psychopathology.

[31] The expression appears above all in *De diff.*, *De caus.*, and *De loc. affect.*, and also in the *Ars medica.*

[32] Compare for example the triad healthy/unhealthy/neutral in the *Ars medica.*

[33] These three categories of disturbance are not peculiar to sicknesses of the soul, but apply to all disturbances of the 'energies' (ἐνέργειαι), as Galen says clearly in *De symptomatum causis* III, c. 1, 7, 210, 8 sqq. K: ἔστι δὲ οὐ μόνον ἐν ταῖς ἀπεψίαις, ἀλλὰ καὶ κατὰ τὰ σύμπαντα τῶν συμπτωμάτων γένη, τὸ μὲν οἷον ἀπώλεια τῆς ἐνεργείας ἢ στέρησις ἢ ὡς ἄν τις ἑτέρως ὀνομάζειν ἐθέλοι· τὸ δὲ οἷον ἀτελὴς καὶ ἐλλιπὴς ἐνέργειά τὸ δὲ μοχθηρά τε καὶ πλημμελής., 'that is true not only for indigestion but for every category of symptom, such as loss of energy or deprivation or whatever you call it, or incomplete or insufficient energy, or for bad and erroneous energy'.

[34] The names of the sicknesses are indicated in *De diff.* at the same time as the three categories of disturbances, in the order 1a, 1b; 2a, 2b; 3a, 3b. In *De caus.* the three categories of disturbance are announced first (1a; 2a; 3a), and each of them is taken up later to give the names of the sicknesses (1b; 2b; 3b), with the addition of remarks about causes.

[35] Galen established, in *De diff.*, a subdivision of hegemonic faculties that is not present in the *De caus.* One of the subdivisions concerns the faculty of representation (φανταστική), and the other is the faculty of thought (διανοητική). The faculty of representation, discussed just before the faculty of thought (224, 10–13 Gundert), contains the same three categories of perturbation and of illness: 1a παράλυσις 1b κάρος καὶ κατάληψις; 2a ἐλλιπὴς καὶ ἄτονος (sc. κίνησις) 2b κώμασι τε καὶ ληθάργοις; 3a πλημμελής τις καὶ μοχθηρὰ κίνησις 3b παραφροσύνη.

1a: The first category of deterioration is a complete loss of 'energy': the term used for this part is παράλυσις in *De diff.* and ἀπώλεια in *De caus.*

1b: The illness corresponding to this complete loss of 'energy' is ἄνοια, 'dementia', in *De diff.* In *De caus.* the names are different: μώρωσις and λήθη (cf. ταῖς καλουμέναις μωρώσεσί τε καὶ λήθαις, 'that which one calls folly and the loss of memory'). This second denomination is restated in the third treatise, *De locis affectis.*

2a: The second category of deterioration is a deceleration of 'energy': the term used in *De diff.* is ἐλλιπὴς κίνησις, 'an insufficient movement'; in *De caus.*, it is simply the term βλάβη, 'damage', 'change' that appears in modern editions. It is tempting to accuse Galen of too little consistency of vocabulary. While the substantive βλάβη designates in *De diff.* any and all changes to 'hegemonic energies', here it designates only one of the three categories. Before accusing Galen of inexactitude, however, one should be certain of the integrity of the text as it exists today. After having enumerated the three types of alteration, Galen restates them, articulating the illnesses that correspond to each type and their causes. The first type is restated by the same word ἀπώλεια (in 1a and 1b), which is satisfactory; as for the second type, it is restated in 1b as αἱ δὲ μέτριαι βλάβαι, which is also satisfactory. It seems to me necessary, then, to reestablish in the initial articulation of this category in 1a, μετρία before βλάβη.[36] When we read the text with this correction in mind, Galen uses two different, but not at all contradictory, denominations to designate this second category of alteration in the two treatises (*De diff.* 'an insufficient movement', *De caus.* 'a moderate alteration').

2b: As to the illnesses that correspond to this second category of alteration, they are called in *De diff.* μωρία τε καὶ μώρωσις, 'foolishness and madness', and in *De causis* οἷον νάρκαι τοῦ λογισμοῦ καὶ τῆς μνήμης, 'one type of numbness of reason and memory'. What is remarkable here is not that the names used to designate the illnesses differ from one treatise to the other, but that the term μώρωσις, used in the singular in *De diff.* to designate an affliction of the second category (2b), appears in *De caus.* in the plural μωρώσεσι as an illness of the first category (1b). This is a genuine contradiction. How can we account for it? This is a question that we should not forget.[37]

One will notice that the same term παραφροσύνη is used to designate the third category of perturbation for both the representative faculty and the faculty of thought.

[36] It will obviously be necessary to check the manuscript tradition.

[37] See below, n. 41.

3a: The third category of alteration is a faulty and adverse movement of 'energies': the term used in *De diff.* is πλημμελὴς (*sc.* κίνησις), the adjective having the sense of 'faulty' (literally, 'off-key'). This adjective belongs to the category of compounds that I have termed 'distancing'.[38] The corresponding expression in *De caus.* is εἰς ἑτέραν ἰδέας ἐκτροπήν or, better, εἰς ἑτέραν ἰδέαν ἐκτροπή, 'the passing into another form'.[39] It is a passing into another state, specifically, it seems, the pathological state. In any case, there is no contradiction between the two expressions in the two treatises defining the third category of alteration (3a), as we will see immediately after examining the illnesses of this third category (3b).

3b: In effect, the same illnesses are assigned to this third category in each text. In *De diff.* we see παραφροσύνη in the singular, and in *De caus.* παραφροσύναι ... πᾶσαι in the plural. The manner in which the παραφροσύναι are qualified in *De caus.*, namely πλημμελεῖς ὑπάρχουσαι κινήσεις τῆς ἡγεμονικῆς δυνάμεως, 'being the faulty movements of the hegemonic faculty', reinforces the analogy between the two treatises, since we reencounter the adjective πλημμελὴς in *De causis*, as in *De diff.*, qualifying the 'faulty' movement of the hegemonic faculty.[40] Thus for this third category of alteration, a perfect coherence exists between the two treatises concerning the definition that is given and the pathology to which it is attributed.[41]

In this new classification, Galen appears to substitute the binary typology used by Hippocrates and Plato with a new tripartite division. I would like to demonstrate, however, that this tripartite typology is no more than a surface structure because, on the aetiological level, a binary explication corresponding to the one first articulated by Hippocrates still abides.

---

[38] See above, p. 98.

[39] One would expect ἐκτροπή in the nominative, since it is parallel to the other terms in the nominative designating the other categories of alteration (ἀπώλεια in 1a/1b and βλάβη-βλάβαι in 2a/2b) in *De caus.* The word ἐκτροπή is frequently used by Galen to designate 'a passage toward' with εἰς+ acc. The most common expression is εἰς τὸ παρὰ φύσιν ἐκτροπή, 'a passing toward a state against nature'.

[40] Another observation about vocabulary arises from this comparison: the word δύναμις is used here to describe 'hegemonic' activity, while the word ἐνεργεία is regularly used earlier in the same passage of *De caus.* and also in the parallel passage from *De diff.* Therefore, δύναμις and ἐνεργεία are synonyms.

[41] The comparison remains above all instructive for minor differences. So, the difference between the singular (*De diff.*) and the plural (*De caus.*) of the name of the 'dementia' makes us notice that the singular παραφροσύνη in *De diff.* is a collective term designating a category of dementias. Galen then articulates the differences of afflictions that are included in this category, but, as he did so in the context of aetiology, we will return to this later.

The three categories of mental affliction described by Galen are not, in fact, of equal intensity. Between categories 1 and 2, there is only a difference of degree. This is a madness of default, whether by a total weakening of mental faculties (category 1, *De caus.* II 7 [7, 200 K]: ἀπώλεια μὲν ἐν ταῖς καλουμέναις μωρώσεσί τε καὶ λήθαις, 'the loss in that which one calls madness and the loss of memory'), or by a partial weakening (category 2, *De caus.* II 7 [7, 201 K]: αἱ δὲ μέτριαι βλάβαι καὶ οἷον νάρκαι τοῦ λογισμοῦ καὶ τῆς μνήμης, 'the moderate lesions and types of numbing of reason and memory'). All of these afflictions are due to the same cause, cold, whether this coldness is due to a cold humor, phlegm, or to an imbalance (*dyscrasia*) of the brain. Regarding the illnesses of the first category, Galen says (ibid.): δῆλον ὡς ἐπὶ καταψύξει γίνεται καὶ μώρωσις καὶ λήθη, 'it is evident that madness and memory loss occur as a result of a chill'. Regarding the illnesses of the second category, he says (ibid.): αἱ δὲ μέτριαι βλάβαι καὶ οἷον νάρκαι τοῦ λογισμοῦ τε καὶ τῆς μνήμης ἐπὶ βραχυτέρᾳ καταψύξει συμβαίνουσι, 'the moderate lesions and the varieties of numbness of reason and of memory are the result of a shorter chill'. The aetiology clearly indicates that the cause is the same, with the difference that the chill is of shorter duration in the second category than in the first.

The third category, however, differs from the preceding two in its very nature. This is a perturbation of inverse motion that culminates in a sudden, uncontrollable craze.[42] This category encompasses the mental illnesses called παραφροσύναι, 'dementias' (*De caus.* II 7 [7, 202 K]). They are produced by an excess of heat, whether from an excess of a mordant and hot humor such as yellow bile, or from an imbalance of the brain in the process of heating (ibid.: ποτὲ μὲν τοῖς δακνώδεσι καὶ θερμοῖς ἐπόμεναι χυμοῖς, ὁποῖος ὁ τῆς ξανθῆς χολῆς ἐστι μάλιστα, πολλάκις δὲ κατὰ τὴν δυσκρασίαν τὴν ἐπὶ τὸ θερμότερον αὐτοῦ τοῦ ἐγκεφάλου συνιστάμεναι). If we consider the aetiology, therefore, we find the same two great types of madness that we met in *On the Sacred Disease*: a calm madness due to a cold humor, phlegm, and an agitated madness provoked by a hot humor, bile.

Galen enriches this binary typology with sub-groups in which he distinguishes particular illnesses. The dementias listed under the title παραφροσύ-

---

[42] This incontrollable character of faulty movement (πλημμελὴς κίνησις) is illustrated by the image of runners on a decline who are not able to stop themselves (*De diff.* 4, 13, 238, 13 sq. Gundert). Thanks to this new view of a tripartite division, we can return to the discordance we remarked upon in the classification of a similar affliction. If the affliction named μώρωσις (singular in *De diff.*, plural in *De caus.*) is attributed to category 2 in *De diff.* and to category 1 in *De caus.*, it is because these two first categories do not differ from each other except by a difference of degree, not nature.

ναι correspond to hyperactive madness, and include madness accompanied by fever, called φρενίτιδες, and madness without fever, called μανίαι (*De caus.* ibid.). Thanks to this redistribution, the word μανία takes, in Galen's work, a more restrained, technical sense than it had in Plato or Hippocrates. Here, it designates no more than a variety of παραφροσύναι corresponding to one of the two great types of madness, hyperactive madness, whereas in Plato's work it signified hyperactive madness in its entirety, and in the Hippocratic texts it could designate any type of insanity.

Because such a diversity of mental illnesses is categorized into two classes of madness according to two opposing aetiological principles, melancholy incontestably poses a problem. Galen places it in the class of παραφροσύναι, mental illnesses caused by heat. Since it is caused by black bile, which differs from yellow bile only in that it is colder, Galen accords it a separate place (*De caus. ibid.*: μόναι δ' αἱ μελαγχολικαὶ παράνοιαι ψυχρότερον ἔχουσι τὸν αἴτιον χυμόν, 'only melancholy dementias have as a cause a colder humor').[43] Following the Hippocratic *Aphorisms* (VI, 23, Littré IV, 568, 11 sq.), Galen characterizes these melancholy dementias with particular symptoms, namely prolonged fear (φόβος) and discouragement (δυσθυμίη) without cause (ἀλόγως). These symptoms, however, also characterize the other type of madness in the Hippocratic treatises and in Plato's work. This redistribution is astonishing, and underlines the ambiguity of melancholy that makes it integrate so poorly into a primitive, binary humoral scheme, in which hot bile was diametrically opposed to cold phlegm, at a time when black bile did not yet exist as a full-fledged humor.

Within the framework of this discussion, it is not possible to treat Galen's last treatise concerning the illnesses of the soul, *De locis affectis*, in detail. Unlike its two predecessors, *De loc. aff.* does not separate aetiology from definitions. In the context of the afflictions of the brain Galen returns to the afflictions of the reasonable soul (*De loc. aff.* III, c. 6, 8, 160 K: τὰ τοῦ λογιστικοῦ πάθη), considering memory, reason, or the two faculties at once. Regarding the loss of intelligence, Galen uses the term μώρωσις, as in *De causis*.[44] And as

---

[43] The aetiology is made precise in the same discussion a little later (*De caus.* II 7, 7, 203, 8–10 K): black bile impairs the principle of the logical soul (ἐπὶ τῇ μελαίνῃ χολῇ καταλαμβανούσῃ τὴν ἀρχὴν τῆς λογικῆς ψυχῆς).

[44] The comparison between the passages from *De causis* and the second passage from *De locis affectis* shows that Galen used the term μώρωσις only to designate the loss of intelligence, which is distinct from the loss of memory (*De causis* II, c. 7 = 7, 200, 15 and 17 201 K and *De loc. affect.* III, c. 7, = 8, 164, K). On the other hand, taken alone, the first passage from *De loc. affect.* could give the impression that Galen took μώρωσις to mean the simultaneous loss of both faculties. The passage is as follows: (*De loc. affect.* III, c. 7 = 8, 160 K): ἅμα μὲν γὰρ αὐτὴ φαίνεται

in the two treatises discussed above, the loss of intelligence, like the loss of memory, is caused by a cold bodily state (*De loc. aff.* III, c. 6, 8, 161 K: ψυχρά τις ἐστιν ἡ δυσκρασία). In this new treatise, we find confirmation that the tripartite division of perturbations of the faculties of the soul presented in both *De diff.* and *De caus.* signifies nothing fundamental. In effect, this tripartite division of the types of alteration is abandoned in *De locis affectis*, where, in a more coherent manner, Galen employs a binary opposition. Two types of madness with opposite symptoms are caused by two opposite bodily states: a cold one provokes the weakening of the spirit, or somnolence, by means of the numbing of psychic faculties (cf. *De loc. aff.* III, c. 6. 8, 161 K: αὕτη γὰρ ὁρᾶται ναρκοῦσα τὰς ψυχικὰς ἐνεργείας), while the hot bodily state leads to insomnia and dementia. And within this framework, we find the opposite effects inflicted on the mind by the hot and cold humors:

> Καὶ μὴν καὶ τὰ χολώδη τῶν νοσημάτων καὶ θερμὰ τὰς ἀγρυπνίας καὶ παραφροσύνας καὶ φρενίτιδας ἐργαζόμενα φαίνεται· τούτοις ἔμπαλιν τὰ φλεγματικὰ καὶ ψυχρὰ νωθρότητάς τε καὶ καταφορά.

> In fact, bilious and hot sicknesses clearly bring on bouts of insomnia, delirium and *phrenitis*; conversely, phlegmatic and cold sicknesses produce slackening (of the spirit) and depression.

This division of afflictions of the mind based on the theory of two opposing humors, hot bile and cold phlegm, thus brings us back to something close to the view we encountered in *On the Sacred Disease*.[45] But Galen, continuing his analysis of different bodily states, adds the secondary characteristics of wetness and dryness to the principal opposition of heat and cold. Wetness has an effect comparable to cold, and dryness to heat. For example, like an excess of cold, an excess of wetness contributes to the deceleration of the spirit (ἀργία ψυχῆς). Abnormal sleep is a symptom of this deceleration, while

---

πολλάκις γενομένη μετὰ βλάβης τινὸς τοῦ λογισμοῦ, καθάπερ γε καὶ ἡ τοῦ λογισμοῦ βλάβη μετὰ τοῦ καὶ τὴν μνήμην βεβλάφθαι, τῆς μὲν διαθέσεως ἀμφοτέροις τῆς αὐτῆς οὔσης, ἐπιτεταμένης δέ, ὁπότε τῇ μνήμῃ συναπόλωλεν ὁ λογισμός, ὅπερ ὀνομάζεται μώρωσις. Daremberg translates: 'Souvent, en effet, elle (*sc.* la lésion de la mémoire) se produit conjointement avec une lésion de la raison, de la même manière que la lésion de la raison est unie à celle de la mémoire, la diathèse étant la même dans les deux cas, mais plus intense lorsque la raison est perdue avec la mémoire, ce qui alors se nomme folie'. According to this translation, the term μώρωσις seems to refer to damage to memory and to reason. It seems better to reestablish a coherence with the other passages by translating the end of the passage as follows: 'the diathesis being the same in both cases, but more intense when, along with memory, reason is lost—a loss of memory that is called μώρωσις.

45 A secondary opposition between dry and wet bodily states is added to the opposition between cold and hot states.

insomnia is a symptom of the agitation of the spirit caused by an excess of heat or dryness. There is an opposition between the afflictions caused by an abnormal slackening of 'hegemonic energies' and those due to the energies' abnormal excitation, even if variations within the two great categories are possible according to the intensity of the elemental qualities. So far, the polarity abides. It is, however, important to signal that Galen envisages a mixed category where the bodily state is at once hot and cold (8, 163 K: καὶ πρός γε ταῖς εἰρημέναις δυσκρασίαις ἐναντίαις ἄλλη τις ἐξ ἀμφοῖν γίνεται μικτή, 'And in addition to the contrary imbalance, there exists a mixed imbalance formed by both at once'). Galen gives as an example the 'waking coma' (ἐν τοῖς ἀγρύπνοις κώμασιν), characterized by the predominance of yellow bile and phlegm, thus by a mixture of an excess of cold and heat. By adding this mixed category to the two simple opposing categories, Galen returns to a triple division of abnormal bodily states, with two simple and one mixed.[46]

Galen's typology of illnesses of the soul can vary according to the context and the perspectives that he adopts. One also encounters a triple classification based on the predominance of a single humor as the cause of a mental illness. Thus, when in *Quod animi mores* he mentions the effects of the body on the soul without always being able to always give an explanation, he declares (c. 3, 4, 776–777 K = 18–19 Bazou):

> ... πολλὰ ζητήσας οὐχ εὗρον ὥσπερ γ' οὐδὲ διὰ τί χολῆς μὲν ξανθῆς ἐν ἐγκεφάλῳ πλεοναζούσης εἰς παραφροσύνην ἑλκόμεθα, διὰ τί δὲ τῆς μελαίνης εἰς μελαγχολίαν, διὰ τί δὲ τὸ φλέγμα καὶ ὅλως τὰ ψυκτικὰ παραίτια ληθάργων, ἐξ ὧν καὶ μνήμης καὶ συνέσεως βλάβαις ἁλισκόμεθα,

> In my extensive research, I have not found much to explain why we are pulled toward dementia when yellow bile is abundant in the brain, but when it is black bile, we tend towards melancholy, and why phlegm and chills in general are the causes of lethargy, with the result that we are equally seized by damage to memory and intelligence.

Galen's text gives the impression of a triple typology based on three of the four humors, in which melancholy seems to occupy a central place, wedged between the two extremes of an excess of heat caused by yellow bile and an excess of cold caused by phlegm.

---

[46] My intention here has been to bring out the typology and the aetiology of mental illnesses in *De locis affectis* and not to enumerate the illnesses themselves. Regarding the different mental illnesses in *De locis affectis*, see Pigeaud 1988b, 153–183. A list of illnesses cannot be made, however, without first taking typology into account. Is it possible to count insomnia and delirium among the illnesses characterized by a combined loss of memory and reason, as Pigeaud does (159)? In reality, they stem from two different types of imbalance.

This opposition between the effects produced by hot yellow bile and by cold phlegm continues even into the period later than Galen, when the theory of four humors and four temperaments predominated. The contrary effects of these two humors appear in the distinction between the mind and the character of bilious and phlegmatic people. In fact, in the classic Greek text on the four temperaments, the anonymous treatise on the *Constitution of the Universe and Man* published in the mid-nineteenth century by J.L. Ideler,[47] the people dominated by yellow bile are described not only as 'angry and bitter' (ὀργίλοι καὶ πικροί), but as 'susceptible to madness' (μανιώδεις). Those on the other hand who are dominated by phlegm are prone to sorrow and forgetfulness (λυπηροί καὶ ἀμνήμονες). But the great difference is that this continuity has become a tradition detached from its origins, since the physicians of this late epoch were no longer directly familiar with the ancient sources, neither the treatises of the Hippocratic corpus nor even those of Galen, all the while continuing to attribute their theories to Hippocrates, master of Galen, or to Galen himself.[48]

Conclusion

A permanent, binary typology composed of a depressive and a hyperactive type of insanity is made apparent by the comparison of these texts, despite evolution over time and despite Galen's superficial tripartite division. The definitions are already set in place in the oldest text, *On the Sacred Disease*, in which we can appreciate the Hippocratic physicians' remarkable spirit of observation. Definitions remain more stable than aetiology. In the first three texts analysed, *On the Sacred Disease, On Regimen*, and the *Timaeus*, we encountered three different explanations, and even two complementary (or concurrent?) explanations within Plato's *Timaeus*. Still, the humoral

---

[47] Ideler 1841, 304.

[48] For the other Greek texts (published and unpublished) regarding the theory of the four temperaments in late antiquity, see Jouanna 2006b. Not all of these texts, however, present the phlegmatic temperaments in the same way: while some writers characterize them according to the tradition that begins with *On the Sacred Disease*, that is with phlegm as the cause of sorrow, forgetfulness, somnolence, and even stupidity (in addition to the *Constitution of the Universe and Man*, cf. Pseudo-John of Damascus, *Quid est homo?*, Pseudo-Galen on *Humors*, Armenian anthology), others present phlegmatics as alert and reflective people (Pseudo-Hippocrates, *On the Formation of Man*, Pseudo-Hippocrates, *On the Pulse and Human Temperament*, the Greek source of Vindicianus' *Epistula ad Pentadium*). On this Hippocrates, the master of Galen, reimagined in late antiquity, whom I have called 'the other Hippocrates,' see also Jouanna 2006a.

explanation of the oldest text, with its opposition between hot bile and cold phlegm, reappears in Galen's work, although it is completely absent from *On Regimen* and Plato's *Timaeus*. This is evidence of a certain permanence even in the domain of aetiology.

The principal question posed in the introduction has been answered. As for the two related 'subterranean' questions, here are some observations:

1. Regarding the vocabulary of madness, there is a spectacular contraction in the scope of the concept of μανία. Although the Hippocratic physicians use this concept to designate either of the two types of madness, Plato uses it for only one, and by Galen's time it is reserved for a single variety of this hyperactive madness, that without fever.[49] The term ἄνοια undergoes a comparable contraction in scope from Plato to Galen. Plato used ἄνοια to designate both types of madness, while Galen uses it for depressive madness alone.

2. Finally, the medical treatise *On Regimen* should find an important place before the *Timaeus* in the history of the genesis of the concept of a 'mental illness.' This is the final essential message of the present paper.

---

[49] These remarks strengthen and complement what Pigeaud (2010) wrote about the evolution of μανία.

GALENIC MADNESS

Vivian Nutton

Whoever wants to understand any aspect of Galen's medicine is faced with two difficult and at times insoluble problems, one external, the other internal. The external problem is to situate Galen's ideas within an appropriate historical context and to identify his debts to others. The internal is to produce a coherent and historically nuanced account of views that might have been expressed at almost any time during sixty or more years of practice as doctor and as writer. A third approach, looking at the way in which Galen's ideas were understood, or misunderstood, over the centuries, is unnecessary here, for, as will become clear, his own views on madness had relatively little influence on subsequent generations beyond their general framework. The Arabs knew their Galen, but added so much of their own to him that it is hardly surprising that medieval scholars depended on Arabic authors rather than directly on Galen.[1] Renaissance doctors enjoyed pointing out Arabic misunderstandings and confusions, but put little in their place, save for a more precise terminology. Nor were medical historians particularly interested in Galen's views on madness, for a long while scarcely venturing beyond the more exciting evidence of fifth and fourth century BC Greece—Johann Ludvig Heiberg's wide-ranging 1927 article, 'Geisteskrankheiten im klassischen Altertumswissenschaft', was a notable exception—and it was not until the 1970s, with Stanley Jackson's article on Galen and mental diseases and Rudolf Siegel's 1973 volume, *Galen on psychology, psychopathology and function and diseases of the nervous system; an analysis of his doctrines, observations and experiments*, that one could point to new insights or to a monograph on the subject.[2] Siegel's book is not without its merits, and it is very much the book that Galen might have written, had he chosen to bring his scattered thoughts together in one place. He did not, and that is one of our difficulties. One might also add, 'That Galen would have written had he been a modern doctor', for as Siegel's long and complicated title indicates, he uses the medical categories of the nineteen fifties to structure his

---

[1] Dols 1992; Pormann 2008.
[2] Heiberg 1927; Jackson 1969 and 1987; Siegel 1973.

discussions. But, lest I appear to be too harsh on this pioneer, it is worth admitting that these categories are far more appropriate to the way Galen thought than those of the Diagnostic and Statistical Manual of mental disorders that are sometimes invoked.

We are fortunate in that Galen acknowledged his debts to others and indicated what he believed were his major contributions more openly when writing about mental diseases than about many other aspects of medicine. He praised the efforts of Rufus of Ephesus, whom he considered the best modern writer on melancholy, and seems to have taken much from him.[3] He is more reticent about his opponents, the Methodists, some of whose psychotherapeutic ideas closely resemble his own. But it is to Hippocrates that he traces his medical ancestry, convinced that he can find Hippocratic precedent for all of his own views somewhere in the Corpus Hippocraticum. But it is not the Hippocrates familiar today from the studies of Bennett Simon and Jacques Jouanna that most attracted Galen's attention, the Hippocrates who in *Sacred Disease* discussed mania at length as well as epilepsy.[4] Galen makes next to no use of that treatise, which came to prominence only in the 20th century. He cites it only a handful of times, for lexicographical, never for medical purposes.[5] Indeed, if a scholium in Marcianus 269 goes back to Galen, he rejected it entirely as a genuine work of Hippocrates or even as one that conveyed reasonable traces of his teaching.[6] Other writers, like Anonymus Parisinus and Caelius Aurelianus, had fewer scruples about citing it.[7] Galen's silence is particularly striking considering that he wrote a large commentary on *Airs, waters and places*, the treatise that most resembles *Sacred Disease*, and which has often been thought to have been written by the same author. It is a pity that we have no clear idea of the reasons for Galen's rejection, given the centrality of this treatise in modern discussions of Hippocratic mental diseases, and its relevance to many other aspects of Galen's medicine.

In its place, Galen appealed to a variety of passages in the *Epidemics* and *Aphorisms* to give the authority of Hippocrates to his own views, and in particular to his conviction that mind and body were so closely interlinked that

---

[3] Pormann 2008, 12.

[4] Simon 1978; Jouanna 2003.

[5] Jouanna, CVI–VII, CXIII–V.

[6] Anastassiou and Irmer 2001, 256.

[7] Anonymus Parisinus, *De morbis acutis et cronicis* III.3: p. 19 Garofalo; Caelius Aurelianus, *De morbis cronicis* I.131: p. 506 Bendz. It was, however, cited by glossographers and by later writers in the Hippocratic tradition, and is found in the best MSS. of our Hippocratic Corpus.

changes in the one had an effect on the other. As he explained it at the end of his long life, the soul's behaviour was dependent on the particular constitution of the body, and how one behaved, whether, as we might say, rationally or irrationally, morally or immorally, followed the humoral balance or imbalance of the body.[8] It was a central tenet of his thought throughout his life, even though he never entirely resolved the ambiguity inherent in a word like 'followed' or 'depended'. On one thing he was clear; this dependence could be scientifically and philosophically demonstrated, and, so he argued, was accepted by adherents of a variety of philosophical and medical thinkers, whatever their views of the essence of the soul, on which Galen maintained an agnostic stance to the end of his days. As Peter Singer will argue in the introduction to his forthcoming translation of *The soul's dependence on the body*, Galen's argument in this tract is that whatever opinion might be held on the substance of the soul—and he cites the views of Hippocrates, Plato and Aristotle as well as those of other less familiar or anonymous thinkers—, all in some way or another acknowledged that mental and moral behaviour was to some extent affected by what was happening to the body, what we ate or drank, whether we were ill or healthy, and so on.[9] The phenomenon was universally accepted, even if the explanations for it that were offered might differ substantially one from another. Galen's view was not materialist in the sense that the soul itself had to be something material; and in that tract he does not commit himself to any specific view of the nature of the soul. He claims only that its workings were in some way, and at times in some obvious ways, affected by what was happening to the body.[10]

This interaction was a two way process, even if not everyone was prepared to acknowledge that it was. Galen time and again asserts that the soul can affect the body's well being. Just as too much food or drink might make one lazy or affect one's judgement, a physical change with consequences for the soul, so in turn the affections of the soul, what we might term the emotions, fear, anger, shame and so on, might have a physical effect on the body. How this might be intrigued Galen for decades, particularly because he was convinced that some of the standard explanations offered for the physical effect of emotions could not be substantiated, but of the phenomenon itself he

---

[8] Galen, *Quod animi mores* 1: IV.767 K. In general, Garcia Ballester 1988.

[9] Singer forthcoming 2013.

[10] This removes the alleged contradiction between Galen's apparent approval of some form of corporeal soul in this treatise and his otherwise universal refusal to pronounce on the nature of the soul.

was totally convinced. In *On prognosis*, in the later sections of the *Commentary on Epidemics VI*, and now in the recently discovered *Avoiding distress*, he provides a series of examples of cases to prove his point that the emotions matter. Some are his own—the lovesick wife of Justus, the slave steward fearing for his life after some dodgy accounting, the grammarian who wasted away through distress at the loss of his library in the fire.[11] Others are universal—we all have experienced some form of physical trembling when looking out over a precipice or climbing a mountain, or worried about some forthcoming test or trial—and still others are *ben trovato* or are ascribed to famous doctors in the past.[12] The love story of Antiochus and Stratonice Galen associates with Erasistratus, although that famous Hellenistic doctor is neither the only nor the most likely candidate for the role of the perceptive physician in this famous story.[13] This interest in what we might term today stress diseases is traced back by Galen to Hippocrates, although Galen's evidence and reasoning are far from compelling. A Hippocratic observation about a throbbing vein in the temples in an angry man hardly proves that the author believed in the direct effect of emotions on the body. But at the same time Galen chides his colleagues for failing to recognise this Hippocratic legacy, stressing at the end of his commentary on *Epidemics VI* that his own unique expertise and interest in such conditions derived ultimately from the example of Hippocrates.[14]

This conviction that mental conditions are closely linked to physical may perhaps go some way towards explaining why Galen, despite his interest in mental states, says remarkably little about madness per se. True, he is not interested in nosography, in distinguishing and describing diseases in the manner of Aretaeus, an equally committed Hippocratic, and, if only for that reason, we would be foolish to expect an account of madness as such.[15] What concerns him is what might be termed the theoretical and intellectual bases of medical practice, from which his therapeutics flow. So, for example, in his treatise *On black bile*, his aim is to establish the existence of that humour, particularly against Erasistratus, and his mention of melancholic diseases,

---

[11] Galen, *On praecogn.* 5–6: XIV.625–626, 630–633 K.; ibid., 6: XIV.633–635 K; *In Epid. VI comm VIII: CMG* V.10,2,2, p. 486 = *De indolentia* 7: p. 4 Jouanna.

[12] Galen, *De motibus dubiis 8.15*: p. 158 Nutton, explaining the importance of imagination, and citing Hippocrates, *De humor*.9: V.490 3–5 L.

[13] Galen, *De praecogn. 6*: XIV.631–635 K. A detailed analysis of the various versions of the story is given by Hillgruber, 2010.

[14] Galen, *In Epid. VI comm. VIII: CMG* V.10,2,2, pp. 483–487, 494–495.

[15] Aretaeus, *De morb. chron.* I.6.

including madness, is largely to point up his opponent's ignorance or, rather deceit. As he says, any educated person knows the story of the daughters of Proteus who were cured of their madness by the shaman-seer Melampus, who purged them with hellebore to evacuate their black bile, a physical cure for a physically determined condition. Erasistratus' refusal to mention the tale is proof of his perversity.[16]

As far as Galen is concerned, all mental disorders are the result of some lesion, some damage to the brain, and particularly to the regent faculty, the *hegemonike dynamis*, that prevents it from functioning properly. It is not that this faculty is removed entirely, as in a complete loss of memory or in *morosis*, what we can perhaps translate as mental deficiency or dementia, but that it is prevented from acting normally. What prevents it from functioning properly is, as with most diseases in Galen, the consequence of some humoral changes and imbalances either in the body in general or in the brain in particular, the latter arising specifically there or by 'sympathy' from some other damaged or diseased part of the body.[17]

In what is the most succinct account of the causes of madness, or perhaps better forms of madness, at the end of Book II of *The causes of symptoms*, Galen offers some very straightforward distinctions.[18] He divides the broader term, *paraphrosynai*, into two categories, *phrenitides* and *maniae*, that differ from one another mainly in one thing, the presence or absence of fever. Almost by definition, the mental disturbances that occur with fever derive from an excess of hot humour, and principally yellow bile, either generally in the body, or more specifically in the brain through either an excess of hot humour or, sometimes, through some inflammation, *phlegmone*, within the brain or specifically in its meninges. In extremely acute fevers, for example, a hot, biting vapour rises up through the body to affect the brain.

There is, however, one exception to this universal ascription of mental disorders to hot humours, with or without fever: melancholic madness, or rather madnesses, for they can take a variety of forms, particularly in the derangement of the imagination. How then does one distinguish a manic madness from melancholic madness? Galen adopts a dual strategy. The first is akin to physiognomy, in that he first identifies those who look as if they would be prone to melancholic diseases, those who are lean, dark and hairy, with large veins, and who are prone to develop these disorders particularly

---

[16] Galen, *De atra bile* 7: V.132 K.
[17] Pigeaud 1988b.
[18] Galen, *De caus. sympt.* III.7: VII.200–204 K.

from a poor life style and if their customary loss of blood through haem-
orrhoids or menstruation has been interrupted.[19] But, more important than
this is the type of behaviour that they display, characterised, as Hippocrates
had long ago declared, by two symptoms, fear and depression, *dysthymia*;
and, given Galen's strong psychosomatism, these two mental conditions
can trigger physical manifestations of melancholic disease.[20] In what may
appear a simile taken too far, Galen twice uses the fact that extreme darkness causes fear in all save the bravest to suggest that the black humour, like
a vapour, obscures and envelops the thinking process to engender fear.[21]

There is also another way in which melancholic diseases can be produced
that does not involve an original imbalance of melancholic humour. In
feverish diseases, the increasing heat cooks the yellow bile within the brain
in ways that become ever more dangerous: pale yellow bile is less harmful
than darker, and both are less violent than the final stage when it turns
into black bile, what later generations knew as 'adust' or burnt melancholy.
It produces the same symptoms as ordinary melancholy, and is equally
dangerous.[22]

All this, one might say, presents Galen at his worst; schematic, combining
categories that should not be combined, and determined to find what he
wants in Hippocrates. His diagnoses, and his underlying theory, do provide,
in his eyes, a clear and logical justification for the therapy that is to be used,
but that is perhaps the best that can be said.

Yet if one leaves these theoretical speculations on one side, Galen's understanding of madness becomes much more impressive. He is interested in
mental illness, and he rightly observes that this can take very many varied
forms. He is well aware that mental disorders that occur during, and perhaps as a result of, other conditions may be temporary concomitants of the
disease, and are thus to be managed within that disease. He recalls his own
experience when in a high fever as a young boy he imagined that there were
dark spots on the bed and his clothes, and tried to tear them off. Only when
he heard his friends talking about his hallucinations did he realise what had
happened, and called on them to cool him down, and even then it took a
little while for his bad dreams to end.[23] Equally he is well aware that mental

---

19 Galen, *De loc. aff.* III.10: VIII.182–183 K.
20 Galen, *De loc. aff.* VIII.190–191 K.
21 Galen, *De loc. aff.* VIII.191 K.; *De caus. sympt.* III.7: VIII.202–203 K.
22 Galen, *De loc. aff.* III.9: VIII.178 K.
23 Galen, *De loc. aff.* IV.2: VIII.226 K.

derangements, *paraphrosynai*, can affect only some of the functions of the brain. The doctor Theophilus was perfectly able to discuss and make judgments about what was in front of him, but was under the illusion that noisy flute-players had occupied his house and made a constant racket day in, day out.[24] Another man stood at his window with kitchen implements, and invited passers-by to encourage him to throw them out. He was sufficiently sane to be able to identify whatever utensil was named, but had no idea why he was throwing them out.[25] This case may or may not be identical with that of a man locked in at home along with a slave who was preparing wool. The man rushed to the window, and began throwing out glass vessels at the crowd's behest. He threw out other things, until, finally, he seized the slave and, in response to the shouting crowd, threw him too out of the building.[26] Laughter turned immediately to silence, and the onlookers rushed to picked up the poor slave. Other instances were less spectacular. A man believed that Atlas was about to drop the world, another that a voice had spoken to him out of a graveyard.[27] Another patient of Galen, while suffering from a fever, imagined that he was in Athens, not Rome, and demanded to be taken to the Ptolemaeum; he told his friends that he was well aware that he was still suffering a little from fever, brought on, he claimed, by the long journey he had made the previous day from Megara to Athens. His hallucinations were only ended by a sudden and copious nose bleed, after which he could not remember anything of his mental aberration.[28]

Given Galen's psychosomatism, it is not surprising that he is prepared to recommend the same sort of humoral remedies for mental as for physical disease, including prophylactic diets. But he is also aware that there may be occasions when one needs to adopt a different approach. Sometimes, as in several of the cases reported in *On prognosis*, it is simple observation that leads him to discover the psychic cause of the illness, and to remove the condition by dealing with the psychological problem. The slave steward is reassured that he will not have to make recompense. In another instance, he cures a woman who believed falsely that she had swallowed a snake, by making her vomit and then slipping a snake into her vomit to make her think that the snake had come out—a trick not much different from the

---

[24] Galen, *De diff. sympt. 3*: VII.60 K.
[25] Galen, *De diff. sympt. 3*: VII.61 K.
[26] Galen, *De loc. aff. 4.2*: VIII.226 K.
[27] Galen, *In Epid. I comm. III*: XVIIA.213 K. = *In Epid. VI comm. VIII*: CMG V.10,2,2,486; *In Epid. II comm.II*; CMG V.10.1, p. 208 = *In Epid. VI comm. VIII*: CMG V.10,2,2,487.
[28] Galen, *De motu musc.II. 6*: IV.446–447 K.

conjuring trick of the Syrian quack who annoyed Galen.[29] More important, in the commentary on *Epidemics VI*, he gives a long list of instances in which he has dealt with those whose physical condition has been damaged by their emotional states. His aim throughout has been to distract the patient from whatever has provoked this emotional state, and by allowing them to do whatever brings them pleasure—hunting, listening to music, going to the theatre, a wrestling match, even drinking. Anything that excites their enthusiasm and distracts them from what has caused their mental disturbance is good—stimulating anger at the wrong done to another may be a good means of treating someone who is wrapped up in his or her own concerns. At other times, tact and discretion may be all that can be offered, but even this may prove to have some value.[30]

These examples are sufficient to disprove Siegel's contention that Galen was not particularly interested in madness and mental diseases as such.[31] Siegel himself seems not to have known the long sections, preserved in Arabic in the *Commentary on Epidemics VI*, where Galen discusses these mental states at length, so his dismissive judgment is not entirely surprising. But it is worth repeating that Galen is not interested in classifying mental illnesses as such—he is not a nosographer—but rather he concentrates on functional disturbances in particular organs.

But there is still a problem, first identified clearly by Michael Dols.[32] Compared with mental aberrations and hallucinations, Galen says very, very little about madness itself, and by madness here I mean what he calls *mania*, less even than melancholia. Is this because he saw mania as something almost incurable, brought about by primarily physical changes? Or is this because, as so often, he never produces a completely systematic account, but follows a trail that leads to a concentration on something slightly different from what may have been his original intention? The latter seems to be at least a possible explanation, and would still allow us to view Galen as a physician the records of whose practice are far more interesting than the traditional theory that underlies them. Galen's friends were surely right in wanting to discover how Galen apparently came to display this expertise in the treatment of emotional disturbances, call them madness if you

---

[29] Galen, *In Epid. II comm. VIII*: CMG V 10,1, pp. 207–208 = In *Epid. VI comm. VIII*: CMG V.10, 2,2, p. 487. For the quack, Meyerhof 1929, 83.

[30] Galen, *In Epid. VI comm. VIII*: CMG V.10,2,2, pp. 494–495.

[31] Siegel 1973, 265.

[32] Dols 1992, 37.

will, for here in particular Galen shows two contradictory tendencies.[33] He combines conservatism and innovation, fidelity to Hippocrates with independent and, to his contemporaries, unusually successful therapeutic practices, and that is no bad epitaph for any doctor.

---

[33] Galen, *De indolentia* 1: p. 1 Jouanna., writes at the request of a friend this treatise on the theme of how one can avoid the distress that may end in physical illness. For wider discussion see Singer 2011, forthcoming 2013.

WHAT IS A MENTAL ILLNESS, AND HOW CAN IT BE TREATED? GALEN'S REPLY AS A DOCTOR AND PHILOSOPHER*

Véronique Boudon-Millot

Exploring the field of mental illnesses, both in modern psychiatry and antiquity, means attempting to penetrate an extremely fluctuating domain where even the definition of illness, not to mention the applicable therapies, is far from being a matter of consensus.[1] In the case of Galen there is the added difficulty of taking into consideration the immense corpus of around 150 treatises written over a period of nearly seventy years, a large part of which has not yet been translated into any modern language. Fortunately the pioneering works of M. Vegetti, L. Garcia Ballester and J. Pigeaud, to cite only these three names, have opened up a number of paths and allowed us to see rather more clearly.[2] My own thoughts, though they sometimes proceed along different lines, are inspired by these scholars.

I will restrict myself to formulating three questions, the apparent simplicity of which covers a very real complexity. What is a mental illness? How should it be treated? And under what conditions can the patient be considered responsible for his/her acts? These are of course modern questions as well.

The object of this study will thus be to try to define the specific characteristics of mental and psychological illnesses in relation to physical illnesses, and at the same time to examine the complex ties which join them together via the mind-body relationship as defined and imagined in Greece by both doctors and philosophers.

1. What Is a Mental Illness and How Can It Be Diagnosed?

The Greek language uses the same words (νόσος, νόσημα and πάθος) to refer to both physical illnesses which are localised in the body and psychologi-

---

* Translated by William Harris.
[1] Moss 1967, Ingleby 1982.
[2] Garcia Ballester 1972; Vegetti 1984; Manuli and Vegetti 1988; Garcia Ballester 1988; Pigeaud 1988b; also Jackson 1969. On the psycho-physiology of Galen see Siegel 1973 and von Staden 2000, esp. 105–116.

cal illnesses (τὰ ψυχικά) which are localised in the brain. Thus in his treatise *How the Faculties of the Mind Follow the Dispositions of the Body* Galen refers to attacks of melancholy, phrenitis and mania without distinction as νοσήματα.[3] Does this mean that the Greeks made no difference between physical and psychological illnesses? Certainly not, but they acknowledged an undeniable link which is demonstrated by the use of a same vocabulary.

Inasmuch as Galen does not use a specific vocabulary to designate psychic illness but has recourse to different terms, themselves interchangeable, it would seem pointless to search amongst medical definitions for a precise vocabulary for mental illnesses. The definition of mental illness is even in modern medicine far from being unanimous. For the purpose of this essay, at least, the expression 'mental illness' will refer to troubles impinging on the cognitive faculties.[4] Galen himself reacts to the lack of precise terminology for such conditions in his treatise *On Affected Places*, when he refers to the cases of amnesia described previously by the physician Archigenes in his works on memory disorders. Galen notes that those who preceded him had not only designated such conditions by different names, lack of memory (ἐπιλησμοσύνη), forgetfulness (λήθη), or the loss of memory (μνήμης ἀπώλεια), but also qualified them indistinctly as damage (βλάβη), affect or illness (πάθος), illness (νόσος), or even symptom (σύμπτωμα) or infirmity (ἀρρώστημα). However, for Galen, as he states clearly himself, 'these discussions about words are in fact the subject of research for the sophists, and contribute not the slightest to actual treatment'.[5]

Leaving aside once and for all the quarrel about words, Galen defines illness, whether physical or psychic, by reference to detectable damage to a function (ἐνεργείας αἰσθητῇ βλάβῃ).[6] The vital functions depend on the principal organs or directive centres (ἀρχαί) such as the brain, the heart, the liver and the testicles, on which other parts of the body are dependant: the nerve system and the spinal cord have their origins in the brain, the arteries in the heart, the veins in the liver, and the sperm canals in the testicles. Thus a lesion affecting one of the directive centres will have consequences, through 'sympathy', for the parts of the body with which it is connected.

---

[3] *Quod animi mores* 5 (*SM* II, 49).
[4] Pigeaud 1988b, 157.
[5] *De loc. aff.* III, 5 (VIII.150 K).
[6] *Ars med.* XXVII, 2 (ed. Boudon-Millot [Budé v.2] 2000, 359).

The approach of a doctor towards a psychic illness will consequently be the same as towards a physical illness. Faced with the need to restore memory to an individual who has lost it, Galen provides us with the following model of reasoning:

> While still young and not having seen any teacher treat this affection (τοῦτο τὸ πάθος), and not having read up the treatment in any of the old authorities, I first attempted to discover which was the affected area (ὁ πεπονθώς τόπος) to which I should apply what are called local treatments (τὰ καλούμενα τοπικὰ βοηθήματα), obviously after providing care for the whole body, for that is necessary with all affections.[7]

The physician not only makes no difference between the treatments of psychic and physical illnesses, but also attempts to treat the two types of 'affection' by applying the same reasoning and by taking care of the body in its entirety. Thus, in the case of the losses of memory already named, Galen endeavours to identify the damaged part of the body and the cause of the damage to its functioning. Therefore the treatment and the place to apply it will depend on whether one situates the memory in the heart like Archigenes, or in the brain like Galen himself.

Galen chooses to situate the memory in the same place as 'what is called the hegemonikon' (τὸ καλούμενον ἡγεμονικόν), the hegemonic part of the 'soul' which he situates in the brain. He points out that the affections called lethargy (λήθαργος) and phrenitis (φρενῖτις) cause suffering of the brain 'when one of its own functions is damaged' (ἔνθα τῶν ἰδίων τις ἐνεργειῶν αὐτοῦ βλάπτεται).[8] The functions of the brain can be affected in a primary way (πρωτοπαθεῖν), as in the case of lethargy or phrenitis, or by 'sympathy' following illnesses such as pleurisy or peripneumonia when they provoke *paraphrosune*. By 'its own functions' Galen understands those functions that are operated by the brain alone as distinct for example from sight which is operated by use of the eyes and from hearing which involves the use of the ears. Only illnesses causing damage to the brain's own functions and affecting its capacities 'to think, to remember, to reason and to choose' are consequently to be considered as psychic and mental.

Galen, who is quite aware that Archigenes situated the hegemonic function not in the brain but in the heart, decided nonetheless to consult his works on the loss of memory, not in order to learn from him where the treatment should be applied, but which type of dyscrasia (τίνα δυσκρασίαν)

---

[7] *De loc. aff.* III, 5 (VIII.147–148 K).
[8] Ibid. II, 10 (VIII.127 K).

is responsible, according to him, for this affection and which types of medicines should be used. Depending on whether cold or dampness, or a combination of the two, or on the other hand dryness and cold, dominate in the brain, it will be appropriate to use medicines opposed to the diathesis present in the brain (τὰ δ' ἰάματα τῇ κατ' αὐτὸν ἐναντία διαθέσει). Great therefore was Galen's surprise on learning that Archigenes, in complete contradiction with his own teaching, recommended applying treatment not to the heart but to the head.

Beyond this polemic with Archigenes, the important point is that the illnesses which affect the memory, and which can be defined as psychic since they are located in the brain, are not to be treated differently from physical illnesses, and are like physical illnesses the result of an unbalanced temperament. In both cases the approach is consequently the same and consists of defining which diathesis can be responsible for the affection which damages areas of the brain and of the meninges (τίς ἦν ἡ διάθεσις ἐν τοῖς κατὰ τὸν ἐγκέφαλον καὶ τὰς μήνιγγας χωρίοις).[9] Thus, so Archigenes apparently thought, if the affection of the brain is cold and damp, the treatment will consist of warming and drying the head. For Galen, however, Archigenes is again mistaken, 'because a similar diathesis in the head could not cause loss of memory' (οὐ γὰρ δὴ κατά γε τὸ κράνιον ἡ τοιαύτη διάθεσις γενομένη τῆς μνήμης ἀφαιρήσεται τὸν ἄνθρωπον).[10] In fact, even though he does not say anything about it here, Galen considers that coldness alone should be considered responsible for losses of memory (as we shall see later).[11]

Nonetheless there is a difference between psychic and physical illnesses, namely that with the former the place affected does not appear as distinctly to the senses as with the latter. Galen deplores the fact that while it is obvious which location is affected in cases of pleurisy, peripneumonia, nephritis, and conditions of the colon, liver, spleen, intestines, bladder, uterus and other such organs, the same does not apply to psychic illnesses:[12]

> in cases of loss of memory, there is no sign of the place affected, no unnatural tumour, no excretion, or anything else. It is the same with melancholy, phrenitis, mania, epilepsy, lethargy, torpidity, and what has been called by modern doctors katoche and catalepsy.[13]

---

[9] Ibid. III, 5 (VIII.152.7–8 K).
[10] Ibid. (VIII.153.16–18 K).
[11] Ibid. III, 6 (VIII.161 K).
[12] Ibid. III, 5 (VIII, 156.1–7 K).
[13] Ibid. (VIII, 156.11–16 K).

It is therefore appropriate, in order to convince those who would still hesitate about where to locate the directive centre of the mind, to appeal to proof (ἀπόδειξις), avoiding the error committed by Archigenes, for whom this view depended purely on 'dogma' and had nothing to do with either reasoning or experience.[14] For as Galen had shown in his treatise *On the doctrines of Plato and Hippocrates*, to which he refers here, there is no doubt that the directive mind resides in the brain:

> as for the general belief that the mind resides in the brain (τὸ λογιζόμενον ἐν ἐγκεφάλῳ), the virile and irascible spirit in the heart (τὸ δ' ἀνδρεῖόν τε καὶ θυμοειδὲς ἐν καρδίᾳ), and the concupiscent part of the soul in the liver (τὸ δ' ἐπιθυμητικὸν ἐν ἥπατι), that is something you can learn any day when you hear it said of a madman that he is brainless (πρὸς μὲν τὸν ἀνόητον ὡς ἀκάρδιος εἴη), or about a pusillanimous or cowardly person that he has no heart (πρὸς δὲ τὸν ἄτολμον καὶ δειλὸν ὡς ἀκάρδιος εἴη).[15]

So when it is the passionate part of the soul, situated in the heart, that is affected, people will have a fierce, choleric and impetuous character, and when it is the concupiscent part of the soul, residing in the liver, they will be envious and jealous. Thus the affections that strike the passionate and concupiscent parts of the soul only influence character (τὸ ἦθος), unlike the lesions of the rational part of the soul, which give rise to melancholy, phrenitis, mania, epilepsy and lethargy, and are responsible for mental illnesses in the strict sense of the term. In fact Galen clearly distinguishes sicknesses of the directive mind that are situated in the brain from characterological problems:

> For clarity of exposition, let the functions of the rational mind (αἱ μὲν τοῦ λογιστικοῦ τῆς ψυχῆς ἐνέργειαι) be called 'directive', and those of non-rational minds (αἱ δὲ τῶν ἀλόγων) 'moral' (ἠθικαί); about the latter I do not intend to speak, or about the affections of the liver or the heart.[16]

We should note that, with this comment, Galen seems to be trying to situate the debate about mental illnesses outside the field of morality (ἠθική). But the tidy boundary that he draws here between what has to do with character features (τοῖς ἤθεσι) and originates in the heart or the liver, and that which on the other hand has to do with problems in reasoning or in the cognitive functions (τὸ λογικόν) does not appear as straightforward or as watertight in the rest of his work. Be that as it may, Galen asserts that rushing into

---

[14] Ibid. (VIII.158.16 K): τοῦτο τὸ περὶ τοῦ τῆς ψυχῆς ἡγεμονικοῦ (δόγμα).
[15] Ibid. (VIII.159–160 K).
[16] Ibid. III, 6 (VIII.163 K).

action, rapid, irascible or tyrannical, has to do with character alone and is caused by the heart's having a temperament that is warmer and drier than is appropriate.[17] Conversely, possessing a timorous character, cowardly and indolent, is the sign of the heart's having a temperament that is more damp and cold.[18]

As for the so-called mental illnesses caused by a lesion to the functioning of the rational mind, the great majority of them are to be explained by 'a cold condition that numbs the psychic functions'.[19] A small number of them, however, are to be explained by a warm condition:

> Bilious and warms illnesses seem to cause attacks of insomnia, delirium, and phrenitis. By contrast, phlegmatic and cold illnesses produce torpidity and drowsiness.

Another disequilibrium, this time between dryness and dampness, can be the origin of such illnesses, but it is secondary in relation to the imbalance of warmth and cold:

> The greatest potential for causing the illnesses that produce insomnia and drowsiness (τῶν ἀγρυπνητικῶν τε καὶ καταφορικῶν νοσημάτων) resides in the imbalance between hot and cold; after that, the imbalance between damp and dry. And in fact baths, by moistening the head, cause sleepiness (ὑπνώδεις ἐργάζονται); it is the same with unmixed wine and with food in general ... All these observations should show that unnatural dampness is less important in causing mental inertia (εἰς ἀγρίαν ψυχῆς), and that cold is more important.[20]

Finally, the imbalance at the origin of this or that psychic illness can occur in different parts of the brain, further complicating the business of diagnosis:

> All affections of this kind are born in the brain, and they differ from each other not only because of the variety in its make-up ..., but also because imbalances sometimes occur in the ventricles, sometimes in the vessels of the whole brain, sometimes in the humour disseminated across the substance of the brain, or finally when the actual mass of the brain becomes unhealthy (δύσκρατον).[21]

This picture can grow still more complicated as a result of the fact that certain affections of the irascible and concupiscent parts of the soul which are not mental illnesses in a strict sense, that is to say are not caused

---

[17] *Ars med.* XI, 1 (ed. Boudon-Millot [Budé v.2] 2000, 306).
[18] Ibid. XI, 5 (ed. Boudon-Millot, 308).
[19] *De loc. aff.* III, 6 (VIII.161.5–7 K).
[20] Ibid. (VIII.162 K).
[21] Ibid. (VIII.164 K).

by a lesion to the rational part of the soul, can nonetheless bring about a disequilibrium of the whole body's temperament and put its health in danger. It is for this reason that it is better to protect oneself against certain passions (τῶν ψυχικῶν παθῶν) such as rage (ὀργή), sorrow or chagrin (λυπή), enjoyment (ἡδονή), temper (θυμός), fear (φόβος), and envy (φθόνος), which are harmful not only to the health of the soul but just as much to the health of the body.[22] And Galen remarks that in general 'all the affections of the soul make the body dry' (πάντα τὰ ψυχικὰ πάθη ξηραίνει τὸ σῶμα).[23]

The best way of diagnosing a mental illness will consist of 'observing the sleep of those who have lost their memories or their intelligence, since madness is a consequence of a loss of intelligence'.[24] According to whether the sick person sleeps a lot or very little, the physician will judge that the condition of his/her brain is cold or warm. It is also useful to examine the residues that come from the head, through the nose or the mouth, to observe whether they are dry or damp. Thus one will observe that 'in cases of loss of memory or serious damage to it, the imbalance is always cold', so that it is appropriate to apply warming medications. This imbalance is not necessarily dry or humid, but if dryness or damp is present too, it is also appropriate to make the head more humid or more dry. One will observe that phrenitis and lethargy are habitually accompanied by fever, while mania and melancholy are free from it. The presence of fever must not lead the physician into error: in spite of appearances, lethargy and mania are caused by a cold temperament. The distinction between calm madness caused by a cold temperament, and an agitated, even violent, delirium caused by a hot temperament continues to constitute the dominant model.

In Galen's eyes, however, it remains easier to observe the effects of cold and heat, and of the humours that are associated with them (phlegm and yellow bile), than to give a satisfying rational explanation of them. And in his treatise *How the Faculties of the Mind Follow the Dispositions of the Body*, he admits his embarrassment:

---

[22] *Ars med.* XXIV, 8 (ed. Boudon-Millot, 351).

[23] Ibid. XXV, 5 (ed. Boudon-Millot, 353). One notes that on this point Galen diverges from Plato (*Timaeus* 43a), who posits a connection between intelligence and dryness. Galen notes in fact in *Quod animi mores* 4 (*SM* II, 42) that Plato maintained that under the effect of bodily humidity the soul begins to forget what it knew before being attached to the body, while conversely bodily dryness is accompanied by intelligence.

[24] *De loc. aff.* III, 7 (VIII.164 K): παραφυλάττειν οὖν χρὴ τοὺς ὕπνους τῶν ἀπολωλεκότων τὴν μνήμην ἢ τὴν σύνεσιν· ἀπώλεια γὰρ τῆς συνέσεως ἡ μώρωσίς ἐστι.

After extensive research I have not discovered why, when yellow bile accumulates in the brain, we are carried along towards delirium (εἰς παραφροσύνην), or in the case of black bile towards melancholia, or why phlegm and cooling substances in general provoke attacks of lethargy which bring on losses of memory and intelligence, or why drinking hemlock brings about dementia (μωρίαν).[25]

Galen takes the example of wine, which 'if it is drunk in moderation, contributes to making our soul gentler and at the same time more courageous, by means evidently of bodily temperament which is produced in turn by means of the humours'.[26] Indeed, the body's temperament is not only capable of modifying our mental faculties, it can also destroy them completely as happens after swallowing poison or after a fatal snake-bite. Galen may have used the following formula to sum up his thinking: 'The substance of the soul is the body's temperament' (τὴν οὐσίαν τῆς ψυχῆς ⟨κρᾶσιν ἢ δύναμιν εἶναι τοῦ σώματος⟩).[27] And in fact the subordination of the soul to the body's ills is all too evident in attacks of melancholy, phrenitis and mania, when 'you recognize neither yourself nor those who are dear to you', even though the visual faculty of sight is not at all affected.

Galen mentions several cases of violent or calm delirium, resulting of course in his view from a hot or cold disposition respectively, and he adopts different strategies to suit the cases. Thus he reports the case of a patient who was delirious (τινα παραπαίσαντα) for thirteen days and thought that he was in Athens though he was actually at Rome. As he was very agitated and his people had been unable to prevent him from going out, he was stricken in public by a violent epistaxis (nasal hemorrhage), followed by sweating, and so got his health back. But he had lost all memory of what had happened to him before, rather like people who have drunk too much, Galen comments, who when they sober up have forgotten all about what they did in a state of inebriation.[28] Apparently in a case like this, the loss of blood, together with sweating, by reducing the excessive heat in the brain, had sufficed to calm the sick person down without the intervention of the physician.

Galen also reports various cases of phrenitis, which he thinks comes in three forms, two simple and a third composed of the first two. In the first

---

[25] *Quod animi mores* 3 (*SM* II, 39, 12–18).

[26] Ibid. 3 (*SM* II, 39, 21).

[27] Ibid. 4 (*SM* II, 44). A formula which he may have borrowed from the Peripatetic Andronicos of Rhodes, that is if the text is correct (the passage suffers from a lacuna, which was filled in by Zeller; see the apparatus criticus).

[28] *De motu muscul.* II, 6 (IV.446–448 K).

type, intellectual judgement is affected but vision is not; in the second, judgement remains sound but the alteration of the senses (sight, hearing ...) leads the sick person to commit insane actions. Finally, certain sick people present the two forms of phrenitis at the same time, with alteration of both the senses and the judgement.[29] Thus Galen reports the case of an individual stricken by phrenitis in his house in Rome, who got out of bed and began to throw out of the window everything that came to hand, before throwing out one of his own slaves, who landed on the ground severely injured.[30] He also recalls that when he was young he was once afflicted with fever and hallucinations. Having understood that his intelligence had not been affected (ἀκριβῶς δὲ παρακολουθῶν ἐμαυτῷ μὴ παραπαίοντι κατὰ τὴν λογιστικὴν δύναμιν), he nonetheless feared that he was developing a case of phrenitis, and asked his friends who were present to come to his help by applying suitable affusions to his head (τὰς προσηκούσας ἐπιβροχὰς): all his symptoms diminished the following day.[31] Presumably these were affusions of cold water meant to reduce the excessive heat of the brain.

But Galen also describes cases of calm delirium like that of the patient who was exhausted by the fear that Atlas would be worn out by his job and would give up supporting the world on his shoulders. Suffering from frequent insomnia and profound anguish, this man developed a severe melancholy. Though Galen mentions this case on two different occasions, he unfortunately does not tell us how he treated this patient, only how he diagnosed his condition.[32]

Rare in fact are the cases in which Galen mentions a precise treatment for a psychic illness. There seem to be two reasons for this: in the first place, the treatment came down to re-establishing heat or cold, or dryness or dampness, with the help of the usual procedures, and was not supposed to be followed by very spectacular effects; and secondly, the more violent patients could only be approached with difficulty. Galen alludes to this difficulty, and to the necessity of carefully observing, in the case of psychic illnesses even more than in others, all the facts and patient's gestures before applying any treatment, in order to make as reliable a diagnosis as possible. This policy makes complete sense when one is aware that such patients, as Galen

---

[29] *De loc. aff.* IV, 2 (VIII.226 K), with the commentary of Pigeaud 1988b, 164.

[30] Ibid. IV, 2 (VIII.225–226 K).

[31] Ibid. IV, 2 (VIII.227 K).

[32] *In Hipp. Epid. 1 comm.* III, 1 (Wenkebach, *CMG* V 10, 1, 107, 24–32), and *In Hipp. Epid. 6 comm.* III, 1 (Pfaff, *CMG* V 10, 2, 2, 486–487).

remarks, can easily mislead one, alternating phases of delirium and periods of calm. Thus Galen mentions a rhetor and a mathematician (or geometer), both of them afflicted with phrenitis, who could nonetheless make coherent remarks about their fields and yet shortly afterwards pronounce the harshest invectives, and could also alternate between astonishing rashness and being terrified for the slightest reason.[33] And no doubt it is not an accident that the author of the little pseudo-Hippocratic treatise *How the Medical Student Should Behave* refers to what the physician has to put up with 'from people who are suffering from phrenitis or melancholic madness' and 'resist us physicians by violent means'.[34] So it is also recommended that the physician 'should make an effort to understand them, because not they but the unnatural nature of their affliction' is responsible for their violent behaviour.

The in a sense natural character of mental illnesses should induce the physician to be understanding and induce his entourage to show patience, always keeping in mind, as Plato knew, that 'the soul is damaged by an unhealthy mixture of the bodily humours'. In these circumstances, how much responsibility could be attributed to the patient, and how far could he collaborate in his own recovery and in his own well-being?[35]

The physical causes of their woes do not exempt the mentally ill from all responsibility. Galen can only deplore that the patient, 'when his mind falls sick and senseless for physical reasons, is erroneously considered to have been deliberately bad rather than unwell'.[36] But that does not lead Galen to exempt him from all responsibility. For the patient has a role to play in preventing illness. And Galen invites all who wish to come to learn from him what they need to eat and drink in order to improve their mental condition:

> For we know perfectly well that every nutriment is first of all absorbed in the stomach, undergoes an initial processing there, is then received into the veins that go from the liver to the stomach, and produces the humours of the body by which all parts of it are nourished including the brain, the heart and the liver. At the moment when they are nourished, these parts become warmer, colder or more damp than usual, in accordance with the humours that are dominant.[37]

---

[33] *In Hipp. Prorrh. 1 Comm.* I, 27 (Diels, *CMG* V 9, 2, 40–41).

[34] [Hippocrates], *Qualem oportet esse discipulum* (ed. K. Deichgräber, 1970). Probably later than Galen, this treatise antedates John Chrysostom, who cites it. See Jouanna 2010.

[35] *Quod animi mores* 6 (*SM* II, p. 49, 12–13).

[36] Ibid. 6 (*SM* II, p. 50), where Galen goes still further, saying that it is not right to praise some for their intelligence and blame others for their stupidity when none of the persons concerned are personally responsible.

[37] Ibid. 9 (*SM* II, 66, 17–67, 2).

For even if some people do not like the idea that nourishment (in so far as it influences the quality of the humours and the temperament of the body and the brain) can make people more or less reasonable and capable of controlling themselves, more courageous or cowardly, more gentle or quarrelsome, such is nevertheless the undeniable reality: 'let them come to me to learn what they ought to eat and drink'.[38]

The modern reader may perhaps be surprised to find listed here traits of character rather than mental disorders properly so called. The reason is that Galen is here in prophylactic mode, giving advice about diet that can improve not only the mental faculties (by modifying the 'temperament' of the brain) but also the moral dispositions of individuals (by modifying the 'temperaments' of the heart and the liver). That explains how Galen can promise his patients that they will profit very greatly from the regimen that he will recommend to them, not only on the ethical plane but on the intellectual plane as well by improving their intelligence and their memory—the first faculties to be affected by mental disorders:

> with regard to the faculties of the rational mind (κατὰ τὰς τοῦ λογιστικοῦ δυνάμεις), they will progress towards excellence (εἰς ἀρετήν) by acquiring more intelligence and more memory (συνετώτεροι καὶ μνημονικώτεροι γενόμενοι).[39]

No question therefore of giving in to bad habits, and in Galen's view (he can seldom resist citing Plato), 'one should try by whatever means to avoid what is bad and to choose the opposite, by means of diet, daily activities and knowledge'.[40]

Galen resorts to the same natural causes (linked to regimen) to explain both psychic illnesses (which affect the rational mind located in the brain) and the 'passions of the soul' (ψυχῆς πάθη) (which depend on the heart and the liver). In doing so, he claims to intervene in both of two areas that are now clearly separated, psychiatry and morals. So we meet here a fundamental difference between Galenic and modern medicine. But Galen is aware of a difficulty here and attempts to justify a physician's intervention in the sphere of morality by reference to the traditional ties between medicine and philosophy and in particular by arguing that a first-rate doctor must also be a philosopher.

---

[38] Ibid. 9 (*SM* II, 67, 2–9).
[39] Ibid. 9 (*SM* II, 67, 9–12).
[40] Ibid. 10 (*SM* II, 71, 22–72, 2), where he cites Plato, *Tim.* 87b.

2. When Psychic Illnesses Endanger the Health of the Body

More subtly, Galen attempts to legitimize his intervention on the basis of the claim that the 'passions of the soul' whose physiological causes he has so clearly set out are in turn harmful to the body: they can threaten its health and even lead to death. In consequence, the physician is justified in involving himself in curing every passion that is capable of threatening the physical integrity of the patient himself or of someone else, notably in cases of violence inflicted on a third party, for example under the influence of anger.

Among these emotions, and next to mental disorders such as delirium, phrenitis and mania, he enumerates in *On the Diagnosis and Treatment of the Passions of the Soul* every kind of passion that sometimes has the effect of rendering the sick person inaccessible to reason. To this category there belong especially dangerous passions such as rage and devoting one-self to 'drinking parties, courtesans and banquets'. Besides these *grandes passions*, there exist smaller ones which, just for this reason, tend to be ignored, such as 'the moderate trouble in the soul that occurs if you lose a lot of money or suffer dishonour, or eat an inappropriate quantity of pastries'.[41]

A little bit later, he gives a still fuller list, claiming that 'the affections of the soul, as everyone knows, are passion (θυμός), rage (ὀργή), fear (φόβος), dismay (λύπη), envy (φθόνος) and excessive desire (ἐπιθυμία)', before adding that excessive hate and love should also be included.[42] Further on still, he clarifies his thinking, saying that quarrelsomeness (φιλονεικία), love of glory (φιλοδοξία) and power-hunger (φιλαρχία) are also passions but to a lesser degree.[43] For it is envy that Galen designates as 'the worst of evils', defining it either as a separate passion or as a variety of sorrow, when it takes the form of 'feeling sorrow (λυπῆται) in the face of another's good fortune'. But still further on again, it is insatiability that is described as 'the vilest passion of the soul'.[44] The list of passions, like their 'hierarchy', is not exactly fixed but evolves within the treatise and from one treatise to another.

---

[41] *De propr. an. aff. cogn. et cur.* I, 2 (De Boer, *CMG* V 4, 1. 1, 5).

[42] Ibid. I, 3 (De Boer, 7).

[43] Ibid. I, 7 (De Boer, 24). The text is corrupt. The translation by Barras, who accepts De Boer's conjecture ἀπληστία and takes the meaning to be that 'insatiability is also a passion, but to a lesser degree', contradicts what is said about insatiability later in the treatise where it is said to be the vilest of all passions of the soul (I, 9 = p. 34).

[44] See previous n.

At all events, given the importance of the passions and their effects on bodily health, the physician will not accept any excuse from a person who gives up on protecting himself from them. Thus Galen remarks that just as old age should not be a pretext for neglecting our bodily health, so it should not lead us to give up improving our 'souls', so as 'not to become as ugly in that respect as Thersites was in his body'.[45] But while he sets the threshold of physical old age at fifty, he lowers the limit to forty as far as the soul is concerned, this being the age beyond which it can no longer be helped or corrected; though in certain cases, in order to avoid being criticized 'for being inhuman' he is willing to push this limit back to fifty.[46] For just as there is no perfect body and no perfect physical health—we have to content ourselves with the second, third or fourth best—, so the impossibility of reaching perfect health of the soul must not discourage us from making efforts in that direction as soon as posssible and ideally from childhood on.

Galen even considers that a person saved from his/her passions should be grateful to the healer 'even more than if he had cured us of a physical illness'. That seems a very strange opinion for a physician. The explanation is to be sought in Galen's childhood memories, and as always in such cases the figure of the father is not far away. Because it was Galen's father who by his example gradually taught him to contain his anger; he said that people inclined to anger 'deserved to suffer convulsions and even to die'. Passions such as insatiability with respect to food are thus likely to degrade the health of the body: gluttony leads to digestive troubles.[47] But there are still worse dangers, when grief brings about the ruin of the body. In *On Avoiding Distress* Galen describes the ill effects of excessive grief on one who had not learned to guard himself against it:

> And you have learned, you said, that even Philides the *grammaticus*, after the loss of his books in the fire, died consumed by discouragement and grief, while others went around for a long time dressed in black, thin and pale, looking like mourners.[48]

This anecdote is parallel to another one about a *grammaticus* named Callistus—they are so close in fact that they have to be about the same person:

> At Rome a short while ago I saw a grammaticus named Callistus whose books were destroyed in the great fire that burned down the Temple of Peace. He

---

[45] *De propr. an. aff. cogn.et cur.* I, 4 (De Boer, 11).
[46] Ibid. I, 10 (De Boer, 35).
[47] Ibid. I, 9 (De Boer, 31).
[48] *De indolentia* 7 (ed. Boudon-Millot and Jouanna, 4).

grieved over that and could not sleep. First he suffered from fevers and soon he declined and died.[49]

Without going to these extremes, insatiability, one of the worst passions as we have seen, can cause minor but real troubles, as in the case of the young man who came to see Galen one morning because he had been unable to sleep all night owing to worry about trivialities.[50] Which got him a long lecture from Galen on the need to master one's desires and passions.

The passions can also cause harm to other persons. It is enough to cite the case of Hadrian, described by Galen: in a rage, the emperor 'struck one of his slaves in the eye with a pen', blinding him. When the emperor regained his reason and asked the slave what he would like as compensation, the latter replied that he simply wanted his eye back, so true is it, says Galen, that bodily health is irreplaceable. A little later he reports the case of the choleric Cretan who struck two of his slaves on the head with the sharp edge of the sheath of his sword, wounding them severely (Galen leads us to believe that he saved their lives).[51]

For the treatment of such passions, Galen recommends never acting under the impulse of anger but always taking time for reflection, putting off a decision to the morrow if need be. Not respecting these instructions means exposing oneself to committing 'acts of real idiocy', and to behaving 'like an animal not a man'.[52] To avoid being reduced to this extreme state, it is advisable 'always to use reasoning after a dispassionate self-examination', in order to defeat 'the irrational faculty of the soul as if it were a savage beast'.[53]

However 'most people let the passions of the soul grow to the point where they become incurable', and one should therefore root them out before they are fully grown. In particular one should distrust the concupiscible faculty of the soul, which grows more powerful through enjoyment itself. To defeat it, one must use the irascible faculty of the soul as an ally. In fact the only way of weakening the concupiscible part of the soul is not to give it what it desires. Galen uses here the example of the sentiment of love, which once one begins to give into it becomes almost invincible, and he recounts the story of the man who came to seek help from him because he had become incapable of eradicating his passion.

---

[49] *In Hipp. Epid. Comm.* VI, 8 (Pfaff, *CMG* V 10, 2. 2, 486), partly extant only in Arabic.
[50] *De propr. an. aff. cogn.et cur.* I, 7 (De Boer, 25).
[51] Both these cases: ibid. I, 4 (De Boer, 13).
[52] Ibid. I, 5 (De Boer, 16).
[53] Ibid. I, 5 (De Boer, 19).

It is therefore necessary to learn to tame one's grief, one of the commonest causes of which is envy, envy of other people's success. Grief has in fact a peculiar status, since it is itself a passion but also results from other passions (envy, insatiability ...). What is more, 'grief is an evil for all, like bodily pain'.[54] The greatest virtue in Galen's eyes, the one which one should really strive for, consists therefore of 'protecting oneself from grief'.[55] 'For who would not like to be protected against grief throughout their life? And who would not choose that over the wealth of Cinyras or Midas?'.[56] The spiritual exercise of *praemeditatio*, which involves one in imagining the worst in order to prepare in case one day it happens, is therefore one of those particularly recommended by Galen in *On Avoiding Distress*.

But Galen goes still further with his claim that psychic health is more important than physical health. For he seems to think that it is enough to make sure that the body enjoys satisfactory health, no more, just allowing it what is necessary. In *On Avoiding Distress*, once again, he asserts that there is no loss that should grieve us as long as we have something to eat and drink and something to wear, in other words the basic means of protecting our physical health from hunger, thirst and cold.[57] Similarly, it is enough to have the money with which to provide for the natural and necessary needs of the body; all the rest is superfluous.

For all that, Galen does not approve the attitude of those individuals who 'are satisfied not to suffer or grieve in their souls', nor does he advocate the ideal of the Wise Man who is insensible to every desire and every emotion.[58] He does not think that he has himself reached the level of total impassibility, and he admits that certain things rightly cause us grief while other things deserve only indifference: thus he confesses that he despises money only as long he is not really hard-up, and that he is fearless about physical suffering as long as it does not turn into torture.[59] The ruin of his country or the loss of a friend are for him serious reasons for grief. And unlike some philosophers, he is far from wishing to experience such misfortunes in order to have a chance to show the strength of his soul. Galen prefers to

---

[54] Ibid. I, 7 (De Boer, 25).
[55] Ibid. I, 8 (De Boer, 29).
[56] Ibid. I, 9 (De Boer, 35).
[57] *De indolentia* 78b (Boudon-Jouanna, 24); the same idea is to be found in *De propr. an. aff. cogn.et cur.* I, 8 (De Boer, 30). See Boudon-Millot 2011.
[58] See *De indolentia* 62 et 68 (Boudon-Jouanna, 19 and 21) on the ἀοχλησία (absence of trouble) advocated by Epicurus.
[59] Ibid. 71 (Boudon-Jouanna, 21–22).

hope that no external event will ever befall him of such seriousness that it would completely ruin his health, or any misfortune so severe that his soul would not be capable of bearing it. Meanwhile he neglects no physical or spiritual exercise that could give his body and soul sufficient strength. He sums up by saying that he scorns losing money as long as he has enough for necessities, and scorns physical pain 'as long as he can still talk to a friend or follow a book being read to him'.[60] As long as these conditions are fulfilled, the health of the soul, which ought to be our first priority, will also be safe.

Conclusion

Galen refuses to envisage a radical natural separation of body and mind, he treats psychological illnesses as illnesses in the full sense of the term, and he identifies them as being capable of influencing a person's thinking, sentiments and behaviour strongly enough to make that person's social integration problematic or to cause him/her to suffer. Thus he escapes from a pernicious dualism such as has been much denounced by the main representatives of modern psychiatry. Similarly, in recognizing the brain as a bodily organ and in assigning a natural and physiological cause to psychological illnesses, Galen anticipates a trend in current psychiatry, the trend towards placing chemical causes at the root of mental illnesses, notably in the case of certain kinds of depression.

On the other hand he includes among psychological illnesses not only behavioural troubles, as modern psychiatry does, but also harmful passions, and thus he invades the field of ethics and unhesitatingly puts forward moral judgements that are altogether alien to his modern counterparts. It is true, however, that modern psychiatry, in Europe at least, seems to hesitate between two opposing tendencies: recognizing a positive role for the passions, which is supposed to make us more sensitive to certain emotions, and even make us more intelligent, and repressing these same passions on the grounds that they are dangerous to society.

But above all, Galen's notion that psychological illnesses have a cultural and intellectual dimension as well as physical causes can contribute to the contemporary debate in the neurosciences of our time about the responsibility of the mental patient. Thus explaining sicknesses of the soul by reference to a bad mixture of temperaments (with Galen), or by the

---

[60] Ibid. 78b (Boudon-Jouanna, 24).

malfunctioning of neurons (with some contemporary neurobiologists), should not lead to the conclusion that the sick person is without responsibility for, or a hold on, what is happening to him/her just because temperament or neurons come into the matter. Galen furthermore agrees with the increasing number of people who are beginning to think that the model of mental illness adopted by the neurosciences is far from self-evident, and that other approaches can be equally legitimate. His assertion that a human being is never a simple aggregate of humours, and his emphasis on the primacy of culture and education and on the need for mutual confidence between patient and doctor, anticipate the positions of some contemporary psychiatrists. For the latter too reject a reductive view of the human being (he/she is not a simple collection of neurons); they prefer a global approach to mental illness and always struggle to combine medicinal treatment aimed at modifying the body's chemistry with an (indispensable) patient-doctor dialogue.

DISTURBING CONNECTIONS:
SYMPATHETIC AFFECTIONS, MENTAL DISORDER,
AND THE ELUSIVE SOUL IN GALEN

Brooke Holmes[*]

Galen's *On Prognosis* reads less like a medical treatise than like a collection of detective stories, more Holmesean than Hippocratean.[1] In one memorable case, Galen, self-consciously following in the footsteps of his Hellenistic predecessor Erasistratus, diagnoses the lovesickness of a woman infatuated with the dancer Pylades. The star performer in the diagnosis, besides Galen himself, is the pulse. That is not to say there is an 'erotically motivated pulse', as some people think. Rather, Galen emphasizes, the pulse loses its natural rhythms whenever the mind is disturbed, an instance of the more general principle that 'the body tends to be affected by mental conditions'.[2] The trick, accordingly, is to figure out what is disturbing the mind, which Galen succeeds in doing by observing fluctuations in the woman's pulse when Pylades' name comes up.

The principle that the body is affected by the mind or, more commonly, the soul had become common by the time Galen was writing in the second century CE. It was often taken as the flipside of another principle—namely, that the mind or the soul is affected by the body. From at least the Hellenistic period and possibly earlier, both tenets fit into the overarching framework of what was called sympathy (*sympatheia*). Galen himself firmly held that the body and, especially, its troubles have an impact on psychic and mental functions, going so far as to write a treatise at the end of his life entitled *That the Faculties of the Soul Follow the Mixtures of the Body*.[3] He also made

[*] I would like to thank the audience at the 'Mental Disorders in Classical Antiquity' conference at Columbia, as well as audiences at the Institute of Classical Studies in London and Stanford University, for helpful comments, criticisms, and suggestions on this paper, especially Serafina Cuomo, Catharine Edwards, Philip van der Eijk, Miriam Leonard, Jake Mackey, Glenn Most, and Reviel Netz; I owe a particular debt to Peter Singer. I am grateful, too, to William Harris and Chris Gill for their responses to the written version.

[1] As Barton 1994, 140–143 observes.
[2] Galen, *Praen.* 6 (XIV 634–635 K = 104, 12–23 Nutton).
[3] I adopt Jacques Jouanna's suggestion (2009, 192) for the translation of the title of the treatise, but I retain the standard abbreviation (*QAM*) for convenience and consistency.

extensive use of sympathy as a pathological concept in his writings, drawing on earlier usage within the learned medical tradition.[4] But what Galen does not do is privilege, at least explicitly, the relationship between the mind and the body as a site of sympathy. Moreover, he is downright wary of implicating the *psychē* in the sympathetic networks that he maps onto a well-defined anatomical landscape. In this paper, I try to account for Galen's bipolar relationship to sympathy in the realm of mental disturbance by asking the following questions: What conceptual and explanatory work does sympathy do for Galen in this realm? Why is he so reluctant to apply it to the soul?

Taking up these inquiries has the advantage of yielding an unfamiliar angle on Galen's psychology and, more specifically, his psychopathology. These topics have attracted a good deal of attention in recent years.[5] Yet analyses of Galen's views on the soul and its relationship to the body have been mostly confined to the obviously psychological works, such as his massive, mid-career opus the *Doctrines of Plato and Hippocrates* and the aforementioned *That the Faculties of the Soul Follow the Mixtures of the Body*. The concept of sympathy brings us into the territory of other texts, most notably *On the Affected Parts*, where the lines between the brain, the rest of the body, and the soul intersect and fail to intersect in ways that shed new light on Galen's ideas about how the body disrupts mental functions.

The inquiry undertaken here also has repercussions for the larger question of the relationship between the mind or soul and the body in antiquity. One of the aspects of sympathy that makes it so intriguing is that the concept posits an affective connection without spelling out how that connection occurs or what ground joins the partners. The open-ended nature of sympathy emerges as particularly significant when the partners are the body and the soul or the mind, for the reason that it can be difficult to grasp the nature of the space where these entities meet (think of the enigmatic pineal gland in the writings of Descartes). In some cases, the language of sympathy is no more than an acknowledgment that two entities, say the body and the

---

On 'mental' faculties—primarily reasoning, memory, and judgment—see, e.g., *Loc. Aff.* 2.10 (VIII 126 K), 3.9 (VIII 174–175 K); *QAM* 2 (IV 770–771 K = 34,16–35,3 Müller). The soul is also responsible for sensation and volitional movement.

[4] The standard study of sympathy in Galen remains Siegel 1968, 360–382, who is primarily interested in reading Galen in light of contemporary medical knowledge, especially neurology. See also the discussion of sympathy and continuities in the body at De Lacy 1979, 361–363.

[5] On Galen's psychology and psychopathology, see García-Ballester 1988; Pigeaud 1988b (with discussion of *On the Affected Parts*); Hankinson 1991a; von Staden 2000, 106–116; Tieleman 2003b; Hankinson 2006; Donini 2008; Jouanna 2009; Gill 2010a.

soul, are affected in tandem, as in the experience of fear. But such language may also set the stage for an exploration of the routes by which affections are trafficked between the body and the soul.

The name of Descartes raises the question of dualism and indeed, the difficulty of understanding how the body and the soul (or the mind) interact presupposes that these are different—and perhaps quite radically different—things to begin with. If we look at our earliest Greek medical texts, we find a proto-sympathetic model of the body as an interior space with communicating parts and migrating affections with little sense of a difference between the *sōma* and the *psychē*, when these terms even appear. The Hippocratic authors largely take it for granted that the functions ascribed by later writers to the *psychē* or the 'hegemonic principle' are damaged alongside bodily functions. By the fourth century BCE, however, the concept of the unified organism found in the Hippocratic writings is being strained by the sharpening contrast between the *sōma* and the *psychē*. It is Plato, of course, who seems to have developed the opposition most extensively, while leaving open the quandary of the *koinōnia*, 'common ground', between them as Aristotle complains a generation later.[6] Aristotle himself, far from solving the quandary definitively, bequeaths an even more complex version of it to subsequent philosophers. He transmits, too, a nascent concept of sympathy as one strategy for negotiating the relationship of the *sōma* and the *psychē*. That concept became part of the Peripatetic philosophical arsenal, acquiring even greater importance in the Stoics and the Epicureans

The post-Hippocratic landscape of psychophysical models is defined, too, by debates about where the hegemonic faculties are located in the body (the problem Descartes was trying to solve with the pineal gland).[7] Aristotle's decision to locate these faculties in the heart is enthusiastically supported by his Peripatetic followers and the Stoics, even as systematic human dissection (and possibly vivisection) in Ptolemaic Alexandria gathers evidence in favor of the brain. The debate is still very much alive centuries later

---

[6] Aristotle, *De An.* 407b13–26. Dillon 2009 analyzes Plato's reticence about the nature of the *koinōnia* of soul and body.

[7] The question of location is raised in some fifth-century treatises, such as *On the Sacred Disease*, whose author forcefully defends an encephalocentric model (although the source of hegemonic power is the air, not the brain itself): see *Morb. Sacr.* 14–17 (VI 386–394 Littré = 25,12–31,15 Jouanna), with Lo Presti 2008. But the lines of the later debate are established decisively in the fourth century BCE, with Aristotle's endorsement of the heart. On the location of cognitive processes in fifth- and fourth-century BCE medical writing and in Aristotle, see van der Eijk 2005a, 206–237.

when Galen enters the fray. Building on the models of articulated networks (arterial, venous, nervous) yielded by Hellenistic anatomical research, he aggressively marshals arguments for the brain as the home of the hegemonic principle by demonstrating its position as the major node in the nervous system.

It is precisely because Galen enmeshes the brain so deeply in the neural and also the vascular networks crisscrossing the body that it is especially vulnerable to affections arising in other parts of the body. Galen, like physicians before him, classified these affections as sympathetic. By privileging the brain as a locus of such affections, Galen, I will argue, generates a new model of mind-body sympathy. More specifically—and significantly for this volume—he tilts that model toward pathology by focusing on how the mental faculties become sympathetically implicated in the disturbances of other parts of the body and especially, as we will see, the gut. One consequence of the shift is that the physician becomes an important player in securing cognitive health.

And yet, as I observed above, for all that Galen embeds the 'ruling part' or mind in the body via the brain, he is conspicuously silent on the sympathetic relationship of the *soul* to the body. His tacit rejection of sympathy in this sense cannot be chalked up to a lack of interest in the major philosophical accounts of psychology. Galen, after all, saw himself as straddling medicine and philosophy, the traditions represented for him by his heroes Hippocrates and Plato. Rather, in Galen's treatment of sympathy we can glimpse divergences and tensions between medicine and philosophy, and especially the difficulties in conceptualizing the human that are raised by dissection. For it is as if the more precise Galen is about the lines joining the brain to the rest of the body, the more elusive the soul, that marker of the truly human self, becomes for him. At the same time, the networks of veins, arteries, and nerves that he uncovers suggest a different tripartite psychology than the one he claims to have inherited from Plato. Galen's engagement with sympathy may give us a glimpse, then, of both the promise and the limits of the anatomical body as a map of the unified human being in the second century CE.

I begin by briefly discussing some Hippocratic passages where the concept of the body as a unity with communication between parts—the language of sympathy does not appear in classical-era medical texts—is broached. In the next section, I sketch the development of the idea of 'suffering together' as part of a larger category of states or processes or events 'common to body and soul' in Plato, Aristotle, and the Hellenistic philosophical schools. In the final section, I examine how Galen uses the concept of sympathy against this medical and philosophical backdrop, concentrating on the susceptibility of the brain to affections originating in the gut. I close by reconsidering Galen's lifelong resistance to locating the soul within the coordinates of the sympathetically webbed body.

The Internally Communicating Body in Early Greek Medicine

Heraclitus famously said that in the circumference of the circle, the beginning and the end are common (Diels-Kranz 22 B103). The fascination with the circle has a long afterlife in philosophy. It found its way into medicine as well. In the opening lines of the Hippocratic treatise *On Places in a Human Being*, the author writes that:[8]

> ἐμοὶ δοκεῖ ἀρχὴ μὲν οὖν οὐδεμία εἶναι τοῦ σώματος, ἀλλὰ πάντα ὁμοίως ἀρχὴ καὶ πάντα τελευτή· κύκλου γὰρ γραφέντος ἀρχὴ οὐχ εὑρέθη.
>
> (*Loc.* 1, VI 276 Littré = 36,1–3 Craik)
>
> It seems to me that there is no beginning point of the body, but every part is beginning and end alike, as the beginning point of the figure of a circle is not found.

The maxim lies behind two significant axioms of the author's theory of diseases. First, each part of the body, upon falling ill, produces disease in another part (e.g., the cavity in the head, the head in the flesh and the cavity).[9] The second is more opaque:

> τὸ δὲ σῶμα αὐτὸ ἑωυτῷ τωὐτόν ἐστι καὶ ἐκ τῶν αὐτῶν σύγκειται, ὁμοίως δὲ οὐκ ἐχόντων, καὶ τὰ σμικρὰ αὐτοῦ καὶ τὰ μεγάλα καὶ τὰ κάτω καὶ τὰ ἄνω· καὶ εἴ τις βούλεται τοῦ σώματος ἀπολαβὼν μέρος κακῶς ποιεῖν τὸ σμικρότατον, πᾶν τὸ σῶμα αἰσθήσεται τὴν πεῖσιν, ὁποίη ἄν τις ᾖ, διὰ τόδε ὅτι τοῦ σώματος τὸ σμικρότατον πάντα ἔχει, ὅσα περ καὶ τὸ μέγιστον· τοῦτο δ' ὁποῖον ἄν τι πάθῃ, τὸ σμικρότατον ἐπαναφέρει πρὸς τὴν ὁμοεθνίην ἕκαστον πρὸς τὴν ἑωυτοῦ, ἤν τε κακόν, ἤν τε ἀγαθὸν ᾖ· καὶ διὰ ταῦτα καὶ ἀλγεῖ καὶ ἥδεται ὑπὸ ἔθνεος τοῦ σμικροτάτου τὸ σῶμα, ὅτι ἐν τῷ σμικροτάτῳ πάντ' ἔνι τὰ μέρεα, καὶ ταῦτα ἐπαναφέρουσιν ἐς τὰ σφέων αὐτῶν ἕκαστα, καὶ ἐξαγγέλλουσι πάντα.   (*Loc.* 1, VI 278 Littré = 36,26–38,3 Craik)
>
> The body is itself identical to itself and composed of the same things, although not in uniform disposition, both its small parts and its large parts, those below and those above. And if someone should take the smallest part of the body

---

[8] See also *Nat. Oss.* 11 (IX 182 Littré = 149,14–18 Duminil); *Vict.* I 19 (VI 492–494 Littré = 138,28–29 Joly and Byl), where the circle is understood literally as a circuit in the body. On the use of the passages to support the (now-discredited) argument that the early medical writers intuited the circulation of the blood, see C.R.S. Harris 1973, 48–49.

[9] *Loc.* 1 (VI 276 Littré = 36,9–15 Craik).

and cause it harm, the whole body will feel the damage, of whatever sort it is, for the reason that the smallest part of the body has all the things that the greatest part has. Whatever the smallest part experiences, it passes it on to its related part, each to that which is related to it, whether it is something good or bad. The body, on account of these things, feels pain and pleasure from the smallest constituent, because in the smallest part all the parts are present, and these communicate with the parts that are their own and inform them of everything.

The figure of a part communicating its pain to the whole will become standard for representing a unified and internally connected cosmos in later philosophy, especially in the Stoics.[10] If the work the figure performs here is more limited, it nevertheless powerfully confirms the author's commitment to the idea that the body is an integrated whole, rather than an agglomeration of parts.

Both these 'proto-sympathetic' concepts assume that affections migrate beyond the point of origin. Yet they offer different perspectives on the relationship between the affected part and the larger structure. The first explains an affection that arises in one part and is transported to another by stuffs—usually fluids—along the generic 'vessels' (*phlebes, phlebia, teuchea*) that connect different parts and flow into one another.[11] Fluids are trafficked through these vessels according to rules of attraction (moving towards the dry part, being drawn downwards naturally).[12] The two affected parts, then, are materially conjoined: permanently by a vessel or a network of vessels; contingently by the transmission of the *materia peccans*. The idea that the same vessels that allow life-giving fluid and air to circulate also enable the movement of noxious stuffs is a fundamental tenet of humoral

---

[10] See Sextus Empiricus, *Math.* 9.80 (*SVF* 2.1013): εἴ γε δακτύλου τεμνομένου τὸ ὅλον συνδιατίθεται σῶμα. ἡνωμένον τοίνυν ἐστὶ σῶμα καὶ ὁ κόσμος (If the finger is cut, the whole body suffers with it. The cosmos, too, then, is a unified body). On the sympathetic cosmos, see below, n. 46. See also Alexander, *Mantissa* § 3 (117,10–22 Bruns), responding to the Stoics.

[11] *Loc.* 3 (VI 282 Littré = 40,30–31 Craik). For the author's understanding of the vascular system, see Duminil 1983, 79–82. See also *Artic.* 45 (III 556 Littré = 107,10–108,5 Kühlewein) on 'vascular' connectivity. On the movement of moisture through the principle by which the body communicates with itself (τὸ σῶμα κοινωνέον αὐτὸ ἑωυτῷ), see *Loc.* 9 (VI 292 Littré = 48,13–14 Craik). It is worth noting, too, that the verb *koineō* is often used with the sense of 'connecting' parts of the body in the surgical treatises: see *Artic.* 13 (IV 118 Littré = 134,8 Kühlewein), 45 (IV 190 Littré = 172,3 Kühlewein), 86 (IV 324 Littré = 243,8 Kühlewein); *Fract.* 9 (III 450 Littré = 62,4 Kühlewein), 10 (III 450 Littré = 62,15 Kühlewein), 11 (III 452 Littré 3.452 = 63,15 Kühlewein).

[12] On the (usually pathological) movement of fluids through the body in various Hippocratic texts, see Gundert 1992, 458–462.

pathology and probably explains the importance of the vessels themselves in Hippocratic concepts of the body.[13]

The second principle puts the migration of an affection in terms of a principle of 'relatedness' (*homoethnie*) that joins the 'smallest parts' of the body to one another. The context is not disease, but rather pleasure and pain, that is, affections thought to be experienced by the body as a whole, rather than in one or more of its parts. The parts in question, moreover, are not the larger structures of the body, such as the head or the cavity, but presumably something like its basic building blocks.[14] These smallest parts participate in a community (*ethnos*) where each 'announces' pain and pleasure to the others.

The idea that the parts of the body form an *ethnos*—a word used of a group of people living together, often, in the medical writers, under the same climactic and environmental conditions—is not found elsewhere in the classical-era Hippocratic writings.[15] The term *homoethnie* does appear once in the gynecological treatises, where a uterine affection results in the swelling of the breasts according to their 'relatedness'.[16] The bond between the womb and the breasts, however, takes us back to the relationship between parts at the macro-level of the body instead of an integrated stratum

---

[13] Duminil 1983, 128–131 argues that as the medico-philosophical understanding of the vascular system improved in the later fifth and fourth centuries, writers were more constrained in imagining the circulation of stuffs within the body. Duminil's account of the development of vascular knowledge in the Corpus seems a bit too neat, but her insight that anatomy can shape an understanding of sympathetic affections is borne out in Galen: see, e.g., *Loc. Aff.* 1.6 (VIII 57, VIII 60–63 K), 3.14 (VIII 208 K), 4.7 (VIII 257 K); *PHP* 8.1.3–4 (V 649–650 K = 480,16–24 De Lacy).

[14] Vegetti 1965, 292, in keeping with his view that the treatise was written by a member of Anaxagoras's circle, sees here the influence of Anaxagorean ideas of mixture (esp. Diels-Kranz 59 B6).

[15] For *ethnos* as a group of people in the Hippocratic Corpus, see *Aer.* 12 (II 52 Littré = 219,12 Jouanna), 13 (II 56 Littré = 222,11 Jouanna), 17 (II 66 Littré = 230,6 Jouanna); *Vict.* II 37 (VI 528 Littré =158,5 Joly and Byl). At *Flat.* 6 (VI 98 Littré = 110,4 Jouanna), it refers to 'species' of living beings. For the *homo-* prefix, see *Nat. Hom.* 3 (VI 38 Littré = 170,10 Jouanna): *homophulos*; *Vict.* I 6 (VI 480 Littré = 130,8 Joly and Byl): *homotropos*.

[16] *Mul.* II 174 (VIII 354 Littré). See also *Epid.* II 1.6 (V 76 Littré) on the 'association' (*koinōnie*) between the chest, breasts, genitals, and voice. On proto-sympathetic affections, see also *Artic.* 41 (IV 180 Littré = 165,14 Kühlewein), 49 (IV 216 Littré = 184,13 Kühlewein), with *koinōneō*; *Glan.* 2 (VIII 556 Littré = 66,8–9 Craik), with *symponeō*; *Prorrh.* II 38 (IX 68 Littré = 284 Potter), with *epikoinōneō*. At *Epid.* VI 3.24 (V 304 Littré = 76,4–5 Manetti-Roselli) and *Hum.* 20 (V 500 Littré), we find references to *hai koinōniai* with the sense of sympathetic affections. For co-affection in Diocles of Carystus, writing in the mid fourth century BCE, see fr. 72 (van der Eijk), where the heart changes its condition (συνδιατιθεμένης καὶ τῆς καρδίας) during an inflammation of the diaphragm—that is, phrenitis; see also fr. 80 (van der Eijk).

at the micro-level. For a self-conscious concept of the integrated whole, we are better off looking to the treatise *On Regimen*, whose first chapters are a veritable paean to the unified and well-structured organism.[17]

The opening discussion is unusual, first, for its degree of interest in the cosmological dimension of medicine and includes a developed account of the mirroring of macrocosm and microcosm, each a blend of fire and water and structurally homologous to the other.[18] What also makes *On Regimen* distinctive is its developed account of human nature in terms of *sōma* and *psychē*.[19] It is worth stressing, however, that the author's approach is not dualistic: the body and the soul enjoy a strongly symbiotic relationship, underscoring a principle of unity that is stressed at the macrocosmic level as well.[20] In particular, the *psychē*, despite being endowed with its own identity, is thought to execute its functions (e.g., sensory, cognitive faculties) most effectively when the blend of fire and water in the body is optimal, free of impurities, and otherwise undisturbed, a state that can be adjusted through proper diet and exercise.[21]

Here, then, we have a psychophysical model that represents soul and body in terms of a unity affected as a whole without sacrificing the sense that soul and body are different domains. The language of sympathy, however, here as elsewhere in the classical-era Hippocratic texts, is not used. Nor is the author much concerned with how the body and the soul share affections: it is enough that both are composed of fire and water. In this respect, the treatise is a good example of the unproblematic holism of most of the Hippocratic texts, despite its apparent dualism.

---

[17] See esp. *Vict.* 16 (VI 478–480 Littré = 128,24–130,17 Joly and Byl), 10 (VI 484 Littré = 134,5–6 Joly and Byl). See also *Vict.* 18 (VI 482 Littré = 132,8–10 Joly and Byl) on *symphōnie*.

[18] On microcosm and macrocosm in the treatise, see esp. Jouanna 1998; in the Hippocratic Corpus more generally, see Magdelaine 1997; Le Blay 2005.

[19] The Hippocratic writers do not speak of the *psychē* very often, and they oppose it to the *sōma* only rarely: see Holmes 2010b, 183, with n. 142.

[20] Cambiano 1980 and Jouanna 1998 rightly reject earlier speculation about the author's Orphic-Pythagorean affiliations to establish the thoroughgoing materialism of his theory of the *psychē*.

[21] For the soul's dependence on the condition of the body, see, e.g., *Vict.* I 35 (VI 518 Littré = 154,20–21 Joly and Byl): ἢν γὰρ ὑγιηρῶς ἔχῃ τὸ σῶμα καὶ μὴ ὑπ' ἄλλου τινὸς συνταράσσηται, τῆς ψυχῆς φρόνιμος [ἡ] σύγκρησις (For if the body is in a healthy condition and is not disturbed by anything, the blend of the soul is intelligent). The condition of the soul does not rely solely on the body, as the author makes clear at *Vict.* I 36 (VI 522–524 Littré = 156,19–32 Joly and Byl), stressing those problems (such as the nature of the 'circuit') that regimen cannot correct. The body depends on the soul, too, to monitor its care, primarily through dreams that communicate incipient diseases, as we see in Book IV.

The idea that the parts of a human being may be neatly split into the body, on the one hand, and the mind (*nous, noos*) or the *psychē*, on the other, was gaining ground in the later fifth century BCE. So, too, was the idea that functions framed as mental or psychic might be impaired by disturbances in the body. By the end of the fifth century, Xenophon's Socrates can ask a student dodging physical fitness training, 'Who doesn't know that many err in the act of thinking because the body is not in good health?'[22] It is not a coincidence that Socrates shows up in this context. For the burgeoning field of philosophical ethics is enthusiastically tackling soul-body relations in this period, including the question of how the soul shares *its* affections with the body.[23] I turn now to the growth of sympathy as a strategy for negotiating the relationship of the *psychē* and the *sōma* in classical and Hellenistic philosophy before considering the philosophical and medical legacies of sympathy in Galen.

Sympathetic Bodies and Souls

The idea of 'suffering together' is a capacious one: as I have already said, it leaves open the nature of the ground shared by the affected parts and the nexus between them. In the philosophical tradition, sympathy can be situated within an even larger, more nebulous class of states, functions, processes, and experiences represented as 'common to body and soul'.[24] The concept of 'common to body and soul' may have appeared for the first time in Plato's *Philebus*, where Socrates describes *aisthēsis* (henceforth translated as 'sensation') as a movement—or, more specifically, a 'shock'—that is not simply 'common' to body and soul but also 'particular to each' (σεισμόν ... ἴδιόν τε καὶ κοινὸν ἑκατέρῳ, *Phlb.* 33d5–6).[25] The movement begins in the body

---

[22] ἐν τῷ διανοεῖσθαι, τίς οὐκ οἶδεν, ὅτι καὶ ἐν τούτῳ πολλοὶ μεγάλα σφάλλονται διὰ τὸ μὴ ὑγιαίνειν τὸ σῶμα; (Xenophon, *Mem.* 3.12.6); see also Herodotus 3.33; [Hippocrates] *Ep.* 23 (IX 394 Littré = 102,9 Smith); Plato, *Phlb.* 66d3–7.

[23] The *psychē* is already seen as causing problems for the *sōma* in the later fifth century, most clearly at Democritus (Diels-Kranz 68) B159, where the *sōma* takes the *psychē* to court for the abuse inflicted on it through the soul's 'love of pleasure'. See Holmes 2010b, 202–206.

[24] For recent essays on the ancient concept of 'common to body and soul', see R. King 2006.

[25] The language of 'shock' is not insignificant. Socrates presents the ideal state in the *Philebus* as one of no disturbance at all (e.g., 33a8–b11). Given that this is impossible for human beings, the next best option is minimal disturbance, still understood as vaguely pathological. On the 'medicalization' of pains and pleasures in the *Philebus*, see D. Frede 1992, 440, 453–454, 456.

(and can end there if it is 'extinguished' before reaching the soul).[26] But
it is properly sensation only when we find 'the soul and the body coming
together in one common affection and being moved in common' (τὸ δ' ἐν
ἑνὶ πάθει τὴν ψυχὴν καὶ τὸ σῶμα κοινῇ γιγνόμενον κοινῇ καὶ κινεῖσθαι, 34a3–4).
The experience of sensation is an event, then, that preserves the boundary
between the body and the soul while allowing for communication between
them. It creates shared suffering but each affection is nevertheless realized
differently in each domain.

The experience of sensation remains a central locus for the meeting of
sōma and psychē in Aristotle's writings. In fact, Aristotle considers a number of states common to body and soul precisely because they participate in
sensation: being awake, pleasure and pain, and desire all fall into this category.[27] Yet Aristotle also departs in some respects from Plato's understanding
of the psychophysical nature of sensation. Whereas in the Philebus, Plato
represents sensation as a 'shock' powerful enough to ripple into the psychē
from the body, in the De Anima Aristotle develops an account of sensation as
a process that, while accomplished through the body, should be understood
as the actualization of a psychic faculty.[28] By assigning the passive role to the
bodily organs of sensing and granting the soul greater agency, he ramps up
the degree of difference between the body and the soul within the shared
experience of sensing. The Aristotle of the De Anima thus represents sensation less as a disturbance, necessary but troubling, and more as an activity
that is natural to ensouled animals.[29]

And yet, Aristotle does speak of affections of the soul. One of the conun-
drums that he raises in the opening pages of the De Anima is whether the
affections of the soul are always shared with that which holds it—namely,
the body (403a3–5). Having briefly entertained the possibility that the soul
acts independently of the body in cognition, he concludes that:

---

[26] On unfelt movements in the body, see Plato, Phlb. 33d2–34a5, 43b7–c6; Ti. 64a2–65b3.
Other experiences, too, do not qualify as common to body and soul. At Phlb. 36b8–9, for
example, the soul and the body have divergent experiences of pleasure and pain. See also
36b12–c1, on a 'double pain' arising independently in the psychē and the sōma; 41b11–d2. On
the psychē-sōma relationship at 33c–d, see Evans 2004; Holmes 2010a, 361–362.

[27] See esp. Aristotle, Sens. 436b1–3. For the expression 'common to body and soul', see also
De An. 433b19–21; Part. An. 643a35; Somn. Vig. 454a7–8. For the koinōnia of body and soul, see
De An. 407b18 and Long. 2, 465a31.

[28] Aristotle does, in some texts, speak of movements in the soul caused, for example, by
pleasure: see Ph. 244b11–12, with Menn 2002, 87–88 (arguing for a developmentalist reading
of the De Anima). See also Menn 2002, 100, 113, 117 on the contrast of the De Anima with the
Philebus.

[29] For the emphasis on the soul as an agent, see Menn 2002; Morel 2006.

ἔοικε δὲ καὶ τὰ τῆς ψυχῆς πάθη πάντα εἶναι μετὰ σώματος, θυμός, πραότης, φόβος, ἔλεος, θάρσος, ἔτι χαρὰ καὶ τὸ φιλεῖν τε καὶ μισεῖν· ἅμα γὰρ τούτοις πάσχει τι τὸ σῶμα.   (Aristotle, *De An.* 403a16–19)

It is likely that all the affections of the soul are with the body: anger, gentleness, fear, pity, courage, and joy, as well as loving and hating. For together with these things the body suffers something.

Shortly thereafter, Aristotle provisionally concludes that it is likely that all the affections of the soul occur *with* the body (μετὰ σώματος, 403a17).

How should we interpret these statements? Aristotle will go on in the *De Anima* to call into question the idea of psychic affections by arguing that emotions are not, in fact, movements occurring in the soul, contrary to the conventional way of speaking.[30] It is difficult to know, moreover, how he understands the terms and modalities of the 'association' or 'partnership' (*koinōnia*) between the body and the soul as it is presented here. Still, without venturing too far into these vexed questions, we can make a few observations about the passage under consideration.

First, to the extent that there is a primary affection at all, it originates with or somehow belongs to the soul, not the body. Moreover, Aristotle speaks in terms of simultaneity and coordination rather than causal interaction without spelling out the relationship between the affections of the soul and the 'something' suffered by the body.[31] Finally, the *De Anima* passage seems to confirm that, in Aristotle's hands, the concept of 'common to body and soul' loses the faintly pathological overtones that it has in the *Philebus*, gravitating instead toward normal events or states (e.g., sensation and states accompanied by sensation like waking and emotion).[32] At the same time, the *De Anima* passage is not the whole story. Elsewhere in his corpus and especially in the biological and physiological writings, Aristotle grants certain states of the body the power to facilitate or disrupt processes such as memory and thought.[33] While he at times speaks in terms of simultaneous events or states, in other cases he uses language indicating that the body *causes* disturbances in the soul.[34]

---

[30] See esp. *De An.* 408b1–15, with Witt 1992, 179–182; Menn 2002, 99–101.

[31] Rapp 2006 emphasizes the absence of causal interaction on the Aristotelian model compared to Hellenistic accounts of psychophysical sympathetic affections.

[32] The *koinōnia* of the *sōma* and the *psychē* also has pathological connotations at Plato, *Phd.* 65a1, c8, 67a3–4; *Resp.* 611b10–c1.

[33] For a discussion of this material, see esp. van der Eijk 2000a, 66–68, 70–77; and, by the same author, 2005 [1997].

[34] On the language of simultaneity, see, e.g., *Ph.* 248a2–6. On causal language, see van der Eijk 2005a, 223–237, esp. 235: 'Passages … in which weight is said to 'make' (ποιεῖν) the soul

In short, Aristotle presents a complex, opaque, and not always consistent picture of the overlap between the affections of the body and the 'affections' of the soul. The fraught nature of the soul's relationship to what the body undergoes and the ambiguous status of psychic affectability *tout court* may help us understand an intriguing situation. By invoking the concept of 'common to body and soul' at crucial moments in his account of the animal as a psychophysical unity, Aristotle seems to play a critical role in endowing that concept with philosophical traction. And yet, he does not habitually use the more specific language of sympathy in his corpus to describe body-soul relations, even in the more biological works. To be fair, both the noun *sympatheia* and the verb *sympaskhein* are relatively infrequent in this period. But it may also be that, for Aristotle, the language of suffering together does not sufficiently differentiate between what happens to a body and a psychic state or function. In other words, on those occasions when Aristotle is puzzling over just how the body and the soul are implicated in one another, difference is as important as coordination—above all in the realm of acting and being acted upon.

It is interesting in this context to observe that when, in the *Prior Analytics*, we do find Aristotle using the verb 'to suffer together' of the co-affection of the soul and the body, the specific nature of their association is not under analysis.[35] The emphasis, rather, is on the association itself as a basis for making judgments about character from appearance. Such judgments are possible, Aristotle says, 'if you grant that body and soul change together in all natural affections' (εἴ τις δίδωσιν ἄμα μεταβάλλειν τὸ σῶμα καὶ τὴν ψυχὴν ὅσα φυσικά ἐστι παθήματα, *An. Pr.* 70b7–8), such as anger and desire. He concludes by restating the assumption that body and soul suffer

slow, or disease or sleep is said to 'confuse' and 'change' the intellect, indicate an *active* role of bodily factors in the operations of the intellect. Thus apart from saying that bodily changes 'correspond with' or 'accompany' psychic activities, which does not commit itself to a specific type of causal relationship, we may go further and say that bodily states and processes *act* on psychic powers or activities just as well as psychic powers may be said to 'inform' bodily structures' (emphasis in original). Yet we must be careful not to overstate the case for a causal relationship. Aristotle himself often prefers the non-committal language of simultaneity and coordination.

    [35] Aristotle is not all that specific about how the association of body and soul works even in the *De Anima* and the *De Sensu*. But in these contexts the nature of the association is at least under reflective consideration. For other instances of sympathy in contexts where the experience of being affected is important, see *Part. An.* 653b5–8, where the heat in the heart is 'most sympathetic' (συμπαθέστατον) with changes elsewhere in the body, 690b4–7; *Pol.* 1340a13; *Somn. Vig.* 455a33–b1. At *De An.* 428b21–23, when we form a judgment that something is frightening, we are immediately affected by it (συμπάσχομεν).

together (70b16–17). What matters, it seems, is the coordination, not the nature of the relationship.

Aristotle, then, was relatively reticent in his use of the language of sympathy. By contrast, such language appears to have become a popular aspect of his difficult account of soul-body relations in later Peripatetic thought.[36] One place where it is especially pronounced turns out to be physiognomy, the backdrop to Aristotle's reference to sympathy in the *Prior Analytics*. The founding maxim of the pseudo-Aristotelian *Physiognomy* (ca. fourth century BCE) is that 'mental dispositions follow bodies and are not unaffected in themselves by the movements of the body' (αἱ διάνοιαι ἕπονται τοῖς σώμασι, καὶ οὐκ εἰσὶν αὐταὶ καθ' ἑαυτὰς ἀπαθεῖς οὖσαι τῶν τοῦ σώματος κινήσεων, 805a1–2). The opposite is equally true—namely, that the body suffers the affections of the soul (τοῖς τῆς ψυχῆς παθήμασι τὸ σῶμα συμπάσχον, 805a5–6; see also 808b12), a claim that the author supports by referring to the emotions. As in Aristotle's own physiognomic remarks in the *Prior Analytics*, what matters here is the fact of co-affection, rather than the differences between what happens in the body and what happens in the soul. The pseudo-Aristotelian *Problemata* also takes soul-body sympathy as a vague working assumption in a chapter that treats sympathy not just between the body and the soul but in a range of contexts.[37]

The concept of things common to body and soul thus functions as an important bridge between two of Aristotle's central commitments: some form of soul-body dualism and the idea that bodies and souls are inseparable halves of a psychophysical (hylomorphic) composite. That concept is not synonymous with the narrower concept of sympathy. Nevertheless, sympathy seems to have become a common way of expressing the association between the body and the soul in writers influenced by Aristotle.

The situation changes significantly when we reach the Hellenistic period. In both Epicureanism and Stoicism, the idea of sympathy not only becomes more visible but acquires a markedly technical sense, grounded in the very premise resisted by Aristotle: the soul *can* be affected by the body and can affect it in turn because it, too, is a body.[38] Despite the fact that we lack

---

[36] On the principle of 'common to body and soul' in Peripatetic thought, see Sharples 2006. Van der Eijk (2005a, 236) stresses continuities between the *Physiognomy* and the *Problemata* and the works ascribed by modern scholars to Aristotle.

[37] See esp. [Aristotle] *Prob.* 3.31, 875b32–33: ὅταν ἡ ψυχὴ πάθῃ τι, συμπάσχει καὶ ἡ γλῶττα, οἷον τῶν φοβουμένων (when the soul suffers something, the tongue suffers in sympathy, as in those who are afraid).

[38] For the Stoics' rejection of Platonic and Aristotelian beliefs about the causal efficacy of incorporeals, see Cicero, *Ac.* 1.39 (*SVF* 1.30).

an extensive corpus of evidence for Hellenistic philosophy, the material
that has come down to us suggests that sympathy played a cardinal role in
establishing the psychophysical holism endorsed, albeit in different ways,
by both the Epicureans and the Stoics.[39]

Given the thoroughgoing materialism of Epicureanism, according to
which everything that is not void is body, it comes as no surprise that Epicurus understood the *psyche* to be corporeal, capable of affecting other atomic
compounds and subject to being affected by them. Yet the soul also has
particular qualities that help account for its specific capacities to act and
be acted upon. In the *Letter to Herodotus*, Epicurus describes the *psyche* as
a body (*soma*) of fine particles distributed through the 'aggregate' (*athro-
isma*)—the term he uses to speak of the atomic composite as a unity—that
closely resembles wind and is mixed with heat. There is, however, a third
element of the soul, still finer than the others, that, precisely because of its
fineness, is 'sympathetic' with the rest of the whole (συμπαθές ... τῷ λοιπῷ ἀ-
θροίσματι, *Ep. Hdt.* 63).[40] One area where sympathy is especially important is,
as we may by now expect, sensation, a task that Epicurus primarily entrusts
to the soul, albeit a soul that must be enclosed in the aggregate in order to
perform its function.[41] The *psyche* also 'gives' sensation to the aggregate 'on
account of its proximity to and sympathy with it' (κατὰ τὴν ὁμούρησιν καὶ
συμπάθειαν καὶ ἐκείνῳ, *Ep. Hdt.* 64).[42]

The doctrinal importance of sympathy within Epicureanism is confirmed
by the role it plays in Lucretius's discussion of the corporeality of the soul in
Book 3 of the *De Rerum Natura*. Lucretius, interestingly, begins by rejecting
the idea that the soul is a harmony, glossed as a 'vital condition of the body'
(*habitum quendam vitalem corporis*, 3.99). He is adamant, rather, that the

---

[39] On the 'psychophysical holism' of both schools, see Gill 2006a.

[40] On the nature of the soul, cf. Lucretius, *DRN* 3.177–287, 425–444, who attributes sensation to an unnamed *fourth* element; see also Aëtius 4.3.11; Plutarch, *Adv. Col.* 1118D–E.

[41] Sensation is thus an example of something 'common to body and soul', as Lucretius *DRN*
3.333–336 suggests: *nec sibi quaeque sine alterius vi posse videtur / corporis atque animi seorsum
sentire potestas, / sed communibus inter eas conflatur utrimque / motibus accensus nobis per
viscera sensus* (And we see that neither the body nor the mind has the capacity to feel on its
own without the help of the other, but by common movements arising from both together
sensation is kindled for us in our flesh). But Epicurus himself does not use such language,
and, as many scholars have observed, the relationship he describes between the *psyche* and
the aggregate seems designed in part to supplant the *psyche-soma* pair.

[42] Note that the language of sympathy is also standard in Epicurus's account of perception,
where it describes how effluences preserve the qualities of the object perceived: *Ep. Hdt.* 48,
50, 52, 53.

mind (*animus*) can withdraw and be *unaffected* by the pains of the body, a position he defends in part by splitting off a thinking soul (*animus*), concentrated in the chest, from a sensing soul (*anima*), distributed throughout the aggregate (3.136–151).

Nevertheless, having established the divergence between the affections of the *animus* and those of the rest of the aggregate, Lucretius proceeds to emphasize the intimacy between the *animus* and the *anima* by pointing out that the *anima* is affected together (*consentire*) with the *animus* in cases of strong emotion (3.158–160). He then goes on to defend the corporeality of both the *anima* and the *animum* (3.161–162), arguing, on the one hand, that the mind and soul must be corporeal if they are to act on the body (for example, to initiate movement), and, on the other hand, that the mind is affected when the body is struck (for example, by a weapon).[43] The mind, in other words, not only communicates its affections to the aggregate but 'suffers along with the body, and shares our feelings together [*consentire*] in the body' (3.168–169). The last point confirms that not only is the *psychē* not unmoved: it is uncommonly sensitive to movement (3.203–205, 243). The mind, despite its capacity to withdraw from the suffering of the aggregate, thus remains vulnerable to the affections of the whole, not just because it is corporeal but because it is especially susceptible to being affected.

The Stoics, for all their differences with the Epicureans, also make sympathy central to their arguments about the nature of the *psychē* and its relationship to the rest of the body.[44] In an argument credited to Cleanthes, sympathy is central to establishing that the soul, in fact, *is* a body:[45]

οὐδὲν ἀσώματον συμπάσχει σώματι οὐδὲ ἀσωμάτῳ σῶμα, ἀλλὰ σῶμα σώματι. συμπάσχει δὲ ἡ ψυχὴ τῷ σώματι νοσοῦντι καὶ τεμνομένῳ, καὶ τὸ σῶμα τῇ ψυχῇ· αἰσχυνομένης γοῦν ἐρυθρὸν γίνεται καὶ φοβουμένης ὠχρόν· σῶμα ἄρα ἡ ψυχή.

(Nemesius, *Nat. Hom.* 2 [21,6–9 Morani] = *SVF* 1.518, in part)

---

[43] Lucretius does not specify why only some of the pains of the body are passed on. It may be that the capacity of the *animus* to withdraw from bodily pain is strengthened by mental pleasures (such as the memories of philosophical conversation Epicurus called upon on his deathbed).

[44] The Stoics actually posited two different forms of *psychē* in a human being: the *psychē* that is responsible for the form of the rest of the body and vital functions (and that is present, too, in other animals) and the hegemonic *psychē*, located in the heart, that functions as a 'ruler' in rational beings. See Sextus Empiricus, *Math.* 7.234, with Long 1996 [1982]. The argument about *psychē-sōma* sympathy implicates both these aspects of the *psychē* in the rest of the body (and vice versa) insofar as they are both corporeal.

[45] For this argument and the two other Stoic classes of argument for proving the corporeality of the soul ('genetic' and 'contactual'), see Long 1996 [1982], esp. 235–236.

No incorporeal interacts with a body, and no body with an incorporeal, but one body interacts with another body. Now the soul interacts with the body when it is sick and being cut, and the body with the soul; thus when the soul feels shame and fear the body turns red and pale respectively. Therefore, the soul is a body.   (Trans. Long and Sedley)

Here, as in Lucretius, affections travel in both directions, from the soul to the body—with the emotions invoked again as a paradigmatic example— and from the body to the soul (e.g., in pain). The argument ascribed to Chrysippus emphatically posits causal relationships designed to prove the corporeality of the soul. The *psychē* is, nevertheless, a specific kind of stuff (a combination of fire and air), perfectly suited to the functions associated with the highest expression of life in human beings.

The sympathetic relationship of the body and the soul shores up, too, the Stoic emphasis on the cohesive unity of bodies (human and non-human), which are held together by the tension of the air or breath (*pneuma*) pervading them. The principle of cohesion extends to the Stoic conceptualization of the cosmos as a whole. The Stoics believed, accordingly, that sympathy operates not just within the microcosm but at the level of the macrocosm as well, between parts and the whole within a continuum of matter.[46] The idea of sympathy is thus central to Stoicism, to the extent that it expresses the dynamic unity of matter, both inside and outside the human being.

Even a cursory overview shows that the concept of psychophysical sympathy has its own history within the ancient philosophical tradition. We glimpse the foundation of this tradition in Plato's understanding of an affection common to body and soul and specific to each. Aristotle appears to have been more ambivalent about the susceptibility of the soul to being moved, but his commitment to understanding the *sōma* and the *psychē* as two halves of an organic whole lays the groundwork for sympathy's entry into the Peripatetic vocabulary. The concept of sympathy seems to truly come into its own in the Hellenistic schools, where it acquires a degree of

---

[46] On sympathy in the cosmos, see Chrysippus in Alexander, *On Mixture* 3 (216,14–17 Bruns; see also 227,8 Bruns) (*SVF* 2.473): ἡνῶσθαι μὲν ὑποτίθεται τὴν σύμπασαν οὐσίαν, πνεύματός τινος διὰ πάσης αὐτῆς διήκοντος, ὑφ' οὗ συνέχεταί τε καὶ συμμένει καὶ σύμπαθές ἐστιν αὐτῷ τὸ πᾶν ([Chrysippus] holds that while the whole of substance is unified, because it is totally pervaded by a pneuma through which the whole is held together, is stable, and is sympathetic with itself … [trans. Todd]). See also Cicero, *Div.* 2.33–34 (*SVF* 2.1211); *Nat. D.* 2.19; Cleomedes, *Caelestia* 1.1.13 (*SVF* 2.534), 1.1.69–73 (*SVF* 2.546); Diogenes Laërtius 7.140 (*SVF* 2.543); [Plutarch], *Fat.* 574E (*SVF* 2.912); Sextus Empiricus, *Math.* 9.78–80 (*SVF* 2.1013). On cosmic sympathy and the continuum, see Sambursky 1959, 41–44; White 2003, esp. 128–133.

technical precision and plays a significant role in establishing the corporeality of the soul and its intimate bond with the larger composite. To speak of *sōma-psychē* sympathy in this context, it would seem, carries a core commitment to the shared materiality underwriting the sympathetic bond.

In sketching this brief history, I have touched only incidentally on mental disturbance and disorder. In some contexts, such as the *Philebus* or Lucretius's arguments about the violent impact of bodily diseases on the mind and the spirit (3.463–469, 487–509), the idea of sympathy leaves mental or psychic functions vulnerable to troubles erupting from within the body. But the body may also be affected by the mind. Moreover, as the concept of things shared by the body and the soul is developed by Aristotle and the Hellenistic philosophers, it comes to describe normal states and processes as often as it describes turmoil. I turn now to the ways in which Galen engages both the philosophical and medical traditions to elaborate an intriguing concept of sympathy, marked, on the one hand, by an emphasis on disturbances of the mind and, on the other hand, by its inability to bridge the domains of the body and the soul.

Sympathy and Mental Disturbance in Galen

Galen was no stranger to the concept of sympathy. He not only invoked sympathy as central to his own understanding of the body as an intelligently fashioned, interconnected unity: he attributed that vision to the divine Hippocrates himself. What is at stake for Galen in laying claim to sympathy is nowhere made clearer than in the treatise *On the Natural Faculties*. There, he declares that, when it comes to the nature of Nature, there are two sects in medicine and philosophy: there are those who believe in a continuum theory of matter and those who adopt a corpuscular or atomist physics.[47]

The division, at first glance, may appear surprising. For, as we have seen, both the Epicureans (atomists) and the Stoics (continuum theorists) use sympathy to describe the interaction of the soul with the rest of the organism or aggregate. But for the Stoics, sympathy is also a macrocosmic principle that bears witness to the absence of void and the tensional unity of the world. It is this larger, philosophically charged concept of sympathy that Galen presumably has in mind in *On the Natural Faculties*.[48] The more

---

[47] *Nat. Fac.* 1.12 (II 27 K = 120,7–11 Helmreich); see also *QAM* 5 (IV 785 K = 46,9–17 Müller).

[48] Galen is often seen as an enemy of the Stoics because of his attacks on their psychology,

global perspective certainly colors the view he ascribes to Hippocrates: 'substance is unified and undergoes alteration and the body as a whole breathes together and flows together' (ἥνωται μὲν ἡ οὐσία καὶ ἀλλοιοῦται καὶ σύμπνουν ὅλον ἐστὶ καὶ σύρρουν τὸ σῶμα, *Nat. Fac.* 1.12, II 29 K = 122,7–9 Helmreich).[49] The grander meaning of sympathy is confirmed by the fact that he sums up the position of his opponents—physicians who defend corpuscular theories of the body and, above all, the first-century BCE physician-theorist Asclepiades of Bithynia—in turn, as the *rejection* of sympathy outside but especially inside the body.[50] Galen's nightmare is a body where interconnectivity is thwarted by fragmentation at the most basic level. To deny sympathy, on his view, is to deny not simply the cohesion but the *coherence* of nature.

The image of Hippocrates as the champion of sympathy that Galen puts forth here and elsewhere has its basis in *On Nutriment*.[51] The treatise is almost certainly Hellenistic, in part because the sympathetically unified body described there betrays such clear Stoic influence. Yet the idea of the body as a unity in which air and fluids circulate through a network of vessels is, as we have seen, not foreign to some of the early medical authors. And despite the serious gaps in our evidence for medicine between the Hippocratics and Galen, there are good indications that some time after the first phase of classical Greek medical writing, the idea of co-affection came to be closely associated with the term *sympatheia*; that term acquired, in turn, a degree of technicality within medicine. Soranus, to take one example, writes that when the womb suffers, it acts sympathetically on the stomach and the meninges (πάσχουσα μέντοι πρὸς συμπάθειαν στόμαχον ἄγει καὶ μήνιγγας); it has, too, he observes, some kind of natural sympathy with the breasts (ἔστι δέ τις αὐτῇ καὶ πρὸς τοὺς μαστοὺς φυσικὴ συμπάθεια, *Gyn.* I 15 [10,27–28 Ilberg]).[52] In a fragment from Rufus of Ephesus's *On Melancholy*,

---

but there are a number of points of contact in their philosophies of nature: see Manuli 1993; Gill 2007a and 2010a. On Galen's relationship with Stoics contemporary with him, see Tieleman 2009.

[49] For similar citations of Hippocrates, see *Caus. Puls.* 1.12 (IX 88 K), *Nat. Fac.* 1.13 (II 38 K = 129,7–9 Helmreich), 3.13 (II 196 K = 243,10–13 Helmreich); *MM* 1.2 (X 16 K); *Trem. Palp.* (VII 616 K); *UP* 1.8 (III 17 K = 1.12 Helmreich), 1.9 (III 24 K = 1.17 Helmreich).

[50] *Nat. Fac.* 1.13 (II 39 K = 129,9–12 Helmreich).

[51] The key passage is *Nutr.* 23 (IX 106 Littré): ξύρροια μία, ξύμπνοια μία, ξυμπαθέα πάντα· κατὰ μὲν οὐλομελίην πάντα, κατὰ μέρος δὲ τὰ ἐν ἑκάστῳ μέρει μέρεα πρὸς τὸ ἔργον (There is one confluence; there is one common breathing; all things are in sympathy. All the parts as forming a whole, and severally the parts in each part, with reference to the work).

[52] For other affections produced sympathetically, often with the womb, see Soranus, *Gyn.* 1.63 (47,16 Ilberg), 1.67 (48,25 Ilberg), 2.11 (58,11 Ilberg), 2.49 (88,22 Ilberg), 3.17 (105,17

preserved only in Arabic, the connection of the head to the stomach may have been framed in terms of sympathy in the original Greek.[53]

The concept of sympathy appears, then, to have developed independently in medicine as a way to describe axes of communication between different parts of the body that leave each part vulnerable to the affections of the others. In *On the Natural Faculties*, Galen outfits this medical concept of sympathy with the larger philosophical connotations it acquires in Stoicism in order to give it a starring role in the confrontation he is staging between the continuum theorists and the atomists. Yet a brief scan of his use of sympathy in his vast corpus suggests that the concept primarily functioned for him as a practical diagnostic tool. Still, we should not be misled into expecting that larger philosophical concerns disappear when we shift to the more pragmatic side of Galen—on the contrary. Galen's diagnostic use of sympathy can tell us something about how the hegemonic principle or mind and, more distantly, the soul, is implicated in the non-conscious, physiological body.

Galen refers to sympathy in a number of treatises (including in commentaries on Hippocratic texts where the term itself is absent).[54] Half a century ago, Rudolph Siegel organized these references into five classes of sympathetic affection according to the means of transmission: two are neural (irritations transmitted via the nerves or through the blockage of nerve

---

Ilberg), 3.20 (106,19 Ilberg), 3.22, *bis* (107,18; 107,27 Ilberg), 3.25 (109,8 Ilberg), 3.29 (113,6 Ilberg), 3.31 (114,6 Ilberg), 3.41, *bis* (120,13; 121,12 Ilberg), 3.49 (127,11 Ilberg), 4.7 (137,7 Ilberg), 4.9 (140,7 Ilberg), 4.15 [1.72], *tris* (145,16; 145,18; 145,29 Ilberg). The verb (συμπάσχειν) is also used to describe women sympathizing with each other's pains: see 1.4 (5,22 Ilberg); a similar (person-to-person) use is found at *Praec.* 14 (IX 272 Littré = 35,6–7 Heiberg). For sympathetic affections, see also Anon. Med., *Morb. Acut.* 7.3.11 (54,27 Garofalo), 22.2.2 (172,5 Garofalo), 37.2.2 (194,1 Garofalo), 40.2.4 (246,19 Garofalo); Cassius, *Quaestiones medicae* 21 (152,3 Ideler), 40 (158,13 Ideler), 83 (167,15–16 Ideler); Severus, *De instrumentis et infusoriis* (24,3–7 Dietz, 30,14–16 Dietz). Maire and Bianchi 2003, I.430–432 list uses of the equivalent Latin terms *consensus* (fifty instances) and *consentire* (thirty-eight instances) in Caelius Aurelianus: see, e.g., *Morb. Acut.* 1.71 (62,17–18 Bendz), 3.140 (376,21 Bendz); *Morb. Chron.* 1.62 (464,24 Bendz), 2.25 (558,18 Bendz), 2.27 (560,3 Bendz), 3.69 (720,16 Bendz). The noun and verb appear frequently in Oribasius as well. Galen refers to earlier treatments of sympathy as a diagnostic concept at *Loc. Aff.* 1.6 (VIII 49 K), 3.11 (VIII 198 K). All this evidence makes it unlikely that Galen was the first physician to establish sympathy as a diagnostic concept, *pace* Siegel 1968, 360–361, although he was no doubt instrumental in installing it in the later medical tradition.

[53] Rufus, *On Melancholy* fr. 8 (Pormann). The Arabic contains the word *mušāraka*, which we can see being used to translate *sympatheia* in medical texts extant in Greek and Arabic: see Holmes 2012. I am grateful to Peter Pormann for the reference and assistance with the Arabic.

[54] Galen's strategic projection of his own theories onto the Hippocratic texts is well known: see von Staden 2002; Flemming 2008, esp. 343–346.

impulses); the others involve the humors, vapors, and contact through prox-imity.[55] Galen himself does not provide such a neat classification, at least in the texts we have, and at times he equivocates on whether all these cases are properly instances of sympathy.[56] Still, Siegel's classification offers a good starting place.

If we read the Galenic system sketched by Siegel together with the 'cir-cular' model that we saw earlier in *On Places in a Human Being*, we notice immediately that Galen has multiplied the possible channels of communi-cation in the body in comparison with his Hippocratic predecessor. More specifically, where the earlier writer focuses on fluids circulating in the body, Galen elevates the nerves to one of the most important routes for the com-munication of affections.

Indeed, despite the fact that Galen himself attributes a sophisticated grasp of neural anatomy to Hippocrates, it is the nervous system that deci-sively divides the Galenic body from that of the classical-era medical au-thors. How information moves between the mind or the soul and the rest of the body was a question increasingly posed by physicians and philosophers in the fourth century BCE. But it is only with the beginning of systematic human dissection at Alexandria in the following century that people came to recognize the role of the nerves in transmitting sensation and motor impulses throughout the psychophysical organism. Galen's model of the body owes much to the anatomical investigations of Herophilus and Erasi-stratus, and he was himself an accomplished anatomist (and a physician to gladiators early in his career).[57] Perhaps most important, he enthusiastically embraced what he saw as one of anatomy's most impressive contributions to the study of human nature—namely, irrefutable proof that the ruling part is located in the head and not in the heart, as the Peripatetics and the Sto-ics believed.[58] He himself undertook vivisectory experiments to demonstrate the control of the brain over the sensory, motor, and mental functions.[59] It is

---

[55] Siegel 1968, 362–370, with examples.

[56] See esp. *Loc. Aff.* 1.6 (VIII 51–51 K), where he doubts whether humoral transmission is really sympathy. On the difference between the transmission of stuffs and the transmission of powers, see De Lacy 1979, 360–361.

[57] On the 'discovery' of the nerves, see esp. Solmsen 1961; von Staden 1989, 247–259. On the cultural context of dissection and its disappearance in the centuries after Herophilus and Erasistratus, see von Staden 1992a.

[58] *PHP* 8.1.3–4 (V 649–650 K = 480,16–24 De Lacy).

[59] On these experiments, see Hankinson 1991a, 219–224; Mansfeld 1991, 129–131; Tieleman 2002. They were often performed in front of large crowds in Rome with the express aim of disproving the positions of opponents: see Debru 1995; von Staden 1995; Gleason 2009.

in Galen's writings that we begin to grasp what the advances in Alexandria meant not only for the concept of sympathetic affections but also for ideas about the implication of the mind or soul in the whole.

The concept of sympathy, as I have already noted, appears throughout Galen's corpus. But he discusses it most extensively in *On the Affected Parts*, which is not surprising given that he believes that a physician has to know *how* a part has come to be affected if he is to administer the proper therapy.[60] In his opening remarks, Galen distinguishes affections that arise through sympathy with another part from those that arise from the damaged condition (*diathesis*) of the part itself ('idiopathy').[61] In theory, he reserves the term sympathy for affections that act as the 'shadows' of affections occurring elsewhere in the body, appearing and disappearing together with them; he introduces the terms 'secondary' or 'later' affection (*deuteropatheia, hysteropatheia*) to describe cases where an affection first triggered by sympathy takes hold in the part itself.[62] In practice, however, terminological precision tends to fall by the wayside. Galen usually uses the term 'sympathy' to refer to *all* affections triggered by suffering elsewhere in the body, while continuing to note when the affection has damaged the sympathetically affected part (creating the need for therapy targeted at that part).[63]

Beyond trying to specify under what conditions an affection arises (that is, whether or not it is caused through sympathy), Galen is interested in *On the Affected Parts* in where and how sympathetic affections most commonly arise. The backdrop to his discussion is the networked body uncovered by anatomy. It comes as no surprise, then, that the major control centers occupy important positions on the map of sympathy. Galen compares the brain at one point to a sun emanating light—that is, psychic *pneuma*—over the rest of the body.[64] The sun's pride of place also means damage to it can trigger a cascade of problems elsewhere.[65] For example, if the brain is

---

[60] For the importance of understanding sympathy in diagnosis and therapy, see esp. *Loc. Aff.* 2.10 (VIII 129 K). See also *Comp. Med. Loc.* 2.1 (XII 559 K); *Loc. Aff.* 3.4 (VIII 146 K), 5.6 (VIII 339 K).

[61] *Loc. Aff.* 1.3 (VIII 30 K). At 2.10 (VIII 129 K), he suggests that such a differentiation, given its therapeutic importance, is the proper topic of the treatise.

[62] *Loc. Aff.* 1.3 (VIII 31 K); see also 1.6 (VIII 48 K). On the shadow, a concept Galen attributes to Archigenes, see *Loc. Aff.* 3.1 (VIII 136–137 K).

[63] See esp. *Loc. Aff.* 3.2 (VIII 138 K), where protopathy and idiopathy appear interchangeable, and 3.7 (VIII 166 K), where Galen refers to two types of sympathy, one that comes and goes with the primary affection and one that fixes in the secondarily affected part. At *Comp. Art. Med.* 15 (I 282 K = 106,12–13 Fortuna), sympathy is opposed to protopathy.

[64] *Loc. Aff.* 1.7 (VIII 66–67 K).

[65] Ibid. 4.10 (VIII 282 K).

corrupted by bilious humors, it can affect the eyes through sympathy: smoky fumes are transmitted through the vessels joining the eyes to the brain and create optical illusions.[66]

But damage can travel the other way, too: not just from the brain but also towards it, and here is where the story becomes particularly interesting. For trouble often arrives in the brain along a path that connects the brain to the stomach and, more specifically, the mouth of the stomach, the *cardia*. It is probably no accident that in his opening remarks on sympathy in *On the Affected Parts*, Galen uses the example of noxious vapors or humors rising up from the stomach cavity to the brain.[67] In his more detailed discussions, too, affections frequently migrate to the brain from the stomach or its mouth. So, for example, when he classifies types of melancholy and epilepsy, he distinguishes between cases that originate with a primary affection of the head and cases that develop in sympathy with the opening of the stomach.[68] Later in the treatise we come across a case of sympathetic epilepsy involving a young student of literature. Galen figures out that the problem is that the young man is too absorbed in his studies to remember to eat; he cures him by enforcing regular meal-times.[69] The problem with the brain, in short, starts in the stomach. Elsewhere we learn that the delirium associated with high fevers is not a primary affection, but a sympathetic condition triggered by the migration of hot vapors from the gut to the brain.[70] Once again, trouble brews at the mouth of the digestive system.

What makes the brain so vulnerable to problems in the gut is the existence of a large nerve (or nerves) connecting it to the opening of the stomach.[71] The nerve in question creates a path upwards for noxious humors, as well as for various vapors that ascend beyond the brain to the eyes.[72] And it

---

[66] Ibid. 4.2 (VIII 227–228 K).

[67] *Loc. Aff.* 1.6 (VIII 48 K).

[68] On types of epilepsy and melancholy, see *Loc. Aff.* 3.11 (VIII 193–200 K). For the role of the stomach in triggering delirium, melancholy, and loss of consciousness, see also *Comp. Art. Med.* 15 (I 282 K = 106,15–17 Fortuna); *Loc. Aff.* 5.6 (VIII 338 K); *Symp. Caus.* 1.7 (VII 128, 137 K).

[69] *Loc. Aff.* 5.6 (VIII 340–342 K).

[70] *Loc. Aff.* 3.9 (VIII 178 K).

[71] See esp. *Loc. Aff.* 3.9 (VIII 178–179 K), where large nerves (identified now as the vagus nerves) connect the brain to the stomach; see also 5.6 (VIII 341–342 K), 6.2 (VIII 381 K); *UP* 9.11 (III 724–731 K = 2.30–35 Helmreich), with Siegel 1968, 362–365. In Galen's view, these nerves do allow movement in both directions (e.g., headaches can trigger gastric trouble), although the majority of the traffic that he describes runs from the stomach to the brain (most of the vagal nerves, in fact, are afferent, relaying information from the gut to the brain). For Galen's identification of the vagus nerve, see *AA* 11.11 (104–105 Duckworth), 14.7 (208–209 Duckworth).

[72] On sympathetic affections of the eyes, see *Comp. Art. Med.* 15 (I 282 K = 106,15–17 Fortuna); *Loc. Aff.* 4.2 (VIII 221–225 K), 5.6 (VIII 342 K).

is not just the brain that falls prey to gastric distress. The heart, too, is easily affected by affections of the stomach—indeed, violently so, often resulting in cardiac syncopes and loss of breath. The reason, once again, is a passage, in this case an artery connecting the stomach and the heart. In *On Causes of Symptoms*, for example, Galen emphasizes the sympathetic relationship of the mouth of the stomach and the heart alongside the relationship between the stomach and the brain. He connects the stomach to the heart by way of the 'great artery'; the stomach and the brain are related, as we have just seen, by way of the vagus nerve.[73]

These lines of sympathy suggest a triangle of sorts involving the heart, the brain, and the stomach. But it is not exactly the triangle that a reader of Galen would expect. That the heart and the brain are included here is no surprise, since each is classified by Galen as a major *archē* in the body and, so, the origin of a major network. What is missing is the liver, the origin of the third network, namely the veins that Galen thinks distribute nourishment through the body.[74] The liver would also complete a triad that replicates— not by accident—Plato's tripartite soul, which Galen defends vigorously against the Stoic theory of a unified hegemonic principle (located in the heart) in his *Doctrines of Hippocrates and Plato* and which he continued to advance throughout his career.[75] The influence of Plato is also strongly felt in Galen's interest in conceptualizing his three *archai* as the origins not just of physiological systems but also of psychological ones: the brain is allied with reason, the heart with emotion and spirit, and the liver with appetitive and sensory desires.

Galen's appropriation of the Platonic soul is, admittedly, not without its problems. Interestingly enough, one of the most pressing is the awkward role of the liver, the only organ we have not seen as a major sympathetic player.[76] Galen himself was aware of the difficulties involved. He openly

---

[73] *Symp. Caus* 1.7 (VII 138 K). The chapter more generally privileges the heart and brain in sympathetic affections with the stomach or the cardia. See also *Hipp. Fract.* (XVIII/2 458 K): ἀλλὰ διὰ μὲν τὰς ἀρτηρίας ἡ καρδία συμπαθοῦσα, διὰ δὲ τῆς τῶν νεύρων οὐσίας ὁ ἐγκέφαλος (But the heart suffers sympathetically on account of the arteries, the brain on account of the substance of the nerves). On sympathetic affections of the heart with the cardia, see also *Loc. Aff.* 5.2 (VIII 302 K), 5.6 (VIII 342–343 K). On sympathy between the heart and brain, see *Loc. Aff.* 5.1 (VIII 300 K); *Praes. Puls.* 4.8 (IX 410 K).

[74] See, e.g., *Loc. Aff.* 5.1 (VIII 298 K); *PHP* 6.3.9 (V 522 K = 374,25–29 De Lacy), 7.3.2–3 (V 600–601 K = 438,28–440,8 De Lacy). Galen also speaks of a quaternary system incorporating the testicles: see Véronique Boudon's remarks in the discussion to Tieleman 2003b, 164–165.

[75] On Galen's Platonism in general, see De Lacy 1972; Singer 1991.

[76] See De Lacy 1988; Hankinson 1991a, 223–231; Tieleman 2002, esp. 266–268 and 2003, 153–154, 158–160; Donini 2008, 193; Gill 2010a, 104–124, 218–220.

admits, for example, that he is unable to demonstrate the liver's importance in the same way that he had used vivisection to prove the roles of the brain and the heart, since damage to the liver does not produce immediately observable effects.[77] And, as contemporary scholars have observed, it is a bit of a leap from the liver's physiological function of regulating nutrition to its purported psychological role as the seat of appetitive and sensory desires.[78] Finally, Galen, for all his interest in the anatomical substratum of the body, never demonstrates how the three parts interact.[79]

The very difficulty of integrating the liver into Galen's anatomo-physio-logical body makes the sympathetic relationship of the stomach to the brain and the heart newly intriguing.[80] For these major lines of sympathy seem to trace an alternative tripartite structure, a structure as much embedded in the networked flesh of the Galenic body as Plato's soul is disconnected from it.[81] What is more, the rival triangle, by shifting attention from the liver to the stomach, suggests a way of seeing the vulnerability of the ratio-nal part of the soul not captured by Galen's Platonic framework. For it grants the stomach considerable power to compromise the rational faculty by disturbing the state of the brain. Recall the image of the brain as a sun emanating its light throughout the body. If we turn to sympathetic affec-tions originating in the gut, that image is quite literally eclipsed by another:

---

[77] *PHP* 6.3.2–6 (V 519–520 K = 372,19–374,8 De Lacy).

[78] Hankinson 1991a, 229–231; Gill 2010a, 107–124.

[79] Singer 1991, 45; Tieleman 2002, 270. Mansfeld also observes the difficulty of seeing the heart and liver as autonomous sources of motion when they lack motor nerves (1991, 141–142). Note, too, that Plato does not locate the third part entirely in the liver but sometimes seems to locate it in the belly as well: see *Tim.* 70d7–71d4. Tieleman suggests that, in privileging the liver, Galen is responding to its role in digestion and growth as it was described by Aristotle (2003, 153–154). See also von Staden 2000, 110, emphasizing the similarity of Galen's system to Erasistratus's model of three sources (of psychic pneuma, vital pneuma, and blood).

[80] The liver is excluded from the discussion at *Symp. Caus* 1.7 (VII 136–138 K), although cf. *MM* 12.5 (X 844 K), where all three *archai* can be led into such sympathetic affections. The liver is not particularly prone to sympathetic affections in *On the Affected Parts*, but see 5.7 (VIII 351–352 K), where humoral imbalance is transmitted to the liver from elsewhere in the body. On sympathy between the heart and the liver, see *Marc.* 7 (VII 693 K); *Loc. Aff.* 5.1 (VIII 299 K); *Praes. Puls.* 4.4 (IX 399–400 K).

[81] It is particularly interesting in this regard that Galen recognizes that hunger and thirst are transmitted to the brain not from the liver but from the stomach, via the large connecting nerve: see *Hipp. Epid.* III 15 (XVII/2 664 K = 118,22–24 Wenkebach); *UP* 4.7 (III 275 K = 1.201,19–202,2 Helmreich), 16.5 (IV 289 K = 2.394,18–24 Helmreich). At *UP* 4.13 (III 308–309 K = 1.226,18–22 Helmreich), Galen tersely notes the small nerve running to the liver. The relationship between the heart and the brain, in contrast, is secured through the anatomical body (in addition to their shared bond with the mouth of the stomach): see Gill 2010a, 120–122.

the image of smoky vapors rising from the gastric cavity to impair the functions of the mind.

Of course, a scenario where the desiring part gains the upper hand over the rational soul is precisely the definition of psychic disease in Plato's *Republic*. Are things really so different in Galen? Perhaps most important, the loose version of the Platonic triangle that sympathy creates in *On the Affected Parts* differs from its philosophical cousin to the extent it is decisively realized in the physiological domain.[82] The stomach that communicates its troubles to the brain is closer to the body in the *Philebus*, whose disruptive motions, as we saw earlier, surface in the soul, than it is to Plato's seat of desire.[83] But even the body of the *Philebus*, which is loosely defined through the rhythms of organic life, is not the same as the webbed inner world described by Galen. For Galen's is an inner world seen through an anatomist's eye—not just 'the body'. In Galen, the relationship between the stomach and the brain made evident by sympathy is embedded in an intricately mapped corporeal landscape. Galen's very anatomical precision in locating the brain as the 'ruling part' of the self means that when things go wrong, it is more firmly subordinated to the forces of the physiological body, especially the digestive body.

To seasoned readers of Galen, the claim that the brain is vulnerable to the functioning of the stomach may seem only natural. After all, Galen's belief that human life, from its lowest to its highest expressions, depends on the state of the body only grew stronger over the course of his life. In one of the most memorable moments of *That the Faculties of the Soul Follow the Mixtures of the Body*, Galen jauntily invites those who scoff at the idea that diet can strengthen the mind to schedule a consultation for a regimen to improve their mental acumen.[84]

Yet Galen's treatment of sympathy alerts us to another, less familiar way of imagining how the physician manages health—and especially mental health—through drugs and diet. When Galen dispatches bitter aloe to

---

[82] The difference between the physiological and the psychological here is also stressed by Singer 1991, 46–47. The difference can be seen as part of a larger divergence between the understanding of psychic disease in medicine and philosophy, on which see Gill 2010a, 300–321.

[83] Singer 1991, 43–46 discusses Galen's tendency to think in terms of bipartition rather than tripartition. What would be contrasted would not be *sōma* and *psychē* but *psychē* and *physis*. For the relevance of the contrast to Galen, see von Staden 2000, 102, 107–111; Tieleman 2003b, 159. See also Gill 2010a, 100–103, 114 on the *psychē-physis* distinction in Stoicism.

[84] *QAM* 9 (IV 807–808 K = 67,2–16 Müller).

corresponding patients in the Roman provinces who suffer from vapors clouding their eyes,[85] he is not so much treating the overall humoral and qualitative mixture, a stance we find already in texts like *On the Sacred Disease* and *On Regimen*. He is targeting the gut as the locus of disturbance. The stomach here emerges as the unruly 'neighbor'—albeit, at a distance— of the brain. From this perspective, what we might call that of the 'body in parts', the physician manipulates diet in order to contain any turbulence at the mouth of the stomach. It is a way of ensuring that power continues to flow from the head downwards, rather than from the gut upwards. Diet, in short, is a considered response to the specific liaison between the stomach and the brain.[86]

Such a scenario casts the physician's role in maintaining health in a new light. One of the quirks of the stomach-brain relationship is its asymmetry. Unlike the liver in Plato, which can be managed by messages from the rational part, the stomach lies beyond the control of the nerves that convey messages from the brain to the rest of the body. At the same time, the stomach easily communicates its own affections to the brain. By telling patients what to put in their mouths, the physician becomes an essential node in a network that determines not just gastric health but the health of the hegemonic principle, which is to say the mind. He becomes, as it were, the mind capable of controlling the stomach. The patient himself still matters, of course. But his appetitive desires fade into the background as the dietary expertise of the physician comes to the fore.

Does such expertise make the physician a doctor of the soul? The question turns out to be rather complicated. For despite the fact that Galen readily implicates the brain in the affections of the stomach, he is unwilling to locate the soul within the sympathetic network that dominates *On the Affected Parts*. Nor does he recognize sympathy between the soul and its corporeal home, that is, the brain. In other words, even as he elaborates a concept of medical sympathy to help account for mental disturbances, he seems to sidestep the concept of soul-body sympathy that gained ground in the Hellenistic period.[87]

---

[85] *Loc. Aff.* 4.2 (VIII 224–225 K).

[86] Such a liaison was assumed in Western medicine for centuries after Galen: see Siegel 1968, 372–377. For a contemporary analysis of the 'brain-gut axis', see E.A. Wilson 2004, 31–47 (who problematizes the idea of a single axial relationship between the two).

[87] The idea of sympathy could be eagerly embraced by a Middle Platonist: see Plut. *Mor.* 142E, 450A, 736A, 1096E.

The sharp contrast between one type of sympathy, enthusiastically embraced, and another, tacitly rejected, comes into particular relief in a passage from *On the Affected Parts*. Galen has just described the sympathetic relationship between the diaphragm and the respiratory organs. He goes on to introduce by way of analogy the involvement in diseases of the ribs and lungs of what he calls 'the place containing the hegemonic principle of the soul in itself' (τοῦ τὸ τῆς ψυχῆς ἡγεμονικὸν ἐν ἑαυτῷ περιέχοντος τόπου), where knowledge, judgment, and understanding are located.[88] Everyone knows, Galen says, that symptoms like delirium do not arise from the lungs directly. The experts recognize, rather, that the part where the hegemonic principle of the soul is located has suffered sympathetically with another part of the body, 'and they try to show the manner of sympathy that agrees with their own doctrine' (καὶ ζητοῦσί γε τὸν τρόπον τῆς συμπαθείας ὁμολογοῦντα δεῖξαι τοῖς ἰδίοις δόγμασιν).[89] Presumably what Galen means by this is that the physicians and philosophers in question outline a connection between the primarily affected part and the place where they locate the hegemonic principle. That is to say, the doctrinal component bears more on the location of the ruling part than on the nature of sympathy itself.

Galen goes on, however, to problematize shared affection of another kind, not between two parts within the body, but between one part and the *archē* or the soul.

ἀλλ' εἰ μὲν οὕτως ἐστὶ τὸ μόριον τοῦτο τῆς ψυχῆς ἐν τῷ περιέχοντι σώματι, καθάπερ ἡμεῖς ἐν οἴκῳ τινί, τὴν μὲν ἀρχὴν ἂν ἴσως οὐδ' ὑπονοήσαιμεν αὐτὸ βλάπτεσθαί τι πρὸς τοῦ χωρίου· θεασάμενοι δὲ βλαπτόμενον ἐζητήσαμεν ἂν ὅπως βλάπτεται· εἰ δ' ὡς εἶδός τι τοῦ σώματός ἐστιν ἀχώριστον αὐτοῦ, συνεχωρήσαμεν ὑπὸ τῆς τοῦ δεδεγμένου σώματος ἀλλοιώσεως βλάπτεσθαι· διαστάντων δὲ τῶν φιλοσόφων περὶ αὐτοῦ, καὶ τῶν μὲν ὡς ἐν οἰκήματι περιέχεσθαι φασκόντων αὐτό, τῶν δ' ὡς εἶδος, ὅπως μὲν βλάπτεται, χαλεπὸν εὑρεῖν, ὅτι δὲ βλάπτεται, τῇ πείρᾳ μαθεῖν ἔστι.

(*Loc. Aff.* 2.10, VIII 127–128 K)

But if this part of the soul lies in the surrounding body just as we might stand in a house, then we probably should not imagine that the *archē* in itself is damaged at all through the part (where it is located). Once we had seen, though, that it does suffer damage, we might have investigated how it is damaged. But if [sc. the soul] as some form of the body is inseparable from it, we have conceded that it is damaged by an alteration of the body that has received it. But while the philosophers dispute about this, some saying that [sc. the soul] is enclosed as in a house, others that it is like a form, [we say] that *how* [sc. the *archē*] *is damaged is difficult to find out, while the fact that it is damaged is learned by experience.*

---

[88] *Loc. Aff.* 2.10 (VIII 126 K).
[89] Ibid. (VIII 127 K).

That the soul (or, here, the *archē*) is damaged by changes in the body is, in Galen's view, an empirical fact, and he goes on to adduce examples of the mind (*dianoia*) being impaired by direct injuries to the head. By contrast, it is difficult to know *how* the soul is harmed. Galen sketches two views that he presents as prominent in contemporary philosophical debates: that the soul resides in the body as one resides in a house and that the soul is some kind of form of the body. But although he implies that he finds it hard to reconcile the idea of the body as a mere house for the soul with the manifest damage done to the soul by the body, he rejects neither position out of hand.[90]

Galen's unwillingness to come down hard on one side of the issue of the relationship of the *archē* to the part where it is located is consistent with the agnosticism about the soul that he maintained to the very end of his career.[91] What I suggest is that it may be in part *because* of his uncertainty about the soul's corporeality that he does not describe the relationship of the soul to the body in terms of sympathy, even in the midst of a discussion awash in sympathy, *despite* his strong belief that the soul can be damaged by changes to the body.[92] For what we saw of the fragmentary Epicurean and Stoic evidence indicates that sympathy in the Hellenistic period was being strategically deployed by philosophers to prove or stress the physicality of the *psychē*. It is likely, then, that by Galen's time, the language of sympathy between the *sōma* and the *psychē* implied a commitment to the corporeality of the *psychē*—the very thing that Galen refrains from affirming or denying.[93]

---

[90] In fact, Galen comes close to an Aristotelian view of the soul as a form of the body at *QAM* 3 (IV 773–774 K = 37,3–38,1 Müller), although for 'form' he reads 'mixture', thereby mitigating the problem of how the body acts on the soul. In general, Galen appears committed to a Stoic notion of cause as bodily: see Hankinson 1991a, 203, 219; Gill 2010a, 54.

[91] Galen categorically restates his agnosticism about the nature of the soul—and, more specifically, whether it is immaterial and immortal—in the late works *On My Own Opinions* (*Prop. Plac.* 3 = 173, 13–18 Boudon-Millot and Pietrobelli) and *That the Faculties of the Soul Follow the Mixtures of the Body* (*QAM* 3, IV 775–776 K = 38,18–39,4 Müller). See also *Loc. Aff.* 3.10 (VIII 181 K). For a discussion of these and other relevant passages, see Hankinson 2006; see also Hankinson 1991a, 201–203; von Staden 2000, 112–116; Tieleman 2003b, 140–141; Donini 2008, 185–186.

[92] The language of sympathy, for example, is remarkably absent from *QAM*, the treatise most devoted to the relationship of soul and body (the verb in the title is *hepesthai*, 'to follow': the faculties of the soul 'follow' the mixtures of the body, an expression that keeps the nature of the interaction vague). On the language of body-soul interaction in the treatise, see Lloyd 1988, 33–39.

[93] See Alexander, *Mantissa* § 3 (117,10–22 Bruns), where Alexander tries to account for sympathy without sacrificing the formal, incorporeal nature of the Aristotelian soul. His argument suggests that sympathy had come to entail a commitment to the corporeality of the soul.

It is impossible to know, of course, why Galen remained agnostic on the nature of the soul (although it is interesting that Descartes occupied a similar position). We might speculate, however, about his reluctance to deploy the soul-body sympathy of the philosophers. Whereas for the major philosophical schools, corporeality was an abstract concept and the inside of a human being was a rather ill-defined space, Galen knew the human body, its parts and its stuffs, with extraordinary intimacy. Perhaps it was this intimate knowledge that made it hard for him to accommodate the soul there. What is clear is that for him, sympathy was a technical concept, validated by the pathways beneath the skin that he had himself verified through dissection. The soul hovers beyond the boundaries of Galen's sympathetically webbed organism, tethered by a line he could map neither anatomically nor conceptually.

Conclusion

Reading Galen on sympathetic affections of the brain, we need to keep in mind at least two different intellectual traditions, one medical and one more philosophical. By elaborating a concept of 'medical' sympathy, Galen confirms early Hippocratic models of the body as a self-communicating web of fluid and air while taking advantage of the networked models of the body developed in the wake of the dissections at Alexandria. In Galen, then, the abstract concept of the body as an interconnected unity acquires a particular texture and specificity. Moreover, by privileging the brain as a locus of sympathetic affection, Galen crosses into the territory of interaction between body and soul (or mind). Such territory had already been colonized by philosophers after Plato, philosophers equipped with their own concepts of sympathy, especially from the Hellenistic period on.

Galen leaves his own mark on this territory. His understanding of sympathy privileges the one-way movement of affections from the gut to the brain (and, to a lesser degree, the heart), affections that are cast as pathological. The pathology can be seen in terms of the old Platonic idea of psychic disease, where the appetites overrule the rational part. Yet despite Galen's own claims of fidelity to Plato, the implicit triangle that emerges in his account of sympathetic affections departs from the model of his master. Galen's triangle does a better job of accounting for how the mind is implicated in the dynamics of the lower order functions and, more specifically, the gut, while grounding the lower order functions firmly in the domain of the body. His triangle also favors the expertise of the physician. Still, even as Galen applies anatomy to map the migration of affections to the brain, the soul's relationship to its physical location remains beyond his grasp. Transformed by the state of the body, even enslaved to it, the Galenic soul is nevertheless not sympathetic with it, its fragile but recalcitrant aloofness a figure of Galen's own resistance to ceding the possibility of escaping the coordinates of the body.

PLATO ON MADNESS AND THE GOOD LIFE[*]

Katja Maria Vogt

What is madness? When does one enter a state of madness? Is it when obsessions, compulsions, moods, or addictions take possession of your motivations, and you no longer decide what you do? Viewed that way, madness is a state that is to be avoided, a state that is irrational in a highly undesirable way: it comes with lack of agency, and thus with a lack of freedom. And yet you might find it boring to be asked to be 'rational'. Excited and enthusiastic about something, you might insist that a certain kind of craziness leads to the best things in life: love, philosophy, art, science, and so on. You find fault with the instinct to draw a line between rationality and madness. Is not some kind of madness a powerful ingredient of a good life, as one might rationally pursue it?

These questions frame Plato's views on madness. It would be naive to consider all madness bad, or to consider madness a remote phenomenon, absent from the lives of most of us. Madness is deeply connected to rationality and to irrationality. Plato's approach has much to recommend it: it addresses madness from the point of view of agents who aim to lead a good life. From this perspective, the relationships between rationality, irrationality, and madness are crucially important. We do not want to lapse into kinds of madness that impede our lives, taking us captive to obsessions, compulsions, mood disorders, and the like. We also do not want to miss out on forms of madness that make life richer and more interesting.

I shall discuss three phenomena—phenomena that, for Plato, all count in one way or another as madness: rational madness (1), god-given madness (2), and disordered desiderative states or mental illness (3). (1) and (2) are beneficial; they increase our powers of agency. (3) is destructive; these conditions are serious impediments to agency. The surface of Plato's discussions, populated by gods and Muses, might appear alien to us. Metaphors

---

[*] I am grateful to William Harris for inviting me to present this paper at a conference on *Mental Illness in Antiquity,* and to the conference participants for lively discussion. Jens Haas read several drafts of the paper and offered most helpful comments.

aside, Plato in effect discusses criteria similar to those scientists employ today, and arguably he offers detail that can help us formulate these criteria in particularly compelling ways.[1]

Most fundamentally, Plato's criteria concern themselves with desire, or, in other terms, with the question of what kinds of things look good—or bad—to agents in a given condition. Throughout many of his dialogues, Plato explores an idea that is known as a Socratic Paradox: everyone desires the good. In being motivated to perform such-and-such an action, one sees the action (or something relating to it, such as its outcome) as good. Otherwise one would not be moved to act. In comparing Plato's accounts of (1) rational madness, (2) god-given madness, and (3) mental illness, I shall pursue the general question of how these conditions fit in with the general directionality of motivation toward the good. (1) and (2) enhance the pursuit of the good; though they add complexity to the theory, they fit perfectly into the general claim that motivation is for the good. (3) raises difficult questions. First, there is the question of whether someone who, say, sees the relief a compulsive action promises as good, is motivated toward the good, even though she herself might be aware that she pursues something harmful. Plato discusses this kind of issue in terms of conflicts between different motivational powers, each with its good. Second, there is the question of what should be said about an agent who no longer pursues the good of any motivational power typically relevant to human action: reason, spirit, and desire. Suppose that a power could grow in an agent that is even lower than desire, and suppose the agent became motivated by the good of that power—a power than Plato characterizes as monstrous. Would there still be a sense in which the agent pursues *her* good, given that the monster is arguably not who she used to be, and that she is inhabited by a force that is alien to the typical patterns of human motivation?

I shall refer to several dialogues—the *Ion, Symposium, Republic, Phaedrus,* and *Philebus*—as making distinct proposals. But I shall not emphasize the differences between these texts. Instead, I am trying to put together a sketch of those states and conditions that Plato associates with madness. My approach should not be mistaken for the view that there is one Platonic

---

[1] Psychiatrists are working with philosophers to advance definitions of central concepts such as autonomy, in the hopes of applying them in court and in other contexts where much hangs on whether a person is assessed as mentally disturbed or not (cf. Bernard Gert's consultant work for the revision of 3rd edition of the *Diagnostic and Statistical Manual* (DSM-III–R) of the American Psychiatric Association, 1987; see also ⟨http://www.guardian.co .uk/education/2010/jun/29/mental-health-patients-decisions⟩).

theory of madness, re-iterated or re-dressed in various dialogues (or even worse, for the view that the dialogues need not be studied as self-standing texts). On the contrary, I assume that Plato thinks through several ways in which the relevant phenomena could be explained. I take these differences, even where they are subtle, to be of great interest. However, I shall focus on an idea that appears to me to be present in dialogues that otherwise differ importantly from each other: the idea that we think about madness in the context of wanting our lives to go well.

Though the relevant dialogues are the subject of an extensive secondary literature, scholars have not focused on this idea. Indeed, as far as I can see, it is not even discussed. Perhaps this is because the intuition that madness is close to home for all of us was unpalatable to a long tradition of scholarship. Perhaps it is also related to the fact that Romanticism embraced the idea that artists are inspired by genius; god-given madness, accordingly, appeared to be a topic exclusively for aesthetics, rather than being interpreted in the larger context of Plato's theory of motivation.[2] Finally, it might also be because in a sense I am saying something obvious. However, I take it that the obvious is often what is hardest to get clear about.

1. Rational Madness

There is an everyday notion of rationality according to which the rational person is the sober-minded person. 'Be rational' means 'don't be such a dreamer,' 'don't be overly enthusiastic,' and so on. Importantly, this is not Plato's notion of rationality. Human rationality includes enthusiasm—it includes a motivational force that is so strong that it is plausibly associated with a god. Typically, human beings desire their own happiness with such fervor that they are, metaphorically speaking, like Eros: hunters who crave their trophy, and who will go to great lengths to get it. Accordingly, rational madness is no oxymoron. A conception of reason that makes no room for positive phenomena of enthusiasm and crazed-ness is too simple.

The *Symposium* contains an account of human motivation that explores this idea.[3] According to Socrates' (and Diotima's) speech, love is not

---

[2] Cf. Asmis 1992.

[3] Only a few scholars read the *Symposium* in this way. Generally, scholars tend to focus on love in the ordinary sense—that is, love for other persons or for ideas, but not love as a general motivational force in the pursuit of a good life. Some contributions relevant to my topic are: Wedgwood 2009; Kahn 1987; Richardson-Lear 2007; Kraut 2008.

primarily about relationships. More fundamentally, love (*erôs*) is a perva-sive motivational force. Love is what drives us in our pursuit of happiness. It motivates the kinds of activities—having children, taking up a craft, engag-ing in politics, and so on—that typically structure human lives, and that we associate with happiness (199–208).[4] In these pursuits, we strive for 'goods' (*agatha*). For example, in having a family, we aim to see our children grow up and flourish; in engaging in politics, we aim to establish improved laws; and so on. To achieve and 'possess' these goods is to be happy. Accordingly, these goods are the principal object of love (205a–206a). Indeed, the desire for these goods—and for being happy—is said to be the greatest and most violent love for everyone (205d).

This proposal contains an under-appreciated idea about human striving for happiness. Love, as the motivator behind this striving, is thought of as a *violent* force. The way we pursue happiness is not measured and sober. On the contrary, it is as if we were love-sick for happiness. We go to great lengths for our children, for political change, and so on. Diotima goes so far as to say that, if one did not understand the nature of human love for happiness—and this includes ideas beyond the scope of this paper, ideas about beauty and immortality—we would have to be puzzled by its *alogia* (208c4). *Alogia*, here, refers to an apparent irrationality. Without an account of love for happiness at our disposal, human behavior would be inexplicable to the observer.

Consider an example. Apollodorus, who reports the conversation of the *Symposium*, is an adherent of Socrates, infected with philosophy as with an illness. He was given the name '*malakos*' on account of following Socrates and pursuing philosophy (173d7). The standard English translation calls him 'crazy.' Literally, '*malakos*' corresponds to derogative epithets that, perhaps, children might use when teasing each other, saying that someone is 'weak-minded' or has gone 'soft in the head'. This, then, is the effect of having had a taste of philosophy by talking to Socrates. Once one begins to pursue phi-losophy, one is 'sold.' One recognizes how good it would be to gain insights, and accordingly one cannot rationally stop pursuing insights, though one realizes that great effort is needed and that one may never get there. Apol-lodorus accepts the designation as *malakos*, admitting that he is mad (*main-omai*) (173e2–3, an expression that connotes Bacchic frenzy) and infatuated (*parapaiô*).

---

[4] On the range of typical human pursuits, cf. 208c–209e and 205d.

His state, however, is a rational kind of madness. Devotion to philosophy is rational, insofar as it reflects the basic structure of human desire for happiness; something good—in this case, knowledge—is associated with happiness and pursued. At the same time, it is a kind of infatuation: philosophers tend to be much like Apollodorus, driven in a way that looks ridiculous to others. Philosophy is just one of the pursuits taken up by people in their quests for a good life. Having children, politics, crafts, and so on, are structurally similar. Something is recognized as good and its pursuit is associated with happiness. It is then aimed at with great fervor.

The madness of desiring happiness is a central component of human motivation toward the good; indeed, it is the greatest motivator in human life, and it is directed toward the good. It is rational in the following sense. First, human beings strive for a good life according to the structures of *human* motivation, and that is, motivation that reflects at once the mortality of human agents and the fact that a person's motivational perspective is not limited to one particular finite life. Second, and relatedly, love for happiness is a general feature of human motivation, rather than an aberration; this is how we rationally respond to what we see as good. Third, it is rational insofar as it is a good feature of human motivation. Love of happiness—associated with the demi-god Eros—makes us better, not worse agents: it drives us into high-gear, and fuels the kinds of pursuits we associate with a life lived to its fullest.[5] What, then, is left of the idea that it is a kind of madness? Only so much: the motivational force of love is a kind of driven-ness and crazed-ness.

2. God-Given Madness

In my reconstruction of rational madness in the *Symposium*, I employed an intuitive notion of madness. Aided by the expressions that Apollodorus and Diotima use, I suggested that madness has something to do with the following states: being in 'high gear' or in a mode of high activity; being 'crazed' or 'driven'; being 'infected' or infatuated with something that one has tasted and now wants more of. Clearly, there can be good and bad versions of

---

[5] Notably, this need not mean that one lives a life of excitement, a life where one is emotionally in high gear. Socrates, devoted to philosophy and driven by its pursuit, is at the same time a rather cool and calm person. In a review of Susan Wolf (2010), Joseph Raz (2010) finds—in my view rightly—fault with Wolf's account of the meaning of life (a topic not unrelated to the *Symposium*'s concern with motivation for a good life). As he sees it, Wolf makes it seem as if only the excited could lead a meaningful life. This is not the idea I suggest we ascribe to the Plato of the *Symposium*.

such states. And clearly, if rational madness is a general feature of human motivation, it counts as madness only in a relatively thin sense. According to another everyday intuition about madness, madness is an extraordinary state. This applies to love only insofar as it is, within everyone's life, the most violent motivation. More robust forms of madness will have to be conditions that are extraordinary in a literal sense, conditions that are rarely found.

In the *Phaedrus*, Plato distinguishes between two such kinds of madness (*mania*), god-given madness on the one hand, and madness as human disease or mental disorder on the other. I shall employ Plato's account of god-given madness in order to generate a list of features of madness, and assign names to them. The features on my list (for which I claim no completeness, and which are closely interrelated) are by themselves neither good nor bad. In god-given madness, they manifest themselves in positive ways; in mental disorder, they manifest themselves negatively.

Throughout the *Phaedrus*, Plato uses two conspicuous expressions for madness: *to aphron* and *paranoia*. Madness is an absence of the usual functioning of the mind (*to aphron*; *Phaedrus* 236a1, 265e4). The mad person is beside herself; what goes on in her mind is past comprehension; or it runs alongside the ordinary functions of the mind. Madness thus is, literally, *paranoia* (266a3), *para* having all these meanings: beside, past, along, beyond, and so on. Moreover, an agent in the relevant kind of state is 'moved' or agitated (*kekinêmenos*, 245b4). Madness is a volatile state.

Platonic madness thus has these characteristics:

APHRON   Madness is a kind of absence or bracketing off of the regular powers of reason.

PARANOIA   The cognitive activities that come with madness can run alongside regular cognitive activities, or go beyond them.

ACTIVITY   Madness is an agitated state, a state with a high level of activity.[6]

Plato does not describe god-given madness as a loss of health (265a9–10). Instead, it is a shifting out of the ordinary and customary (*exallagês tôn eiôthotôn nominôm*), effected through divinity (265a10–11). What is removed is the condition we are used to, and that we associate with ordinary ways of doing things. This is an important point. Madness is not, qua madness, immediately a disease. At bottom, madness is a state that differs from what we are used to. Here, then, is a fourth characteristic of madness:

---

[6] Plato does not seem to think of mood disorders that come with motivational inertia.

CUSTOM   Madness is not primarily the opposite of health, but of ordinary states and customary ways of doing things.

God-given madness is, like motivational love as discussed in the *Symposium*, a good phenomenon. Divine inspiration figures in the greatest achievements: creation of poems, healing of diseases, rescue from disaster, philosophical insight. In the phrase that is the ancestor of 'enthusiastic', Plato says that in such conditions, a god is in the agent—the agent is *enthousiazôn* (*Phaedrus* 241e, 249e, 253a, 263d). Alternatively, the agent is in-spired—a 'spirit' (*daimon*) is 'in' her. It is hard to assess how literal Plato wants us to take these formulations. Is he seriously suggesting that a divine being inhabits a human agent's mind?

A deflationary reading, which sees talk about divine inspiration as metaphorical, would have to capture the following ideas. First, in order to be in agreement with Plato's core theological commitment, reference to divine inspiration must mean that something positive influences an agent's mind. This is Plato's most central claim about god or the gods: that he or they are good.[7] That is, where Plato refers to divine intervention, he means to suggest that the relevant phenomenon is—at least in important respects—good. Second, insofar as Plato, though he rejects much of traditional religiosity, consistently expresses reverence for the divine, it means that something takes place that is superior to ordinary events. Third, something goes on in the mind that is typically experienced as not deriving from the agent's own thought-processes. The relevant experience might be that of the cognizer herself: she does not know how she arrived at a given idea, and thus sees it as something that was put into her mind. Alternatively, it might also be the experience of on-lookers. Suppose a poem is found to be deep and beautiful. The poet, however, is found to be silly and unable to say anything coherent about the poem. In response, one might be tempted to say that the poem must derive from cognitive powers beyond the poet's own.[8]

---

[7] Cf. *Republic* II, 379a–b. Cf. Bordt 2006.

[8] This seems to be Plato's attitude in the *Ion*. The protagonist Ion is a professional reciter and interpreter of Homeric poetry. At the end of the dialogue, Socrates says to Ion 'you must be divine' (542b). This pronouncement is a response to Ion's proposal that the Athenians should hire him as military leader for their next war: qua Homeric expert, he is an expert on everything Homer writes about, and accordingly he is a military expert. Quite likely, Socrates makes fun of Ion in calling him divine. Ion greatly prefers this idea to Socrates' earlier claim that he is out of his mind (535d). The implication, throughout the dialogue, is that Ion is ignorant in a baffling way: though able to recite Homer and to talk about Homer, he understands nothing—neither any of the topics that come up in Homer, nor his own thought-processes.

I shall not argue for this deflationary reading; this would lead to questions too far afield from the topic of this paper. Given that Plato does not hold traditional theological views—for which his core premise 'god is good' serves as sufficient evidence—it is unlikely that his talk about divine intervention fits into a conventional, religious perspective. Admittedly, more would have to be said. For present purposes, however, focus on the impression that a superior power adds something to a cognizer's thought processes is legitimate. The question of whether this impression is well-interpreted by literal reference to divine intervention can be left open.

In sum, the proposal seems to be that there is a *positive* version of finding oneself with cognitive activity that does not appear to result from one's ordinary thought-processes. In these states, human beings can accomplish something extraordinarily good (244a): they can make predictions, find cures, create poetry, and be philosophical lovers of the Forms. These agents are mad without being irrational. For example, the poet comes up with verses the meaning of which might be obscure to her. Someone or something else seems to think through the agent. And yet, the cognitive powers of the poet are not diminished or otherwise negatively affected. Though the production of poetic verse happens in the heightened mode, she is herself when she turns back to mundane tasks. Here is, accordingly, a fifth features of madness:

ALIEN   In madness, something alien to the agent's own mind is experienced as affecting cognitive activity.

Consider Socrates' claim that sometimes a divine spirit warns him.[9] For example, he wants to step into a river, but has a premonition, one that he does not perceive as originating in his own mind, but rather ascribes to a good demon; the premonition makes him stop in his tracks (*Phaedrus* 242b8–d2). Why does this qualify as a positive case of having one's reason overruled? First, that which overrules one's reason is better rather than worse than one's reason. It is divine reason, not one's desires; it is a good spirit who warns Socrates, not a bad spirit. Second, while one's reason is overruled, it is not inhibited in its activities. Socrates retains his cognitive powers. He appropriates the divine sign as something for him to take into consideration. Socrates' condition is not one of madness, but it displays one

---

[9] Cf. Long 2006. Long's discussion is in the spirit of my paper. He takes seriously that Socrates, otherwise known for his commitment to reason (in a sense that excludes 'mad' phenomena) takes the voice of his *daimon* seriously, and considers it a positive force.

aspect of god-given madness: he finds himself with thoughts that he ascribes not to himself, but to a higher being. Socrates' divine sign appears to be at the end of a spectrum of cases, some of which might go significantly further. A human agent's reason might be altered in a way that cannot be integrated into ordinary reasoning. The foreign element can 'take over,' so much so that the agent is out of her mind, and therefore in a more literal sense mad.[10]

In the *Phaedrus*, god-given madness is discussed in celebratory terms. In an earlier discussion of inspiration and poetry, in the *Ion*, Plato makes fun of the poets. Their lack of comprehension tends to come with presumptions: when they utter grand and beautiful sentences, they feel as if they 'owned' them, or, in other words, as if the poetic verses were their thoughts, and as such, were transparent to them.[11] A singer like Ion, who does not create poetry, but recites and interprets it, greatly misunderstands his own expertise. He considers himself an expert on all topics that figure in Homer's epic poetry (and that is, virtually everything, from chariot-building to speech-making to medicine to military strategy).

Poets and rhapsodes can fail to realize that in fact the poetic verses they formulate are not their thoughts. It is not a failure of rationality to be divinely possessed, and in this sense out of one's mind. But it is a failure of rationality not to be able to distinguish between the divine influence and one's own cognitive activities. Scholars have sometimes suggested that the *Phaedrus* and the *Ion* offer substantially different outlooks on inspiration.[12] But in spite of the many differences between the two dialogues, it would seem that the point from the early dialogue *Ion* could survive in later Platonic philosophy. Divine inspiration is a good thing insofar as its results are concerned. When it comes to assessing a particular agent's state of mind, it is good only if is recognized for what it is.[13] The inspired person should be able to distinguish

---

[10] Cf. Bortolotti (2010) on the question of integration. For example, it is a sign of serious disturbance if a delusional belief is not reflected in one's actions—say, someone thought 'I am dead,' but continued to go through ordinary activities. Bortolotti argues for a point that is related to this paper: that such rather extreme cases are on a continuous spectrum with more ordinary cases of irrationality.

[11] Though Ion does not think of himself as the author of the thought, he thinks of himself as owning it: as having come to think it as one of his thoughts. Both authorship and ownership of thoughts are core things to get wrong in phenomena of irrationality and mental disorder.

[12] See for example Pappas (2008).

[13] It is sometimes assumed that Plato, by not ascribing expertise to an artist, de-values poetry. However, it is important to keep apart the high regard for the results of god-given madness, and the assessment that those who voice a given poem lack knowledge. Indeed, the move to god-given madness enables Plato to hold artistic products in high esteem, and yet criticize the states of minds of artists. For an interpretation of the *Ion* that conflates the

her own thoughts from the thoughts instilled in her by a superior power. We can thus derive a sixth feature of madness from the *Ion*:

LACK OF OWNERSHIP   Mad cognitive activity is not properly 'owned' by the agent; the agent's thoughts are in some sense not her thoughts, and should be recognized for what they are.

God-given madness thus poses challenges to those who experience it. A cognizer should aim to assess correctly what goes on in her mind. On the whole, however, god-given madness is a positive phenomenon. It fits perfectly into the framing premise of Plato's theory of motivation, namely that it is for the good: in god-given madness, agents pursue the good with heightened powers.

3. *Madness as Disease*

Mental disorders, as I shall call the kinds of madness that are diseases, are not ascribed to superior powers, and they do not lead to good things. In discussing these phenomena, I shall continue to refer to the *Phaedrus*; additionally, I shall draw on the *Republic* and the *Philebus*. Most generally speaking, mental disorders, according to these dialogues, are messed-up motivational states, and they are destructive. They are largely the negative effect of indulgence in excessive pleasures; such pleasures infect the soul with madness (*Phil.* 63c and 45e–23).[14]

In Book IV of the *Republic*, Plato famously conceives of three motivational faculties. Motivational conflict, so the argument goes, can only be explained if the soul—that aspect of human beings associated with cognitive and desiderative capacities—has several such powers.[15] Plato distinguishes between three sources of motivation: reason, spirit, and the ap-

two issues, see Jannaway 1995, 14. A study of great influence is Scharper 1968; Scharper makes Plato the ancestor of Romantic aesthetics. For valid objections, see Stern-Gillet 2004.

[14] Another idea, equally important, focuses on directionality: towards what kinds of objects does the soul turn? Much of the *Republic*'s discussion of education is framed in terms of a turning (*peritropê*) of the soul, away from particulars and toward intelligible objects. Mathematics is a core and long-term aspect of education, precisely because it helps one develop the ability to engage with intelligible objects (cf. Burnyeat 2000). The positive development of *Republic*-style education has its negative corollary: decline is a turning toward perceptible particulars. The question of directionality and the question of which pleasures are sought out are intertwined. In turning, say, to the abstract objects of mathematics, one tastes and comes to appreciate the pleasures of reason.

[15] On Platonic tripartition, cf. Cooper 1999, ch. 5. On the desiderative part of the soul, cf. Lorenz 2006; see also Moss 2006 and 2005.

petites. Each of these motivational faculties has its good: each sees something as 'good-for-it,' desires it, and takes pleasure in it. Reason sees learning as its good, desires it, and takes pleasure in it; spirit sees honor as its good, desires it, and takes pleasure in it; the appetites see money and bodily pleasures as good, desire them, and take pleasure in them (*Rp.* IV; cf. IX, 580d–581c).

Though the tripartite soul reappears in rather similar terms in the *Timaeus* (69c5–72d3), tripartition cannot be simply treated as a Platonic doctrine. Indeed, it is not even clear that Plato presents a unified account of tripartition in the *Republic*. Later divisions in this same dialogue (*Rp.* 602c–603a, 603e–605c) have been thought to differ from the Book IV account, or to explore further angles.[16] The *Phaedrus* offers yet another version of the *Republic*'s trias: a charioteer drives a wagon with two horses, one of them noble, the other wild (246a–254e). The *Philebus* is devoted to a comparison between lives—the life of reason and the life of pleasure—and eventually to distinctions between different cognitive activities on the one hand, and kinds of pleasures on the other, as they figure in lives that go better or worse. For present purposes, we need not discuss the differences between these approaches. Instead, we can assume that Plato is interested in a range of related contrasts between reason and non-reasoning powers; between aspects of us that adhere to reason and others that cling to appearances; and between different kinds of pleasures associated with different parts of the soul. It is this set of intuitions that we need in order to put together a sketch of Platonic mental disease.

Mental disorders involve a failure by the agent's reason to assert power over her desires, and a failure to adopt desires that are good for her. Notably, this failure is not something for which Plato blames the agent. On the contrary, Plato thinks that much depends on how one is brought up, and what kinds of pleasure are on offer in a given society.[17] Insofar as blame is assigned, it goes to political systems.[18] Perhaps even more importantly, it goes to the nature of pleasure itself. As Plato emphasizes in the *Philebus*, pleasure is a

---

[16] Cf. Moss 2008.

[17] The story Plato tells about decline of one's motivations is a generational story (*Rp.* VIII–IX): he looks at young people growing up with parents of such-and-such a kind, and in a society with such-and-such values. The dynamic unfolds between children who object to their parents' way of life, fall victim to temptations offered by others who are ostensibly more successful (richer, more powerful) than their parents, and so on.

[18] For a similar point on the relationship between an individual's psychology and the societal setting, cf. Lear 1998, 219–246.

manifold (*poikilon*) phenomenon: pleasures differ deeply from each other (*Phil.* 12c4–8).[19] This multiplicity and many-facedness is a symptom of a dangerous nature. Figuratively speaking, one pleasure will lead to the next. Once tasted, pleasures become easily the object of desire. This process is inherent in the nature of pleasure, rather than being a function of the presumed weaknesses of particular agents. It is a further fact about the workings of pleasure that relatively lowly pleasures are a kind of entry-path towards even lowlier and more dangerous pleasures. Plato thinks of agents living in societal contexts that are seductive, and having to ward off as best as they can what is, after all, a rather likely downhill development.

Education that shields one against these temptations must begin early. In his discussion of childhood education in the *Republic*, Plato makes an interesting proposal. Children ought to be raised with stories, music, and athletic exercises. How do these components of education interrelate? A good physical condition, Plato says, does not make the soul good; but a good psychological condition will eventually be reflected in a person's body. More care must go into the psychological than into the physiological aspects of raising a child: if a person has the right affective attitudes and well-trained cognitive faculties, she will be able to shape her physique accordingly (403d). However, before this can happen, childhood education must make sure that the body is well-configured (403e–404d).

Though Plato's discussion of athletics qua physical education is short, movement receives great attention as a part of the education that addresses the soul. Musical education is, to a significant extent, concerned with dances and games (*Rp.* 376c8f.). According to Plato, a child needs to develop love for the good (and that includes a directionality toward the right pleasures), and she can do this only if she listens to the right songs and stories, and plays the right games, moving her body in ways that induce order, discipline, beauty, and gracefulness (*euschêmosunê*). *Euschêmosunê* is, literally, a 'well-configured state': in part through the right kind of movement, the soul is shaped and formed well.[20] Plato casts this process as a kind of

---

[19] Pleasures are not, qua pleasures, essentially the same. Though all pleasure is pleasant, pleasures have particular properties that make them differ crucially from each other. A similar claim is made for cognitive activities; they come in rather different forms (*Philebus* 13d4–14a3). Pleasure and cognitive activity (*phronein*) are each one, and many (12c–19b). However, in the case of pleasure, Plato thinks of an inherently problematic multiplicity; in the case of our reasoning faculties, he simply proposes that there are several of them.

[20] I agree with Burnyeat that, in the early books on education of the *Republic*, gracefulness is presented as the core virtue (1997, 220). Burnyeat's focus is on the musical part of early

feeding (*trophê*): our bodies and souls need to taste the right things, and to digest the right things, for us to become attuned to pleasures that are good for us. Interestingly, exercise is here not understood as sports; it is understood as something we must do for our psychological balance and well-being. Plato conceives of the structured movements of games as something that directly translates into the states and attitudes of the soul. What we might think of as physical education, for him, is immediately and primarily about the shaping of our motivations.

In the later books of the *Republic*, then, Plato is concerned with mental disorder as a condition into which a young adult or grown-up person may gradually slide. For the agent who is trying to lead a good life, it is imperative to avoid settings in which destructive pleasures are tasted, and become newly-acquired predilections. A central feature of Plato's account of psychological decline is the following: the worst pleasures, those that derange and enslave us, do not follow the patterns of 'regular' tripartite motivation. They belong to an aspect of human beings that need not figure in ordinary action, and that most people succeed to banish from their waking lives.

Notably, even a person who pursues the good of the appetites leads a relatively stable life (551a and 553b–c). As lover of wealth, this kind of person is careful not to acquire expensive tastes. She sees how costly everything is, and she wants to keep her money. Accordingly, though she is ruled by lowly desires, her desires do not spiral out of control. In making this point, Plato distinguishes between necessary and non-necessary pleasures. The stingy person has a piece of cheese and a glass of water for dinner, returning to work the next morning without a hang-over. In being so motivated, she pursues wealth, one of the goods of the appetites. This person may not lead the kind of life Plato admires, and her soul is not well-ordered. But she is not in a state of mental disease.

Someone else will engage in non-necessary pleasures, buying expensive wines and imported delicacies (558d–560a). This person too is ruled by her appetites, but by another aspect of them: by their pursuit of bodily pleasure. Due to the nature of bodily pleasure, this agent crosses a line. Bodily pleasures, if there is no self-imposed discipline, lead toward increasingly intense and violent desires. A person who develops such desires will be in temporary states of madness. In the *Philebus*, Plato says that the greatest bodily pleasures come with a kind of madness: at least for some intense moments, they

---

education; as I see it, Plato is serious about the role of physical movement. On the importance of education for shaping motivation, cf. also Burnyeat 2000.

make people 'freak out', leaping and kicking, with distorted features (*Phil.* 47a–b).[21] In the *Republic*, unrestrained pursuit of such pleasures is associated with liberty (*eleutheria*, *Rp.* 562b12). Liberty here is a kind of chaos, a lack of discrimination with respect to which pleasures are sought (564a4–5). A person who leads this life is, in a way, motivated by her appetites; but she is not guided by appetites that are in their unadulterated state. Rather, she is ruled by appetites that have been enlarged, through a kind of growth that involves diversification. In a well-known metaphor, Plato thinks that, in this degenerative process, one's appetites become a many-headed monster, with ever more heads (588c). This monster was raised and fed by the agent. It makes a value-judgment: it regards liberty, or lack of restraint and excessive variety, as good. On her downhill path, the agent develops ever more disastrous desires. Wild and excessive pleasures come to control her. If these pleasures are tasted and cultivated, they persistently rob a person of her agency: there is no sense in which *she* is still in control. These pleasures, which Plato describes as lawless (*paranomoi*, 571b6), are tyrants (577b–580c).

The lawless pleasures are not strictly speaking alien to our natures. Plato proposes that they have an echo in everyone's psychological make-up: it is not outside of the realm of human motivation to have dreams in which tabus are violated, even for those who would never seriously entertain such thoughts when awake, and are disgusted by having such a dream (571b–572b). But in the perverted life that we are imagining now, lawless pleasures are available. On her downward spiral, the agent is set up for tasting them, and coming to depend on them. Lawless pleasures are the domain of serious mental disorder (*mania*, cf. 573a–c). The agent lives as if in an on-going dream—the kind of dream that breaks tabus and vividly presents actions that, for any ordinary person, are unthinkable (576b).

---

[21] Bodily pleasures, Plato argues, come with pain and a semblance of pleasure, rather than real pleasure. From the point of view of bodily pain, the removal of pain looks like pleasure. This is a perspectival mistake: when you are in pain, then relief from it appears so desirable that you falsely consider it pleasure (*Rp.* 583b–585a, cf. *Phil.* 51a and 42a–b on perspectival mistakes). But it is only the relief from physical pain, not yet pleasure. Bodily pleasures and pleasures of anticipation are merely perceived pleasures; really, they are the cessation of pain. There is a better kind of pleasure, namely pleasure which is not the cessation of pain, so-called 'pure pleasure,' and that is, the pleasure of reason. This argument involves a three-stage model of pain and pleasure, the third stage being a neutral, in-between stage. Plato defends the three-stage model in *Philebus* 43d f., where he ascribes a two-stage model—pleasure is the removal of pain—to harsh people who have an inordinate hatred against the power of pleasure and do not acknowledge anything healthy in it (44c5–d1).

Plato proposes that this dimension of ours, shared by everyone, need not and ordinarily does not figure in motivation. It can be banned from our waking lives, and perhaps even extirpated from one's sleeping mind (571b–572b). Tripartite motivation does not draw on this source of desire: ordinary agents pursue the good of reason, of spirit, and of the appetites, without accessing this sub-region of motivation. The mentally ill agent, however, whose waking life has the quality of a nightmare, is in a no-man's land of motivation, neither directed by reason, nor by spirit, nor by a recognizable version of the appetites. The monster-heads that have grown out of a tamer set of desires are not literally foreign to our natures, and yet they are an alien force. In a slightly altered metaphor, one might say that the relevant sub-region of motivation houses a monster that, if things go well, is asleep. If it is woken up, it shows itself to be unmanageable: it takes over one's whole being. What does this mean for the basic assumption about human motivation, namely that agents are motivated by what they see as good? Mentally ill motivation, according to Plato's proposal, still fits the pattern of pursuing the good. However, it is no longer the agent, or her regular motivational powers, who pursue the good. It is a sub-agential force in the agent that pursues its good.

Mental illness, thus, displays negative versions of the features discussed above. The agent's life is bare of rationality (APHRON). The agent is 'beside' herself (PARANOIA), or in other words, has lost her former, rational self. Hers is a driven way of life, she is constantly in 'high gear' (ACTIVITY). Her behavior violates all customs and ordinary ways of life (CUSTOM). What rules her is alien to her insofar as it resides below her tripartite soul (ALIEN). The agent finds herself with thoughts and desires that do not originate in either of the regular three motivational powers; instead, they originate in a sub-region of motivation, that does not properly represent a human agent (LACK OF OWNERSHIP).

4. Conclusion

In the *Phaedrus*, Socrates cites the Delphic injunction 'know yourself' (229e5–6) and explains that it is a core aspect of his quest for self-knowledge to find out whether he is a monster (229e6–230a8). Socrates worries whether he is a wild animal, worse even than Typhon, a monster with a hundred dragon-heads. He would like to be a tamer and simpler animal, one that naturally has some divine part to it. As of now, he does not know which kind of being he is. This passage highlights that, for Plato, the worry whether one might be a mad person is central to the quest for a good life. In dealing with ourselves, we want to make sure that our life is not ruled by a monster, a monster that, in effect, would be 'who we are' if it ruled us. The fact that even Socrates has to worry about this, not being sure whether he is tame, reminds us that the danger of becoming a monster is real for everyone.

Plato explores madness from the point of view of a person who aims to lead her life well, and who aims to be well. Rational madness is an essential part of the good life—the pursuit of happiness is, when adequate, not engaged in with an attitude of thorough soberness. But since irrational madness is dangerous, it is imperative for us to keep things apart; importantly, this involves that we understand the manifold nature of pleasure. Because these matters are so central to our lives, it is essential to define the boundaries between rational and irrational madness. These boundaries are difficult to understand, a point which reflects the fact that madness is deeply related both to rationality and to irrationality.

PART III

PARTICULAR SYNDROMES

MENTAL DISORDER AND THE PERILS OF DEFINITION: CHARACTERIZING EPILEPSY IN GREEK SCIENTIFIC DISCOURSE (5TH–4TH CENTURIES BCE)*

Roberto Lo Presti

Introduction

This paper will approach the general theme of mental illness in Antiquity from quite an eccentric angle, as it will investigate how the Greek scientific discourse[1] of the fifth and fourth centuries BCE dealt with epilepsy (the so-called 'sacred disease'), that is to say with a disease whose primary forms contemporary medical culture tends not to include in the list of the psychiatric, viz. mental, disorders.[2] For this and other reasons, which I am going to elucidate in this introduction, this kind of investigation requires some historical-epistemological *prolegomena*.

* I am most grateful to the Alexander von Humboldt-Stiftung for its financial and institutional support, and to Philip van der Eijk, for the care with which he follows and encourages my work. I am also grateful to William Harris and the other participants in the New York conference for their questions and critical remarks, to Maria Michela Sassi, with whom I discussed various versions of this paper, and to the colleagues of the Institut für Klassische Philologie of the Humboldt-Universität, who read and commented the final version of this paper. Special thanks are due to Anna-Maria Kanthak, whose remarks have been of great help in clarifying some crucial points of my argument.

[1] By adopting the notion of 'Greek scientific discourse of the classical period' I deliberately avoid drawing any rigid distinction between such forms of intellectual enterprise as medicine and philosophy, whose boundaries at that time were far from being defined. For a definition of 'science' and 'scientific text' I refer to Asper 2007, 11: 'Unter dem für Anachronismen anfälligen Begriff "Wissenschaft" verstehe ich einerseits Wissen, das in allgemeine Sätze gefasst werden kann und einer bestimmten Gruppe als konsensfähiger Faktenbestand gilt, andererseits die wissensorientierten Praktiken dieser Gruppe'. On the social, cultural, intellectual, epistemological factors that determined the constitution of the disciplinary fields as well as their fluidity in classical Greece extensive research has been carried out by G.E.R. Lloyd (1979, 86–98 and 126–169; 1990, 39–72; 1991, 249–260), van der Eijk, 2008b, 385–412. On the structural, rhetorical, and stylistic features of the Greek scientific discourse see also van der Eijk 1997, 77–129.

[2] Epilepsy is not included in the latest version of the *Diagnostic and Statistical Manual of Mental Disorders* (DSM-IV-TR).

First of all, it must be said that in the ancient texts the term 'epilepsy' can indicate both the disease as a well-defined morbid entity and the single attack,[3] and that the label 'epileptic' is frequently used with reference to a wide range of convulsive attacks, many of which would not be classified as 'epileptic' according to modern nosological criteria. But also when speaking of 'epilepsy' today we must not forget that we are making reference to a somewhat slippery nosological entity, or rather clinical diagnosis.[4] For, although it is now generally acknowledged that epilepsy is basically a *biological* disorder of the nervous system, characterized by intermittent and recurrent alterations of the electrical activity of the brain,[5] and although significant progress has been made in the fields of both neurological and psychiatric research toward a differentiation and classification of the various forms of epileptic disorder[6] as well as of the so-called psychogenic *non*-epileptic seizures,[7] what O. Temkin wrote more than half a century ago still remains largely valid: 'There is no unanimity about the range of the concept of epilepsy, and the nature of the disease is as yet obscure [...] The broader the point of view from which epilepsy is studied, the more the condition tends to lose its identity and merge into the domain of convulsive states, encompassing many 'epilepsies' of different origin'.[8]

In spite of, or more probably because of, the difficulty of reaching an exact and comprehensive definition,[9] the concept of epilepsy has ended up with

---

[3] Temkin 1971², 28: 'The distinction between symptomatic epilepsy, i.e., a syndrome which might be associated with various diseases, and the possible existence of an 'essential' or 'genuine' disease, epilepsy, is of relatively modern origin and was of little importance in Antiquity'.

[4] Johnston and Smith 2008, 7.

[5] See Levy 1993, 713, and Johnston and Smith 2008, 7: 'Seizures are sudden and usually transient stereotyped clinical episodes of disturbed behaviour, emotion, or motor or sensory function that may or may not be accompanied by a change in consciousness level. They result from abnormal excessive but synchronized discharges from a set of cerebral neurons. [...] Epilepsy is the tendency to experience recurrent unprovoked seizures. A single seizure is not epilepsy'.

[6] For a brief survey of the most important forms of epileptic seizure see Levy 1993, 715–716.

[7] The psychogenic non-epileptic seizures are a class of events that are not associated with the electrical discharges characteristic of epilepsy, while superficially resembling an epileptic seizure. Clinicians (see Mellers 2005, Levy 1993, 714) also define these attacks as 'psychologically mediated episodes' or 'dissociative seizures'.

[8] Temkin 1971², X. Cf. Levy 1993, 713: 'It is misleading to think of epilepsy as one disease. There are many causes of this symptom cluster, just as there are for the symptom cluster of nausea and vomiting. A better term would be "the epilepsies"'. See also Friedlander 2001, and Eadie and Bladin 2001.

[9] Doctors were aware of this difficulty already in antiquity. See Aretaeus, *SA*, I, 4 (p. 38, 12

passing across different ages and a variety of medical paradigms and cultural frames.[10] It has even survived to the triple epistemological shift that resulted from the rise of anatomopathology, the development of neurophysiology as an autonomous branch of medicine, and Sigmund Freud's invention of the modern 'scientific' concept of psyche and redefinition of the boundaries between the domain of the neurological disorders—viz. disorders caused by a clear, definite, and detectable lesion of one or more regions of the brain—, and that of the mental diseases—viz. disorders which do not seem to have an organic basis but are ascribed to a 'functional' alteration of intentionality, of the faculty of judgment, as well as of the mechanisms of categorisation and of formation of the qualia.[11] The interesting point is that epilepsy as a nosological category has not survived through all the Modern Age until present day just as a residual of a traditional medical mentality, or as part of the popular lexicon to indicate a disease associated to, or associable with, insanity, as has been the case, to different extents and in different terms, with other ancient medical concepts such as *mania, hysteria, phrenitis, melancholia*. There is, in fact, quite a remarkable continuity between the ancient and the modern *clinical* accounts of the epileptic seizure, and this proves to be evident in spite of the etiological and cultural frameworks of reference of these accounts being largely incommensurable.

The same tension between continuity and incommensurability also characterizes the fields of intellectual forces, to use Pierre Bourdieu's category, that have historically developed around the so-called falling sickness. The history of the conceptions of the epileptic disorder, or better to say of *the epilepsies*, can be represented as the history of a centuries-long struggle between mystifying and demystifying approaches to the disease (divine vs. natural etiology) and between stigmatization (the epileptic as a madman and a mentally impaired) and destigmatization (the epileptic as a sane subject whose body and not mind, or psyche, or soul, is affected by the disease).[12]

Hude): 'Epilepsy is an illness of various shapes and horrible' (Ποικίλον ἠδὲ ἀλλόκοτον κακὸν ἡ ἐπιληψίη).

   [10] An excellent analysis of how the modern narratives of epilepsy have developed and interacted with the 'scientific discourse' on epilepsy has been recently provided by Stirling 2010.

   [11] For a critical discussion of Freud's distinction between physical and functional disorders see Edelman 1992, 179.

   [12] As remarked by Baker et al. 1997, 353, even in modern culture epilepsy remains 'a stigmatizing condition par excellence'. See also Baker 2002, 26–30; Jacoby 2002, 10–20; Jacoby and Austin 2007, 6–9; de Boer et al. 2008, 540–546.

In this paper I shall investigate whether, in which terms, and by what
theoretical tools and explanatory strategies the Greek scientific discourse
drew a distinction, or vice versa accounted for the intertwinement, between
the somatic and the cognitive/behavioural manifestations of epilepsy. I shall
consequently pose the question whether and to what extent epilepsy was
represented in classical antiquity as something that *we* would label as a
'mental' disease and the epileptic as a mentally impaired subject.

The first texts at stake will be two medical treatises of the Hippocratic
corpus, namely *On the Sacred Disease* and *On Breaths*. Of course, many other
texts of the Hippocratic corpus contain references to epilepsy or, more generally, to 'epileptic subjects' or 'epileptic attacks' (but the adjective *epilep-
tikos* can also indicate any kind of fit and the adjective *epileptos* someone
who suffers from the 'attack' of a disease).[13] *On the Sacred Disease* and ch. 14
of *On Breaths* represent, however, the only texts of the Hippocratic Corpus to provide an in-depth etiological account of the epileptic seizure. I
will then take into account two passages from the physiological section of
Plato's *Timaeus*: in the first (85a1–b2) Plato briefly indicates the cause of the
'sacred disease' (this being included among the diseases of the body), in the
second (86e3–87a7) he considers the physical causes of some manifestations of psychic pain. I will also draw attention to a passage of Aristotle's
De somno et vigilia,[14] which draws a parallel between the physiology of sleep
and the physiopathology of the epileptic fit; to a passage of the *Anonymus
Parisinus*,[15] in which Diocles' and Praxagoras' views on epilepsy are briefly
sketched; and, finally, to ch. 30.1 of the *Problemata Physica*,[16] a collection of
peripatetic knowledge that postulates an interesting link between epilepsy,
melancholic temperament and genius.

Phlegm, Blood, Black Bile: Epilepsy and the Debate on the Causes

The two Hippocratic treatises *On the Sacred Disease* and *On Breaths* provide an account of epilepsy by adopting quite a similar explanatory pattern, although this pattern develops into substantially different theories on
the seat of cognition and the cause of epilepsy. Both treatises conceive of

---

[13] Cf. *Acut.Sp.* 7; *Epid.* VII, 1; *Aph.* II, 45, III, 16 and 20, V, 7; *Prorrh.* I, 131; *Mul.* II, 151, and
various aphorisms of *Coan Prenotions* (157, 339, 445, 450, 511, 587).

[14] Aristotle, *Somn.Vig.* 3, 457a1–14.

[15] *Anonymus Parisinus* 3 (p. 18, 10–20 Garofalo).

[16] Pseudo-Aristotle, *Pr.* 30.1, 953a10–955a40.

cognition as the result of a harmonious spreading of some 'consciousness-bearing' substance over the whole body—air, according to *On the Sacred Disease*, blood, according to *On Breaths*—, and explain both the impairment of the cognitive faculty and the rise of other somatic disorders as a consequence of the blockage or perturbation of such ordered and continuous flow. *On the Sacred Disease*'s argument is entirely concerned with the nature, the origin, and, so to say, the phenomenology of epilepsy, and provides an explanation of the disease as well as of the single attacks of epilepsy.[17] This treatise describes the brain as a cognitive centre, which serves as a mediator (*hermeneus*) between the consciousness-bearing materials carried by the air and the organs deputed to movement and sense perception:

> For these reasons I hold that the brain is the most powerful part of the human body, for when it is healthy it is an interpreter (ἑρμηνεύς) of the things which come from the air. But it is the air that provides it with consciousness (τὴν δὲ φρόνησιν αὐτῷ ὁ ἀήρ παρέχεται). Eyes, ears, tongue, hands and feet carry out what the brain knows.[18]   (ch. 16, p. 29, 4–10 Jouanna; tr. is mine)

This account puts forward the idea that epilepsy is caused by an accumulation of phlegm in the vessels that get to the brain from both sides of the body and that make it possible for the vital *pneuma* to circulate throughout the whole body. This accumulation and the subsequent obstruction of the vessels are due to an insufficient prenatal or postnatal purification (*katharsis*) of phlegm in the brain (ch. 5),[19] but, along with this internal remote cause, there are a number of external, environmental, factors that play an essential role in determining and influencing the whole pathological

---

[17] Temkin 1971, 55.

[18] On the role played by the brain in *On the Sacred Disease*'s account of cognition see Lo Presti 2008 and 2011, Jouanna 2003, LX and 118–121, van der Eijk 2005a, 126–127, Anastassiou 2007, Roselli 1996, 26–28, Gundert 2000, 21–22, López-Morales 2002, 509–522, Pigeaud 1980, 420–422, and 1981, 33–31, Manuli and Vegetti 1977, 45.

[19] *Morb.Sacr.* 5 (12,21–14,2 Jouanna): 'This disease attacks the phlegmatic, but not the bilious. Its birth begins in the embryo while it is still in the womb, for like the other parts, the brain too is purged (καθαίρεται) and has its impurities expelled before birth. [...] But if the flux from all the brain be too abundant, and a great melting take place, he will have as he grows a diseased head [...] Should the purging not take place, but congestion occur in the brain, then the infants cannot fail to be phlegmatic. If while they are children sores break out on head, ears and skin, and if saliva and mucus be abundant, as age advances such enjoy very good health, for in this way the phlegm is discharged and purged away which should have been purged away in the womb. Those who have been so purged are in general not attacked by this disease. Those children, on the other hand, that are clean, do not break out in sores, and discharge neither mucus nor saliva, run a risk of being attacked by this disease, if the purging has not taken place in the womb'. (Tr. Jones).

process.[20] According to the different places of the body in which it occurs, this obstruction results in different symptoms: palpitations and asthma, when the fluxes of phlegm gather around the heart;[21] diarrhoea, if the belly is affected;[22] foaming at the mouth, grinding of teeth, clenched hands, rolling eyes, disorders in consciousness, and lack of bowel control, if the obstruction occurs in the veins.

This last series of symptoms forms the 'clinical' picture of the epileptic fit as the author describes it in ch. 7:

> If the phlegm be cut off from these passages, but makes its descent into the veins I have mentioned above, the patient becomes speechless and chokes; froth flows from the mouth; he gnashes his teeth and twists his hands; the eyes roll and intelligence fails, and in some cases excrement is discharged. I will now explain how each symptom occurs. The sufferer is speechless when suddenly the phlegm descends into the veins and intercepts the air, not admitting it either into the brain, or into the hollow veins, or into the cavities, thus checking respiration. For when a man takes in breath by the mouth or nostrils, it first goes to the brain, then most of it goes to the belly, though some goes to the lungs and some to the veins. From these parts it disperses, by way of the veins, into the others. The portion that goes into the belly cools it, but has no further use; but the air that goes into the lungs and the veins is of use when it enters the cavities and the brain, thus causing intelligence and movement of the limbs, so that when the veins are cut off from the air by the phlegm and admit none of it, the patient is rendered speechless and senseless. The hands are paralysed and twisted when the blood is still, and is not distributed as usual. The eyes roll when the minor veins are shut off from the air and pulsate. The foaming at the mouth comes from the lungs; for when the breath fails to enter them they foam and boil as though death were near. Excrement is discharged when the patient is violently compressed, as happens when the liver and the upper bowel are forced against the diaphragm and the mouth of the stomach is intercepted; this takes place when the normal amount of breath does not enter the mouth. The patient kicks when the air is shut off in the limbs, and cannot pass through to the outside because of the phlegm;

---

[20] The most important of these factors is the sudden and violent change of the winds, especially when the hot and wet winds from the South alternate with the cold and dry winds from the North. See ch. 13, 23,6–11 and 25,1–8 Jouanna, and ch. 17, 31,8–13 Jouanna. On the semantic field of 'change' in the Hippocratic collection see Demont 1992, 305–317.

[21] *Morb.Sacr.* 6 (p. 14,3–11): 'Should the discharge make its way to the heart, palpitation (παλμός) and difficulty of breathing (ἄσθμα) supervene, the chest becomes diseased, and a few even become hump-backed; for when the phlegm descends cold to the lungs and to the heart, the blood is chilled; and the veins, being forcibly chilled, beat against the lungs and the heart, and the heart palpitates, so that under this compulsion difficulty of breathing and orthopnoea (ὀρθόπνοιαν) result.' (Tr. Jones).

[22] *Morb.Sacr.* 6 (p. 14,18–20): 'Such are the symptoms when the flux goes to the lungs and heart; when it goes to the bowels, the result is diarrhoea.' (Tr. Jones).

rushing upwards and downwards through the blood it causes convulsions and pain; hence the kicking. The patient suffers all these things when the phlegm flows cold into the blood which is warm; for the blood is chilled and arrested. If the flow be copious and thick, death is immediate, for it masters the blood by its coldness and congeals it. If the flow be less, at the first it is master, having cut off respiration; but in course of time, when it is dispersed throughout the veins and mixed with the copious, warm blood, if in this way it be mastered, the veins admit the air and begin taking part in consciousness again (ἐδέξαντο τὸν ἠέρα αἱ φλέβες καὶ ἐφρόνησαν).[23]

(p. 14,21–16,23 Jouanna; trans. Jones, with adjustments)

From this long passage it is clear that the brain is identified as the cause (*aitios*) of epilepsy,[24] insofar as the seizure is accounted for as the final result of a concatenation of pathophysiological processes that originates in an overproduction or an insufficient purification of the phlegm that naturally tends to form in the brain cavities.

Air plays a substantial role also in *On Breath*'s etiology of epilepsy (as well as of many other forms of impairment of consciousness and of intelligence), but as the obstructing factor rather than as the substance whose course in the body is obstructed.[25] Consciousness, says this author, remains stable insofar as blood remains in a stable condition. But when blood undergoes change, consciousness proportionally changes and becomes subject to more or less severe forms of alteration. Interestingly, the same rationale applies to explaining a physiological state 'common to all the living beings' like sleep (it arises from the blood being chilled and its stream becoming sluggish), a transitory disease-like condition like drunkenness (the author's conviction that the blood becomes more abundant when someone is drunk is probably grounded on the belief, attested also elsewhere in the Hippocratic collection, that during digestion the so-called 'black' wine changes

---

[23] See Jouanna 2003, 79–80 n. 10, on the points of contact between this account of the symptoms of the epileptic fit and the later medical accounts of epilepsy: Aretaeus (I,5, III,4, V,5, VII,4), Celsus (III,23), Galen (*Loc.Aff.* III,11 = VIII,193 K), Caelius Aurelianus (*Chron.* I, 4), Alexander of Tralles (I,15), Aetius (VI,13–21), Paul of Aegina (III,13). On the relationship between this account of the epileptic fit and the tragic representations of madness—and especially the Euripidean representation of Heracles' and Medea's madness (respectively, v. 934 and v. 1173 ff.), in which a tragic author for the first time includes foaming as a sign of an attack of madness—see von Staden 1992, 131–150, and Guardasole 2000, 196–204.

[24] See *Morb.Sacr.* 3 (11, 6–8 Jouanna): 'For it is the brain that is responsible of this affection (ἀλλὰ γὰρ αἴτιος ὁ ἐγκέφαλος τούτου τοῦ πάθεος), as of the other most important diseases'; 17 (31, 6–8 Jouanna): 'That is why the heart and the diaphragm are most sensitive; nevertheless none of them takes part in consciousness, but the organ that is responsible (αἴτιος) for all these things is the brain.'

[25] Van der Eijk 2005a, 133.

into blood, whose colour for the Greeks was also 'black'[26]), and a chronic disorder characterised by sudden acute attacks like the so-called 'sacred disease':

> I hold that the sacred disease is caused in the following way. When much wind has combined throughout the body with all the blood, many barriers arise in many places in the veins. Whenever therefore much air weighs, and continues to weigh, upon the thick, blood-filled veins, the blood is prevented from passing on. So in one place it stops, in another it passes sluggishly, in another more quickly. The progress of the blood through the body proving irregular, all kinds of irregularities occur. The whole body is torn in all directions; the parts of the body are shaken in obedience to the troubling and disturbance of the blood; distortions of every kind occur in every manner. At this time the patients are unconscious of everything (ἀναίσθητοι πάντων εἰσίν)—deaf to what is spoken, blind to what is happening, and insensible to pain. So greatly does a disturbance of the air disturb and pollute the blood. Foam naturally rises through the mouth. For the air, passing through the veins, itself raises and brings up with it the thinnest part of the blood. The moisture, mixing with the air, becomes white, for the air being pure is seen through thin membranes. For this reason the foam appears completely white. When then will the victims of this disease rid themselves of their disorder and the storm that attends it? When the body exercised by its exertions has warmed the blood, and the blood thoroughly warmed has warmed the breaths, and these thoroughly warmed are dispersed, breaking up the congestion of the blood, some going out along with the respiration, others with the phlegm. The disease finally ends when the foam has frothed itself away, the blood has re-established itself, and calm has arisen in the body. (ch. 14, 122,16–124,10 Jouanna; trans. Jones)

It was Plato in the *Timaeus* who introduced the soul into this inquiry. Plato here provides a full account of the structure of the human body and of the faculties of the tripartite soul, and also describes in full detail the embryological and physiological processes that govern the generation of the body, its development and decadence until death. After that, he turns to classifying the diseases that can affect a human being. A first general distinction is made between the diseases of the body, which are discussed and further sub-divided into three groups (82a1–86a8),[27] and the diseases

---

[26] Cf. *Vict.* II, 52 (172, 18–28 Joly CMG). See Jouanna 1988, 122 n. 1, Jouanna and Demont 1981, 197–209.

[27] The first group of the diseases of the body includes the diseases caused by an excess, scarcity, or displacement from their natural seats of the four primary elements (earth, fire, water, air) which a body is composed of (82a1–7). On the theory of the four elements in Plato's *Timaeus* see Black 2000 (especially pp. 5–8); Reale 2000, 25–27. The second group includes those diseases that affect the secondary structures of the body, that is to say those homogeneous parts consisting of a combination of the four elements (bones, flesh, nerves,

of the soul (86b1–87b8). Now, we should be very careful not to treat this distinction in too simplistic and rigidly dualistic terms. For Plato clearly states that his aim is to show in which way the diseases of the soul are brought on by the condition of the body (τὰ δὲ περὶ ψυχὴν διὰ σώματος ἕξιν τῇδε). Such a statement, while implying an actual difference between soul and body, also recognizes the existence of a *direct* link of causation that makes the states of the mind depend on the condition of the body. For, as recently argued by L. Grams, according to the medical theory of Plato's *Timaeus* 'bodily disease has an immediate effect on the soul when the flow of nutrition into marrow where the soul is located is reversed, or when fever caused by trapped bile burns up the marrow. However, the body can affect the soul in other ways, which mirror the three main classes of bodily disease'.[28] It is therefore in the light of this wider interpretative problem concerning the ontological structure of the relationship between soul and body in the physiology of the *Timaeus* that we must take into exam the passage in which Plato deals with the cause of epilepsy:

> White phlegm, also, is dangerous when it is blocked inside because of the air in its bubbles [...] And when this phlegm is blended with black bile and spreads over the revolutions of the head, which are the most divine, and perturbs them, its action is more gentle during sleep, but when it attacks persons who are awake it is harder to shake off; and because it is a disease of the sacred substance it is most justly termed the 'sacred disease'.[29]
>
> (85a1–b2)

Plato includes epilepsy in the third group of the diseases of the body, i.e. of the diseases caused by the air breathed in, or by phlegm, or by bile.[30] In particular, epilepsy is attributed to a mixture of white phlegm and bile that pours out into the brain, interfering with and altering the circular

---

marrow, and blood), when the process of generation of the tissues turns into a process of degeneration (82b8–c7); the third group includes the diseases caused by the phlegm or the bile (84c8–d2). On the processes of composition of the body from the four elements see Joubaud 1991, 52–63. On the definition, causation, and classification of the diseases of the body in Plato's *Timaeus* see Miller 1962, 175–187 (with a remarkable analysis of the pathophysiological processes underlying the second group of diseases); Joubaud 1991, 88–101; Grams 2009, 161–192. On Plato's classification of the diseases of the body see also Ayache 1997, 57–58.

[28] Grams 2009, 183.

[29] Τὸ δὲ λευκὸν φλέγμα διὰ τὸ τῶν πομφολύγων πνεῦμα χαλεπὸν ἀποληφθέν ... μετὰ χολῆς δὲ μελαίνης κερασθὲν ἐπὶ τὰς περιόδους τε τὰς ἐν τῇ κεφαλῇ θειοτάτας οὔσας ἐπισκεδαννύμενον καὶ συνταράττον αὐτάς, καθ᾽ ὕπνον μὲν ἰὸν πρᾳΰτερον, ἐγρηγορόσιν δὲ ἐπιτιθέμενον δυσαπαλλακτότε-ρον· νόσημα δὲ ἱερᾶς ὂν φύσεως ἐνδικώτατα ἱερὸν λέγεται.

[30] See *supra*, n. 27.

movements that the immortal soul makes in it and that Plato describes as
the very source of rational thinking for man.[31] Plato also points out that, this
being the cause of epilepsy, it is perfectly understandable, and even reasonable, that this disease is called 'sacred', since it results from a perturbation
in the movement of that part of the soul that represents what is most divine
in the human being, as it consists of the same non-material stuff of which
the cosmic soul is made (41d4–42e4) and has been implanted in the body
by the gods created by the Demiurge.[32] We have therefore quite a complex
and problematic picture, in which epilepsy is counted among the affections
of the body, being prompted by an entirely physical cause (the mixture of
phlegm and bile), but is at the very same time defined as a disease of the
'sacred nature' (νόσημα ἱερᾶς φύσεως)—viz. the rational soul—consisting in
a perturbation of the spatial movements that the soul accomplishes in the
brain.

The characterisation of epilepsy as a disease of the body proves to be even
more problematic in the passage on the diseases of the soul in which Plato
accounts for some forms of psychic pain:

> For whenever the humours which arise from acid and saline phlegms, and
> all humours that are bitter and bilious wander through the body and find
> no external vent but are confined within, and mingle their vapour with the
> movement of the soul and are blended therewith, they implant diseases
> of the soul of all kinds, varying in intensity and in extent; and as these
> humours penetrate to the three regions of the soul, according to the region
> which they severally attack, they give rise to all varieties of ill-temper and
> despondency, and they give rise to all manner of rashness and cowardice, and
> of forgetfulness also, as well as of stupidity.[33]
>
> (86e3–87a7) (trans. Bury, with modifications)

---

[31] For an in-depth analysis of the *Timaeus*' theory of the 'revolutions of the soul' (περίοδοι
τῆς ψυχῆς) and of their perturbations as the source, respectively, of intelligence and of mental
impairment see Jouanna 2007, 34–38 (this contribution is central to the understanding of
Plato's theory as it raises the question of its relationship with the theory of intelligence of
the Hippocratic treatise *On Regimen* by putting in evidence several theoretical and lexical
commonalities between these two texts).

[32] On the characterization of the rational soul in the *Timaeus* see Sassi's contribution to
this volume, p. 417.

[33] Ὅπου γὰρ ἂν οἱ τῶν ὀξέων καὶ τῶν ἁλυκῶν φλεγμάτων καὶ ὅσοι πικροὶ καὶ χολώδεις χυμοὶ
κατὰ τὸ σῶμα πλανηθέντες ἔξω μὲν μὴ λάβωσιν ἀναπνοήν, ἐντὸς δὲ εἱλλόμενοι τὴν ἀφ᾽αὑτῶν
ἀτμίδα τῇ τῆς ψυχῆς φορᾷ ξυμμίξαντες ἀνακερασθῶσι, παντοδαπὰ νοσήματα ψυχῆς ἐμποιοῦσι,
μᾶλλον καὶ ἧττον, καὶ ἐλάττω καὶ πλείω· πρός τε τοὺς τρεῖς τόπους ἐνεχθέντα τῆς ψυχῆς, πρὸς ὃν
ἂν ἕκαστ᾽αὐτῶν προσπίπτῃ, ποικίλλει μὲν εἴδη δυσκολίας καὶ δυσθυμίας παντοδαπά, ποικίλλει δὲ
θρασύτητός τε καὶ δειλίας, ἔτι δὲ λήθης ἅμα καὶ δυσμαθίας.

Here we have the indication of various kinds of intellectual and behavioural impairment that are explicitly defined by Plato as diseases of the soul (νοσήματα ψυχῆς). What is interesting is that, according to Plato's account, these forms of mental distress, which range from ill-temper to despondency, from rashness to cowardice, from forgetfulness to stupidity, are prompted by a cause very similar to that of epilepsy, that is to say a flow of vapours that arises from the phlegmatic and/or the bilious matter and perturbs, alters or impedes the movements of the soul by attacking one of its three regions.[34] Such a coincidence of causes, in and by itself, is not entirely surprising, because Plato had already clearly explained how the diseases of the soul are prompted by physical causes, so that, as C. Joubaud has observed, 'il n'y a pas de maladie de l'âme désincarnée, cela est impensable';[35] moreover, Plato conceives two of the three principles of the soul (the passionate and the appetitive) as mortal and as particularly affected by passions (this is why the *Demiurgos* has separated this principle of the soul from the divine and immortal one by locating them in different regions of the body),[36] even if no specific description of their composition is provided.

But what to my mind really makes epilepsy a sort of liminal *nosema* within the *Timaeus'* theoretical framework[37] is 1) the fact that this affection, while being included among the diseases of the body, is located in the head, that is to say in the seat of that immortal and immaterial principle of the soul that Plato describes as the very centre of the highest cognitive faculties and thus of the rational life of man,[38] and 2) the fact that Plato explains epilepsy as a result of the same perturbed spatial movements of the soul, and of the same perturbing factor, to which he attributes a number of declaredly 'mental' disorders.[39]

---

[34] See Taylor 1928, 617, and Tracy 1969, 123–136, who have extensively discussed the rationale of this section of the *Timaeus* and put it in the wider context both of Plato's theory of the soul as expounded in other Platonic dialogues and of the earlier and co-eval medical literature. According to Tracy's analysis, forgetfulness and stupidity are to be seen as affections of the rational soul and must therefore be prompted by a flow toward the head; rashness and cowardice are accounted for as affections of the affective soul and must be caused by a flow toward the chest; ill-temper and despondency are thought to affect the nutritive soul, which thing implies a flow of humoral matter toward the region of the liver. For the location of the affective and nutritive soul see, respectively, 69c1–70a7, and 70d7–71a2.

[35] Joubaud 1991, 179.

[36] 69d6–e4. See Pigeaud 1981, 48–50.

[37] Joubaud 1991, 95–96.

[38] Joubaud 1991, 134–135.

[39] In this regard see Sorabji 2003, 161: 'Plato in the *Timaeus* allows the body a major role in affecting even the rational part of the soul, partly because the soul's movements are spatial'.

In the passage of the *De somno et vigilia* in which he makes reference to epilepsy (3, 457a4–11),[40] Aristotle further develops an idea that had been already sketched by the author of *On Breaths*, namely the idea according to which epilepsy is somehow associated, or comparable, with sleep:

> Sleep arises from the evaporation (ἀναθυμίασις) due to food ... Young children sleep deeply, because all the food is borne upwards. An indication of this is that in early youth the upper parts of the body are larger in comparison with the lower, which is due to the fact that growth takes place in the upward direction. Hence too they are liable to epilepsy, for sleep is like epilepsy (Διὰ ταύτην δὲ τὴν αἰτίαν καὶ ἐπιληπτικὰ γίγνεται· ὅμοιον γὰρ ὁ ὕπνος ἐπιλήψει); indeed, in a sense, sleep is a type of epileptic fit (καὶ ἔστιν τρόπον τινὰ ὁ ὕπνος ἐπίληψις). This is why in many people epilepsy begins in sleep, and they are regularly seized with it when asleep, but not when awake. For when a large amount of vapour is borne upwards and subsequently descends again, it causes the blood vessels to swell and it obstructs the passage through which respiration passes.   (trans. van der Eijk 1994b)

Aristotle's views on the link between sleep and the epileptic fit seem to be much more elaborate than those ascribable to the author of *On Breaths*, as Aristotle does not limit himself to affirm that sleep and epilepsy can be explained as *different* outcomes, let's say different actualizations, of the same very general causal schema, but he goes so far as to say that 'sleep is like epilepsy; indeed, in some way, sleep *is* a seizure', which also explains, in the eyes of Aristotle, why epileptics are often seized while being asleep.[41]

But how does Aristotle account for epilepsy, and for this kind of epilepsy, which is sleep? He explains that sleep results from the digestion of food, which, after ingestion, is carried to the centre of the body and 'cooked' or digested by the heat of the heart. This process culminates in the evaporation of food and the consequent saturation of the internal *pneuma* with

---

[40] For a discussion of the unity and the rationale of the *De somno* and, more in general, of Aristotle's treatment of sleep see Enders 1923, Everson 2007, Hubert 1999, Lowe 1978, Marelli 1979–1980, Repici 2003, Sprague 1977, van der Eijk 2005a (especially 175–179), Wiesner 1978, Wijsenbeek-Wijler 1976.

[41] Aristotle's association of epilepsy with sleep is anything but a unique example in the history of the medical representations of epilepsy. As a matter of fact, from the second half of the nineteenth century onwards the relations between sleep and epileptic phenomena have become a subject of increasing interest for experimental physiologists and neuropathologists, as testified by the seminal works of Féré 1890 and Gowers 1885. But it is since the second half of the twentieth century, with the research carried out by P. Passouant and his Montpellier School of Neurophysiology, that the study of epilepsy in sleep has been systematically undertaken on an experimental basis and has significantly contributed to better understand the arousal mechanisms both of human epilepsy and of sleep as well as the organisation of the neural patterns of the human brain: see Sterman et al. 1982, Degen and Niedermeyer 1984.

hot vapours. The air so saturated tends toward the brain, where it is chilled and redirected to the heart. Thus the heart is chilled, which is what actually causes the sensory faculties to fail.[42] As far as epilepsy is specifically concerned, Aristotle's explanation is consistent with his idea that the region of the heart is the source of sensation and movement. He explains that the epileptic fit occurs as a consequence of the vapours obstructing the airways and perturbing the regular course of respiration during their descent from the brain to the heart.

We find in this brief account no mention of the motor disorders nor of the spasms, which instead are described in full detail in the accounts that we find in the Hippocratic collection:[43] the only points in which Aristotle seems to be interested are the temporary failure of consciousness, which is a typical feature both of sleep and of epilepsy, and the natural proneness of young children to the epileptic fits.[44] This of course can be interpreted as a result of Aristotle's well-known habit of selecting empirical data according to his theoretical and argumentative purposes. But it could also indicate a capacity of Aristotle or of his (medical?) sources[45] to identify some

---

[42] *Somn. Vig.* 456b17–28: 'Yet, as we said, not every capacity of the perceptual part is sleep; rather this affection comes about from the exhalation involved in nutrition (ἐκ τῆς περὶ τὴν τροφὴν ἀναθυμιάσεως). For it is necessary that what is exhaled must continue to some point and then turn back and change course, like the Euripon. Now in every animal the hot matter naturally rises upwards; but when it has reached the upper areas, it turns back again in a mass and moves downwards. That is why episodes of sleep occur especially after food; it is because the matter, both liquid and solid, rises in a dense mass. This, then, while static, weighs down and causes nodding. But when it has descended again, and by returning has repelled the hot matter, at that point sleep ensues and the animal falls asleep'; 458a25–32: 'What is the cause of sleep has, then, been stated: it is the recoil of the solid matter, carried upwards by the connatural heat, *en bloc* onto the primary sense-organ. Also what sleep is: it is a seizure of the primary sense organ (τοῦ πρώτου αἰσθητηρίου κατάληψις), making it incapable of activity. It occurs of necessity (for it is not possible for an animal to exist unless the causes which produce it occur), and is for the sake of the animal's preservation, since rest does preserve it.' (trans. Everson).

[43] It is interesting to note that a text like *Epid.* V, 22 (14, 1–18 Jouanna), which reports the case of a patient who was seized by epileptic attacks only at night and after falling asleep, also makes a clear reference to spasms and contractions in the face and in both sides of the patient's body (at first in the right side, and then also in the left side). This clinical description has been praised for its accurateness by Souques 1936, 77. For their part, Grmek 1992, 193, and Jouanna and Grmek 2003, 135 n. 9, have suggested a retrospective diagnosis of 'hemiplegic Bravais-Jackson epilepsy'. On the genesis and the further developments of this nosological category see Temkin 1971, 305–311, and Eadie 2010, 1–6.

[44] See Debru 1982, 25–41.

[45] On the empirical basis of the physiology of the *Parva naturalia* see Lloyd 1978, 215–239. For a discussion of the influence of the medical tradition on Aristotle see Oser-Grote

non-convulsive states as epileptic episodes, in some way prefiguring the contemporary nosological category of 'absence seizure' (le *petit mal* so frequently described by 18th century French doctors), which, indeed, mainly applies to forms of epilepsy characteristic of childhood and adolescence.[46]

Two medical authors who were more or less contemporaries of Aristotle, Diocles and Praxagoras, expressed opinions about epilepsy, as is reported by the *Anonymus Parisinus* (ch. 3, p. 18, 10–20 Garofalo):

> Praxagoras says that [epilepsy] arises around the thick artery from phlegmatic humours that gather in it; by producing bubbles, they stop the passage of the psychic pneuma out of the heart and so this vibrates and induces spasm in the body. When afterwards the bubbles subside again the affection ceases.[47]
> (trans. Fuchs)

> Diocles also thinks that there is an obstruction in the same place and explains the other matters as Praxagoras does.[48]   (trans. Fuchs)

It seems from such evidence as we have that Diocles and Praxagoras shared a cardiocentric view on the seat of the cognitive processes, but also attributed an important role to the brain and to the mediation between the two by what they seem to have called 'psychic *pneuma*' (this expression is used by the later anonymous writer who reports Diocles' and Praxagoras' views by using the terminology of his own time, but we cannot be entirely sure that the two physicians had not somehow developed such a concept).[49] Diocles and Praxagoras both said that epilepsy occurs when phlegmatic humours accumulate around the thick artery and form bubbles, which obstruct the passage of the psychic *pneuma* coming from the heart; as a consequence of its passage being obstructed, this *pneuma* provokes the spasms

---

2004. For a discussion of the empirical elements in Aristotle's treatment of sleep see van der Eijk 2005a, 177–178.

[46] See Penfield and Jasper 1954, cited in Daly 1968, 176: 'Minor petit mal consists of a complete lapse of consciousness without significant motor accompaniment ... there is, however, little impairment of motor functions. The patient may remain standing or walking'; Passouant 1982, 3: 'A second epileptic manifestation during REM sleep consists of petit mal paroxysms and of brief generalized myoclonic discharges. The petit mal paroxysms are comparable to those seen during waking. Their frequency can be greater than that during waking, although duration remain comparable'.

[47] Πραξαγόρας περὶ τὴν παχεῖαν ἀρτηρίαν φησὶ γίνεσθαι φλεγματικῶν χυμῶν συστάντων ἐν αὐτῇ· οὓς δὴ πομφολυγουμένους ἀποκλείειν τὴν δίοδον τοῦ ἀπὸ καρδίας ψυχικοῦ πνεύματος καὶ οὕτω τοῦτο κραδαίνειν καὶ σπᾶν τὸ σῶμα· πάλιν δὲ κατασταθεισῶν τῶν πομφολύγων παύεσθαι τὸ πάθος.

[48] Διοκλῆς δὲ καὶ αὐτὸς ἔμφραξιν περὶ τὸν αὐτὸν τόπον οἴεται· συμβαίνειν καὶ τὰ ἄλλα κατὰ τὰ αὐτὰ ἃ Πραξαγόρας φησὶ γίνεσθαι·

[49] Van der Eijk 2005a, 134.

characteristic of the epileptic seizure; when the bubbles have disappeared, the attack is over.

The last text I shall take into account is the chapter 30.1 of the *Problemata Physica* (954b20–955a1). Let us start by saying that, although we do not have sufficient elements to ascribe it directly to Aristotle,[50] this short text appears to be quintessentially Peripatetic both in the rationale and in the structure of the explanation and seems to be wholly consistent, or at least very well acquainted, with Aristotle's own concept of melancholy.[51] In this text epilepsy is mentioned among the 'diseases of the black bile' (τὰ μελαγχολικὰ νοσήματα) that can affect this or that part of the body of a subject with a melancholic nature:

> such men are very melancholic, and if the mixture is of a certain kind, they are abnormal. But if they neglect it, they incline towards melancholic diseases, different people in different parts of the body; with some the symptoms are epileptic, with other apoplectic, others again are given to deep despondency or to fear, others are over-confident, as was the case with Archelaus, king of Macedonia. The cause of such force is the mixture, how it is related to cold and heat. For when it is colder than the occasion demands it produces unreasonable despondency; this accounts for the prevalence of suicide by hanging amongst the young and sometimes amongst older men too. But many commit suicide after a bout of drinking. Some melancholic persons continue to be despondent after drinking; for the heat of the wine quenches the natural heat. But heat in the region with which we think and hope makes us cheerful.
> (trans. H. Rackham)

An association of epilepsy with the melancholic nature seems to be established also at the very beginning of the text—so, in a particularly emphatic position—, when the author explains Heracles' madness as a result of the hero's melancholic nature and, at the same time, seems to identify this 'heroic' disease with epilepsy:

---

[50] Recent scholarship has attributed the theory expounded in this chapter to Theophrastus. The most important piece of evidence adduced in support of this attribution is a passage of Diogenes Laertius (5.44) in which it is said that Theophrastus wrote a treatise 'On Melancholy'. The chapter of the *Problemata physica* would therefore be a summary or a reworked version of this lost text. On the plausibility of this attribution see van der Eijk 2005a, 167 n. 91. If van der Eijk is sceptical about the possibility that the question of the authorship of this chapter can get to a solution, Pigeaud 1988c, 54–56, on the contrary, seems to endorse the attribution to Theophrastus. Other relevant literature: Müri 1953, 11; Flashar 1962, 111–114; Flashar 1966, 61. On the contrary, both Marenghi 1966 and Louis 1991–1994, vol. 3, have included this text among Aristotle's authentic works.

[51] The most systematic attempt at analyzing the relationship between Aristotle's own concept of melancholy and the theory expounded in the ch. 30.1 of the *Problemata physica* has been made by van der Eijk 2005a, 139–168; see also Flashar 1962, 111–122.; Klibansky et al. 1990, 81–87.

> Why is it that all men who have become outstanding in philosophy, states-
> manship, poetry or the arts are melancholic, and some to such an extent that
> they are infected by the diseases arising from black bile (τοῖς ἀπὸ μελαίνης
> χολῆς ἀρρωστήμασιν), as the story of Heracles among the heroes tells? For Her-
> acles seems to have been of this nature, so that the ancients called the illnesses
> of those who get seized 'Sacred disease' after him.[52]   (953a10–17)

The same association had been already suggested in the Hippocratic corpus,
in a short aphorism of the sixth book of *Epidemics* (*Epid. VI*, 8, 31, pp. 192–194
Manetti-Roselli = V, 354 L.): 'Melancholics tend to become epileptic generally and epileptics melancholic. Each of these develops more according
to what the weakness inclines towards: if towards the body, epileptics, if
towards the mind (ἐπὶ τὴν διάνοιαν), melancholics'. While the Hippocratic
author seems to draw quite a clear distinction between a somatic and a
mental outcome of the same pathogenic factor—epilepsy being defined as
a disorder of the body—, things become sensibly more complex in the case
of this *Problema*. Here the melancholic subject is described as someone in
whom the 'mixture of the black bile' (*krasis tes melaines choles*)[53] is dominant. According to this account, the melancholic nature shares with wine
a sort of 'ethopoietic' faculty: both wine and black bile are responsible for
the states of mind of a subject being extremely unstable and alterable, and
for the same person being capable of embodying different behavioural pat-

---

[52] Scholars have long debated this identification of Heracles' disease with epilepsy. Temkin 1971, 20–21, has argued that it is not possible to affirm with an acceptable degree of
certainty that this passage suggests such an identification nor that, more in general, the other
accounts of 'Heracles disease' that we find in other Greek texts (for example in *Diseases of
Women* I, 7 = VIII, 32 Littré) actually refer to this disease as a case of epilepsy. A different
stand is taken by Pigeaud 1988c, 109 n. 4: he admits that the ancient popular label 'Sacred
disease' embraces a wider spectrum of phenomena than what we would define as an 'epileptic attack' (cf. Pigeaud 1987, 48; Grmek 1983, 70), but he nonetheless affirms that this passage
very probably refers to epilepsy. On the 'disease of Heracles' see also von Staden 1992.
[53] The problem is to establish whether the expression 'the mixture of the black bile'
indicates a mixture of qualities which the black bile consists of, or a mixture of humours
in which the black bile is predominant. However, on the basis of textual evidences taken
both from ch. 30.1 (954a11–14: 'such melancholic humour is already mixed in nature; for it
is a mixture of hot and cold; for nature consists of these two elements') of the *Problemata
physica* and from other works of Aristotle (see especially *Ph.* 246b4–5, and *Pr.* 954a15), van
der Eijk has argued (2005a, 151 and 159–160) that 'as Aristotle makes no mention of a mixture
of humours anywhere else, but does mention a particular mixture of heat and cold as the
basis for a healthy physical constitution, it is appropriate to think of a mixture of heat and
cold. In this theory, melancholics are characterised by a mixture of heat and cold (either
too heat and too cold) that is permanently out of balance, something which Aristotle clearly
regards as a sign of disease.'

terns according to the quantity of wine ingested or to the changes of the black bile inside him[54] (the mixture of the black bile, says the author, can easily pass from being too hot to being too cold and vice versa, as it participates of a mixture of hot and cold that is constantly out of balance[55]). These states of mind can vary from depression to euphoria, from calm to maniacal excitement, and their unstableness is considered as the source of creativity and genius. The only difference between the 'ethopoietic' action of wine and that of the melancholic nature is that the first is occasional and temporary, while the second is permanent and connatural to the melancholic subject.[56] According to this view, melancholy is thus to be conceived as a natural temperamental instability and as a disposition to disease rather than as a disease in itself. However, it is a form of physiological instability that can, and actually *must*, reach a 'mean' by adopting an appropriate regimen. Yet, when the 'mixture of the black bile' is not kept at the most proportioned possible state within its innate instability, this natural disposition easily turns into a number of physical as well as behavioural and what we would define as psychic disorders, which range from apoplexy to delirium, from numbness and obtuseness to aggressiveness, from ulcers to epilepsy, but which are all ascribable to the same melancholic disease.[57]

Now, it is clear from this list of diseases that in this text we cannot find any definition of the 'mental disorder' as opposed to the physical diseases, all the diseases of the black bile being defined as affections of this or that part of the body. It is important to remark, however, that such a definition only tells us that the 'psychic' disorders are also conceived as *embodied* affections, but does not give any indication as to whether epilepsy is or is not to be counted among the disorders of the cognitive and behavioural sphere of man. Actually, the only passage that gives us some useful information

---

[54] 953a33–36: 'For wine in large quantities seems to produce the characteristics which we ascribe to the melancholic, and when it is drunk produces a variety of qualities, making men ill-tempered, kindly, merciful or reckless'.

[55] 954a14–15: 'So black bile becomes both very hot and very cold'; 954b8–10: 'The melancholic temperament is in itself variable, just as it has different effects on those who suffer from the diseases which it causes; for, like water, sometimes it is cold and sometimes hot'.

[56] 953b17–21: 'Wine endows man with extraordinary qualities, not for long but only for a short time, but nature makes them permanent for so long as the man lives; for some men are bold, others silent, others merciful and others cowardly by nature. So that it is evident that wine and nature produce each man's characteristic by the same means; for every function works under the control of heat'. See Pigeaud 1988c, 25–34; van der Eijk 2005a, 157–159. In other contexts Aristotle uses the same analogy between the melancholic nature and wine: *Insomn.* 461a22; *Eth. Nic.* 1154b10.

[57] van der Eijk 2005a, 156.

on this point is 953b4–6, in which, while discussing the effects of wine on one's character, the author establishes a link between epilepsy and a state of obtuseness/madness by affirming that 'a very large quantity [of wine] relaxes them and makes them stupid (μωρούς), like those who are epileptic (ἐπιλήπτους) from childhood, or also those who are heavily affected by the diseases of the black bile (ἢ καὶ ἐχομένους τοῖς μελαγχολικοῖς ἄγαν)'.[58]

Explaining and Characterizing Epilepsy:
The 'Physical' and the 'Mental' Intertwined

It is now time to try to answer the question what kind of relations between cognitive faculties and pathophysiological processes the Greek doctors and philosophers of the classical period establish in accounting for epilepsy, and whether, and in which terms, we can refer to these faculties by using the concept of 'mind', and to their impairment by adopting such a category as 'mental disorder'.

Let us start by saying that all the accounts I have considered identify a physical origin of epilepsy, as they explain the epileptic fit as the conse-quence of an alteration, corruption, or overproduction of some material substance(s) present in the body as well as of the troubling or disruption of some physiological process. From this point of view, and insofar as these texts seem to regard the body as a psychophysical continuum, we can affirm that epilepsy was conceived as an entirely *somatic* disease.[59] Still, the prob-lem of determining what the etiological accounts of epilepsy tell us about the actual constitution of this psychophysical continuum remains. In order to cope with this problem, it is necessary to raise a couple of methodolog-ical points. On the one hand, when we find ancient definitions of epilepsy

---

[58] The adjective μωρός, the verb μωραίνω, and the abstract noun μωρία occur many times in Greek literature, and especially in tragedy, to indicate a state of foolishness, obtuseness or madness: see Aeschylus, *Pers.* 719, *Ag.* 1670; Sophocles, *Ichn.* 353, *El.* 890, *Ai.* 594; Euripides, *Med.* 614, *Andr.* 674, *Her.* 682, *Bac.* 369. In this passage the use of the disjunctive particle ἤ might be taken as the sign of a distinction drawn between epilepsy and melancholic disease, so opening the field to a contradiction in the theoretical structure of the text. But, to my eyes, this is not the case, as the contextual use of the adverb ἄγαν may simply suggest the author's will of differentiating various diseases that all have the same etiological principle according to a scale of intensity (in this case the intensity of a disease would correspond to the degree of instability of the mixture of the black bile by which it is prompted).

[59] Temkin 1971, 51 ('It remains a cause for wonder that [the Greek philosophers and physicians] attempted a theory of psychic afflictions which was not only rational and natural but was mainly based on somatic factors ...'). See also Hankinson 1991, 206–208.

as a 'disorder of the body' (as, for example, in Plato's *Timaeus* and in Hipp. *Epid.* VI, 8, 31) or as a disorder 'that impairs both the body and the leading functions' (this second definition becomes canonical from Erasistratus onwards),[60] we should be very circumspect about understanding these as explicit attempts to frame the definition of epilepsy within what a scholarly tradition which dates back to what B. Snell has described as a rough opposition between the inert *soma* and the active *psyche* in ancient Greek culture, or even within what modern philosophy and science have traditionally conceived as the dichotomous approach to the 'mind-body' problem.

For, in order for ancient doctors and philosophers to conceive of the mind-body dichotomy in the same way as we usually tend to do, they would have had to have a definite concept of mind as a real thing *entirely* distinct from the body, 'pure thought' opposed to, and ontologically independent from, pure (or mere) physicality. But a well-established scholarly tradition in the fields of ancient and early modern philosophy has shown that such a concept appeared relatively late and became hegemonic in Western culture only with the advent of the Cartesian psychology.[61] Even a clearly dualistic psychology like that expounded in Plato's *Timaeus* does not seem to imply a disembodiment of the rational part of man in such terms as the Cartesian and post-Cartesian dualistic theories of mind would do, if it is true, as remarked by Th. Johansen and, in this volume, by M.M. Sassi, that

---

[60] 'Epilepsy is a convulsion of the whole body together with an impairment of the leading functions' is the definition, attributed to the Alexandrian physician Erasistratus, which we find in Fuchs 1895, p. 598. See also Galen, *De symptom. differ.* 3, VII.58–59 K: 'Yet if there is not only convulsion of the whole body, but also interruption of the leading functions, then this is called epilepsy' (εἰ δὲ μὴ μόνον σπασμὸς εἴη τοῦ παντὸς σώματος, ἀλλὰ καὶ τῶν ἡγεμονικῶν ἐνεργειῶν ἐπίσχεσις, ἐπιληψία τὸ τοιοῦτον προσαγορεύεται). For other medical authors, it is the impairment of the leading function, and not convulsions, that distinctively characterize the epileptic fit: see Caelius Aurelianus, *Morb. Chron.* I.4, par. 60: 'Epilepsia vocabulum sumpsit, quod sensum atque mentem pariter apprehendat'; Pseudo-Galen, *Definitiones medicae*, 240, XIX.414 K: 'Epilepsy is a seizure of the thinking faculty and the senses together with a sudden fall, in some with convulsions, in others, however, without convulsion. Besides, in these patients froth flows through the mouth, when the evil is abating and past its height'. We find substantially the same definition in Celsus, *De medicina*, III.23 (I.332–334 Spencer). For his part, Paulus of Aegina (Paul.Aeg. III.13, p. 153, 1–3 Heiberg CMG) also describes the phenomena that precede and announce an epileptic fit: involuntary tension of the body and the soul (σώματος καὶ ψυχῆς τάσις ἀπροαίρετος), despondency (δυσθυμία), loss of memory (τῶν προσεχῶν λήθη), dreadful visions at night (ἐνυπνίων ὄψεις ταραχώδεις).

[61] This is the opinion put forward, for example, by Putnam 1995, 3. For a historical-epistemological introduction to the mind-body problem and a survey of the main contemporary theories of mind see Cellucci 2005, 383–410, and Eckert 2006.

for Plato the soul, while being immaterial, has spatial extension and there-fore is not *ontologically* different from the body.[62]

On the other hand, the fact that none of these texts propounds a concept of soul, or of 'psychic' or 'mental' activity, that can be considered as entirely equivalent to and consistent with that concept of 'disembodied mind' that sounds so familiar and even intuitive to us does not necessarily imply that their authors were not aware of the problem of recognizing and accounting for the differences between certain bodily diseases whose outcomes are entirely physical and certain other diseases that also touch the spheres of perception, consciousness, behaviour, emotion, intentionality and thinking, but are nevertheless as bodily as the former with respect to the cause and the seat.[63]

At this point it should be clear that we should read the ancient accounts of epilepsy, as well as the theories of cognition which these accounts belong within, through the lenses of, and in the light of some thought patterns provided by the so-called 'embodied mind' theories.[64] These are a set of the-ories that have been elaborated for the last decades by neurophysiologists, anthropologists, cyberneticists, and philosophers of mind such as G. Edel-man, G. Bateson, A. Damasio, and F. Varela and that have ended up with providing a very attractive and innovative scientific paradigm of the men-tal. This paradigm seems to me particularly interesting as it explicitly aims at bypassing Descartes' dualism and at 'putting the mind back into nature', to use a happy expression of G. Edelman.[65] I will mention five claims put for-ward by the 'embodied mind' theories that can be of some use when address-ing the ancient accounts of mental disorder: 1) the sensory-motor faculties are to be encompassed within the notion of mind, which implies that differ-ent kinds, and different degrees, of mental activity are shared between man and other forms of life;[66] 2) As the sensory-motor faculties, as well as many

---

[62] Johansen 2000, 87–111, and 2004, 142; Sorabji 2003, 161 (cf. *supra*, n. 38); Sassi, in this volume.

[63] For a brave and happy attempt to rewrite the traditional story of the rise of body-soul dualism in ancient Greece and to shed new light on the constitution of the *soma* as a subject of physical inquiry in Greek culture see Holmes 2010 (especially 29–37, 192–227).

[64] The main assumption of the 'embodied mind theory' is, to put it somewhat roughly, the nature of the human mind is largely determined by the form of the human body. They argue that all aspects of cognition, such as ideas, thoughts, concepts, and categories are shaped by aspects of the body. These aspects include the perceptual system, the intuitions that underlie the ability to move, activities and interactions with our environment and the native understanding of the world that is built into the body and the brain.

[65] Edelman 1992, 9–15.

[66] The necessity of integrating the sensory-motor faculties into a definition of 'cognitive'

other basic faculties (such as respiration) are based on mainly unconscious or involuntary mental processes, it is wrong to affirm that mental activity entirely coincides with consciousness;[67] 3) Since the sensory-motor faculties are also a vehicle for emotions, these must be part of a definition of 'mind';[68] 4) A mind is a system consisting in the internal processes of a cognitive subject coupled to the external processes with which it interacts;[69] 5) the 'mental world' is the world of information processing, that is to say a domain in which effects are caused by the perception and codification of a *difference which makes a difference*.[70]

I am not suggesting that these five claims identify the *only* conditions to fulfil in order for a process be defined as 'mental' within the embodied cognition framework, nor am I affirming that any definition of 'mind' and 'mental activity' which wants to be consistent with such framework must necessarily make *explicit* reference to all these five principles.[71] I am not even trying to argue that any of the theories of cognition discussed in this paper can be taken as a sort of *avant-la-lettre* actualization of the 'embodied mind' paradigm, which would be anachronistic and somewhat anti-methodological as well. Rather what I would like to suggest in the last part of the paper is that these claims, when abstracted from their experimental context and taken as heuristic and, so to say, comparative tools, can help us to get fresh understanding as to how the Greek scientific discourse of

---

and or 'mental' activity has been proved by a number of recent studies in the fields of the neurophysiology and neuro-engineering. Suffice here to mention Alain Berthoz's pioneering, experimentally grounded, works on the physiology of movement and of action: Berthoz 1997 and Berthoz and Petit 2006.

[67] The points that (1) cognition does not coincide with consciousness, and (2) there are in nature many forms of cognitive life that are in-, or pre-, or even a-conscious, are among the main corollaries of the theory of the 'self-organisation' of the biological systems put forward by H. Atlan 1972 and further developed into the theory of the 'autopoietic organisms' by F. Varela and H. Maturana (see Maturana and Varela 1980 and 1987).

[68] See LeDoux 1986, De Sousa 1991, Damasio 1994 and 1999.

[69] The concept of 'mind' as the result of a coupling between internal and external processes is at the basis of the 'extended mind theory' formulated by A. Clark and D.J. Chalmers in their seminal paper 'The Extended Mind' (Clark and Chalmers 1998, 10–23) and recently developed by Logan 2007. Also G. Edelman's theory of neuronal group selection (see Edelman 2006, 27–31) rests on the idea that the 'matter of the mind' is determined both by the anatomy of the brain and by one's experience f the external world.

[70] G. Bateson has provided this definition of 'the mental' in an article entitled 'Form, substance, and difference' (Bateson 1972, 454–471).

[71] Of course the outline I propose here is not intended to be prescriptive, as it represents just one of the many possible schematization of the Embodied Cognition paradigm. M. Wilson 2002, 625–636, for example, has singled out six claims as the main common features of the theories that refer more or less explicitly to this paradigm.

the classical period dealt with the question why such a great variety of cognitive/behavioural, perceptual, and motor impairments are to be observed as co-occurring phenomena in epileptic disorders.

The first important thing to observe is that all the ancient texts I have examined associate the cause or the origin of epilepsy with what they identify as the seat of, or the vehicle for, the intellectual or, more generally, the upper forms of the cognitive activity of man—be it the brain,[72] the blood, the region of the heart (where Aristotle seems to locate the *sensorium commune*), or the psychic pneuma—or with a 'character-affecting' substance (*to ethopoioun*), as is the case with the black bile in chapter 30.1 of the *Problemata Physica*.[73] In so doing, these texts do not account for epilepsy just as a disorder of some bodily processes whose outcomes *coincidentally* reverberate in the psycho-cognitive sphere, but as a *systemic* disorder whose whole phenomenology *primarily* depends on a physical derangement of the main centre, or source, of man's consciousness and perceptual faculties. In Aristotle's *De somno et vigilia*, for example, the systemic character of the epileptic disorder is suggested by the definition of sleep as an interruption of the *sensorium commune*[74]—this being the centre of, and the point of junction between, man's perceptual faculties and voluntary movement—and the subsequent assimilation of sleep to 'a kind' of epilepsy.[75] Even more interestingly, Aristotle further specifies that not all the affections of the *sensorium commune* can be equated with sleep—he mentions, in this regard, unconsciousness (*eknoia*), faintness (*leipopsychia*), and throttling (*pnigmos*)—, as they do not result, as the epileptic fit does, from a physiological process comparable to that from which sleep has its origin.[76]

But the characterisation of epilepsy as a systemic disorder of the 'physiology of consciousness', so to say, emerges in its clearest terms from the

---

[72] This is the case both of the *On the Sacred Disease*'s theory of the *enkephalos-hermeneus* and of the *Timaeus*' account of the brain as the seat of the revolutions of the rational soul.

[73] *Pr.* 30.1, 955a29–35: 'The melancholic are not equable in behaviour, because the power of the black bile is not even; for it is both very cold and very hot. But because it has an affect on character (διὰ δὲ τὸ ἠθοποιὸς εἶναι)—for heat and cold are the greatest agents in our lives for the making of character—, just like wine according as it is mixed in our body in greater or less quantity it makes our dispositions (ποιεῖ τὸ ἦθος) of a particular kind.'

[74] *Somn. Vig.* 455b3–13.

[75] See *supra*, p. 206.

[76] *Somn.Vig.* 456b9–19: 'For sleep, as has been said, is not any and every incapacity of the sensitive faculty (ἡτισοῦν ἀδυναμία τοῦ αἰσθητικοῦ); for such incapacity is produced by unconsciousness (ἔκνοια), throttling (πνιγμός), and faintness (λιποψυχία) [...] But as we have said, sleep is not every incapacity of the sensitive faculty. This affection arises from the evaporation due to food.'

accounts of *On the Sacred Disease* and *On Breaths*. In *On Breaths*, the account of the so-called sacred disease follows the statement according to which 'consciousness is *entirely* destroyed (παντελέως ἡ φρόνησις ἐξαπόλλυται) if blood is *entirely and deeply* perturbed (παντελέως ἅπαν ἀναταραχθῇ τὸ αἷμα)' (p. 122, 12–13 Jouanna), and seems actually to exemplify such a statement, insofar as the seizure is said to result from 'much air mixing with all the blood through the entire body' (κατὰ πᾶν τὸ σῶμα παντὶ τῷ αἵματι μιχθῇ) (p. 122, 17–18 Jouanna).

For the author of *On Breaths* the disruption of the state of consciousness does not represent just *one* of the possible manifestations of the epileptic fit, but constitutes the fundamental event in the light of which any other concurrent form of impairment (both of the sensory-motor faculties and of the basic physiological functions of the body) must be understood. Moreover, while the state of being *anaisthetos* engendered by another affection such as apoplexy is described in very generic terms and consists more in a lack of sensibility than in a proper state of lack of consciousness,[77] the epileptic fit is characterised by a complete loss of consciousness, and this is in turn regarded as a multifaceted phenomenon consisting of a complex combination of perceptual and cognitive impairments: by making reference to the concurrence of insensibility to sensorial stimuli, blindness, deafness and inability to feel pain (ch. 14, p. 123, 8–10 Jouanna), the author clearly aims to lay stress on the complete interruption of both lower as well as higher, of both passive as well as active, forms of cognitive interaction between the epileptic and his surroundings.[78]

We find a similar structure of the explanation in *On The Sacred Disease*. This treatise also makes a clear distinction between disorders caused by *local* accumulations of phlegm and the epileptic fit, whose cause is a generalized overflow of phlegm from the brain into the vessels that impedes the spread of consciousness (*phronesis*) over the *whole* body.[79] Moreover in

---

[77] *Vent.* 13 (120, 11–121, 2 Jouanna): 'Apoplexy, too, is caused by breaths. For when they pass through the flesh and puff it up, the parts of the body affected lose the power of feeling. So if copious breaths rush through the whole body, the whole patient is affected with apoplexy'. As remarked by Jouanna 1988, 120 n. 3, 'l' apoplexie est une paralysie qui frappe soudainement le malade; il peut s' agir d' une paralysie locale ou généralisée'. On apoplexy in the Hippocratic collection see also Souques 1936, 73–75; Clarke 1963, 301–314.

[78] This description of the state of unconsciousness has interesting points of contact with two other descriptions that we find in the books of *Epidemics* (none of them, however, is concerned with a case of epileptic fit): see *Epid.* V, 2 (3, 2–4 Jouanna): ἐν δὲ τῷ ὕπνῳ οὐκ ἐδόκει τοῖσι παρεοῦσιν ἀναπνεῖν οὐδὲν ἀλλὰ τεθνάναι, οὐδ᾽ ἠσθάνετο οὐδενὸς οὔτε ἔργου; *Epid.* V, 14 (9, 8–9 Jouanna): πρὸς τὴν ἑσπέρην οὔτε ἐφθέγγετο οὔτε ἠσθάνετο οὔτε ἔργου οὔτε λόγου;

[79] It is controversial whether the author of *On the Sacred Disease* identifies the brain as the

this treatise we also find the idea that all the sensory-motor disorders that are observable during the seizure are to be understood in the light of a systemic loss of *phronesis*. This is clear, for example, from the structure of ch. 7, which I have extensively quoted above: after accounting for all the physical impairments characteristic of the epileptic fit, the author explains that all the symptoms cease once the natural movements of the air and the blood are restored in the vessels and these start taking part in *phronesis* again (ἐ-φρόνησαν).[80]

It seems, therefore, that some of the most crucial assumptions on which many if not all the accounts of epilepsy (and their underlying theories of cognition) of the fifth and fourth centuries are based are somehow comparable with the first three claims I have singled out as characteristic of the embodied cognition paradigm. For, as we have seen, the clinical descriptions of the states of consciousness and unconsciousness tend to associate elementary forms of sensation, motor functions and the highest forms of perceptual interaction with one's own surroundings within the same explanatory framework.

Similarly the Pseudo-Aristotelian *Problemata Physica* encompasses emotions within a broader definition of cognitive activity and even attempts to outline a psychophysiology of the emotional states. And *On the Sacred Disease* states that:

> Men ought to know that our pleasures, joys, laughter, and jests come from no other source than the brain, from which also come our pains, sorrows,

---

only seat of *phronesis* (as Jouanna 2003, 120–121, has suggested) or whether the whole body takes part in it, although in different degrees and to different extents. The problem is that, as far as this specific point is concerned, the author's stand proves to be not very clear and in fact somewhat contradictory, as both the interpretative options I have just mentioned are supported by textual evidence. In order to appreciate the degree of contradictoriness of the text, it is enough to examine ch. 16: we see that the statement according to which 'throughout the body there is a degree of consciousness (τῆς φρονήσιος) proportionate to the amount of air which it receives' is immediately followed by another statement, according to which air leaves behind in the brain 'its best portion and whatever contains consciousness and thought (φρόνιμόν τε καὶ γνώμην ἔχον)'. A key-passage to solve this problem is to be found in ch. 7 (p. 15, 17–20 Jouanna), when the author affirms that 'the air that goes into the lungs and the veins is of use when it enters the cavities and the brain and in this way provides the limbs with intelligence and movement (καὶ οὕτω τὴν φρόνησιν καὶ τὴν κίνησιν τοῖσι μέλεσι παρέχει)'. I therefore agree with Ph. van der Eijk, when he points out that 'in this context *phronesis* clearly means more than 'thinking' or 'intelligence', as the word is commonly translated. It means 'having one's senses together' and refers to a universal force by which a living being can focus on its surroundings and can undertake activities; it also implies perception and movements. *Phronesis* can be found throughout the body' (van der Eijk 2005a, 127). See also Hüffmeier 1961, 58; H.W. Miller 1948, 168–183.

[80] *Morb.Sacr.* 7 (16, 24–23 Jouanna).

anxieties, and tears. Through it, in particular, we have consciousness and think, and see, and hear, and discern the ugly and the beautiful, the bad and the good, the pleasant and the unpleasant, distinguishing some things by custom, perceiving some other things according to what is useful, but some other times also distinguishing pleasures and unpleasantness according to opportunity.[81]   (ch. 14; 25, 12–26, 4 Jouanna)

Finally, we have seen that some texts, such as the *De Somno et vigilia* and *On Breaths*, beside characterizing epilepsy first of all as a generalized loss of consciousness, also admit the existence of a physiological interruption of consciousness such as sleep[82] that is somehow connected to or comparable with epilepsy. In so doing, these texts—and especially Aristotle's *De somno*—suggest the idea that there must exist 'unconscious' forms of cognitive activity,[83] in order for this activity to be successfully carried on, and that it is the task of medical investigation to clarify in what, and to what degree, the physiological and the pathological forms of unconsciousness differ from each other.

---

[81] In the following section of ch. 14 (26, 4–13 Jouanna) the author explains that 'with the brain we also become mad and delirious, and both fears and dreads occur to us, some during the night, but some other also during the day, and nightmares, and inopportune wanderings, and aimless worries, and ignorance of the real things and feelings of unaccustomedness. We suffer from all these things because of the brain, when it is not healthy, but becomes or warmer than normal, or colder, or wetter, or drier, or when it comes to be in any other unnatural state, to which it is not accustomed'. He passes then (26, 13–29, 3 Jouanna) to refer each of the mental/behavioural disorders mentioned to its physical cause, which is always traced in an alteration of the brain.

[82] There was a strand in Greek thought, which can be traced back to some of the inquiries *peri physeos* of the sixth and fifth centuries BCE, in which sleep was conceived in mainly negative terms 1) as a half pathological suspension of a number of activities that are characteristic of the waking life and, more specifically, of the rational life of man, and consequently 2) as a phenomenon which, in an ideal scale of biological normativeness, is somehow equidistant from both life and death (see Marelli 1979–1980, 123–127; Brillante 1986, 51–53; van der Eijk 2005a, 171–172). As I have argued elsewhere (Lo Presti forthcoming, with bibliography), this 'negative' representation of sleep was first strongly brought into question by parts of the fifth/fourth century medical tradition (the books of the 'Hippocratic' *Epidemics* provide ample evidence of this process of re-conceptualization and redefinition) and ended up with being replaced by Aristotle's 'positive' approach to sleep as a physiological process necessary for maintaining the life of any living being endowed with a sensitive soul.

[83] That sleep cannot be regarded as a mere suspension of the cognitive activity *tout court* is proved by the fact the people have dreams while being asleep. This is what Aristotle argues in *De ins.* 1, 459a1–6. In this regard, the physiological account of sleep and waking provided by Aristotle in the *De somno et vigilia* must be taken as the fundamental premise of his theory of dreams as expounded in the *De insomniis* and in the *De divinatione per somnum*. On the connection between the *De somno et vigilia* and the two treatises on dreams see Düring 1976, p. 637; Gallop 1996, 19–21; Repici 2003, 10–11; van der Eijk 2005a, 174–179.

As far as the claims 4 and 5 of the embodied mind paradigm are concerned, it is my impression that they are heuristically useful especially when put in relation to *On the Sacred Disease* and when used as a key to better appreciating some of the most interesting, but also controversial, aspects of its theory of cognition.

Unlike the other texts taken into exam in this paper, *On the Sacred Disease* does not limit itself to individuate *one* bodily seat, main source, or main agent of cognition. Rather, it individuates a *system* consisting of two distinct elements—an external source (air) and a bodily seat of cognition (the brain)—whose interaction gives rise to a process of *diakrisis* (cf. embodied mind claim (4)) This 'discerning' or, so to say, 'diacritical' process has both a semantic outcome, insofar as it is directed toward the 'consciousness-bearing' materials provided by air, and a physiological one, insofar as it acts upon the humoral matter that gathers in the brain. It is through this process that the system air/brain is said to prompt the perceptual, emotional, and cognitive life and to shape the motor faculties of a body as a coherent perceiving unity.

Now, one of the reasons why I consider the category of 'mental process' suitable for describing the structure and the outcome of this interaction between the air and the brain is that the role played by the brain seems definitely more complex than a simple *reaction* to a number of environmental impulses. For *On the Sacred Disease* ascribes to the physiology of the brain the power to engender a coupling of bodily and environmental processes, that is to create a system of correspondences and to reproduce, at an intra-somatic level and with both a physical and a cognitive outcome, a morphogenetic phenomenon in which phases of compaction and thickening of matter alternate with phases of loosening and moistening, and whose effects are also observable at a wider scale in the whole environment. This is what we can infer from ch. 13, which contains an account of the impact that winds and seasonal changes have on the human brain as well as on the other natural (and even celestial) bodies. According to this account the morphogenetic process through which the matter of the brain undergoes cyclical modifications is always prompted by the perception of a difference, more specifically of a change of the quality, properties, and direction of the winds (cf. embodied mind claim (5)). The brain, says the author, is particularly sensitive to this specific kind of change as it is the first part of the body to come into contact with air, and in fact is the part which receives its purest and most active part (*akme*), which lets him explain both why the brain is the main centre of man's cognitive life (here the term 'cognitive' is to be intended in the broadest sense) and why it is prone to the greatest diseases:

As therefore it is the first of the bodily organs to perceive the intelligence coming from the air, so too if any violent change (μεταβολὴ ἰσχυρή) has occurred in the air owing to the seasons, the brain also becomes different (διάφορος) from what it was. Therefore I assert that the diseases too that attack it are the most acute, most serious, most fatal, and the hardest for the inexperienced to judge of.[84]   (ch. 17, p. 31, 8–15 Jouanna; transl. Jones)

On the one hand, and at a physical level, this theory describes a system in which the *perception of a difference* (the changes of the winds) *makes a difference* (the cyclical modification of the brain shape); on the other hand, and at an intellectual, perceptual and emotional level—this system of difference-based correspondences established between the brain and the environment results in a capacity to discern—viz., *to recognize, establish and codify differences between*—things, a capacity which the author of *On the Sacred Disease* accounts for in ch. 14 (see *supra*).

Now, it is interesting to note that, when considered as a whole, this frame of causal relations seems to be in many regards compatible with the last theoretical claim, which I referred to in this paper, and which also provides the basis for G. Bateson's technical definition of 'mind'. But it is even more interesting to observe that epilepsy, as well as many other affections, is said to arise when some physical factor perturbs or even breaks the system of correspondences between the changes that the brain *perceives* from the environment, the changes that it undergoes in its own matter, and the power of the brain of engendering changes (in form of sense perceptions and voluntary motion) and of codifying differences between things (in form of judgements, knowledge, emotions).[85]

Conclusions

I have tried to show that the question of the definition of epilepsy in the Greek medical texts of the classical period is far from being solved. No serious attempt to understand how ancient physicians perceived and accounted

---

[84] Immediately afterwards (ch. 18 = 31, 16–32, 1 Jouanna), the author reaffirms the same concept, this time with specific reference to the sacred disease: 'This disease called sacred comes from the same causes as others, from the things that come to and go from the body, from cold, sun, and from the changing restlessness of winds'. The existence of a causal link between epileptic attack and wind and, more in general, climate changes (especially if these changes are sudden and violent) is suggested also in ch. 10 (20, 16–18 Jouanna), in ch. 11 (21, 6–9 Jouanna), and in ch. 13 (23, 6–7 Jouanna).

[85] For a broader discussion of the biological rationale behind *On the Sacred Disease*'s theory of cognition see Lo Presti 2008, 159–194, and 2011.

for the psychophysical manifestations of the epileptic disorder can be made without clarifying what *we* actually mean when speaking of 'body' and 'mind' as well as of 'somatic' and 'mental' disorders. If we adopt these concepts as roughly dichotomous, the only conclusion we will be allowed to draw is that all the texts taken into exam have an unequivocally 'somatic' approach to epilepsy, as they trace the cause of the seizure in an alteration of some physiological processes. But, as I have tried to argue, the very same texts prove to be open to more complex and heuristically fruitful readings that may pave the way for a better appreciation of the body and its properties as subjects of physical inquiry and ultimately for a rethinking of the whole problem of the relationship between 'the physical' and the 'psychic' in classical antiquity.

To my mind, the first and most essential condition that has to be met in order for this interpretative shift to happen is to escape from the limitations imposed on us by the modern, Cartesian and post-Cartesian notion of mind as pure thinking substance independent, and ontologically distinct, from the body, and to adopt a concept of 'mind' as an emergent property of the body consisting of perceptual, behavioural, emotional and motor faculties interconnected with each other, and, so to say, as the expression of the body's *intrinsic* capacity to act within, and be aware of, its own bio-cognitive domain. If we look at the fifth and fourth century ancient medical accounts of epilepsy through the lenses of this second, more complex, definition of mind, it will be perhaps easier to achieve two aims: to get to a fresh understanding of the theoretical and argumentative strategies through which the Greek scientific discourse of the classical period accounted for the epileptic seizure as a 'systemic' disorder whose origin is to be traced in the main centre of man's cognitive faculties, and to show that there does not exist any natural/universal definition of 'mind' and 'mental disorder', but different and sometimes even antithetical definitions whose premises and corollaries must always be made explicit and framed in a definite historical and epistemological context before being used as heuristic tools by the historian of medical ideas.

MEDICAL EPISTEMOLOGY AND MELANCHOLY:
RUFUS OF EPHESUS AND MISKAWAYH

Peter E. Pormann

Madness and other mental disorders have clear epistemological implications. When people hallucinate, thinking that they are earthen jars, or seeing things that do not actually exist, their judgments are obviously impaired. Therefore, their opinions about the outside world cannot be relied upon, nor do they correspond to reality. But more fundamentally, madness poses an even greater problem, as the madman often does not realise that he is mad: he constructs his own, alternative reality that possesses internal cohesion and therefore remains unchallenged. A vivid example for this phenomenon is provided in the novel *Shutter Island*, recently turned into a blockbuster film.[1] The protagonist has taken refuge in an alternative reality owing to the traumatic experience of finding his own children killed by his delusional wife, and then killing her in an act of desperation. Both in the novel and the film, one only discovers gradually that the protagonist's alternate reality is a phantasy, a fabrication from which he cannot escape. But if this is the case, how can we then be certain that the reality that we experience is not also a similar fabrication?

This question underlies the arguments made by an anonymous opponent and refuted by Miskawayh (d. 1030), the great historian and Neo-Platonic philosopher. Interestingly, these arguments centre around the notion of scholarly melancholy as Rufus of Ephesus developed it in his treatise *On Melancholy*. In the present article, I propose to investigate Miskawayh's melancholy, so to speak, in both medical and philosophical terms. In order to do so, it will be necessary to provide some background information about Rufus of Ephesus' scholarly melancholy first, and then turn to Miskawayh's anonymous opponent and Miskawayh's own conception of melancholy as he uses it to confute this opponent's ideas.

---

[1] Lehane 2003.

Rufus of Ephesus' Scholarly Melancholy

Rufus of Ephesus, who lived towards the end of the first century AD, wrote many medical monographs on a wide variety of topics.[2] He had a particular interest in Hippocrates, and generally adhered to the principles of humoral pathology, that is, the theory of the four humours that includes black bile. Rufus wrote a monograph in two books on the topic of melancholy, but unfortunately, it has only come down to us in fragments in Greek, Arabic, and Latin.[3] According to Rufus, the disease melancholy is unsurprisingly caused by black bile (*mélaina cholé* in Greek), which occurs both naturally and as a product of yellow bile being burnt.[4] It is a type of madness that occurs in different manifestations, ranging from general despondency and fear to hallucinations, ravings, and aggressive streaks.[5] But Rufus also records a case where melancholy is caused by the traumatic experience of drowning.[6] And, famously, he claimed that too much thinking leads to melancholy.[7] It is this last point around which the argument between Miskawayh and his anonymous opponent hinges.

In the famous Aristotelian problem 30.1, the author links great achievements in philosophy, politics and the arts to melancholy. Rufus draws on this Aristotelian tradition,[8] but also develops it further. 'Abū Bakr Muḥammad ibn Zakarīyā' ar-Rāzī (d. 925) reports Rufus as saying:[9]

قال وأصحاب الطبائع الفاضلة مستعدّون للمالنخوليا لأن الطبائع الفاضلة سريعة الحركة كثيرة الفكر.

He [Rufus] said: People of excellent nature are predisposed to melancholy, since excellent natures move quickly and think a lot.

Rufus thus postulates a causal link between excessive thought, to which great people are prone, and melancholy. To put it differently, their excellent nature (*ṭabīʿa fāḍila*, corresponding to Greek εὐφυΐα) involves also an extreme use of their mental faculties, which in its turn leads to melancholy.

---

[2] See Sideras 1994 and Ullmann 1994.

[3] Pormann 2008 and Pormann, forthcoming for a number of new fragments; see also Fischer 2010, 180–183.

[4] Pormann 2008, 4–5.

[5] F 11 § 24 ed. Pormann 2008. All subsequent references to Rufus are to this edition.

[6] F 69.

[7] FF 33–36.

[8] van der Eijk 2008b.

[9] F 33; the fragment also appears in a later author, al-Qumrī (fl. 960–980s), who probably quoted from ar-Rāzī rather than having direct access to the Arabic translation here (F 34).

Another quotation by ar-Rāzī expresses this causal link explicitly:[10]

قال: وقد يوقع فيه [أي :المالنخوليا] شدّة الفكر والهمّ.

He said: Violent thoughts and worries may make one succumb to it [sc. melancholy].

The expression used here is *šiddat al-fikr*, literally meaning 'violence of thought', which appears here next to the more general 'worries (*hamm*)'.

Unfortunately, in the extant fragments of Rufus' *On Melancholy*, we do not have a description of how the melancholy caused by violent or excessive thinking manifests itself. But we do have the case notes of one of Rufus' patients suffering from melancholy brought about by 'constant contemplation of geometrical sciences (*mudāwamatuhū 'alā l-nazari fī 'ulūmi l-handasati)*'.[11] This thought activity led to the blood of the patient being burnt. Because of the wrong treatment by another physician, this burning intensified, and resulted in madness (*ǧunūn*) and eventually death. This case suggests that scholarly melancholy could result in delusional states—the madness mentioned by Rufus—, and even death. From other fragments, we also know that symptoms of melancholy included delusions of thinking that one is an earthen vessel; that one does not have a head; that the sky will fall down, as Atlas gets tired; or that one is a cock.[12] It was probably this kind of delusion that the anonymous opponent had in mind when challenging the foundations of Neo-Platonic epistemology.

Miskawayh's Anonymous Opponent

Miskawayh wrote a number of works in which he expounds his views on the human soul, the intellect, and the different kinds of knowledge.[13] Among them is his treatise *On the Soul and the Intellect, this Being an Answer to Someone who Asked* [*sā'il*] *about Them, and a Solution for Doubts Which He Had about the Simple Essence Subsisting through Itself* [*al-qā'im bi-nafsihī*].[14]

---

[10] F 35.

[11] Ullmann 1978, 72; F 68 Pormann.

[12] F 11 §§ 3–5; F 13a and F 13b. The last two examples occur in the new fragments first discovered by Fischer 2010; see Pormann, forthcoming. They confirm that much of what Galen says about melancholy in *On the Affected Parts*, iii. 9–10, comes from Rufus.

[13] See Adamson 2008.

[14] Both the first edition of this treatise by Arkoun (1961/2, 65–20) and the new edition by 'Abd ar-Raḥmān Badawī (1981, 57–97) are based on the same unique manuscript and suffer from a number of misprints and problems. Adamson and Pormann 2012b have recently

As the title already indicates, Miskawayh refutes in this treatise a person who challenged him and whom he does not name. This refutation takes the form of Miskawayh's first quoting from the letter in which his opponent challenged him. Then he discusses the points made by the opponent one by one, generally arguing against them, or pointing out inconsistencies. In this way, Miskawayh proceeds until the end of his opponent's epistle. This technique of quotation followed by refutation had already been employed by the Christian philosopher Yaḥyā ibn 'Adī (d. 974) when countering the arguments of al-Kindī (d. after 870) against the doctrine of the trinity.[15] In ibn 'Adī's case, it is likely that he preserved the whole of al-Kindī's epistle, and this also seems likely for Miskawayh and his anonymous adversary.

Be that as it may, the quotations preserved in Miskawayh's *Treatise on the Soul and the Intellect* allow us to reconstruct the main points of the adversary's argument.[16] It runs roughly along the following lines. One can only grasp universals through intellection on the basis of having perceived particulars through sensation. Therefore, if the sensation is impaired or wrong, then so is the intellection. The anonymous adversary does not state explicitly that many Neo-Platonic philosophers like Miskawayh would argue that intellection without sensation is the only way that can lead to the truth. Against this view, in any case, the adversary offers an argument based on Rufus' idea of scholarly melancholy. Intense mental activities can trigger delusions. Therefore, the idea of pure thought without sensation cannot work, as the results of these thought processes may be delusional. The adversary emphasises this point by more cosmological considerations. Heat is the all-pervading principle of the world, and therefore also the material out of which the soul is made. This is illustrated by the fact that we perceive particulars through the heat of fire and the sun, and universals through the heat, as the perception of universals depends on that of particulars. Moreover, the intellect is light: just as the light of the sun, moon, or fire makes sense perception possible, so the light of the intellect brings about intellection. Therefore, again, the adversary insists that only sensation and intellection, both based on material principles (light and heat) in combination allow us to avoid the

---

translated this important text into English for the first time. The quotations from this work given here are taken from their translation. The epistle has previously been translated into French and studied in an undergraduate thesis by Harika 1993.

[15] Périer 1920; see also Rashed and Jolivet 1998, 123–127; an English translation of al-Kindī's *Refutation of the Trinity* and further discussion is available in Adamson and Pormann 2012a, 76–81.

[16] Adamson 2008, 50–52, provides an English translation of all the quotations culled from Miskawayh's epistle in appendix I to his article.

delusional states of which Rufus speaks. The danger of wrong imagination is illustrated by Galen. He once became delusional and also talked about the wool-carder who thought that a carpet could feel pain. Heat produces the movement of the celestial spheres, and heat and light together are the only principles that can be safely perceived as true. Any idea of spiritual beings beyond this material world are fantasies of the kind that Rufus talked about and that affected Galen. Even divine powers and prophecy must be explained in these terms, and not through recourse to spiritual entities.

This summary already shows that Miskawayh's anonymous adversary adhered to a philosophical position that is *sui generis*. To date, no probable candidate has been identified who could be this adversary, and it is likely that he will remain anonymous. Of interest to us here specifically is the use that he makes of Rufus' notion of scholarly melancholy.

In the first passage quoted by Miskawayh, the opponent says the following:[17]

ويحكى عن روفس الطبيب أنه قال: «ليس أحد يمعن في الفكر في علم ما إلا وينتهي به ذلك إلى
مالنخوليا» فما يؤمننا، إذا اعتقدنا أوهاما ليس لها جزئيات مشاهدة بالحس، أن (لا) تكون بهذه
الصفة ؟ وإذا كان الحس يكذب ويغلط أحيانا كثيرة، وكان التخيل في ذلك على أضعاف ما عليه الحس
من الغلط والكذب في المنى والوسوسة وحديث الناس وأجناس الخوف والأماني والعلل العارضة،
وكان العقل إنما يأخذ ما يأخذه إن كان على جهة التذكير أو على جهة الانقداح عن أحد هذين كيف
نأمن فما نعتقد في هذه الجواهر التي نعتقد أنها روحانية إذا لم ندرك لها جزئيات.

It is reported that Rufus, the physician, said the following:[18] 'No-one who devotes too much effort to thinking about a certain science (*ʿilm*) can avoid ending up with melancholy.' How can we be certain, if we firmly believe in illusions (*ʾawhām*) with no particulars for them, that this description does not apply to us? Sense-perception lies and errs much of the time. Imagination (*taḥayyul*) errs and lies many times more than does sense-perception when it comes to desires, insinuations (*waswasa*), the rumours people spread, different kinds of fears, wishes and diseases which befall [us]. Finally, the intellect can only grasp things—be it by remembering or by being incited (*inqidāḥ*) by one of these two [sc. sensation or imagination].' If this is so, what confidence can we have in our beliefs about these substances assumed by us to be spiritual, if we do not even comprehend their particulars?

The opponent argues two main points in this passage. First, since sensation is prone to error, and intellection is based partly on sensation, then

---

[17] Ed. Arkoun 1961–1962, p. 57, last line—p. 58, line 6; tr. Adamson, Pormann 2012b, p. 487. All subsequent references are to this edition and translation; for a discussion of variant readings and emendations, see the notes to Adamson, Pormann 2012b.

[18] F 36.

intellection is prone to error as well. Second, intellection itself is even more unreliable than sense perception. For this second point, Rufus provides evidence: too much thinking leads to melancholy, to be understood here as a delusional state.

The adversary returns to Rufus again twice more throughout his attack against Miskawayh, and the context of these passages provides us with a better understanding of how the adversary understood Rufus. In the first one, the adversary reiterates his point:[19]

فإن لم نفعل واعتقدنا في النفس أنها جوهر روحاني لطيف لا ندرك لها كليا ولا جزئيا، فما يؤمننا مما قال روفس و (هو) أن يكون هذا ضربا من الوسوسة لا حقيقة له؟

But if we do not do this, and adhere to the doctrine that the soul is a spiritual, subtle substance which is grasped neither universally nor as particular, then what would make us feel safe from what Rufus has said, namely that this is a kind of madness (waswasa) with no truth to it?

The second quotation reaffirms points made earlier, but also introduces interesting new elements:[20]

وإن أضربنا عن هذا وتوهمنا شيئا روحانيا، هو العقل في العالم الصغير وهو غير هذا النور فمن أين نأمن ما قال روفس؟ وإذا كان أشرف ما ينتهي إليه الشرف فيما أدركناه وعرفناه هو هذه الأنوار التي بها الوصول إلى الإدراكات والحرارة التي هي سبب كل فعل وانفعال في العالمين فلم لا نقف عند هذين ولا نتجاوزهما لنكون على ثقة ويقين وبصيرة أنا لسنا نعتقد ما هو وسوسة وأنا تخلصنا مما قال روفس؟

وقد كان جالينوس فسد تخيله، وحُكِيَ في «الجوامع» أن التفكير يجري مجرى الرداءة. وإن مشاطا للصوف فسد تفكره حتى ظن أن البساط يألم، فرمى به من فوق إلى أسفل ليؤلمه لما غضب عليه.

But if we reject this [that the intellect is light], and imagine a spiritual thing that is intellect in the microcosm [sc. the human being], but is not this light, then what would make us feel safe from what Rufus said? If the most noble and ultimately exalted thing in what we perceive and know is these lights, through which we arrive at perceptions, and heat, which is the cause for all acting and being acted upon in the two worlds [i.e., the microcosm and the macrocosm], then why do we not stop at these two things, without going beyond them, in order to have confidence, certitude, and insight that we do not believe things that are mad [mā huwa waswasa] and are free from what Rufus said?

Galen's imagination (taḥayyul) had once been corrupted, and he relates in the Summaries (al-Ǧawāmiʿ) that his thinking functioned badly; and that the wool-carder's thinking had corrupted so much that he thought that the carpet suffered pain, so that he threw it down from above in order to hurt it, because he was very angry with it.

---

[19] Ed. p. 70, last line—p. 71, line 1; tr. p. 500.
[20] Ed. p. 74, last line—p. 75, line 7; tr. p.

The adversary begins by restating that only when one accepts his materialist world view in which heat and light play a major role, can one really know things. Anything spiritual would be beyond our comprehension, but also probably does not exist. The anecdote about Galen and the wool carder comes from the chapter on *phrenîtis* in Galen's *On the Affected Parts* (book 4, chapter 2).[21] Galen describes how he himself was affected by the disease when he was a young man (μειράκιον). He had delusions of seeing straws on his bed and threads on his gown; he tried to pick them, but to no avail. The case of the wool-carder is quite famous. Galen tells the story quite differently from Miskawayh's opponent. A man had a wool-carder slave. One morning, he became affected by *phrenîtis*. As a result, he went to the open window, and threw out various earthen vessels, each time asking the crowd below whether he should do so. The people were amused by this, and encouraged him. Finally, he demanded whether he should also throw out the wool-carder. They said yes, and he did so. This dampened the mood, and we do not know whether the slave survived.

How then could the opponent provide such a distorted and very short version of the episode, with a carpet feeling pain at the centre? The first indication may come from the source reference provided by the opponent: he says that the episode occurs in the 'Summaries (Ǧawāmi')'. This is presumably a reference to the so-called *Alexandrian Summaries (Ǧawāmi' al-'Iskandarānīyīn)*, a famous group of texts produced in Late Antiquity and only extant in Arabic and Hebrew.[22] There the episode is summarised in the following terms:[23]

في العلة التي يقال لها فرانيطس.

ربما كانت الآفة من الدماغ في التخيل فقط كما عرض لجالينوس. ويستدل على ذلك بأن صاحب هذه العلة يتخيل أشياء ليست بموجودة. ومن أجل ذلك صار أصحابها يَلْتُطُون الزئبر من الثياب والتبن من الخيطان. وربما كانت هذه العلة في الفكر فقط بمنزلة ما عرض لمشاط الصوف. ويستدل على ذلك بأن العليل لا يفهم ما يؤمر به. وربما كان فيها جميعا. ويستدل على ذلك بأن صاحب العلة يلتقط الزئبر والتبن ولا يفهم ما أُمِرَ به.

On the disease called *phrenîtis*.

Sometimes the ailment of the brain occurs only in the imagination [*at-taḫayyul*], as happened to Galen. This is indicated by the fact that the patient suffering from this disease imagines things that do not exist. Therefore, the

---

[21] See the discussion by McDonald 2009, 128–135.

[22] See, for instance, Savage-Smith 2002; Pormann 2004; Garofalo 2007.

[23] Sezgin 2001 published a facsimile of these *Summaries*; the episode quoted here can be found in volume ii., p. 300, last line—p. 301, line 6.

patients collect rags and worn out threads [*yalquṭūna z-zi'bara mina ṯ-ṯiyābi wa-t-tibna mina l-ḫīṭāni*]. Sometimes, this disease occurs in the thinking [*al-fikr*] only, as for instance what happened to the wool-carder. This is indicated by the fact that he does not understand what he is ordered [to do]. And sometimes, it occurs in both [i.e., imagination and thinking]. This is indicated by the fact that the patient collects rags and worn-out threads and does not understand what he is ordered [to do].

We have a brief mention of the wool-carder (*maššāṭ aṣ-ṣūf*) here, but nothing that would explain the carpet (*bisāṭ*) that feels pain, mentioned by the opponent.

This incident constitutes one of the cases where a scribal error triggered a fruitful misunderstanding. This scribal error and corruption must have occurred in the Arabic, not the Greek. For the Arabic words for 'wool-carder (*maššāṭ*)' and 'carpet (*bisāṭ*)' are extremely close from a palaeographical point of view (بساط مشاط), especially when one takes into account that diacritical dots are often omitted or sloppily written in manuscripts. Somewhere along the textual transmission, the second mention of the wool-carder must have been turned into the carpet by inadvertence. This led to the episode being further embroidered by the element of the rug feeling pain.

Whatever the vagaries of transmission may be, Miskawayh's adversary clearly uses Rufus' concept of scholarly melancholy to show that pure thought cannot be relied upon. This view obviously represents a major challenge to Neo-Platonic epistemology. How, then, did a major representative of this current in late tenth- and early eleventh-century Baghdad refute this opponent? And, more to the point, how did he conceive of melancholy and madness in this context?

Miskawayh's Melancholy

To answer these questions, it will be necessary to conduct a close reading of Miskawayh's description of melancholy in his *Epistle on the Soul and the Intellect*. As this text will not be familiar to many classicists, it is useful to paraphrase the salient points in this description, and to quote a number of key passages. In each case, I shall also offer some initial interpretation and analysis, and then provide a more detailed critical discussion in the concluding part of this section.

Miskawayh begins his refutation by addressing the first point of his opponent: that intellection has to be based on sensation. Miskawayh states that the opponent is gravely mistaken. Sense-perception occurs before intellection in temporal terms: we have sensation before being able to comprehend complex ideas. This, however, does not mean that sensation is essentially prior to intellection. Moreover, intellection can also occur without any reference to sensation. On the contrary, sensation requires intellection, as it is only through intellection that the right sensations are separated from the wrong ones. According to Miskawayh, Aristotle and his commentator Themistius were also of this view: for instance, in the case of vision, the sensation needs to be validated by the intellect. One may think here of Aristotle's discussion in *On the Soul* about whether sensation can be false, with the famous example of the sun looking as if it were a foot wide.[24] 'Aristotle', however, could also be more broadly understood, as not only the genuine works, but also many other writings were attributed to him, the two most famous being the *Theology of Aristotle*[25] and the *Book on the Pure Good*, known in Latin as *Liber de Causis*.[26] Miskawayh continues that the active intellect exists by necessity, since only this intellect is able to actualise the various functions of the soul. And obviously, intellection is superior to sensation, since the latter often goes wrong: for example, our vision plays tricks on us, or the sense of touch is not objective, as a cold hand finds things warmer.

Miskawayh then turns to the topic of melancholy. His argument runs as follows:[27]

فأما قول روفس الطبيب: «إنه ليس يمعن أحد في الفكر في علم ما إلا وينتهي ذلك إلى مالنخوليا» فإذا ظن أن هذا الاسم في تلك اللغة التي تخصص بها ليس بمطلق على المرض وحده، بل هو اسم لكل فكر، وإلا لزم بحسب قول روفس أن الآراء الصحيحة التي تصدر عن الأفكار الطويلة الزمان تكون مرضا عظيما. ونحن نعلم أن الفكر الذي يمعن فيه صاحب الهندسة حتى يستخرج به أمرا نافعا في العالم من نحو استخراج ماء إلى وجه الأرض أو رفع طريق أو تحريك شيء ثقيل بقوة ضعيفة يسيرة والفكر الذي يمعن فيه مدبر الجيش وسائس المدينة حتى تتم له عمارة أو غلبة عدو مفسد، ليس بمرض. وكيف يكون مرضا، والإنسان إنما يطلب الصحة من جسده وتدبيره لبدنه ليتم له بها الفكر الصحيح الذي يؤديه إلى كل خير مطلوب من دنيا وآخرة.

Rufus, the physician, said: 'Those who devote too much effort to thinking about a certain science (*'ilm*) end up suffering from melancholy.' As regards this quotation, if he [the opponent] thinks that this word in that language

---

[24] 428b2–4: 'There are, however, also false appearances, in connection with whose objects true supposition simultaneously occurs. For instance, the sun appears to be a foot across. Yet we are convinced that it is greater than the inhabited world. (φαίνεται δέ γε καὶ ψευδῆ, περὶ ὧν ἅμα ὑπόληψιν ἀληθῆ ἔχει, οἷον φαίνεται μὲν ὁ ἥλιος ποδιαῖος, πιστεύεται δ᾽ εἶναι μείζων τῆς οἰκουμένης)' (trans Lawson-Tangred 1986, p. 199).

[25] See Adamson 2002, and, most recently, Belo 2010.

[26] D'Ancona 1995.

[27] Ed. p. 64, lines 1–10; tr. pp. 492–493.

in which he specialises [Greek] does not specially designate one illness, but rather is a name for thought in general, [then he is wrong]. For otherwise, it would follow according to Rufus' exposition that true opinions which derive from thought-processes over a long period of time generate a powerful disease. We know that the thinking to which a geometer (ṣāḥib al-handasa) assiduously applies himself to arrive at something useful in the world, such as extracting water to ground level, or raising a road, or moving something heavy with little force; and the thinking to which a general (mudabbir al-ǧayš) and the manager of a city (sāʾis al-madīna) assiduously apply themselves to accomplish a building or victory over an evil foe, are not a disease. How could they be a disease, given that man strives for physical health and trains his body only in order to reach fulfillment in true thought, which leads to every good sought in this world and the next?

Miskawayh thus addresses the main point made by the opponent: that intense thought leads to melancholy and delusion. Miskawayh is aware that malinḫūliyā is a Greek word. Interestingly, he says that the opponent 'specialises (taḫaṣṣaṣa)' in the Greek language, one of the few indications about the opponent's background. But, Miskawayh continues, the word melancholy is not applied to all mental activities, but only to a specific disease, namely the delusional melancholy about which Rufus talks. Miskawayh then provides some examples of people who think a lot, but who clearly do not go mad in the process. They include the engineer, the governor, and the general, all of whom apply their thinking to complex problems with beneficial results. The inclusion of the engineer or geometer (ṣāḥib al-handasa) in his list of examples is quite remarkable. For this figure is later identified with the figure of the melancholic thinker, as it appears for instance in Dürer's famous copperplate Melencolia I.[28] And, as we have seen, Rufus recorded the case notes of a patient suffering from melancholy because of excessive contemplation of the geometrical sciences.[29]

Miskawayh then remarks that a healthy mind resides in a healthy body; here again, his implication appears to be that healthy individuals can think in a non-delusional way, and that striving for physical health does not necessarily impair mental health. This raises the question of the relationship between body and soul, between bodily health and mental well-being, that is of crucial importance for the understanding of melancholy. Miskawayh goes on to talk about thought separating man from beast, and compares the skills of a physician to those of a carpenter. Both have a notion of correct

---

[28] See Toohey 2008, 221–243.
[29] F 68; see above p. 225.

tools and procedures, specific to their art (ṣinā'a, téchnē). Our author then addresses another objection to his anonymous opponent:[30]

ونقول أيضا على سبيل المعارضة لهذا المتشكك: هل إمعان روفس في الفكر وبلوغه من الطب ذلك المبلغ وهو الذي صيره فاضلا في صناعته مالنخوليا؟ وفكره في قوله هذا الذي حكيته عنه هو على حكمه أيضا مالنخوليا؟ فكيف يجب أن نحكم عليه؟ وما الذي نقول فيه؟ إلا أنا نتدارك نصرة كلام هذا الرجل الفاضل بتخريج وجه لكلامه صحيح، هو أن روفس أومأ إلى العلوم الوهمية والأوهام بأسرها إذا أمعنت في الحركة، انتهت إلى المالنخوليا على هذه الجهة.

> We also say the following by way of refuting this sceptic. Does Rufus' excessive thinking and his attainment of such a high station in medicine—this being what made him so outstanding in his art—constitute melancholy? And is his thinking in this quotation which you related—and also according to his [Rufus'] own judgement—melancholy? How should we judge him, and what should we say about him? Should we not leave [intact] the victory of this excellent man's words by taking what he says in a correct way? Namely, that Rufus refers to instances of imaginary knowledge ('ulūm waḥmīya), and acts of imagination in general (al-'awhām bi-'asrihā); if they [the acts of imagination] are aroused in excess, they finally lead to melancholy in this way.

In this passage, Miskawayh argues that Rufus himself as a medical thinker would be prone to melancholy, if one were to follow the opponent's argument. But this would be a contradiction: one cannot trust Rufus' authority, if he is affected by melancholy resulting form his medical thinking. The solution to this conundrum is easy: Rufus did not talk about all acts of thinking leading to melancholy, but only 'instances of imaginary knowledge ('ulūm waḥmīya), and acts of imagination in general (al-'awhām bi-'asrihā)'. It is important to note that 'imaginary' and 'imagination' here translate words derived from the Arabic root w-h-m. This root often has negative connotation in the sense of fanciful and wrong imaginations. To put it differently, Greek phantasía, frequently translated into English as 'imagination', denotes at least two things: first, the activity or ability of representing to oneself an image or an idea; and the fanciful and wrong imagination. In the former sense, it is mostly translated into Arabic by the root ḫ-y-l; and in the latter by the root w-h-m, although the distinction is not always clearcut.[31] For instance, in his letter On the Definitions and Descriptions of Things, al-Kindī

---

[30] Ed. p. 64, line 5 from the bottom—p. 65, line 1; tr. p. 493.

[31] See Ullmann 2006–2007, under φαντασία; Ullmann quotes a number of examples from Aristotle where taḫayyul translates φαντασία in the former sense, but also two instances (from Nemesius of Emesa and Galen) where it is rendered as tawahhum; and he adduces one instance (from Dioscorides) where φαντασία in the sense of delusion is rendered as ḫayālāt.

equates *phantasía* in the former sense with *tawahhum*, and gives *taḥayyul* as a possible synonym.[32]

Miskawayh exploits this ambiguity in his discussion. His explanation of imagination illustrates in quite some detail how he understands melancholy:[33]

والوهم تابع للحس. وإذا أخذ صورة طبيعية فإنما يجعلها عن طبيعة ثم تركب منها تركبات لا نهاية لها،
وليس لواحدة منها وجود طبيعي بوجه من الوجوه. ومثال ذلك أن الوهم يأخذ صورة الجسم، أعني
الأبعاد الثلاثة، فيأخذها في غير جسم، ثم يتوهمها موجودة من خارج الوهم، معتقدا من ذلك الخلاء
وأنه مسكوب حول العالم موجود لا محالة. ثم يشكل في وهمه أيضا أنواع الأشكال التي ليس لها وجود
ويسأل عنها سؤال ما هو موجود، وأعني أنه يتصور شخصا خارج العالم جالسا على سطح الكرة
القصوى، ثم يسأل كيف يكون حال هذا الوهم المحال سؤال من ظنه موجودا. وكذلك حاله في الأوهام
التي تجري هذا المجرى. وكلما أمعن في هذا الضرب، كان أبعد من الأمر الموجود. وهذه حال الوهم
والعلوم الوهمية. وتتبعها التخيلات الباطلة والوساوس المكروهة. وربما ترقى إلى المحالات من الأماني،
واستشعار مخاوف ومهالك لا حقائف لها: وهذه هي صورة المالنخوليا.

> Imagination [*wahm*] depends on sensation. When it [imagination] forms a natural image, it produces [that image] from nature, and then puts together innumerable combinations on this basis. Nor does any one [of these combinations] have a natural existence in any way. For example, imagination takes the image of a body, that is, something three-dimensional, and applies it to something non-corporeal. Then it imagines that this exists outside the imagination, firmly believing in the void, and that it [the void] is poured around this world and exists—which is impossible. Then in his imagination he conceives of forms which have no existence. He asks about them as if they existed, that is to say that he imagines an individual outside the world, sitting on the surface of the outermost sphere. Then he asks how this absurdly imagined situation occurs, posing the question as if he really thought that it exists. His situation is similar with regard to other such imaginations. As long as he 'devotes too much effort ['*am'ana*]' to this sort [of thinking], he is very remote from reality. This is the state of imagination and instances of imaginary knowledge [*al-wahm wa-l-'ulūm al-wahmīya*], which are followed by futile fantasies [*taḥayyulāt bāṭila*] and despicable delusions [*wasāwis makrūha*]. Sometimes it gets as far as absurd desires, or a feeling of dread and doom [*istiš'ār maḥāwif wa-mahālik*] without any basis in reality. This is the idea [*ṣūra*] of melancholy.

Miskawayh thus links imagination to sensation. He begins by talking about the process of combining different images derived from sense perception in a way that creates an image of something that does not exist at all. One such

---

[32] Al-Kindī, *On the Definitions and Descriptions of Things*, no. 21 in Adamson and Pormann 2012a, 301.

[33] Ed. p. 65, lines 1–11; tr. pp. 493–494.

example is the void which, according to Aristotle and many of his followers, cannot exist.[34] Then Miskawayh cleverly shifts from the imagination in the first sense—the representation to oneself of images—to the imagination in the second sense—i.e., that of delusions. Imagination (*wahm*) sometimes allows one to conceive of images that do not exist in reality, but are based on real images; for instance, when one imagines a centaur, one combines the image of a man with that of a horse. Sometimes, however, one is not aware that one's imagination conceives of unreal objects. It is in this last sense that he defines imagination as a characteristic symptom of melancholy. Too much thinking in the sense of imagining too many things that do not exist leads to the delusions, fancies, and desires that characterise melancholy. Put differently, imagination in the first sense produces imagination in the second sense. One could summarise Miskawayh's main points here as follows: Rufus did not mean that all thinking would lead to melancholy, but only the imaginary thinking that would then result in imaginary delusions.

Miskawayh further explains the difference between correct thinking (*fikr ṣaḥīḥ*) and delusional melancholy through an analogy with vision. For just as vision can be blurred because the instrument of vision, that is, the eye, is damaged or diseased, so thought processes can be flawed when the instrument of thought, the brain, is impeded. Miskawayh states:[35]

وكما تعرض للبصر أحوال تسمى أمراضا فتعالج حتى يعود إلى صحته فكذلك للعقل الهيولاني أمراض
تعالج حتى يعود إلى صحته. فأحد أمراضه المالنخوليا، وهو الفكر الذي لا يؤدي إلى حقيقة ولا يأخذ
إلى مطلوبه على سمت صحيح صحيح فيضطرب إلى أن يعالج بفكر صحيح من ذي عقل سليم. والذي يفكر
في استخراج علته ثم دوائه ليس بذي مالنخوليا ولا بموسوس.

Just as states called 'diseases' that affect vision [*baṣar*] are treated until it [the vision] returns to health, so the material intellect (*al-ʿaql al-hayūlānī*) suffers from diseases that are treated until it [the intellect] returns to its [state of] health. One of its [the material intellect's] diseases is melancholy; it is thinking that does not lead to truth [*al-fikru l-laḏī lā yuʾaddī ʾilā ḥaqīqatin*], nor does it follow the right path to what it seeks, so that it becomes confused until it is treated through correct thinking by someone who has a sound intellect. Someone who thinks about how to remove his disease and conceive a remedy for him is not someone suffering from melancholy, nor is he delusional (*muwaswis*).

---

[34] Aristotle famously considers this question in *Physics* iv. 6–9; for later developments in the Greek world, see Sorabji 2004, II, 251–252; and for a discussion of the developments in Arabic, see Nony forthcoming 2013. Miskawayh may echo al-Kindī's discussion of void in his *On First Philosophy*, section two, IV. 8–9; see Adamson and Pormann 2012a, pp. 15–16.

[35] Ed. p. 72, line 4 from the bottom—p. 73, line 2; tr. p. 502.

Aristotle already compared thinking to seeing in his *On the Soul*. For instance, he stated that just as sense-perception does not take place without objects of sensation (*aisthémata*), so intellection requires images (*phantásmata*).[36] Likewise, in the famous chapter iii. 5 of *On the Soul*, Aristotle compares the active intellect (*noûs poiētikós*) to the light: the light actualises potential colours.[37] Miskawayh's opponent also saw similarities in the two processes as both require the same essential component of the universe, namely light. And yet, the way in which Miskawayh constructs his analogy between vision and intellection is quite remarkable. For he introduces the notion of the 'material intellect (*al-ʿaql al-hayūlānī*)' to create this analogy: just as vision (*baṣar*) can be affected by disease, so can the material intellect be. There appears to be a certain unevenness in this analogy, as vision, the activity brought about with the help of the visual instrument, the eye, would, strictly speaking, correspond to intellection, the activity brought about by the intellect. We shall return to this difficulty shortly. Before that, one should note that Miskawayh further constructs his analogy by saying that melancholy is the disease of the material intellect. Then Miskawayh plays with the notion that treating melancholy does not in and of itself result in melancholy. In other words, he reaffirms his idea that physicians (such as Rufus) do not become melancholic just by thinking about melancholy.

In order to understand what Miskawayh meant exactly by his idea of the 'material intellect', we need to consider the next paragraph that follows on immediately from the previous one:[38]

ولعمري إن الفكر الصحيح محتاج إلى آلة صحيحة ومزاج ما في جزء من الدماغ خاص به واعتدال من
الدم الذي يجري في الشرايين التي بين أجزاء الدماغ، وإن هذه آلات الفكر. وكما أن طبقات العين
واعتدالاتها آلات للقوة الباصرة، فإذا لحقتها آفة ساء البصر. حتى إذا عولجت، رجعت إلى الصحة
وأبصر بها المبصر. فكذلك حال الدم الرقيق الذي يجري من القلب في الشرايين الدقاق التي تتخلل
الدماغ: له اعتدال في رقة، وله بخار لطيف في تجويف الشريان: فمتى انحرف عن اعتداله وتكدر ذلك

---

[36] Aristotle, *On the Soul*, iii. 7 (431a14–17): 'For in the thinking soul, images play the part of percepts, and the assertion or negation of good or bad is invariably accompanied by avoidance or pursuit, which is the reason for the soul's never thinking without an image (τῇ δὲ διανοητικῇ ψυχῇ τὰ φαντάσματα οἷον αἰσθήματα ὑπάρχει, ὅταν δὲ ἀγαθὸν ἢ κακὸν φήσῃ ἢ ἀποφήσῃ, φεύγει ἢ διώκει· διὸ οὐδέποτε νοεῖ ἄνευ φαντάσματος ἡ ψυχή).' (trans Lawson-Tangred 1986, p. 208).

[37] Aristotle, *On the Soul*, iii. 5 (430a14–17): 'And indeed there is an intellect characterized by the capacity to become all things, and an intellect characterized by that to bring all things about, and to bring them about in just the way that a state, like light, does. (For in a way, light also makes things that are potentially colors colors in actuality.) (καὶ ἔστιν ὁ μὲν τοιοῦτος νοῦς τῷ πάντα γίνεσθαι, ὁ δὲ τῷ πάντα ποιεῖν, ὡς ἕξις τις, οἷον τὸ φῶς· τρόπον γάρ τινα καὶ τὸ φῶς ποιεῖ τὰ δυνάμει ὄντα χρώματα ἐνεργείᾳ χρώματα.)' (trans Lawson-Tangred 1986, p. 208).

[38] Ed. p. 73, lines 3–10; tr. p. 502.

البخار، حدث في الفعل الصادر عن قوة النفس بهذه الآلة نقصان واضطراب حتى يعالج ويرد إلى
اعتداله فيصدر حينئذ الفاعل بهذه الآلة فعله على التام.

Upon my life, correct thinking [al-fikr aṣ-ṣaḥīḥ] requires [a)] a sound instrument ['āla ṣaḥīḥa], [b)] a certain mixture [mizāǧ] in the relevant part of the
brain, and [c)] a balance [i'tidāl] of the blood that flows in the blood vessels between the parts of the brain. For these are the instruments of thought.
The tunics of the eye and their balance [i'tidālātuhā] are instruments for
the visual faculty ['ālāt al-qūwa al-bāṣira]. If damage ['āfa] affects them, the
vision is impaired. Then, when it [the damage] is treated, it [the visual faculty]
returns to health, and one can see through it again. The case of the thin blood
that flows from the heart through the thin blood vessels and permeates the
brain is similar. It has a balance in thinness, and it has a subtle vapour in the
cavity of the blood vessel. When it departs from its balance and this vapour
becomes turbid, then deficiency and confusion occur in the action that proceeds from the faculty of the soul through this instrument [bi-hāḏihi l-'ālati],
until it is treated and returned to its balance. Then that which acts through
this instrument [bi-hāḏihi l-'ālati] performs its functions perfectly.

We have hinted above at the problem of the somewhat skewed analogy
between vision and the material intellect. This paragraph potentially solves
this difficulty, but unfortunately, it also offers a number of interpretative
problems that need to be solved. The paragraph begins with a statement that
sound thinking requires: a sound instrument; a certain mixture in relevant
part of the brain; and a balance in the blood flowing in the rear of the brain.
The next sentence is particularly puzzling: 'These are the instruments of
thought (wa-'inna hāḏihī 'ālātu l-fikri)'. The antecedent of 'these (hāḏihī)' is
probably the three things mentioned in the first sentence, for there is no
other plural or feminine singular word that would fit. But then, Miskawayh
would say in a somewhat tautological fashion that 'a sound instrument
('āla ṣaḥīḥa)' is one of the instruments of thought. Now what is this 'sound
instrument'?

The remainder of this paragraph sheds some light on this issue, but does
not resolve it. Miskawayh specifically compares the tunics of the eye and
its balances to the thin blood that also contains vapour and flows through
the brain. The tunics are 'instruments of the visual faculty ('ālāt li-l-qūwati
l-bāṣirati)', and likewise the vapour is an instrument ('āla). In other words,
the things that are clearly identifiable as instruments of thought are the
blood and the vapour flowing in the blood vessels of the brain. Therefore,
we are still left with the question what Miskawayh meant by the 'sound
instrument' in the first sentence. Could it be the material intellect that was
the topic of discussion of the previous paragraph? Leaving this question
aside for a moment, it is clear that the 'instruments of thought ('ālat al-fikr)'

can be affected by disease: when the mixture of the blood that flows in them having come from the heart is balanced, then correct thinking occurs; if, however, an imbalance supervenes, then the instrument is impaired, and thinking hampered. Likewise when the vapour (*buḫār*) flowing with the blood becomes imbalanced, it turns turbid (*takaddara*), thus impairing the thinking. In these cases, just as in the impairment of vision, one needs to employ a treatment that reestablishes the balance. Once this is done, the thinking returns to normal.

However one answers the question of what the 'sound instrument' is, this and the previous paragraph show that the material intellect can be affected by disease. Since Miskawayh explains the process of how disease occurs—namely through an imbalance in the blood and vapour in the brain—, the disease of the material intellect has a clear physiological component: it is located in the blood vessels of the brain, especially the small ones in its rear. These physiological ideas that Miskawayh mobilises here to explain melancholy are truly exceptional. To be sure, Nemesius of Emesa (late fourth century AD) had already developed some Galenic concepts and located specific activities of soul such as imagination, thinking, and memory in specific parts of the brain, namely the frontal, central, and posterior ventricles respectively.[39] But it seems that no-one before Miskawayh had situated the material intellect in the blood vessels of the brain. This idea of localisation is linked to the concept of melancholy, as the next quotation will illustrate.

A little bit later in his discussion, Miskawayh comes back to the comparison between vision and thought. The opponent had made light one of the main sources of intellection; moreover, light also constitutes, together with heat, one of the essential building blocks of the universe, conceived in materialistic terms. The opponent then draws a parallel between the 'eye of the head ('*ayn ar-ra's*)' and the 'eye of the soul ('*ayn an-nafs*)' which he says are in the same class (*ǧins*).[40] Miskawayh attacks this idea vehemently. Vision, he argues following standard Aristotelian theory,[41] depends on light: the presence of light actualises potential vision. He then explains the physiology of vision in a somewhat cryptic, yet crucial passage:[42]

---

[39] See Nemesius of Emesa, *On the Nature of Man* (trans. Sharples and van de Eijk 2008), chapters 6 ('imagination'), 12 ('thought'), and 13 ('memory'). For the whole question of the localisation of these faculties, see Rocca 2003, appendix 1.

[40] Ed. p. 74, line 2; tr. p. 503.

[41] Aristotle, *On the Soul*, 418b19–20; see now Polansky 2007, 263–274.

[42] Ed. p. 74, lines 13–21; p. 504.

فأما الحركة الإرادية، فإنها تكون بالجزء من الدماغ الذي تنشأ منه الأعصاب. وما يكون بجزء الدماغ
جرما يكون بالجرم الصقيل المستشف، وكذلك ما يكون بالبخار الذي يكون في تجويف الشريان،
وذلك أن العصبة المجوفة التي تنشأ بين الدماغ إنما تتم بها ضروب الحركات الإرادية في بؤبؤ العين. فأما
القوة الباصرة فإنها تكون بالبخار النافذ في ثقبي هاتين العصبتين المنتهيتين إلى طبقات العين، أعني
الجليدية والعنبية والقرنية وسائر الطبقات، والرطوبة التي يتم بها البصر. وإذا صادفت النفس هذه
الآلات معدة سليمة، أدركت المبصرات. وإذا عرض لأحدها آفة، لحقها من نقصان الإدراك بحسب تلك
الآفة. فإذا عولجت الآفة حتى تزول، عادت النفس إلى الإدراك باستعمال ما استقام من آلاتها.

Voluntary movement is brought about by the part of the brain out of which
the nerves come. What arises through the part of the brain [is itself] a body,
and is a polished, transparent body. Likewise for what arises through the
vapour in the hollow space of the blood vessel. For it is only through the
hollow nerve that comes out from between the brain that the [different]
kinds of voluntary motion of the pupil of the eye are accomplished. The visual
faculty [al-qūwa al-bāṣira] is brought about by the vapour that passes through
the two openings of these two nerves which end at the tunics of the eye,
namely the crystalline [tunic], the 'grape-like ['inabīya]' [tunic], and the other
tunics; and the moisture through which vision is accomplished. When the
soul meets these instruments whilst they are deemed to be healthy, it grasps
the visual objects. If, however, an ailment befalls one of them, then it [the
soul] becomes deficient in grasping [them] in accordance with this ailment.
When the ailment is cured so that it disappears, the soul returns to grasping
[them] by using its instruments that are in order [again].

Miskawayh discusses how the images produced in the eye are transferred
to the brain, presumably the part of the brain responsible for sensation.
Although the second sentence in this passage is difficult to understand, it
is clear that Miskawayh thinks of a vapour transferred through the hollow
nerves as the vehicles mediating between the brain and the eye: it brings
about the movement of the eye, but also conveys the images from the eye to
the brain. Whereas Miskawayh talks of 'vapour (buḫār)', Galen believed that
a pneuma was passing through the nerves linking the brain to the eyes; this
is the 'luminous pneuma (augoeidès pneûma)',[43] called rūḥ nayyir in Arabic.[44]

---

[43] Galen, On the Usefulness of the Parts (IV.275–276 K): Therefore, if, in an hour of leisure,
you wanted to test the propositions that we set out among other places in the thirteenth
[book] On Demonstration about the fact that the instrument of vision has a luminous pneuma
(augoeidès pneûma) flowing through everything from the brain, you would be astonished
about the disposition of the optical nerves, for they are hollow inside in order to receive the
pneuma, and they stretch to the ventricle of the brain itself for the same reason. For it is there
that one of the two anterior ventricles ends on the side; the optical nerves grow out [of there];
and this is the thalamus of these ventricles that is there because of them.

[44] Ullmann 2006–2007, under αὐγοειδής.

What occasioned the shift from *pneuma* to vapour (*buḫār*), for which the underlying Greek is *anathymíasis* or *atmós*? Although it is not possible to give a definitive answer to this question, it is clear that the concept is certainly not Galenic, as Galen rejects the idea that vapour or air flows in the blood vessels.[45] It may well be the case that the disease of melancholy itself played a large role here. For vapours rising from the stomach to the brain are one of the explanations for this disease that we find in a variety of sources, from Rufus of Ephesus to Isḥāq ibn ʿImrān (d. c. 904) and beyond. Rufus once mentions 'vapours' obliquely in the context of melancholy.[46] Isḥāq ibn ʿImrān, who often draws on Rufus, specifically talks about vapours (*buḫārāt*) rising from the stomach to the brain, where they 'corrupt the intellect (*yufsid al-ʿaql*)'.[47] Moreover, in the commentary tradition on *Aphorism* vi. 23—'If fear and despondency last for a long time, this is something melancholic ("Ην φόβος ἢ δυσθυμίη πουλὺν χρόνον διατελέῃ, μελαγχολικὸν τὸ τοιοῦτον)'—the idea of a vapour rising to the brain and impairing the psychic pneuma (*ar-rūḥ an-nafsānī*) appears as early as the eleventh century.[48]

Be that as it may, in this and the previous passages, we find the idea that melancholy, the disease of the material intellect, can be cured. We need to return to the example of the carpet that feels pain in order to see what kind of treatment Miskawayh envisions:[49]

وأما ما حكاه عن جالينوس من فساد الفكر والتخيل، وعن مشاط الصوف، يعني ثاوسيس، فقد
بينا طريق الصواب في الفكر والطريق الخطأ. وإنما يعالج الفكر الخطأ بالفكر الصحيح وتستخرج العلة
التي (لها) ظن المريض أن البساط يألم، ويبين (له) أن ما لا حس له لا يألم. فإن الحس إنما يكون
بالعصب الذي ينشأ من دماغ الحي. فما لا عصب له ولا حياة فيه، فلا حس له. وما لا حس له فلا
ألم له.

He [the opponent] talked about Galen whose thought and imagination was corrupted, and about the wool-carder, that is, Thessalus.[50] In this regard, we have already shown the correct and incorrect way of thinking. The incorrect

---

[45] See e.g., Galen, *An in arteriis natura sanguis contineatur*, IV.707 K: 'Yet in isolation by itself, neither vapor, nor air, nor aether, nor any pneuma whatever is seen to be contained in them [sc. the arteries] (οὐ μὴν αὐτός γε καθ᾽ ἑαυτὸν ἀτμὸς ἢ ἀὴρ ἢ αἰθὴρ ἢ ὅλως πνεῦμα περιεχόμενον ἐν αὐταῖς [sc. ταῖς ἀρτηρίαις] φαίνεται).' (ed. and trans Furley and Wilkie 1984, p. 148, lines 24–26; p. 149).

[46] F 62.

[47] ed. Omrani 2009, p. 45, lines 6 from the bottom—last (Arabic text); p. 57 (French translation).

[48] Joosse and Pormann 2012, 224–225, 244, 246.

[49] p. 76, lines 6–2 from the bottom.

[50] *Ṭwʾsys* in the manuscript; Thessalus is one possible, but uncertain reading.

thinking is treated by correct thinking; the disease through which the patient thinks that the rug feels pain is removed. One has to show [the patient] that what has no sensation cannot feel pain. Pain is only brought about through the nerves [*bi-l-ʿaṣab*] emerging from the brain of the living being. What does not have nerves and does not have life, cannot have sensation; furthermore, without sensation, it cannot feel pain.

Therefore, Miskawayh advocates a treatment through reasoning with the patient; after all, he already stated that melancholy 'is treated through correct thinking [*fikr ṣaḥīḥ*] by someone who has a sound intellect [*ʿaql salīm*]'.[51] This person needs to correct the incorrect opinions by pointing out inconsistencies. In fact, Miskawayh here provides an example where a syllogistic argument is used to refute a false opinion. Talking to patients suffering from melancholy has been one of the options in the therapeutic arsenal of the physicians.[52] Likewise, the idea that philosophy can cure certain states of the mind is an old one: in Stoicism, for instance, the passions (*páthē*) result from wrong opinions (*dóxai*) that need to be rectified.[53]

Miskawayh combines here the ideas of medicine and philosophy in an interesting way to offer a treatment for melancholy. We have seen above that one of Rufus' patients contemplated the geometrical sciences so much that it led to the blood being burnt.[54] In other words, a mental process had a physiological result. This physiological situation was then made worse by a bodily treatment: the patient was given purging drugs by an incompetent physician. This then led to the patient suffering from a mental problem: he became mad. In the case of Rufus, we do not know how he conceived of this interaction between mental and bodily processes in the human being. Miskawayh appears to have solved this problem by locating the material intellect in the blood vessels of the brain. The blood and vapours there seem to interface with this material intellect: it can thus be affected by disease when they are imbalanced. For, as Miskawayh stated, 'the material intellect suffers from diseases' just as the eye does, and, like the eye, it can be treated.[55] And melancholy, one of these diseases, is clearly caused by certain physiological processes in the brain.

The term 'material intellect', known in Greek as *hylikòs noûs*, goes back to Alexander of Aphrodisias.[56] Alexander calls material intellect the potential

---

[51] p. 72, last line—p. 73, line 1; quoted above p. 235.
[52] Starobinski 2011, 71–76.
[53] See Inwood 1985, 197–201; Forschner 1981, 165–171; see also Gourinat 2005.
[54] Ullmann 1978, 72; F 68.
[55] See above, p. 235.
[56] Bruns 1887, p. 81, lines 22–25; see Tuominen 2010.

intellect that Aristotle appears to postulate in *On the Soul*, iii. 5, and further develops this concept. This material intellect is able to receive the objects of sense-perception, and Alexander used this term it in order to solve the problem of how the higher intellectual processes, devoid of matter, can have access to sense-perception that is based on matter. In other words, the material intellect bridges the gap between sensibles and intelligibles. For Alexander, the material intellect was not corporeal.[57] Al-Kindī, who often had a great impact on Miskawayh's thought, also talks about different types of intellect, notably in his treatise *On the Intellect*.[58] There, he discusses the concept of the potential intellect without using the term 'material intellect'; and he certainly does not situate the potential intellect in any specific part of the brain. Other authors such as al-Fārābī (d. 950), and Avicenna (Ibn Sīnā, d. 1037) also wrote profusely on the subject of the intellect, but it was only Averroes (Ibn Rušd, d. 1198) who uses the term 'material intellect' again.[59] This makes Miskawayh's ideas even more intriguing, and shows that they deserve further study, especially their relationship with and contributions to notions of the potential intellect and the body-mind dichotomy.[60]

Conclusions

Rufus of Ephesus linked the philosophical tradition of the Aristotelian *Problem* xxx.1 and the medical tradition beginning with the Hippocratic *Aphorism* vi. 23 to create the notion of scholarly melancholy. Jacques Jouanna has shown that the former did not have any significant direct impact on the later medical tradition from Galen onwards.[61] Therefore, it was through Rufus of Ephesus that the link between intense thinking and melancholy became known in the later medical tradition. But, as the example discussed here shows, it is also Rufus' scholarly melancholy that became the object of intense philosophical debate in Baghdad of the late tenth and early eleventh century. Rufus was not a very philosophically inclined physician, as Philip

---

[57] Tuominen 2010, 172.

[58] McCarthy 1964; Jolivet 1971; Ruffinengo 1997; Adamson and Pormann 2012a, 93–106.

[59] See H.A. Davidson 1992, especially 258–313.

[60] See Adamson 2008, 43–44, who discusses how Miskawayh explained the Platonic tripartition of the soul and its relation to organs of perception and thinking such as the eyes and the brain, notably as they are developed in other philosophical writings by Miskawayh. I believe, however, that much more can be said about this topic. For a discussion of the mind-body dichotomy in Avicenna (with special references to the inner senses), see Pormann 2013, 102–107.

[61] Jouanna 2007.

van der Eijk rightly remarked, but his medical thought did have, for instance, epistemological implications.[62] The case history of the patient dying of contemplating the geometrical sciences also raised the issue of how the activities of the soul are linked to the mixtures of the body, and more specifically, how the physiological and psychological aspects of thought interrelate.

Miskawayh's anonymous opponent focussed on the epistemological implications of melancholy as described by Rufus. He quoted the latter's notion of scholarly melancholy to illustrate that pure thought can never be a reliable way to arrive at incontrovertible truths. This opponent adduced not only Rufus as an authority, but also Galen and Hippocrates.[63] He adhered to a materialist worldview, and is said to have specialised in the Greek language. One would really like to know who this opponent was. It appears likely that he either belonged to the large group of intellectual personalities in the medieval Islamic world who were both physicians and philosophers, or that he had, at least, strong medical interests.

Miskawayh refuted the epistemological reservations of this opponent: not all thinking would lead to melancholy, but only one specific type, that linked to imagination. In this way, Miskawayh offered a solution to the problem of what causes this scholarly melancholy. He also pondered the issue of how it can be cured: through intelligent discussion. And although he did not tackle the subject directly of how the bodily and mental functions of thinking interact and interrelate, his analogy between vision and thought reveals a theory of this interaction and interrelation that is both novel and startling. For Miskawayh, the material intellect can become affected by disease through the blood and vapours in the small veins that crisscross the brain, and especially those located in its rear part. Therefore, the 'dialogue' that took place between Rufus of Ephesus and Miskawayh in Baghdad—separated by one millennium, as well as different languages and cultures—proved extremely fertile in the conception of scholarly melancholy and its consequences.

---

[62] Van der Eijk 2008b.

[63] For Rufus and Galen, see above; Hippocrates is mentioned twice at ed. p. 81; tr. pp. 509–510.

'QUEM NOS FUROREM, ΜΕΛΑΓΧΟΛΙΑΝ ILLI VOCANT': CICERO ON MELANCHOLY

George Kazantzidis

Melancholy, Greek μελαγχολία, as we first find it in a number of literary and philosophical texts of the classical period, means something quite different from depression; from Aristophanes (*Av.* 14; *Eccl.* 251; *Pl.* 12) to Plato (*Phdr.* 268e2; *Rep.* 573c9) to Aristotle (*Eth. Nic.* 1150b25–26; 1151a1–1152a19), the linguistic evidence we have shows that the word is used at that time to indicate rather an aggressive form of madness.[1] While the case seems to be the same with the majority of the Hippocratics (5th–4th cent. BC),[2] melancholy in the sense of depression is not entirely absent from medical discourse: one can find it associated with a pathological state of lasting sadness (δυσθυμίη) and fear (φόβος) in [Hippocrates] *Aphorismi* 6.23 [4.568 Littré].[3] However the exact relation between these two aspects of melancholy (a manic and a depressive one) remains, for some time, unclear since both are for the most part explored in early medical writings independently from each other.[4] The first author to display a more inclusive attitude is not a physician but a philosopher of the late 4th cent. BC:[5] in a treatise which sets out

---

[1] See Harris 2001, 16–17. For 'melancholia' as 'a coarse synonym' for madness in antiquity see also Padel 1992, 24, and 1995, 48.

[2] See e.g. [Hippocrates] *De morbis* 1.30 [6.200 Littré]: προσεοίκασι δὲ μάλιστα οἱ ὑπὸ τῆς φρενίτιδος ἐχόμενοι τοῖσι μελαγχολώδεσι κατὰ τὴν παράνοιαν· οἵ τε γὰρ μελαγχολώδεις, ὅταν φθαρῇ τὸ αἷμα ὑπὸ χολῆς καὶ φλέγματος, τὴν νοῦσον ἴσχουσι καὶ παράνοοι γίνονται, ἔνιοι δὲ καὶ μαίνονται. See the medical evidence collected in Müri 1953, 33.

[3] Ἢν φόβος ἢ δυσθυμίη πολὺν χρόνον διατελέῃ, μελαγχολικὸν τὸ τοιοῦτον.

[4] See, however, the interesting description of the patient Parmeniscus in [Hippocrates] *Epidemiae* 7.89 [7.446 Littré]: Τῷ Παρμενίσκῳ καὶ πρότερον ἐνέπιπτον ἀθυμίαι καὶ ἵμερος τῆς ἀπαλλαγῆς βίου, ὁτὲ δὲ πάλιν εὐθυμίη. Ἐν Ὀλύνθῳ δέ ποτε φθινοπώρου ἄφωνος κατείχετο, ἡσυχίην ἔχων, βραχύ τι ὅσον ἄρχεσθαι ἐπιχειρέων προσειπεῖν· εἰ δὲ δή τι καὶ διαλεχθείη, καὶ πάλιν ἄφωνος. Ὕπνοι ἐνῆσαν, ὁτὲ δὲ ἀγρυπνίη, καὶ ῥιπτασμὸς μετὰ σιγῆς, καὶ ἀλυσμός, καὶ χεὶρ πρὸς ὑποχόνδρια ὡς ὀδυνωμένῳ· ὁτὲ δὲ ἀποστραφεὶς, ἔκειτο ἡσυχίην ἄγων. Parmeniscus' catatonic state (Jouanna 2000, 39 n. 1, describes it as a case of 'mélancholie stuporeuse'; cf. Montiglio 2000, 232) alternates with fits of delirium (ῥιπτασμὸς, ἀλυσμός). Nonetheless, there is nothing in the text to positively suggest that the patient is a melancholic or that black bile lies at the origin of his disease.

[5] While traditionally referred to as ps.-Aristotle, most scholars agree that this philosopher is Theophrastus. See e.g. Flashar 1962, 711–714, and Sharples 1995, 5–6.

to explain the exceptional intelligence of melancholics (*Problemata Physica* XXX.i), ps.-Aristotle discusses melancholy as a disease which can manifest itself *either* as madness *or* as depression, depending on the temperature of black bile (μέλαινα χολή). When turning too hot, black bile is described as giving rise to ἐκστάσεις (953a25), a term which is used elsewhere in the text to describe the madness of (Sophocles') Ajax (953a22); when turning too cold, it is said to cause ἀθυμίας and φόβους (954a23–24). Rather than treating them separately, ps.-Aristotle thus unites madness and depression as the two sides of one and the same disease.[6]

In what follows, I set out to discuss Cicero's translation of μελαγχολία with *furor* at *Tusculanae Disputationes* 3.11—the first attempt made in Latin literature to investigate the meaning of the Greek term. In the first section of my paper I will demonstrate that this is by no means a passing linguistic remark but should rather be situated within the context of Cicero's critical engagement with ps.-Aristotle's text and ideas, as this becomes evident at other points of his philosophical work (*Tusc. Disp.* 1.80; *De divinatione* 1.81). I will then proceed to argue that, while Cicero's translation is not followed by the observation that μελαγχολία can also have the meaning of depression (*tristitia*),[7] his allusion to ps.-Aristotle's treatment of Bellerophon as a *depressive* melancholic (953a21–25) at *Tusc. Disp.* 3.63 (a part of the treatise which discusses the results of extreme sorrow) reveals that Cicero is familiar with both sides of the disease.

Cicero and Ps.-Aristotle

Cicero's discussion of μελαγχολία runs as follows (*TD* 3.11):

> Graeci autem μανίαν unde appellent non facile dixerim: eam tamen ipsam distinguimus nos melius quam illi; hanc enim *insaniam*, quae iuncta stultitiae

---

[6] Cf. Menander, *Aspis* 306–309: μελαγχολῶ τοῖς πράγμασιν· μὰ τοὺς θεούς, / οὐκ εἴμ' ἐν ἐ-μαυτοῦ, *μαίνομαι* δ' ἀκαρὴς πάνυ· / ὁ καλὸς ἀδελφὸς εἰς τοσαύτην ἔκστασιν/ἤδη καθίστησίν με τῆι πονηρίαι. But see also *Aspis* 329–339: δεῖ τραγωιδῆσαι πάθος/ἀλλοῖον ὑμᾶς ... / δόξαι σε δεῖ νῦν, εἰς ἀθυμίαν τινὰ/ἐλθόντα τῶι τε τοῦ νεανίσκου πάθει ... / ... τὰ πλεῖστα δὲ/ἄπασιν ἀρρωστήματ' ἐκ λύπης σχεδόν/ἐστιν· φύσει δέ σ' ὄντα πικρὸν εὖ οἶδα καὶ/μελαγχολικόν.

[7] Contrast Celsus *De medicina* 3.18.17: 'alterum insaniae genus est ... consistit in *tristitia*, quam videtur *bilis atra* contrahere'. Celsus has identified *atra bilis* earlier in the text (*De medicina* 2.1.6) as the Latin equivalent to Greek 'melan-cholia' ('bilis atra, quam μελαγχολίαν [Graeci] appellant'). Furthermore, it is worth noting that the first time that Celsus speaks of black bile in association with sadness, it is in the context of a short statement which is clearly modeled (not, however, without some suggestive additions) on [Hippocrates] *Aphorismi* 6.23 (cited above in footnote 3): 'si longa tristitia cum longo timore et vigilia est, atrae bilis morbus subest' (*De medicina* 2.7.19).

patet latius, *a furore disiungimus*. Graeci volunt illi quidem, sed parum valent verbo: *quem nos furorem, μελαγχολίαν illi vocant*. Quasi vero atra bili solum mens ac non saepe vel iracundia graviore vel timore vel dolore moveatur, quo genere Athamantem, Alcmaeonem, Aiacem, Orestem furere dicimus.

I cannot easily say how the Greeks came up with the term 'mania'. We distinguish this concept better than they do, for we differentiate unsoundness of mind, which has a wider application, due to its association with folly, from madness. The Greeks want to do this, but their word is not strong enough: what we call madness they call 'melancholia', as if it were true that the mind is moved by black bile alone and not often by a stronger anger, or fear, or sorrow, in the way in which we say that Athamas, Alcmaeon, Ajax, and Orestes are mad.[8]

Cicero makes a sharp distinction between *insania*, on the one hand, and *furor* on the other.[9] The first is clearly suggested to apply to any mental condition that falls short of the ideal of peace of mind and wisdom[10] and is, therefore, said to have a 'wider application' (*patet latius*) than the second, which should be taken, in its turn, to refer specifically to a clinical condition which requires proper medical treatment. These two kinds of mental aberration should not be confused with each other, although Cicero leaves enough space to suggest that *insania*, in the form of a strong and violent emotion, can have on occasion a long-lasting effect which may in the end lead to clinical madness. Madness, so Cicero means to claim at this point, can also have a psychological origin[11] and one should not therefore restrict

---

[8] Translation in Hershkowitz 1998, 11.

[9] On this distinction see Graver 2003.

[10] Cicero clearly has the Stoics in mind at this point; see Graver 2002, 81. On the Stoic doctrine of the affections of the soul see Inwood 1985, 127–181, and Frede 1986. On Stoicism and emotion in general see Graver 2007.

[11] It is important to notice that Cicero does not entirely dismiss the idea of a biological origin of melancholic madness at this point; he rather means to emphasize that black bile is not its only cause; see Flashar 1966, 80–81. Stok 1996, 2360–2362, on the other hand, believes that Cicero suggests that black bile should be left entirely out of discussion (see also Pigeaud 1981, 264) and invites a connection here with the medical theories of Asclepiades of Bithynia, who is known to have 'preserved some of the traditional language of humoral pathologies, while totally abandoning the causal analyses of disease which came with them' (Vallance 1990, 102 n. 33); see also Vallance 1993, 701, and Nutton 2004, 190–191. Asclepiades spent a considerable part of his life in Rome, establishing himself as the most important medical practitioner of the Late Republic; some believe that this period lies between 120–190 BC; see Rawson 1982; 1985, 171; Gourevitch 1987 and Pigeaud 1991, 42–47. But the evidence is not conclusive and it may as well be the case that he lived into the 70s, the 60s or, even, the 50s; see Nutton 2004, 167. For a recent attempt to establish Asclepiades' dates see Pollito 1999. In any case, Cicero appears to have been familiar with his work (see e.g. *De oratore* 1.14.62) and some of the Latin poets (Lucretius) have been shown to display an interest in his medical theories; see Pigeaud 1988a.

its aetiology to black bile alone,[12] which is in other words what the exclusive Greek term 'melan-cholia' seems to suggest.

Although in speaking of 'melancholia' as madness Cicero refers to the 'Greeks' in general, it is possible that he has in mind a particular text. One plausible source of information in this case would be Chrysippus' discussion of Orestes' hallucinations in Euripides as a characteristic example of 'non-cataleptic' impressions (*SVF* II.54),[13] that is, of empty images that correspond to no real objects and to which one is attracted under the influence of madness. What is important about Chrysippus' account is that, while none of the surviving tragedies attests to the use of μελαγχολία or μελαγχολικός, Chrysippus describes Euripides' character as both 'manic' and 'melancholic' (ταῦτα δὲ γίνεται ἐπὶ τῶν μελαγχολώντων καὶ μεμηνότων· ὁ γοῦν τραγικὸς Ὀρέστης ὅταν λέγῃ ...), in a way which suggests that the two words should be counted synonymous.[14] This seems to fit well with Cicero's list of melancholic heroes at *TD* 3.11 (Athamas, Alcmaeon, Ajax, Orestes), where emphasis is clearly laid on instances of tragic madness.

---

[12] An 'anti-humouralist' reading of Cicero's text can be found in Caelius Aurelianus, *De morbis chronicis* 1.6.180: 'Melancholy ('melancholia') derives its name from the fact that the patient often vomits black bile ('nigra fella'), the Greek word for 'black' being 'melan' and for 'bile', 'cholen'. The name is not derived ... from the notion that black bile is the cause or origin of the disease. For such notion would be put forward only by those who guess at, rather than observe, the truth ... Thus Cicero speaks of black bile in the sense of profound anger ('nam Tullius atram bilem dixit, velut altam iracundiam'); translation in Drabkin 1950, 561. It is evident that Caelius at this point projects his own anti-humouralist views into Cicero's text; Flashar 1966, 80. The Methodist school of medicine, to which Caelius belongs, advocates that bodily humours should be irrelevant to treatment (not without some exceptions though; van der Eijk 1999a, 326 n. 113); for a 'humoural pathologist must not only make complicated evaluations of bodily evacuations ... he must' also 'assume etiologies of disease that are hidden from sense perceptions' (Hanson and Green 1994, 1000). On the Method see Frede 1982; Gourevitch 1991 and Nutton 2004, 187–201. On Caelius' epistemology see van der Eijk 1999b. On Caelius' (puzzling) reference to Cicero as one that has been added on Soranus of Ephesus' text (whose work Caelius translates in Latin) see Pigeaud 1981, 125 n. 453; Vázquez-Buján 1991, 90; Urso 1997, 113–114, and Stok 1999, 24 n. 65.

[13] On this text see Graver 2003, 42–44; 2007, 112–114, and Tieleman 2003, 183–184.

[14] Cf. Sextus Empiricus, *Adv. Math.* 7.247–249: μυρίοι γὰρ φρενιτίζοντες καὶ μελαγχολῶντες ἀληθῆ μὲν ἕλκουσι φαντασίαν, οὐ καταληπτικὴν δὲ ἀλλ' ἔξωθεν καὶ ἐκ τύχης οὕτω συμπεσοῦσαν ... ἔνιαι γὰρ πάλιν ἀπὸ ὑπάρχοντος μέν εἰσιν, οὐκ αὐτὸ δὲ τὸ ὑπάρχον ἰνδάλλονται, ὡς ἐπὶ τοῦ μεμηνότος Ὀρέστου μικρῷ πρότερον ἐδείκνυμεν. εἷλκε μὲν γὰρ φαντασίαν ἀπὸ ὑπάρχοντος, τῆς Ἠλέκτρας, οὐ κατ' αὐτὸ δὲ τὸ ὑπάρχον· μίαν γὰρ τῶν Ἐρινύων ὑπελάμβανεν αὐτὴν εἶναι. On the whole, Sextus disagrees with Chrysippus in that he finds that even a hallucination may draw its origin from something 'existent' (in the case of Orestes in Euripides that would be Electra) and should therefore be taken to create an impression which is 'both false and true'. Even so, Sextus' account remains consistent with describing Euripides' hero as a 'melancholic'.

This having been said, the first writer to speak of tragic madness (μανία) in close association with (or, rather, as one of the sub-categories of) 'melancholia' is ps.-Aristotle.[15] As we read at the opening of his treatise (953a10–22):

Διὰ τί πάντες ὅσοι περιττοὶ γεγόνασιν ἄνδρες ἢ κατὰ φιλοσοφίαν ἢ πολιτικὴν ἢ ποίη-
σιν ἢ τέχνας φαίνονται μελαγχολικοὶ ὄντες, καὶ οἱ μὲν οὕτως ὥστε καὶ λαμβάνεσθαι
τοῖς ἀπὸ μελαίνης χολῆς ἀρρωστήμασιν, οἷον λέγεται τῶν τε ἡρωϊκῶν τὰ περὶ τὸν
Ἡρακλέα· καὶ γὰρ ἐκεῖνος ἔοικε γενέσθαι ταύτης τῆς φύσεως, διὸ καὶ τὰ ἀρρωστή-
ματα τῶν ἐπιληπτικῶν ἀπ' ἐκείνου προσηγόρευον οἱ ἀρχαῖοι ἱερὰν νόσον … ἔτι δὲ
τὰ περὶ Αἴαντα καὶ Βελλεροφόντην, ὧν ὁ μὲν ἐκστατικὸς ἐγένετο παντελῶς, ὁ δὲ τὰς
ἐρημίας ἐδίωκεν.

Why is it that all men who have become outstanding in philosophy, politics, poetry or the arts turn out to be melancholics and some of them to such an extent as to be affected by diseases arising from black bile, as the story of Heracles among the heroes tells? For Heracles seems to have been of that nature, so that the ancients called the disease of epilepsy the 'sacred disease' after him … The same is true of Ajax and Bellerophon; the former went completely insane, and the other craved for desert places.[16]

This passage, which counts both Euripides' Heracles and Sophocles' Ajax as 'melancholics', is one that Cicero knows well. In fact, a straightforward reference to it can be found in the first book of the *Tusculan Disputations* (1.80). At this point of the dialogue, one of the discussants has just given a brief account of Panaetius' two arguments intending to prove that the soul is mortal. According to the first of these arguments, anything that is sensible of pain, as the soul is, is also liable to disease and, therefore, subject to death. The second and most important argument runs as follows: the soul has been born and that which has been born will die; and the fact that the soul has had a beginning is indicated by the resemblance of a child's soul (one may also call it 'character') to that of the parent, as though the soul of the child had been born from that of the parent.[17]

It is in the context of the refutation of this second argument that a reference to melancholics (in connection with Aristotle) crops up in Cicero's text (*TD* 1.80):

Iam similitudo magis apparet in bestiis, quarum animi sunt rationis expertes; hominum autem similitudo in corporum figura magis exstat et ipsi animi magni refert quali in corpore locati sint; multa enim e corpore existunt quae acuant mentem, multa quae obtundant. *Aristoteles quidem ait omnes*

---

[15] See von Staden 1992, 148.
[16] Translation in Radden 2000, 57; modified at points.
[17] On this text see Inwood and Gerson 2008, 100–101 with n. 17.

ingeniosos melancholicos esse, ut ego me tardiorem esse non moleste feram. Enumerat multos, idque quasi constet, rationem cur ita fiat adfert. Quod si tanta vis est ad habitum mentis in iis, quae gignuntur in corpore—ea sunt autem, quaecumque sunt, quae similitudinem faciant—nihil necessitatis adfert, cur nascantur animi, similitudo.

Then as to resemblance, this is more obvious in animals whose souls have no trace of reason; likeness in men consists more in the configuration of the bodies: and it is of no little consequence in what bodies the soul is lodged; for there are many things which depend on the body that sharpen the soul, many which blunt it. Aristotle, indeed, says that all men of great genius are melancholics and so makes me less distressed at being slow-witted. He gives an extended list of them, and, as if his claim was a matter of fact, brings his reasons for it. But if the things begotten in the body exert such an influence upon the mind (for they are the things, whatever they are, that occasion this likeness), still that does not necessarily prove why a likeness of souls should be generated.[18]

Cicero argues at this point that, in contrast with animals, resemblance in people, as conveyed from generation to generation, applies more to their bodies. Still, it is conceded that one's body, or otherwise, what the body consists of and contains within it, can also affect one's soul; a certain likeness in mind and spirit can thus be occasioned within two bodies that share common physical characteristics as a result of heredity, but this by no means amounts to saying that a likeness of souls is a matter of engenderment: on the contrary, it amply demonstrates that, however strong a likeness of that kind might be, one should trace its origins to the body and its commonly shared elements and not independently and directly to the soul.

In support of the thesis that one's body can affect one's soul, and, in that case, the capacities of one's intellect, Cicero cites Aristotle's thesis that all men of genius have been of a melancholic constitution (*omnes ingeniosos melancholicos esse*)—the implication here being, when taken in the context of the present argument, that black bile can give 'an edge' to the soul or mind. Nonetheless, it is worth noting that, while cited as supporting evidence, Aristotle's thesis is also met with some strong criticism and elicits a certain degree of irony. This is at least what one surmises from the speaker's subsequent remark that, if this hypothesis of the melancholic genius holds true, then he is not displeased at being somewhat dull himself.

As we have seen above, ps.-Aristotle's text opens with a question and it is evident that this question contains part of its answer; for it states as a fact,

---

[18] Translation in Yonge 1880; slightly modified.

which seems to admit of no exception, that all (πάντες) outstanding men, be it in poetry, philosophy or the arts, fall into the category of (natural) melancholics (a claim which is then reversed at the end of the text (955a36–40), at which point all melancholics are presented as people of an exceptional nature).[19] Cicero's critical comment that Aristotle first introduces his thesis and then proceeds to explain it as if it were a matter of fact (*idque quasi constet, rationem cur ita fiat adfert*) seems to be responding precisely to this kind of logical inconsequence.[20] This also tells us, of course, that at least insofar as its opening section is concerned, Cicero must have been familiar with this text in the form that we have it.[21] Equally revealing in this respect is the fact that in the same context of critique Cicero speaks of a long list of melancholics (*enumerat multos*), which is in fact what one finds in ps.-Aristotle with his references to Heracles, Ajax and Bellerophon but also, later in the text, to Empedocles, Socrates and Plato (953a27).

Regarding now Cicero's sarcastic statement that, if to be a genius means that one should also be a melancholic, he is then not distressed at not being a genius himself, this seems to emerge as a critical response to ps.-Aristotle's central claim that one's powers of the intellect depend on black bile, also the material cause of a serious disease. This is already evident in the opening section of ps.-Aristotle's cited above; in fact less emphasis is laid there on the exceptional nature of melancholics than on the diseases affecting them (… φαίνονται μελαγχολικοὶ ὄντες, καὶ οἱ μὲν οὕτως ὥστε καὶ λαμβάνεσθαι τοῖς ἀπὸ μελαίνης χολῆς ἀρρωστήμασιν). As regards the rest of the treatise, ps.-Aristotle

---

[19] … περιττοὶ μέν εἰσι πάντες οἱ μελαγχολικοί, οὐ διὰ νόσον, ἀλλὰ διὰ φύσιν. See van der Eijk 2005a, 157 n. 64.

[20] See Flashar 1966, 67–68.

[21] It should be noticed at this point that, after its publication in the late 4th cent. BC, ps.-Aristotle's text leaves no distinct traces on subsequent medical and philosophical sources, at least up to the point that Cicero 're-discovers' it (as one of Aristotle's genuine writings). See Flashar 1962, 715, and Jouanna 2006, 56. This certainly has something to do with the increased availability of Aristotelian texts at that time in Rome, which led eventually to the so called 'Roman edition' of Aristotle by Andronicus of Rhodes; see Flashar 1966, 67. The exact date of this edition remains a matter of considerable debate; Gottschalk 1987, 1083–1097. As Barnes 1997, 24, observes, 'it cannot be dated before 65; it is implausible to date it before Cicero's death [because Cicero nowhere mentions it]; and it need not be dated before the 20s'. The fact that Cicero nowhere mentions the Roman edition of Aristotle by Andronicus of Rhodes or even the fact that he did not live to see it published does not necessarily entail that he was unaware of its preparation nor that he was ignorant of its contents. As van der Eijk 1993, 225 n. 8, points out, '[t]he date of Andronicus' edition is disputed … but it is questionable whether this should be regarded as providing the terminus post quem for Cicero's (or any other contemporary writer's) familiarity with Aristotle's school treatises'; on Cicero and Aristotle in general see Gigon 1959; Görler 1989 and Long 1995.

proceeds to explain that one's genius requires a natural excess of black bile (954a22–23) and a balance between warm and cold (954a39–954b4), two of the qualities of the melancholic humour, or melancholic mixture (κρᾶσις) as he calls it (954a13). Yet, black bile, as ps.-Aristotle tells us, is unpredictable by its very nature and can easily change its temperature (954b8–9); when turning too hot, it causes melancholic madness; when turning too cold, it becomes the cause of depression (954a13–26). Being a natural melancholic, in other words, comes with a price; for while one is thus naturally predisposed to becoming a genius, one's liability to all sorts and kinds of melancholic disease also becomes considerably higher.

This is something that Cicero finds hard to accept since, in his mind, it contaminates the language of genius with that of disease. While not that evident at *TD* 1.80, this hypothesis finds strong support in Cicero's next reference to melancholics, as found this time at *De divinatione* 1.81. At this point of the text Quintus[22] is stressing the idea that the gods do not normally communicate through direct epiphanies, but rather through divination, either natural or artificial. In Quintus' mind, there is a divine power that is diffused far and wide into the natural world around us but can also be imparted directly to human nature. As his prime example Quintus mentions the case of the Sibyl, but he also proceeds to include in the same context instances of poetic inspiration, thereby invoking the authorities of Democritus and Plato on the subject (1.80). It is at the end of this section that a reference to melancholics occurs. Let it be noticed in advance that, as is the case with Cicero's earlier mention of them, this reference implicates the name of Aristotle; and, as happens there, it elicits again a great deal of criticism, only this time of a more revealing kind (*De divinatione* 1.81):

> Aristoteles quidem eos etiam qui valetudinis vitio furerent et melancholici dicerentur censebat habere aliquid in animis praesagiens atque divinum. Ego autem haud scio an nec cardiacis hoc tribuendum sit nec phreneticis; animi enim integri, non vitiosi est corporis divinatio.

> Aristotle thought that even those who rave because of illness and are called 'melancholics' have in their souls some divine, prescient power. But I have my doubts whether this [kind of gift, as it were] should be attributed to those with disordered stomachs or minds; for divination is a quality of a healthy soul, not of a sick body.[23]

---

[22] Cicero's interlocutor, speaking in defense of divination in book 1. For some comprehensive discussions of Cicero's treatise see Denyer 1985; Beard 1986; Schofield 1986 and Wardle 2006.

[23] Translation in Wardle 2006, 72.

As Philip van der Eijk suggests,[24] to find the principal source for Quintus' statement at this point, one should look at Aristotle, *De divinatione per somnum* 463b12–22:[25]

Ὅλως δὲ ἐπεὶ καὶ τῶν ἄλλων ζῴων ὀνειρώττει τινά, θεόπεμπτα μὲν οὐκ ἂν εἴη τὰ ἐνύπνια, οὐδὲ γέγονε τούτου χάριν (δαιμόνια μέντοι· ἡ γὰρ φύσις δαιμονία, ἀλλ' οὐ θεία). σημεῖον δέ· πάνυ γὰρ εὐτελεῖς ἄνθρωποι προορατικοί εἰσι καὶ εὐθυόνειροι, ὡς οὐ θεοῦ πέμποντος, ἀλλ' ὅσων ὥσπερ ἂν εἰ λάλος ἡ φύσις ἐστὶ καὶ μελαγχολική, παντοδαπὰς ὄψεις ὁρῶσιν· διὰ γὰρ τὸ πολλὰ καὶ παντοδαπὰ κινεῖσθαι ἐπιτυγχάνουσιν ὁμοίοις θεωρήμασιν, ἐπιτυχεῖς ὄντες ἐν τούτοις ὥσπερ ἔνιοι ἀρτιάζοντες· ὥσπερ γὰρ καὶ λέγεται 'ἂν πολλὰ βάλλῃς, ἄλλοτ' ἀλλοῖον βαλεῖς', καὶ ἐπὶ τούτων τοῦτο συμβαίνει.

On the whole, forasmuch as certain of the other animals also dream, it may be concluded that dreams are not sent by God, nor are they designed for this purpose [that is, to act as a medium of divine communication and inspiration]. They have a mysterious aspect, however, for nature [that is, the nature of those dreaming, be it men or, even, animals] is daemonic, though not divine. A proof is this: the power of foreseeing the future and of having vivid dreams is found in persons of an inferior type, which suggests that God does not send their dreams; but merely that all those whose physical temperament is, as it were, loquacious and melancholic, see visions of all kinds. For it is because they experience many movements of every kind that they just happen to encounter sights resembling real events, being fortunate in those, like certain people who play at odds and evens. For the principle which is expressed in the gambler's maxim, 'if you make many throws your luck must change', holds good in their case also.[26]

Aristotle states as a fact at this point that melancholics do have prophetic dreams but it is important to notice that, in so doing, he also points out that, daemonic as these dreams might be, one should not associate them with the divine as such.[27] In fact, Aristotle chooses the case of a melancholic precisely as that of an *inferior* kind of person, both biologically and mentally impaired, so as to prove that the divine could not be implicated in the process. This being so, what is accorded in the end to a melancholic dreamer is not the possibility of 'divine' but rather that of a statistical,[28] as it were,

[24] See van der Eijk 1993, 225–228; see also Repici 1991, 184 n. 23. On Aristotle and dreams see Harris 2009, 252–261.

[25] For a detailed discussion of this text see van der Eijk 1994, 289–301.

[26] Translation in Barnes 1984 I, 737; slightly modified.

[27] See Gallop 1996, 44–46, and Holowchak 1996, 420–422.

[28] Cf. Cicero, *De divinatione* 2.121: 'iam ex insanorum aut ebriorum visis innumerabilia coniectura trahi possunt, quae futura videantur. Quis est enim, qui totum diem iaculans non aliquando conliniet? Totas noctes somniamus, neque ulla est fere, qua non dormiamus; et

prescience.[29] On the whole, this seems to create a problem with stressing the connection with Quintus' statement too far; for it is clear that, in Quintus' understanding, Aristotle finds something truly divine in the soul (and nature) of a melancholic who foretells the future—and this he is suggested to be doing in a positive rather than a negative context. It is true, of course, that Quintus' *aliquid divinum* ('something divine') sounds somewhat vague and one cannot thus disregard the possibility that it might have evolved as a paraphrase of what one finds in Aristotle's text as an emphasis on the 'daemonic' nature of melancholic dreaming.[30] Nonetheless, whatever its exact implications, the case remains that this daemonic element is starkly distinguished there from the divine. This pressing distinction and, on the whole, Aristotle's insistence on stressing that any hypothesis about the divine origin of these dreams should be dismissed make it hard in the end to fully reconcile this text with Quintus' phrasing and choice of words in Cicero.[31]

This having been said, another possible source for Quintus' statement at this point would have been that of ps.-Aristotle, 954a28–38,[32] in which case a clear line of connection is established between black bile, frenzied enthusiasm and divination.

---

miramur aliquando id quod somniarimus evadere? Quid est tam incertum quam talorum iactus? Tamen nemo est quin saepe iactans Venerium iaciat aliquando, non numquam etiam iterum ac tertium. Num igitur, ut inepti, Veneris id impulsu fieri malumus quam casu dicere?'.

[29] See Kany-Turpin and Pellegrin 1989, 225, and van der Eijk 2005a, 144. Later in the same text one finds a considerably different explanation for the prophetic dreams of melancholics, which again does not raise the implication of divine inspiration. This time it is not just the number of images which melancholics encounter in sleep but also a certain ability to associate objects that are far apart which makes them have this kind of dreams (464a27–464b1). See Croissant 1932, 38–40; Pigeaud 1978, 28–29, and van der Eijk 2005a, 144–145.

[30] See van der Eijk 1993, 227 and Wardle 2006, 307.

[31] Although Aristotle does not explicitly claim that there is something divine in the souls of melancholics, he nonetheless leaves enough space to suggest that these people entertain a special relationship with some kind of 'divine movement' (*Ethica Eudemia* 1248a34–41): καὶ τούτων φρονίμων καὶ σοφῶν ταχεῖαν εἶναι τὴν μαντικήν, καὶ μόνον οὐ τὴν ἀπὸ τοῦ λόγου δεῖ ἀπολαβεῖν, ἀλλ' οἳ μὲν δι' ἐμπειρίαν, οἳ δὲ διὰ συνήθειάν τε ἐν τῷ σκοπεῖν χρῆσθαι· τῷ θεῷ δὲ αὗται. τοῦτο καὶ εὖ ὁρᾷ καὶ τὸ μέλλον καὶ τὸ ὄν, καὶ ὧν ἀπολύεται ὁ λόγος οὗτος. διὸ οἱ μελαγχολικοὶ καὶ εὐθυόνειροι. ἔοικε γὰρ ἡ ἀρχὴ ἀπολυομένου τοῦ λόγου ἰσχύειν μᾶλλον. In comparing this passage with *De divinatione per somnum* 463b12–22, van der Eijk 1993, 226, observes that, 'a fundamental connection between the two accounts' is that 'the divine working is not conceived as a form of divine dispensation ... but as an interaction between a divine movement and a particular human state of receptivity: melancholic people 'use' ... a general and universal divine movement, to which they are more susceptible than other people because of their physiological constitution, which weakens their intellectual powers'. See also van der Eijk 1989.

[32] See Flashar 1962, 715; 1966, 68 n. 13; Pigeaud 1981, 263, and Schäublin 1991, 325. Wardle 2006, 307, does not rule out the possibility.

ὅσοις δὲ ἐν τῷ φύσει συνέστη κρᾶσις τοιαύτη, εὐθὺς οὗτοι τὰ ἤθη γίνονται παντο-
δαποί, ἄλλος κατ' ἄλλην κρᾶσιν· οἷον ὅσοις μὲν πολλὴ καὶ ψυχρὰ ἐνυπάρχει, νωθροὶ
καὶ μωροί, ὅσοις δὲ λίαν πολλὴ καὶ θερμή, μανικοὶ καὶ εὐφυεῖς καὶ ἐρωτικοὶ καὶ εὐκί-
νητοι πρὸς τοὺς θυμοὺς καὶ τὰς ἐπιθυμίας, ἔνιοι δὲ καὶ λάλοι μᾶλλον. πολλοὶ δὲ καὶ
διὰ τὸ ἐγγὺς εἶναι τοῦ νοεροῦ τόπου τὴν θερμότητα ταύτην νοσήμασιν ἁλίσκονται
μανικοῖς ἢ ἐνθουσιαστικοῖς, ὅθεν Σίβυλλαι καὶ Βάκιδες καὶ οἱ ἔνθεοι γίνονται πάντες,
ὅταν μὴ νοσήματι γένωνται ἀλλὰ φυσικῇ κράσει.

But those with whom this temperament exists by nature, at once develop the
greatest variety of characters, differing according to their different temperaments; for example, those who posses much cold black bile become dull
and stupid, while those with whom it is excessive and hot become frenzied
or clever or erotic or easily moved to anger and desire, while some become
more talkative. But many because this heat is near to the seat of the intellect, are affected by diseases of frenzy and possession, which accounts for the
Sibyls, soothsayers, and all inspired persons, when their condition is due not
to disease but to a natural mixture.[33]

It has been noticed that, while ps.-Aristotle does attribute the ecstatic power
of divination to people with a melancholic temperament, his explanation
remains physiological and he never appears to commit himself to the idea of
a divine power at work inside them.[34] Nonetheless, it is important to notice
that, although suggesting that divination is, in essence, a matter of hot black
bile affecting the seat of the intellect, ps.-Aristotle's text still allows considerable space for the use of some rather strong language relating to divine
inspiration and possession (e.g. ἔνθεοι);[35] this is at least what one surmises
from his emphasis towards the end of the text on the manic and 'enthusiastic' diseases (νοσήμασιν ... ἐνθουσιαστικοῖς) which affect melancholics who
foresee the future. One cannot thus rule out the possibility that, in his reading of ps.-Aristotle, Quintus, for whom natural divination and the gods exist
and are directly connected to each other, would not have found the idea of
a melancholic temperament at this point irreconcilable with that of divine
dispensation.[36]

---

[33] Translation in Radden 2000, 58.
[34] See van der Eijk 1993, 225–226.
[35] See Screech 2004, 35.
[36] See also Cicero, De divinatione 1.18.34 (Quintus on the seminal distinction between
natural and artificial divination): 'eis igitur assentior, qui duo genera divinationum esse
dixerunt, unum, quod particeps esset artis, alterum, quod arte careret. est enim ars in eis
qui novas res coniectura persequuntur, veteres observatione didicerunt. carent autem arte ei
qui, non ratione aut coniectura observatis ac notatis signis, sed concitatione quadam animi
aut soluto liberoque motu futura praesentiunt, quod et somniantibus saepe contingit et
non numquam vaticinantibus per furorem, ut Bacis Boeticus, ut Epimenides Cres, ut Sibylla

However, in order to connect Quintus' comments on melancholic divination with the text of ps.-Aristotle, one may also follow a different line of argument, one that would take into account Cicero's criticism of the concept of melancholic genius at *TD* 1.80. As I have argued, Cicero finds it in that case hard to accept Aristotle's thesis, since in his mind this seems to bring the idea of genius too close to that of disease. Likewise, in Quintus' understanding of things, the hypothesis of melancholic divination does not work, since it confuses a state of divine inspiration with that of a mental and physical disorder:

> ego autem haud scio an nec cardiacis hoc tribuendum sit nec phreneticis.[37]

> I for my part don't know whether this is to be attributed to the mentally ill.

Prior to this statement, and in the context of discussing natural divination, Quintus has also mentioned poetic inspiration precisely as another instance of a divine power being directly imparted to human nature (1.79–80). Quintus invokes in that case the authority of Democritus and Plato and proceeds to add that *furor* can be used as a word for inspiration in Latin so long as it is 'praised' in the way that Plato does it in his *Phaedrus* ('Quem, si placet, appellet furorem, dum modo is furor ita laudetur ut in Phaedro Platonis

---

Erythrea'. Even if it is the case that by the time of ps.-Aristotle terms such as ἔνθεος and ἐνθουσιαστικός do not implicate the notion of divine possession but rather that of an affection of the human soul (see e.g. Aristotle, *Rhet.* 1408b1; *Pol.* 1340a11 with van der Eijk 1993, 226 n. 12), it is hard to believe that Quintus would have disassociated the image of a melancholic Sibyl, as found in ps.-Aristotle's text, from the idea of possession. Wardle 2006, 196 suspects that by referring to Bacis and Sibyl side by side, Quintus is keeping an eye at this point on ps.-Aristotle, XXX.i 954a 36. On Bacis and his oracles see Prandi 1993. On Sibyl as an inspired prophet see Stumfohl 1971 and Lightfoot 2007, 8–14.

[37] Cicero's choice of 'phreneticis' at this point might be related to the close association drawn in earlier medical sources between 'melancholic' and 'phrenetic' derangement (van der Eijk 2008b, 171–172). See e.g. [Hippocrates] *De morbis* 1.30 [6.200 Littré]: προσεοίκασι δὲ μάλιστα οἱ ὑπὸ τῆς φρενίτιδος ἐχόμενοι τοῖσι μελαγχολώδεσι κατὰ τὴν παράνοιαν. As regards now his reference to 'cardiacis', it should be mentioned that this is a condition which affects not the heart, as its name suggests at first sight, but rather the orifice or the upper part of the stomach (see e.g. ps.-Galen, *Introductio seu medicus* 13 [14.735 K]: ἡ δὲ καρδιακὴ διάθεσις οὐκ ἀπὸ τοῦ περὶ καρδίαν εἶναι τὸ πάθος οὕτως ὠνομάσθη, ἀλλ' ἐπεὶ καρδίαν οἱ παλαιοὶ τὸν στόμαχον ἐκάλουν. Cf. [Hippocrates] *Prorrheticon* 1.72 [5.528 Littré] with C.R.S. Harris 1973, 114). With that in mind, it might not be a coincidence that already Diocles of Carystus (4th cent. BC) associates an affection of the abdominal region with what others before him have called a 'melancholic' disease (Galen, *De locis affectis* 3.10 [8.185 K] ~ Diocles fr. 109 in van der Eijk 2000): ἄλλο δὲ γίγνεται μὲν περὶ τὴν κοιλίαν, ἀνόμοιον δ' ἐστὶ τοῖς προειρημένοις, καλοῦσι δ' αὐτὸ οἱ μὲν μελαγχολικόν, οἱ δὲ φυσῶδες. ἕπονται δὲ τούτῳ μετὰ τὰς ἐδωδὰς, καὶ μάλιστα τῶν δυσπέπτων τε καὶ καυστικῶν, πτύσεις ὑγραὶ καὶ πολλαὶ, ὀξυρεγμίαι, πνεύματα, καῦμα πρὸς ὑποχονδρίοις. See van der Eijk 2008b, 168.

laudatus est'). There is no doubt that Quintus refers at this point to the fact that Plato, while designating poetic inspiration as an instance of madness (*mania*), makes it clear that this is not madness in its clinical sense but rather a privileged state of divine possession or, as Socrates calls it, 'a divine disruption of our conventions of (normal) conduct' (*Phdr.* 265a9–11). Ps.-Aristotle's concept of melancholic genius has long been seen to respond to and in effect to radically revise this thesis, thereby suggesting that the sort of condition which allows for good poetry to be written (a) has nothing to do with the divine (as it is more a matter of physical constitution and temperament) and (b) can very easily take a distinctly pathological form, one that extends beyond the established limits of madness (μανία) and comprises a wide range of other mental and physical disorders.[38] It is with this revisionist attitude that Cicero disagrees, hence his remark that if to be a genius means that one should also be a melancholic, that is, diseased and imperfect, he is then not distressed at not being a genius himself. In Cicero's mind genius clearly has nothing to do with disease and this is precisely what Quintus also means to stress when saying that *furor* is an acceptable choice of word for poetic inspiration so long as it is 'praised' (*laudetur*) and is distinguished, one may add, from *furor* in its pathological sense (which is how Cicero uses the word at *TD* 3.11). In essence, Quintus' subsequent critique of melancholic divination relates to the fact that Aristotle fails in that case to do what Plato does with poetic 'madness', namely to establish that his subject of discussion does not implicate disease in its pathological form. This, in a way, points back to Cicero's critique of the idea of melancholic genius (*TD* 1.80) and suggests, in the end, that there is a good chance for Quintus to respond at *De divinatione* 1.81 to that same text of ps.-Aristotle.

Finally a point needs to be raised with regard to the text we started with (*TD* 3.11) and Cicero's emphatic statement that the importance of black bile as a pathogenic cause should not be overestimated in cases of melancholic madness (... *quasi vero atra bili solum mens ac non saepe vel iracundia graviore vel timore vel dolore moveatur*). In the other two cases that I have examined in detail (*TD* 1.80; *De divinatione* 1.81), Cicero has been seen to respond to ps.-Aristotle's text with a blend of criticism and irony, his discomfort with it emerging from his belief that black bile should not be associated as a *cause* either with one's powers of the intellect or with one's competence in foretelling the future; and while Cicero recognizes black bile as a cause of disease (in fact this his reason for dismissing the idea of a

---

[38] See van der Eijk 2005a, 156. For a general discussion see Flashar 1956.

melancholic genius in the first place), it is, I would suggest, as if to sustain
this rhetoric of disassociation, that he attempts to downgrade its importance
also as a possible *causal* explanation for melancholic madness. In other
words, to the extent that *TD* 3.11 forms part of a wider network of allusions
to ps.-Aristotle, then arguing that madness is not just about black bile can
be seen to stress, once again, that the latter's possible range of effects and
connection to the mind (regardless of whether this connection is found to
have a positive or a negative outcome) should not be overrated.

Cicero and Melancholic Depression

As has been noticed above, ps.-Aristotle conceives of black bile as something
that can become either too hot or too cold and therefore as the possible
material cause of both madness and depression.[39] As one reads for instance
at 954a11–26:

περὶ οὗ δὲ ἐξ ἀρχῆς προειλόμεθα διελθεῖν, ὅτι ἐν τῇ φύσει εὐθὺς ὁ τοιοῦτος χυμὸς ὁ
μελαγχολικὸς κεράννυται· θερμοῦ γὰρ καὶ ψυχροῦ κρᾶσίς ἐστιν· ἐκ τούτων γὰρ τῶν
δυοῖν ἡ φύσις συνέστηκεν. διὸ καὶ ἡ μέλαινα χολὴ καὶ θερμότατον καὶ ψυχρότατον
γίνεται. τὸ γὰρ αὐτὸ πάσχειν πέφυκε ταῦτ᾿ ἄμφω, οἷον καὶ τὸ ὕδωρ ὂν ψυχρόν, ὅμως
ἐὰν ἱκανῶς θερμανθῇ, οἷον τὸ ζέον, τῆς φλογὸς αὐτῆς θερμότερόν ἐστι, καὶ λίθος καὶ
σίδηρος διάπυρα γενόμενα μᾶλλον θερμὰ γίνεται ἄνθρακος, ψυχρὰ ὄντα φύσει ...
καὶ ἡ χολὴ δὲ ἡ μέλαινα φύσει ψυχρὰ καὶ οὐκ ἐπιπολαίως οὖσα,[40] ὅταν μὲν οὕτως
ἔχῃ ὡς εἴρηται, ἐὰν ὑπερβάλλῃ ἐν τῷ σώματι,[41] ἀποπληξίας ἢ νάρκας ἢ ἀθυμίας ποιεῖ
ἢ φόβους, ἐὰν δὲ ὑπερθερμανθῇ, τὰς μετ᾿ ᾠδῆς εὐθυμίας καὶ ἐκστάσεις καὶ ἐκζέσεις
ἑλκῶν καὶ ἄλλα τοιαῦτα.

But to return to our original subject, that such a melancholic humour is
already mixed in nature; for it is a mixture of hot and cold; for nature consists
of these two elements. So black bile can become both very hot and very
cold, for one and the same substance can naturally be affected by both these

---

[39] For a different explanation of the two sides of melancholy, which though again concentrates on the elements of hot and cold, see Rufus of Ephesus fr. 11 §§ 22–25 (Pormann 2008,
34): For a discussion of this text see Dandrey 2005, 120 n. 1 and Jouanna 2006, 48; 2009, 255.
On Rufus of Ephesus and ps.-Aristotle see van der Eijk 2008b.

[40] καὶ οὐκ ἐπιπολαίως οὖσα: this is a difficult phrase. Klibansky et al. 1964, 23 translate it
as 'and not superficially so', which seems to suggest that black bile is fundamentally cold;
but Pigeaud 1988b, 118–119, argues convincingly that reference is made to the fact that, for
melancholic depression to take over, black bile needs to remain on the inside, that
is, with melancholic madness and the outward direction of black bile (ἐκ-στάσεις/ἐκ-ζέσεις)
when it is heated. See also Louis 1994, 32.

[41] Although emphasis is laid at this point on the excessive quantity of black bile one may
assume that its excessive coldness is also important. See Müri 1953, 23, and Flashar 1962, 720.

conditions, as for instance water, which although in itself cold, yet when sufficiently heated so as to start boiling is hotter than the flame itself. And stone and iron when heated in the flame become hotter than charcoal, though by nature they are cold .... Now black bile, which is naturally cold and does not reside on the surface, when it is in the condition described, if it is in excessive quantity in the body, produces apoplexy or torpor, or depression or fear; but if it becomes overheated, it produces cheerfulness, bursting into song, and ecstasies and the eruption of sores and the like.[42]

This dichotomy pervades the text and in the end establishes melancholy as an essentially two-sided disorder.[43] Ps.-Aristotle underlines its importance when dealing, for instance, with the unpredictable temperature of black bile (954b8–18) and its varied effects on one's mood and highlights it once again at the part of the text which introduces suicide as a result of melancholic depression (954b28–35):

ῥέπουσι δ᾽, ἂν ἀμελῶσιν, ἐπὶ τὰ μελαγχολικὰ νοσήματα, ἄλλοι περὶ ἄλλο μέρος τοῦ σώματος· καὶ τοῖς μὲν ἐπιληπτικὰ ἀποσημαίνει, τοῖς δὲ ἀποπληκτικά, ἄλλοις δὲ ἀθυμίαι ἰσχυραὶ ἢ φόβοι, τοῖς δὲ θάρρη λίαν ... αἴτιον δὲ τῆς τοιαύτης δυνάμεως ἡ κρᾶσις, ὅπως ἂν ἔχῃ ψύξεώς τε καὶ θερμότητος. ψυχροτέρα μὲν γὰρ οὖσα τοῦ καιροῦ δυσθυμίας ποιεῖ ἀλόγους ...

And melancholics, if not careful, incline towards diseases related to black bile, different individuals being affected in different parts of the body: some people suffer from epileptic seizures, others from apoplectic ones; some are given to deep sadness and fear while others become overconfident; the cause of such force is the melancholic mixture, how it is related to cold and heat; for when it is colder than the occasion demands it produces irrational sadness ...[44]

---

[42] Translation in Radden 2000, 57–58; modified at points.

[43] In essence ps.-Aristotle is the first writer to explicitly attribute both madness and depression to the same humoural cause; earlier medical writers distinguish between what one may refer to as manic and depressive states of mind but in that case one has two different humours to account for each state; see e.g. [Hippocrates] De morbo sacro 15 [6.388 Littré]: γίνεται δὲ ἡ διαφθορὴ τοῦ ἐγκεφάλου ὑπὸ φλέγματος καὶ χολῆς ... οἱ μὲν γὰρ ὑπὸ τοῦ φλέγματος μαινόμενοι ἥσυχοί τέ εἰσι καὶ οὐ βοῶσιν ... οἱ δὲ ὑπὸ χολῆς κεκράκται καὶ κακοῦργοι καὶ οὐκ ἀτρεμαῖοι. An intriguing example, which in a sense lies closer to ps.-Aristotle's text, comes from [Hippocrates] De diaeta 1.35 [6.518–520 Littré]: εἰ δὲ κρατηθείη ἐπὶ πλεῖον τὸ πῦρ ὑπὸ τοῦ ἐόντος ὕδατος, τούτους ἤδη οἱ μὲν ἄφρονας ὀνομάζουσιν, οἱ δὲ ἐμβροντήτους. ἔστι δ᾽ ἡ μανίη τοιούτων ἐπὶ τὸ βραδύτερον· οὗτοι κλαίουσί τε οὐδενὸς λυπέοντος ἢ τύπτοντος, δεδίασί τε τὰ μὴ φοβερά, λυπέονταί τε ἐπὶ τοῖσι μὴ προσήκουσι ... εἰ δέ τινι πλέον ἐπικρατηθείη τὸ ὕδωρ ὑπὸ τοῦ πυρός, ὀξείη ἡ τοιαύτη ψυχὴ ἄγαν, καὶ τούτους ὀνειρώσσειν ἀνάγκη· καλέουσι δὲ αὐτοὺς ὑπομαινομένους· ἔστι γὰρ ἔγγιστα μανίης τὸ τοιοῦτον. Jouanna and Boudon-Millot (in this volume) distinguish at this point between a 'folie dépressive' and a 'folie agitée'.

[44] Translation in Radden 2000, 59; strongly modified at points.

It should be noticed that, on the whole, ps.-Aristotle's concept of the melancholic differs significantly from the one found in the Hippocratic writings.[45] Although black bile is believed to be an integral part of one's natural constitution (954b20), and not a 'residue', as Aristotle, for instance, would have it (*De partibus animalium* 677a13–18),[46] there is nothing in the text to suggest that it is also conceived as part of a wider humoural system, which involves either phlegm or, in its most complete and elaborate form, phlegm, yellow bile and blood.[47] The idea of 'mixture' (κρᾶσις) crops up often in the text (e.g. 954a13) but, again, this refers to a mixture of heat and cold (the two essential qualities of black bile) and raises no implication of an interaction with a different humour.[48] Even so, the case remains that when it comes to the symptoms of a melancholic disease, whether in its manic or depressive form, ps.-Aristotle evidently relies on the earlier medical tradition;[49] and for what concerns us here, it is worth noting that this point of contact becomes most evident in the case of melancholic depression: for instance the emphasis laid on fear and sadness, a sadness which ps.-Aristotle designates as 'groundless' (ἄλογος) and 'unreasonable' (954b35) in the sense that it is disproportionate or even unrelated to external events,[50] finds a close parallel in [Hippocrates] *Aphorismi* 6.23 [4.568 Littré] (Hippocrates' definitive word on the subject, according to Galen at least),[51] which sets out to speak of a melancholic affection in similar terms:

---

[45] See Jouanna 2006, 50–54. For some comprehensive discussions of this text, especially within its Aristotelian context, see Gravel 1982; Roussel 1988 and van der Eijk 2005a, 155–168. See also Massimiliano 2006.

[46] On bile as a 'residue' (περίττωμα) with no final cause in Aristotle see Bostock 2006, 89, and Lloyd 1996, 47. Cf. ps.-Aristotle, *Problemata Physica* I 861b14–20: ἐὰν οὖν μὴ ἐν τοῖς ἄνω, καθάπερ εἴρηται, τὰ περιττώματα εὐθὺς ἀνέλῃ, καταβαίνουσιν εἰς τὰς κοιλίας ἄπεπτα ὄντα ... ἡ γὰρ τοῦ ἀπέπτου ὑπόστασις μονιμωτάτη ἐστὶ καὶ σύντονος γίνεται τῷ σώματι, καθάπερ ἡ μέλαινα χολή. The fact that our author speaks of his exceptional melancholics as περιττοί (e.g. 953a10) suggests a line of connection with the idea that black bile is a kind of (material) excess in its own right. See Pigeaud 1988b, 18–20. On the notion of περιττώματα in general see Thivel 1965.

[47] See Jouanna 2006, 118–119.

[48] See van der Eijk 2005a, 159; see though Pigeaud 1988b, 19, on ps.-Arist. XXX.i 955a14.

[49] For some points of agreement between ps.-Aristotle and the Hippocratic tradition see Jouanna 2006, 52 n. 27, and Angelino and Salvaneschi 1981, 35–36.

[50] See Horwitz and Wakefield 2007, 58, and Radden 2009, 183–184.

[51] See e.g. Galen, *De locis affectis* 3.10 [8.190–191 K]: διαφέρονται δὲ ἀλλήλων οἱ μελαγχολικοί, τὸ μὲν φοβεῖσθαι καὶ δυσθυμεῖν καὶ μέμφεσθαι τῇ ζωῇ καὶ μισεῖν τοὺς ἀνθρώπους ἅπαντες ἔχοντες ... ὥστε ὀρθῶς ἔοικεν ὁ Ἱπποκράτης εἰς δύο ταῦτα ἀναγαγεῖν τὰ συμπτώματα αὐτῶν πάντα, φόβον καὶ δυσθυμίαν.

Ἢν φόβος ἢ δυσθυμίη πολὺν χρόνον διατελέῃ, μελαγχολικὸν τὸ τοιοῦτον.[52]

If fear or sadness persist for a long period of time, this indicates a melancholic affection.[53]

Equally revealing in this respect is ps.-Aristotle's insistence on associating depression with 'apoplexy' (954a23; 954b30–31), by which one should understand a fit of paralysis which strikes suddenly and leaves someone unable to move or even speak; again the evidence that we have shows that apoplectic fits can be closely associated in earlier medicine with a melancholic condition, and this in a context which suggests a catatonic state pointing towards depression rather than madness. As one reads this time at [Hippocrates] *Aphorismi* 7.40 [4.588 Littré]:

Ἢν ἡ γλῶσσα ἐξαίφνης ἀκρατὴς γένηται, ἢ ἀπόπληκτόν τι τοῦ σώματος, μελαγχο-λικὸν τὸ τοιοῦτο γίνεται.[54]

If the tongue is suddenly paralyzed, or a part of the body suffers a stroke, the affection is melancholic.

Overall, it seems then safe to argue that while ps.-Aristotle acknowledges that black bile can in fact cause strong fits of madness this by no means entails that he disregards its strong associations with melancholic depression; in fact one may go so far as to say that ps.-Aristotle's extensive discussion of suicide as the result of depression (954b34–955a22), along with an elaborate section on post-coital sadness that follows (955a22–29),[55] indicate that our author finds depression more intriguing than madness (or at

---

[52] As Pigeaud 1988b, 58–59, points out, the syntax of this short aphorism remains ambiguous (perhaps deliberately so) and does not allow us in effect to reach a definite conclusion as to whether it is a melancholic affection (in the sense of black bile) which leads to sadness and fear or, conversely, whether it is feelings of that nature which give rise to a melancholic affection; see also Pigeaud 1981, 122, with (the objections in) Jouanna 2006, 49.

[53] As Radden 2009, 183, points out, '[t]he reasoning here appears to be that since in most people such states are short-lived, prolonged fears and despondencies must be ungrounded, unfounded, or without sufficient cause' and therefore symptomatic of a pathological condition.

[54] Apoplexy can either be local ([Hippocrates] *Coa Praesagia* 353 [5.658 Littré]) or affect the entire body ([Hippocrates] *Coa Praesagia* 490 [5.696 Littré]). Interestingly enough, in one of its earliest occurrences in the Hippocratic corpus, it is connected with an excessive state of coldness (which though is attributed to air in the body and not specifically to a humour). See [Hippocrates] *De ventis* 13 [6.110 Littré] with Jouanna 1988, 120 n. 3. Cf. [Hippocrates] *Aphorismi* 6.56–57 [4.576–578 Littré]. On apoplexy in the Hippocratic writings and Galen see Clarke 1963 and Karenberg 1994 respectively.

[55] Ps.-Aristotle XXX.i 955a22–29. Cf. ps.-Aristotle IV.30 880a30–33 (on the aphrodisiac nature of melancholics) with Jouanna 2006, 56 n. 42.

least worth exploring). Assuming then that this is a text which Cicero, as I have argued, knows well, his translation of μελαγχολία with *furor* looks one-sided.[56] This is of course not to say that Cicero would not have been familiar with the fact that μελαγχολία in Greek can also have the meaning of depression. In fact, a third allusion to ps.-Aristotle's text suggests quite the opposite. This allusion concerns the figure of the Iliadic Bellerophon, mentioned alongside Heracles and Ajax at the opening of ps.-Aristotle's text (953a21–25):

> ... ἔτι δὲ τὰ περὶ Αἴαντα καὶ Βελλεροφόντην, ὧν ὁ μὲν ἐκστατικὸς ἐγένετο παντελῶς, ὁ δὲ τὰς ἐρημίας ἐδίωκεν, διὸ οὕτως ἐποίησεν Ὅμηρος "αὐτὰρ ἐπεὶ καὶ κεῖνος ἀπήχθετο πᾶσι θεοῖσιν, ἤτοι ὁ κὰπ πεδίον τὸ Ἀλήϊον οἶος ἀλᾶτο, ὃν θυμὸν κατέδων, πάτον ἀνθρώπων ἀλεείνων."

The same is true of Ajax and Bellerophon; the former went completely insane, and the other craved for desert places. so that Homer wrote of him: 'but the day soon came when even Bellerophon was hated by all the gods; across the Aleian plain he wandered, all alone, eating his heart out, a fugitive on the run from the beaten tracks of men' [= *Iliad* 6.200–202].[57]

For ps.-Aristotle, these last three lines cited from Homer describe an essentially melancholic pathology, which, however, is not explicitly identified as either manic or depressive. Yet later medical writers clearly tend towards the latter; one reads, for instance, in ps.-Galen, *Introductio seu medicus* 13 [14.740–741 K]:[58]

> τῆς δὲ περὶ τὴν διάνοιαν ἐκστάσεως, δύο μὲν τὰ ἐξέχοντα εἴδη μανία τε καὶ μελαγχολία. πολλαὶ δὲ καὶ ἐν τούτοις αἱ διαφοραὶ .... αἰτία δὲ τῆς μὲν μανίας ξανθὴ χολή. διὰ τοῦτο ταραχώδεις καὶ ἔκφοροι καὶ πρόχειροι ὑβρισταί τε οἱ τούτῳ ἐχόμενοι τῷ πάθει. τῆς δὲ μελαγχολίας αἰτία μέλαινα χολή, ψυχρότερος χυμὸς καὶ ζοφώδης. διὸ ζοφοειδεῖς τέ εἰσι καὶ δύσθυμοι οἱ τοιοῦτοι. ὕποπτοι δὲ εἰς πάντα καὶ μισάνθρωποί τε καὶ ἐρημίαις χαίροντες, οἷος ὁ Βελλοροφόντης ἱστορεῖται. ἤτοι ὁ καππεδίον τὸ Ἀλήϊον οἶος ἀλᾶτο, ὃν θυμὸν κατέδων, πάτον ἀνθρώπων ἀλεείνων.

Regarding the distraction of the mind, madness and melancholy present its two most prominent forms. The differences between the two are many ... the cause of madness is yellow bile; and this explains why people afflicted with this kind of disease cause troubles, are carried astray, and are impetuous and abusive. As for the cause of melancholy, this is black bile, a humour colder (than yellow bile) and dark; this is the reason why melancholics have a dark complexion and get depressed; they also are suspicious towards everything, and hate the company of people and take pleasure in isolated places, just as

---

[56] See Toohey 2004, 34.
[57] Translation in Radden 2000, 57; strongly modified at points.
[58] A late text of the 2nd cent. AD. See Nutton 2004, 185.

the story goes for Bellerophon: 'across the Aleian plain he wandered, all alone, eating his heart out, a fugitive on the run from the beaten tracks of men'.[59]

As it is, Bellerophon does not find a place in Cicero's list of (manic) melancholics at *TD* 3.11 (Athamas, Alcmaeon, Ajax and Orestes), and this might be telling us that, to his mind (as to that of ps.-Galen later on), Bellerophon's case does not qualify as a typical instance of melancholic madness. Nevertheless, one can find Bellerophon's name mentioned towards the end of the same book of the *Tusculans*, significantly enough alongside the grieving figure of Niobe, and while discussion has now moved on to the consequences of extreme sorrow and, more specifically, to the (mis)conception that it is appropriate for someone to grieve at the death of relatives (*TD* 3.61–63):

> Sed ad hanc opinionem magni mali cum illa etiam opinio accessit, oportere, rectum esse, ad officium pertinere ferre illud aegre, quod acciderit, tum denique efficitur illa gravis aegritudinis perturbatio. Ex hac opinione sunt illa varia et detestabilia genera lugendi: pedores, muliebres lacerationes genarum, pectoris, feminum, capitis percussiones ... Ex hoc evenit ut in animi doloribus alii *solitudines captent* [cf. ps.-Aristotle XXX.i 953a22: τὰς ἐρημίας ἐδίωκεν], ut ait Homerus de Bellerophonte: '*Qui miser in campis maerens errabat Aleis, / ipse suum cor edens, hominum vestigia vitans*'; et Nioba fingitur lapidea propter aeternum, credo, in luctu silentium.

> But when our belief in the seriousness of our misfortune is combined with the further belief that it is right, and an appropriate and proper thing, to be upset by what has happened, then, and not before, there comes about that deep emotion which is distress. It is this latter belief that gives rise to all those despicable forms of mourning such as smearing oneself with dirt, scratching at one's cheeks like a woman, and striking oneself on the chest, head and thighs ... it is this belief that causes some people to seek out lonely places when their minds are grieved, as Homer says Bellerophon did: 'Sadly he wandered in the Aleian fields, eating his heart for sorrow, shunning every human track'. Niobe, too, observed a perpetual silence in her grief, and this is no doubt the reason she is supposed to have turned into stone.[60]

One cannot fail to notice that in illustrating Bellerophon's grief (*aegritudo, dolor animi*) Cicero cites two of the three Homeric lines which one finds already quoted in ps.-Aristotle's text;[61] what is more, there is no doubt that the mental suffering of which Cicero speaks at this point is that of a deep grief and distress: Bellerophon's association with Niobe, the archetype of silence and sorrow, is quite revealing in this respect; as is also the fact that

---

[59] My translation.
[60] Translation in Graver 2002, 28.
[61] Fischer 2011, 42.

line 201 of the Iliadic text is considerably changed in Cicero's translation precisely to the effect of stressing this idea of sorrow and mourning further—
miser and *maerens* have no equivalent in the Greek original. It is therefore
safe to conclude that if it is indeed ps.-Aristotle's Bellerophon (that is, a
melancholic Bellerophon) that Cicero has in mind at this point, our author
is then familiar with the fact that, apart from its established connections
with madness (*TD* 3.11), 'melancholia' can also be used in Greek as a word
for depression.

To sum up: Cicero's translation of 'melancholia' with *furor* at *TD* 3.11 should
not be treated as an isolated linguistic remark on the Greek language of mental illness; it should rather be seen as forming part of a wider network of allusions to ps.-Aristotle's treatise on the subject. On the one hand, this would
help to explain Cicero's interest in instances of tragic madness, considering
that ps.-Aristotle is the first writer to speak of the mad heroes of tragedy as
'melancholics'. On the other hand, Cicero's insistence on downgrading the
importance of black bile as a pathological cause in cases of mental illness
falls in line with his critique of ps.-Aristotle's ideas at other parts of his work
(*TD* 1.80; *De divinatione* 1.81), where emphasis is primarily laid on the observation that black bile cannot affect one's mental capacities. Finally, while
Cicero's translation of 'melancholia' with *furor* looks one-sided, his allusion
to ps.-Aristotle's Bellerophon in his discussion of the consequences of sorrow at *TD* 3.61–63 shows that our author is aware that the Greek word is not
exclusively associated with madness but can also have in it the meaning of
depression.

FEAR OF FLUTE GIRLS, FEAR OF FALLING*

Helen King

Within the texts of the Hippocratic corpus, in both *Epidemics* 5 and 7, we read of two men who sought treatment for what we would now call phobias. Forming two of the 54 chapters that are shared by both collections,[1] their case histories are given consecutively, apparently not because the writer grouped them together due to their similarity,[2] but because they approached him together; the second man, Democles, is 'ho met' ekeinou', 'who was with him'. It is noteworthy that these patients meet the physician together; normally only one case at a time is described in a Hippocratic case history.[3] Both cases are striking. The first man, Nicanor, suffers from 'fear of flute girls' or, more specifically, symptoms brought on by hearing the *aulos* play at the symposium; he has no symptoms if he hears this instrument in the daytime. This appears to be a very culturally-specific, or indeed idiosyncratic, phobia.[4] The second case contrasts in its apparent universality:[5] a fear of heights and

---

* My thanks to the audiences at the conferences 'Mental Disorders in Classical Antiquity II' (Columbia University, October 2010), 'The *aulos* in ancient music: celebrating the Reading *aulos*' (March 2011) and at the Bristol Anglo-Hellenic Society (February 2011) for their interest and their suggestions, and above all to Oswyn Murray for reading the penultimate draft of this paper.

[1] Langholf 1977 argued that the parallel texts derived from the library at Cos.

[2] [Hippocrates] *Epid.* 5. 81 and 82: 7. 86 and 87. The cases are in a section along with patients suffering from delirium, visual disturbances, and depression.

[3] While those at the 'Mental Disorders' conference speculated that the men may have been homosexual partners, and Jandolo translates the case of Democles as 'che viveva con lui' and later glosses this as 'faceva abitualmente vita in comune con un certo Nicandro' (1967, 45 and 47–48), there is nothing in the text to suggest we should go this far; the form *meta* + genitive pronoun is a common one, with *ho meta tinos*, for example, meaning 'his companion' in a non-sexual sense. LSJ points here to examples such as Herodotus 1.86 and Plato, *Protagoras* 315b. There are few other examples of *meta* + genitive in the Hippocratic corpus in the sense of 'una cum aliquo', the only other one in *Epidemics* being 1.11 (Loeb I.164, Littré 2.636), a reference to the patient working 'along with the doctor' against the disease. Jouanna and Grmek 2000, 38 n. 3 speculate that the two men 'renforçaient peut-être leurs obsessions' but correctly point out that there is no way of telling whether they lived together, or simply came to visit the doctor together.

[4] Jandolo 1967, 48: 'una particolare forma di idiosincrasia fobica'.

[5] Jandolo 1967, 47 presents this as 'un caso di classica vertigine psiconevrotica'. Doctor et al. 2008, xiii, amalgamate the two Hippocratic individuals into a single 'highly phobic

bridges, so severe that, even if the bridge is over a very low ditch, Democles is compelled to get off the bridge and walk through the ditch to the other side.

These two books of the *Epidemics* were dismissed in the Galenic tradition as late, and so were not considered the genuine works of Hippocrates; book 5 was attributed by Galen to Hippocrates the younger, son of Draco.[6] As there was no Galenic commentary on them, both books were relatively neglected by Renaissance and early modern readers.[7] However, as Jouanna and Grmek pointed out, they were rehabilitated by the nineteenth-century editor Émile Littré, who admired their detailed comments on individual cases.[8] Claims for the nature of the texts as pure observation were however challenged from Langholf's work of 1990 onwards, and they are now considered to be 'filtered reality', the observations being guided by prior theory and assumptions.[9]

Here are the two case histories in the recent Loeb translation of Wesley Smith, using the versions in *Epidemics* 5:

> Nicanor's affection, when he went to a drinking party, was fear of the flute girl. Whenever he heard the voice of the flute begin to play at a symposium, masses of terrors rose up. He said that he could hardly bear it when it was night, but if he heard it in the daytime he was not affected. Such symptoms persisted over a long period of time.

> Democles, who was with him, seemed blind and powerless of body, and could not go along a cliff, nor on to a bridge to cross a ditch of the least depth, but he could go through the ditch itself. This affected him for some time.

In these Hippocratic case histories, it is worth noting that in the first 'he said' features; in the *Epidemics* 7 version of Democles, the text includes 'he said' too, to read 'he said he could not go along a cliff ...'. We are apparently receiving the patients' voices,[10] rather than a medical diagnosis. Patient voices come through elsewhere in the *Epidemics* collections. For example, in *Epidemics* 7 there are also two cases in which a woman patient's own feelings or beliefs about her condition are flagged up. In 7.28, the wife of Polemarchos 'said she felt as though there was a gathering about her heart'. In 7.11, the wife of Hermoptolemos, sick with a fever in the winter, 'said that her heart had been damaged'.

---

individual'; they use Errera's article, on which see further below, although they name him 'Errara'.

   [6] Galen, *De difficultate respirationis* 2, 8 (7.854–855 K).

   [7] Nutton 1990, 425–427; Graumann 2000, 22.

   [8] Jouanna and Grmek 2000, xvii.

   [9] Langholf 1990, 208; current scholarship usefully summarised by Graumann 2000, 59.

   [10] Jouanna and Grmek 2000, 38 n. 2.

To the modern reader, it may seem striking that no diagnosis or treatment is given, simply a description of what the patients experienced; however, this pattern is typical of the *Epidemics* collections. In terms of treatment, elsewhere in *Epidemics* fear is considered something that the physician should be willing to induce 'for the sake of restoring colour and humours'.[11] As fear is not always bad, perhaps these men would not have been treated, merely talked with, about the effects of the fear on their bodies. The lack of diagnoses has not prevented modern commentators from adding their own. For example, Corvisier suggested that Nicanor's diagnosis combines 'an obsession, and alcoholism'.[12] I will argue here that this is a misunderstanding of the symposiac context of Nicanor's fear, and that these cases need to be replaced within their cultural context. The most common retrodiagnosis offered for them in the period from the Renaissance to the nineteenth century was 'melancholy' and then, from the nineteenth century until the present, 'phobia'. A recent textbook on psychiatric and mental health nursing correctly notes that there is little discussion of ancient anxiety disorders in modern literature, and quotes in full these two cases as examples of phobia;[13] classical texts are widely cited in modern works on phobia, to give authority and a sense of continuity. Before considering their original meaning, I will first examine how the texts have been used within these two diagnostic categories.

Writing the History of Phobia I: Melancholy, Mania and Social Phobia

Until the development of the category of 'phobia', the diagnosis for both our cases was one of 'melancholy', mania and melancholy being the two main diagnoses of conditions of the mind in ancient medicine.[14] In particular, *Aphorisms* 6.23, 'Fear (*phobos*) or depression (*dysthymia*) that is prolonged means melancholia', encouraged readers familiar with the rest of the Hippocratic corpus to see Nicanor and Democles in this way. As *Aphorisms* was central to medical education from the Middle Ages onwards,[15] and had the status of a genuine work of Hippocrates, the statement in 6.23 was taken very seriously; 'prolonged' fear could be read as applying to both Nicanor and

---

[11] *Epidemics* 2.4, 4.
[12] Corvisier 1985, 106. For a summary of recent diagnoses, see Graumann 2000, 242–243.
[13] Elder et al. 2009, 38.
[14] For an overview of ancient texts on melancholy, see Flashar 1966.
[15] H. King 1993, 57–60.

Democles, as their symptoms endured 'for some time'. Renaissance commentators, such as Anuce Foës, whose edition of the Hippocratic corpus was
particularly widely used, readily made this connection.[16] Francisco Valles
linked the case of Nicanor to another section of the *Aphorisms*, 4.9, which
advises purging in melancholics, seeing a link between his symptoms being
worse at night (a time which, Valles notes, is full of fear for everyone) and
the darkness of the fluids of melancholia.[17]

There is one further Hippocratic reference to the story of Nicanor: it
features in the pseudepigrapha, which date from the Hellenistic period, as
part of the series of 'letters' in which Hippocrates diagnoses the madness of
Democritus. Nicanor is not named, but is clearly intended in Letter 19 'On
madness', which ends as follows: 'And there was another who was seized,
when he went to a symposium, by fear of the flute girl if he heard her playing.
But when he heard it in the daytime he suffered no effect'.[18] The case is given
after a discussion of the preceding chapter of *Epidemics* 5, the fatal case
of Androthales (5.80), which suggests that bile is the cause of this man's
delirium. The pseudepigraphic writer assumes that madness is due either
to phlegm, or to bile, affecting the brain: madness from phlegm is a quiet
form, while that from bile is a violent form. He links 'fearful dreams' (*enypnia
phobera*) and terrors (*phoboi*) to the heating effects on the brain of excess
bile, *cholê*. The suggestion, then, is that Nicanor suffers from too much bile;
not, it may be noted, specifically the 'black' bile of melancholy.

The modern concept of phobia dates from the nineteenth century; Westphal's *Die Agoraphobie* (1872) is usually cited as the classic text from which
modern approaches derive.[19] In DSM-IV, phobia is described as excessive or
unreasonable fear in the presence of, or in anticipation of, a specific object
or situation; the diagnosis involves the affected person's acknowledgement
that the fear felt is indeed excessive or unreasonable. The sufferer will either
avoid the stimulus or endure it 'with intense anxiety and distress'.[20] The fact
that they are speaking to a doctor suggests that these two men believe their
fear to be 'excessive'.[21] Democles avoids: he has given up on bridges. But
Nicanor endures: he keeps going back to symposia.

---

[16] Foës 1595, 253.

[17] Valles 1554, 546.

[18] L 9.386; W.D. Smith 1990, 94–96. Jouanna and Grmek 2000, lvi point out that *Letter* 19 is
based on the version in *Epidemics* 5.

[19] E.g. Thorpe and Salkovskis 1997, 83.

[20] Davey 1997, xiii–xiv.

[21] Gourevitch and Gourevitch 1982, 888.

To today's reader, Nicanor's behaviour may resonate with the rise of therapy for phobia based on controlled and increasing exposure to the stimulus, popular in the late 1960s/early 1970s, although it is clearly not working for him; in the later 1970s and 1980s, cognitive approaches to phobia were preferred.[22] Psychiatrists in the 1960s and early 1970s, familiar with the approach of gradually exposing the sufferer to the stimulus, could find an extreme version of this treatment in another ancient source, Celsus, who wrote on how to treat hydrophobia,

> ... throw the patient unawares into a water tank he has not seen before. If he cannot swim, let him sink under and drink, then lift him out; if he can swim, push him under at intervals so that he drinks his fill of water even against his will; for so his thirst and dread of water are removed at the same time.[23]

This is given by Celsus as the only remedy for hydrophobia, if it has progressed to the point that cauterisation of the dog bite, followed by sweating the patient, will not help. The water tank treatment is followed by a bath in hot oil.

The key feature of modern phobia diagnosis, that the level of fear is unreasonable, has its own classical counterpart in Caelius Aurelianus who, in his discussion of mania in *On Chronic Diseases* 1.5, notes that the impairment of rationality in mania can show itself 'as some relate, in an overpowering fear of things that are quite harmless'.[24] He expands on this by stating that the affected person 'will be afraid of caves or will be obsessed by the fear of falling into a ditch';[25] while Democles is not mentioned here, his case may come to mind, as he can manage ditches only by walking through them, rather than over them.

The reference to mania in this context is interesting. In Hippocratic texts, as we have just seen, it is melancholy, rather than mania, which is associated with fear. Caelius Aurelianus shows that this was not the only view taken in antiquity, as he explicitly distances from the diagnosis of melancholy his own discussion of irrational fears, stating that, while Apollonius Mus says that melancholy is a form of mania, 'we distinguish melancholy from mania'.[26] Caelius Aurelianus' section on melancholy is far

---

[22] Davey 1997, xiv.

[23] Celsus 5.27c; tr. Grieve 1814, cited by Thorpe and Salkovskis 1997, 82–83, who consider that 'Celsus ... appears to have invented flooding as a therapeutic technique'.

[24] ... *nunc timore comminante inanium rerum, sicut quidem memoraverunt*; Drabkin p. 539.

[25] ... *ut nunc speluncas timeant, nunc lacunas, ne in easdem concidant.*

[26] Drabkin p. 539.

shorter than that on mania, and differentiates the two conditions by saying that in melancholy the *stomachus* (oesophagus) is affected the most, while in mania it is the head.[27] He further separates melancholy from hydrophobia, on the grounds that melancholy is chronic but hydrophobia acute;[28] here he sets himself up against Eudemus, a follower of Themison, who saw them both as the same condition. He insists that hydrophobia is a disease of the body rather than of the soul, even though fear is normally an affection of the soul; fear, he states, arises from a 'sympathetic accord between body and soul'.[29] He opposes the advice to immerse patients in water to force them to drink, a therapy which he associates not with Celsus, but with Artorius.[30] We can see here that the ancient texts were in dialogue, and in disagreement; there was no agreed position on irrational fear, so that later commentators were able to weave together the ancient materials to produce different results.

Where the stories of Nicanor and Democles feature in the current literature of phobia, the source is usually the article on 'Some historical aspects of the concept, phobia' published by Paul Errera in 1962. Errera regarded Nicanor and Democles as sufferers from phobia, making them 'two of the earliest clinical descriptions of men who feared 'that which need not be feared'. He quoted both cases in full, and believed that the Hippocratic diagnosis would have been one of melancholy, which he described as 'one of the three major Hippocratic types of insanity'.[31]

While Robert Burton's *The Anatomy of Melancholy* (1621) mentioned neither Nicanor nor Democles, in modern works this classic text on the condition is often elided with these Hippocratic accounts. In a section on "Symptoms or signs in the mind", Burton describes a man who

> through bashfulness, suspicion and timorousness will not be seen abroad, loves darkness as life, and cannot endure the light, or to sit in lightsome places, his hat still in his eyes, he will neither see, nor be seen by his good will ... He dare not come in company for fear he should be misused, disgraced, overshoot

---

[27] 1.6, Drabkin p. 563.

[28] *Acute Diseases* 4.12, Drabkin p. 369.

[29] ... *timor enim per consensum animae corporis compatientis nasci perspicitur*, 4.13, Drabkin pp. 368–371.

[30] Drabkin p. 385.

[31] Errera 1962, 327. Errera is also responsible for another standard part of modern accounts of the history of phobia; the origin of the term in the Greek *Phobos*, and Phobos as a god. Here Errera cites LSJ and Roscher's 1884 Lexicon (1962, 326); this material is repeated in, for example, Davey's introduction to his 1997 work on phobia, as well as in chapter 4 of that volume, by Thorpe and Salkovskis (1997, 82).

himself in gesture or speeches, or be sick; he thinks every man observes him, aims at him, derides him, owes him malice.[32]

Burton cites here the pseudo-Hippocratic *De insania et melancholia*, which he refers to elsewhere as the Calvi edition.[33] This passage has been used in modern work as an example not just of phobia, but of 'social' phobia 'from the time of Hippocrates'[34] or even less plausibly as 'seen by Hippocrates'.[35] Social phobia, in which the sufferer avoids social situations due to fear of embarrassment, is the most-researched of all the phobias, but is currently seen as having a psychopathology that is very different from that the others.[36] In DSM-IV terms, it is not in fact a 'phobia' at all because a phobia is defined as 'inappropriate fears to *relatively specific* stimuli or events [my italics]',[37] while social phobia is much broader. Yet it has drawn into its net not only the Burton/Hippocrates description, but also the case of Nicanor, becoming the most common retrospective diagnosis of his condition.[38]

Writing the History of Phobia II: Nicanor and Democles in the Nineteenth and Early Twentieth Centuries

It was in 1869 that Nicanor and Democles entered nineteenth-century discussions of mental illness: this was when Armand Semelaigne picked up Etienne Esquirol's linking of symptoms and social change, arguing that the history of madness was interesting precisely because of 'ses intimes rapports avec la civilisation et les doctrines philosophiques régnantes'. He cited Esquirol's *Des maladies mentales*: 'Les idées dominantes dans chaque siècle influent puissament et sur la fréquence et sur le caractère de la folie'.[39] He proposed that Hippocrates established the foundations of psychiatry, and that the main divisions found in his works still formed the basis of the classifications used, even if theories explaining these categories had changed over

---

[32] Burton 1989.1.386.25–30.
[33] Burton 1989.1.382.5–9.
[34] Heckelman and Schneier 1995, 3.
[35] Mannuzza et al. 1990, 41.
[36] Pers. comm. Graham Davey, 11 August 2010.
[37] Davey 1997, xiii.
[38] E.g. Mannuzza et al. 1990; Heckelman and Schneier 1995, 3.
[39] Semelaigne 1869, 6 citing Esquirol 1845, 43. In the 1845 English translation this appears on p. 39; 'The prevailing sentiments of every age, exercise a powerful influence, over both the frequency and character of insanity'.

time.[40] Using Littré's translation, Semelaigne discussed Nicanor and Democles in his chapter on melancholy, based on the remark in *Aphorisms* 6.23
that, if fear or sadness persists for a long time, then this is a melancholic
condition.[41] He prefaced the case histories with a discussion of *Regimen* 1.35,
on those who fear what does not need to be feared.[42] In this Hippocratic
treatise, melancholy is said to derive from situations in which fire is over-
powered by water.

One further contribution from the French tradition, and one which was
rapidly transmitted to the English-speaking world, should also be mentioned here. In 1934 Alexandre Souques published two articles in the journal
Revue Neurologique. Here he described the cases of Nicanor and Democles from *Epidemics* 5.[43] His main point was that, despite only a sketchy
knowledge of the anatomy and physiology of the brain and the nervous
system, Hippocrates' clinical understanding was excellent, as he knew how
to observe, how to collect facts and how to compare them.[44] He praised
one case history, for example, as representing 'une admirable observation'
and as 'cette irréprochable observation'.[45] When he gave the case histories
of Nicanor and Democles, he presented them in a section on depressive
states of nervous origin; specifically, as 'des exemples d'obsessions et de phobies'.

Souques's first 1934 article was summarised in *Archives of Neurology and
Psychiatry* in the following year by 'Freeman of Washington DC'; this has
to be Walter Jackson Freeman, head of neurology at George Washington
University, who was to become infamous after he began performing frontal
lobotomies in 1936.[46] Freeman believed that many psychiatric conditions
had organic origins, so that treatment should take place on the brain itself;
ancient medicine, in which the mind/body divide was placed very differently to that of modern medicine, was thus of interest to him.[47] In the

---

[40] Semelaigne 1869, 7.
[41] Semelaigne 1869, 33. Rufus fr. 73 Pormann, preserved in Galen's commentary on Book 6
of *Epidemics* (which may itself have been based on Rufus), also cites the Hippocratic linking
of fear and melancholia.
[42] Semelaigne 1869, 36–37.
[43] Souques 1934, 197; he repeated this material in his 1936 book, *Étapes de la neurologie
dans l'antiquité* (1936, 92–93).
[44] 'Autant son anatomie est superficielle et sa physiologie imaginaire, autant sa clinique
est profonde et réelle', Souques 1936, 50–51.
[45] Souques 1936, 72.
[46] Freeman 1935.
[47] El-Hai 2005, 70.

abstract of Souques' article, Nicanor and Democles are included;[48] however, Freeman, in translating Souques, omits 'le festin', and therefore loses entirely the symposiastic context of the condition.

The Symposium and the Aulos

This omission of the symposium by Freeman reflects the historical lack of interest in this feature of ancient society as a social ritual. Scholarly attention only turned to it in the late 1960s, as the result of a greater interest in Greek and Roman social customs, and the influence of social anthropology on the classics.[49] An appreciation of the symposium is based on an understanding of how, in agricultural societies, 'culture ultimately derives from the various modes of the ritualized use of an economic surplus'.[50] The symposium is now understood as 'in many respects a place apart from the normal rules of society, with its own strict code of honour in the *pistis* there created, and its own willingness to establish conventions fundamentally opposed to those within the *polis* as a whole'.[51] The size of the group would be between 14 and 30 men, two to a couch.[52] At the end of the symposium, the participants would take part in the *komos*, a public drunken riot done to demonstrate the group's power; this disorder was, however, of a very controlled type, with a steady build-up during the rest of the symposium, and although it is a group activity it is 'a group activity with everyone on his own'.[53] Not every symposium was an elite occasion; recent scholarship shows that these dining events occurred lower down the social scale too, including 'the mercantile, artisan or peasant classes'.[54] As an event combining the consumption of wine, jokes, discussions of politics and of the nature of love, singing and music, with specific types of pottery and of extempore songs associated with it, and creating both homosexual bonds and an atmosphere for uninhibited heterosexual activity with the entertainers, the symposium—at least in its elite manifestations—could certainly be stressful. It would thus appear to be an important focus for what John Oliver, in a paper read to the American Psychiatric Association meeting in Richmond, Virginia in 1925, described as

---

[48] Souques 1934, 656.
[49] O. Murray 1990, 8.
[50] O. Murray 1990, 4.
[51] O. Murray 1990, 7.
[52] O. Murray 1990, 7.
[53] Frontisi-Ducroux and Lissarague 1990, 227.
[54] Pellizer 1990, 180–181.

the 'elements of emotional stress and strain' in ancient Athens; as Pellizer put it, 'the actual guests put themselves to the test in front of the group'.[55]

But what exactly was an *aulos*, and what was its role within the symposium? Although the usual English translation is 'flute', it is in fact a double reed instrument, so it is played more like an oboe. The two pipes, each normally with six holes, are entirely separate.[56] A halter could be worn to support the pipes and also to prevent the cheeks from distorting; it has been suggested that this meant the player breathed in through the nose, and out through the mouth, possibly through what is now known as circular breathing.[57] While it is not clear from two dimensional representations on vase paintings whether the two pipes would normally be identical in length and width, archaeological evidence suggests that one would be around 3 cm longer than the other.[58] The fact that the sound is referred to in the singular as 'the sound of an *aulos*' could be taken to suggest that only one pipe is heard at any one point, but as Stefan Hagel has demonstrated on reconstructed instruments, both can be played together.[59] References to the 'maiden *auloi*' (*parthenioi*) and the 'wedding *auloi*' in which a 'male' and a

---

[55] Oliver 1925, 111; Pellizer 1990, 183. But the two parallel passages in which Nicanor's affliction is described are the only references to the symposium in the Hippocratic corpus. If we look back even before Semelaigne and Littré, we can see that the symposium had already been lost in translation. In Latin versions of the *Epidemics*, it had become a simple *conuiuium*, a banquet, or just 'drinking' (e.g. Valles 1554, 546, *quum in conuiuium progrediebatur*; compare the edition of 1652, 271, *Nicanoris passio cum in potum progrederetur ... Foës 1595, 252: Nicanor cum ad conuiuium prodiret ...*). In eighteenth-century English translations of *Epidemics* 5 and 7, not only the context of the symposium, but even the female gender of the flute player, went unnoticed. In Francis Clifton's 1734 translation of Nicanor's story, 'when he was oblig'd to go to a drinking-bout, he was always afraid of a flute; and, when the piper began to play, the musick immediately threw him into such a great fright, that he was not able to bear the disorder of it, if it was night' (Clifton 1734, 231). In Samuel Farr's 1780 version, 'when he went to a feast he took an aversion to the sound of the trumpets' (Farr 1780, 165). This version was dismissed as a poor one by both Adams 1849 and Jones 1923; see Graumann 2000, 25 n. 131.

[56] Psaroudakes 2008.

[57] Bundrick 2005, 35. However, Stefan Hagel has shown on reconstructed instruments that it is possible to inhale while playing the *aulos*, and demonstrated this for example on http://www.oeaw.ac.at/kal/agm/ (accessed 12 February 2011).

[58] Gentili and Luisi 1995, 19 and 31; Hagel 2004, 375; Bundrick 2005, 35. As for the contribution of archaeology, a complete pair was found in 1996 in Pydna, with one pipe 34.2 cm and the other 37 cm. Other complete instruments include the 'Elgin *aulos*'; see Psaroudakes 2008; Hagel 2010, 329.

[59] The film *Agora* (2009) includes a scene in which the *aulos* is played, with one pipe being used rather like a drone. The track in which this features, 'Orestes' Offering', can be heard on http://www.youtube.com/watch?v=SI0AXE0O4Bs, accessed 8 January 2013. Stefan Hagel's attempts to reconstruct the sound can be found on http://www.oeaw.ac.at/kal/agm/ accessed 12 February 2011.

'female' pipe appear suggest that there were different instruments for different occasions, and an analogy may be drawn here with the Bolivian pan-pipes, where different types existed and were played seasonally, for example to make it rain.[60]

As Peter Wilson noted, the *aulos* was 'everywhere' in classical Athens.[61] It was used to accompany the army and to keep rowers in time.[62] While it could play music in any of the modes, it is particularly associated with the Phrygian mode, the one that arouses emotion.[63] It was associated with certain mystery cults, being played at Eleusis and in Dionysiac rites, and Proclus specifically comments on the effect of the *aulos* on the emotions of someone undergoing initiation.[64] In mystery cults, as in the symposium, the player would be female.[65] In classical Athens, it also featured in state religion, being played while sacrifices were offered, and accompanied athletic competitions.[66] It featured at weddings and funerals.[67] It was also part of Greek drama. The choruses and solo songs of Greek plays were accompanied by an aulete,[68] who would be a 'dignified, formally costumed' figure; as we shall see, this makes him quite unlike his female counterpart at the symposium.[69]

It was also a sexualised instrument. In a scene from Aristophanes' *Thes-mophoriazusae*, a Scythian archer—one of the police force at Athens—refers to the carrying case in which his arrows were kept (the *sybênê*, a term also used for the carrying case for the *aulos*). He puns on *binein* (to fuck), to come out with a line translated in Sommerstein's version as 'I've lost my shaft-case by shafting'—the woman in this case, conveniently, being a flute-girl.[70] Both the penis and the *aulos* were seen as difficult to control.[71]

While not every woman playing a flute was immoral—plenty of 'deco-rous' scenes exist on vase paintings[72]—it appears that women did not play at public events. The *aulêtris*, who sets off Nicanor's reaction, is in a category on her own. At the symposium, the *aulos* was used to set the rhythms by which

[60] Wilson 1999, 70; Stobart 2000, 40–42.
[61] Wilson 1999, 58.
[62] Wilson 1999, 80–81; Wallace 2004, 261–262; Bowie 1990, 227.
[63] Hagel 2010, 412.
[64] Hardie 2004, 16–17.
[65] Barker 2004, 198.
[66] Landels 1999, 3 and 5; Wilson 1999, 79.
[67] Wilson 1999, 80.
[68] Wilson 1999, 76; Barker 2004, 200.
[69] Barker 2004, 203.
[70] *Thesm.* 1215; Sommerstein 1994, 236–237.
[71] Wilson 1999, 72.
[72] Bundrick 2005, 41.

the wine was prepared, served and drunk.[73] Davidson associated this instrument with 'music for working and moving', in processions and marches;[74] in the symposium, it was first played at the start of the drinking. The halter was not worn by an *aulêtris*, so her cheeks were distorted.[75] Bearing in mind how the sound was produced, Clifton's 'piper' may indeed be a better translation than 'flute-girl', but 'flute-girl' (Gk *aulêtris*) is a term that says much about the player, as well as the instrument (see above, n. 55).

So what exactly is an *aulêtris*? Frontisi-Ducroux and Lissarague suggest that the flute-girl is 'herself an instrument', and they have shown how many images of her on 'Anakreontic' vases of the period 510–460 BC present her as static while she plays, with a man dancing next to her.[76] As many texts and vase paintings clearly show, the *aulêtris* had what Andrew Barker, discussing Aristophanes, *Birds* 667–668, calls a 'tawdry image'; 'the all too familiar, degraded figure of the slave-girl hired out to play the pipes and to double as a prostitute'.[77] Landels writes 'the connection was so firmly established that the Greek word for a female aulos-player, *aulêtris*, was regularly used to mean a high-class prostitute'.[78] Pellizer notes that the symposium could include '(and perhaps fairly frequently) activities which might cause a modest classical scholar to blush' and refers coyly to 'the extramusical activities of flute-girls'.[79] He has in mind here references to their extensive oral skills; what Henderson, basing himself on Aristophanes' *Wasps* 1335–1381, calls 'the polite ritual of symposiac fellation', and what Wilson described as 'the likely overlap of sexual and musical services'.[80] Another famous passage used in discussions of the status of the flute-girl is Athenaeus 607d, where it is claimed that she was usually auctioned off at the end of the night. Wilson also reminds us that, according to the *Constitution of Athens* 50.2, the city officials (the *astyonomoi*) charged with ensuring that the fee for a flute-girl's services does not exceed two drachmas were also those who dealt with blocked drains and collecting dung from the streets; 'the rougher edges of the line between public and private'.[81]

---

[73] Wilson 1999, 82.

[74] Davidson 1997, 81.

[75] Bundrick 2005, 35.

[76] Frontisi-Ducroux and Lissarague 1990, 224.

[77] Barker 2004, 198. See also Serghidou 2001, 63, for the flute-girl as a 'prototype of depravity and debauchery'.

[78] Landels 1999, 7.

[79] Pellizer 1990, 181.

[80] Henderson 1991, 81, cited by Starr 1978, 408; Wilson 1999, 83.

[81] Wilson 1999, 83. In Plato's far-from-standard symposium, the flute-girl is sent out of the

As for the effect of hearing her instrument, views on the *aulos* shifted over the course of Athenian history. Like its female player, it was usually seen negatively by Athenians, as an instrument from other *poleis*—it was originally linked to Boeotia and Sparta—bringing in disorder. However, scholars such as Wallace have argued for an early fifth century '*aulos* revolution' in Athenian culture, in which this instrument was adopted in Athens 'both by citizen players and by serious students of music'.[82] In 490, Pindar even claimed that Athena was its inventor.[83] While sixth-century vase paintings featured the *aulos*, almost all showed it in the context of the *symposion/komos*, or in Dionysiac ritual; however, in the early fifth century, scenes in which a young male citizen is taught to play the *aulos* started to feature.[84]

A reaction against the *aulos* took place in the mid-fifth century, at a period when the Athenians were defeated by the Boeotians (457), and then lost the battle of Coronea to Thebes (446); this would not have helped the image of an instrument originally associated with Boeotia. The *aulos* was rejected in favour of stringed instruments.[85] In art, after 450 scenes of Athena appear in which she is throwing away the *aulos* in disgust after seeing the reflection of her distorted face playing it; the instrument was then picked up by the satyr Marsyas.[86] Athenaeus (616e–617b) preserves a comment of Melanippides, a mid-fifth-century poet, who in his *Marsyas* had Athena saying 'Away, shameful things, defilers of my body! I do not give myself to ugliness'. According to two lives of Alcibiades, in his youth the Athenian general (born around 450) did not want to learn the instrument because it made him look ugly; it was 'a sordid thing, not becoming a free citizen';[87] however, ancient authorities were not agreed on Alcibiades'

---

room when the intellectual conversation begins (Pl. *Symp.* 176e), while, if it was not an elite event, I suspect she would have stayed put. In the *Protagoras* (347c–d), Socrates contrasts the symposium of the *kaloikagathoi*, where no flute girls feature, with those of ordinary people, where the voice of the *aulos* substitutes for that of intelligent conversation. But not everyone has seen the flute girl as a prostitute: Chester Starr once defended her honour, regarding her as a 'true professional', 'trained to play a difficult instrument and to learn the music composed for it, which became much more complex in the fifth century' (Starr 1978, 403 and 404).

[82] Wallace 2003, 76.

[83] *Pyth.* 12; Wallace 2003, 79.

[84] Wallace 2003, 81.

[85] Wallace 2003, 82.

[86] Serghidou 2001, 60–61 notes that Athena is the inventor, not the player, of this instrument. For an example of this scene see the 4th c mosaic on http://www.nytimes.com/2007/04/11/arts/design/11mosa.html?_r = 1.

[87] Ps-Plato, *Alcibiades* 1.106e and Plutarch, *Alcibiades* 2; Starr 1978, 401–402; Vickers 1990, 114.

opposition to the instrument, and Athenaeus 184d quotes from Duris, who said that he did indeed learn to play it.[88]

As for its continued history into the period of *Epidemics* 5 and 7 and beyond, these collections of cases appear to date to the mid-fourth century. This dating is supported by a reference to a catapult injury sustained at the siege of Datum in 358–357 by Philip of Macedon (5.95 = 7.121),[89] and by references to Olynthus, destroyed by Philip in 348.[90] How would the *aulos* have been understood at that time? While it was less likely to feature in elite male education after 450, respectable women were shown on vase paintings playing it, and it continued to accompany dramatic performances and religious rituals, and to be played at parties.[91]

The *aulos* was thought to have the power to take over those who heard it due to its 'enticing' sound;[92] as Davidson puts it, 'when the *aulos* played, men forgot themselves ... all flutes were half way to being magic ones'.[93] Indeed, in Euripides' *Herakles*, performed in 416 BC, it is 'the instrument of madness'.[94] In his *Quaestiones conviviales* Plutarch asked whether flute girls should be allowed at feasts, and described a party getting out of control precisely because of the effects of the *aulos* music.[95] Aristotle's objections to the instrument, probably dating to just after the cases in *Epidemics* 5 and 7,[96] also see the *aulos* in terms of loss of control. At *Politics* 1341a26–35, he states that the instrument used to be prohibited for the young and for free men, then draws on this historical evidence to support his case against using *auloi* in schools because 'they produce a passionate rather than ethical experience in their auditors and so should be used on those occasions that call for catharsis rather than learning' (1341a17–24).[97] Wilson makes a good case that the *aulos* was always an ambiguous instrument. While essential to the city, it was usually played by foreigners, and often slaves. In the city of

---

[88] Wallace 2003, 83.

[89] Graumann 2000: 53; Jouanna and Grmek 2000, xlii, point out that Littré preferred to link this to an earlier siege in 453, which would make these books of *Epidemics* pre-date Hippocrates.

[90] Jouanna 1999, 390.

[91] Wallace 2003, 87 and 91.

[92] Pollux, *Onomasticon* 4.72 and 73; West 1992, 105–106, n. 101.

[93] Davidson 1997, 81.

[94] Lines 871, 879, 897; Wallace 2003, 88.

[95] *Quaest. Conv.* 704c–706e.

[96] If we assume that *Politics* is part of the project on the constitutions of Greek cities composed by Aristotle's pupils, then perhaps 335–322.

[97] Ford 2004, 325–326.

logos, its sound was 'the antithesis of *logos*', a threat to self-control and the cause of distortion in the aesthetics of the body.[98]

Nicanor and Democles

In contrast to the *Pseudepigrapha* version, the *Epidemics* give us the story of Nicanor in conjunction with that of Democles, and reading the stories together can provide further suggestions. Both concern loss of control. Both are chronic conditions. But there is another link between these two men. In each case, the symptoms strike at a point of transition; for Nicanor, the moment when the symposium starts, and for Democles, when he is literally 'on the edge' of a cliff or bridge. Reading Democles' story helps us to appreciate that Nicanor too experiences an 'edge', as night starts, and as the symposium begins.

But what exactly is the *pathos* of Nicanor? Does it centre on the girl, the flute, or what the sound of the flute heralds? Despite Corvisier's attempt to suggest alcoholism is involved, Nicanor's symptoms are not brought on by too much wine; it is when he starts to drink, rather than when he has been drinking, that the symptoms start.[99]

The point that a symposium is much more than a drinking-bout (Greek *potos*, the first term for a *symposion* used in Nicanor's case history) or a feast suggests that Nicanor's fears derived from the competitive male context of the event, with the flute girl's music reminding him of a past failure, sexual or otherwise, during a symposium. This would explain why he was fine if he heard the flute in the day, but not if he heard it at night. But the cultural belief in its enticing sound, conducive to disorder, suggests that although the problem does not lie with the *aulos* itself—since he is not affected when he hears it in the daytime—the cultural baggage that surrounds this musical instrument leads him to fix on the moment when it starts to play as the moment when his fears rise up.

A final question concerning Nicanor revolves around his status at the symposium. Not everyone present there was invited. The *akletoi* or 'uninvited' turn up hoping for some food, and join in the activities by imitating the paid professional dancers, and generally making the invited guests feel superior: *akletoi* 'perform themselves as physically and morally imperfect',

---

[98] Wilson 1999, 58.
[99] Corvisier 1985, 106.

displaying to the guests 'the exhilarating assurance of their own physical and moral inferiority'.[100] Maybe Nicanor was not an elite guest, but one of these. Davidson regards them as the 'male counterparts' of the *aulêtrides*,[101] which would make Nicanor's reaction to the *aulêtris* particularly poignant. Fehr associates the presence of *akletoi* above all with the fourth century BC, although he also finds a concern about 'hangers-on' in the late archaic period.[102] He argues that the *akletoi* were in competition with each other, and would dance or fight 'to make the invited guests laugh, so as to get a meal or a drink'.[103] Competition, whether elite or not, could lie at the heart of the phobic reaction.

What of Democles and his fear of heights? Democles 'seemed' (*edokei*), in Wesley Smith's translation, 'blind and powerless of body'. The use of 'seemed' may suggest that the writer is simply describing what was presented, while reserving judgement as to whether or not Democles could really see. However, a further possibility is that Democles does not have these symptoms when the Hippocratic writer observes him, but is instead describing what happens when he is exposed to the stimuli. Within the text, his impaired vision and weakness are in a comparable position to Nicanor's fears, as subjective experiences which could not be witnessed by the writer.[104] This would explain why the term Smith translates as 'powerless of body', *lysisômatein*, is not found elsewhere in Greek, with LSJ simply suggesting 'relaxed'. Is this the word used by the patient, made up in order to convey how it feels to him when he is on the edge of a cliff or a bridge?

On first reading, this story recalls the blinding of Epizelos at the battle of Marathon, where Herodotus tells us that this soldier lost his sight in both eyes when an enormous armed figure passed by him and killed the man beside him.[105] I have argued that, by attributing his blinding to a divine act in the context of a battle that quickly attained mythic status, Epizelos became a hero, and so could not easily recover later on. One question these case histories raise is why these two men decide to consult a physician about their symptoms; what is their *self*-diagnosis? Democles' consultation of a doctor suggests that he believed that his blindness had a physical origin, rather than being due to divine intervention.

---

[100] Fehr 1990, 187 and 192.
[101] Davidson 1997, 93.
[102] Fehr 1990, 188.
[103] Fehr 1990, 191; e.g. 'beggar envies beggar', Hesiod, *Erga* 26.
[104] I owe this point to Elizabeth Warren.
[105] Herodotus 6.117; H. King 2001.

However, Smith's translation is not without its problems. The verb used here, *amblyôssein*, features in other Hippocratic texts not with the meaning 'blind', but rather as 'to see unclearly'. Earlier translations may give a better sense of this; even Farr has 'seemed to be affected with a sort of blindness' while Clifton gives 'seem'd to be dim-sighted'.[106] In one Hippocratic case in which this word is used, it is clear that the sufferer is able to see, because he has double vision.[107] In another, the doctor is advised to ask the patient if he has this symptom; unlike blindness, then, it is not immediately apparent to someone else.[108]

Democles is not 'blind'—so any suggestion that he comes with Nicanor because he is unable to walk without a guide must be rejected—but his vision blurs and his body becomes weak when he is exposed to cliffs or bridges. In this, his reactions recall those of Sappho in fr. 31, where she states 'sight fails my eyes' alongside symptoms of palpitation, sweating, and a whirring noise in her ears.[109] This passage has been seen as describing an 'anxiety attack'. The psychiatrist George Devereux put forward an interpretation of this kind in 1970, but Marcovich correctly noted that this is not an 'attack' because the problem is chronic; Sappho's use of the subjunctive *idô* in line 7 should be translated as '*each* time I look at you ...'.[110] For Democles and Nicanor too, these are chronic conditions.

In exploring these two cases in *Epidemics*, we have seen further evidence for the image of Hippocrates promoted by the history of western medicine, as keen observer and comprehensive guide; this image is as common in modern psychiatry as in other aspects of medicine. The diagnosis of melancholy provides an excellent example of how later readers of the ancient medical texts wove together different comments from different treatises to make a disease. As for the diagnosis of phobia, while this is no less susceptible to the temptation to massage the sources to create a better story, it is

---

[106] Farr 1780, 165; Clifton 1734, 231.

[107] *Diseases* 2.15 (Littré 7.28).

[108] *Prognostics* 7 (L 2.128). In contrast, the term used for Epizelos is *typhlos*; 'from that time on he spent the rest of his life in blindness (*eonta typhlon*)'. The word was first used in Homer, and denotes somebody with no sight whatsoever (Rose 2003, 80). It is used twice in the *Epidemics*, to identify a person ('the wife of blind Maeandrios', *Ep.* 4.8, L 5.148; 'As for blind Echecrates', *Ep.* 7.57, L 5.422). This does not necessarily imply that these people had been blind from birth; the same word is used in the sense of 'going blind' in *Prorrhetic* 2.1 (L 9.6), and in *Epidemics* 7.26 it features when the son of Antiphanes goes blind in one eye and then the other, dying a few days later (L 5.398). On one occasion, it is used metaphorically; in *Breaths* 14 the patient becomes blind to what is happening (L 6.112).

[109] ... *oppatessi d'ouden orêmm'*.

[110] Devereux 1970; Marcovich 1972.

interesting not only how far these two stories can illustrate features of DSM-IV, but also how this diagnosis places emphasis on different parts of the texts, so that 'this affected him for some time' seems to hold less interest once the diagnosis of 'melancholy' fades.

For Nicanor, I have argued that what is important is to recover the context of the symposium, historically lost in translation. This is not just a feast, but a very specific competitive male event. Nicanor's condition is thus not 'social phobia' but rather something closely tied to a particular cultural context. Whether he is an elite diner or another type of performer, it is a form of performance anxiety, stimulated by a musical instrument that, for a Greek of this period, already came with its own emotional baggage. Democles' fear of heights is not culturally specific, but it is interesting that he too is affected at an 'edge', in his case spatial rather than temporal. His appearance alongside Nicanor suggests that, from the patients' perspective, these men had discussed their symptoms, recognised similarities, and were sufficiently aware of Hippocratic medicine to think that there was a physical reason, probably an excess of bile, to account for their reactions to these very different stimuli.

PART IV

SYMPTOMS, CURES AND THERAPY

GREEK AND ROMAN HALLUCINATIONS

W.V. Harris

One possible approach to studying mental disorders in antiquity is to take relatively familiar symptoms and consider how the ancients understood them (without any assumption that the symptoms were completely identical). Hallucinations are an obvious case to choose, since the evidence, though not voluminous, is fairly extensive. A major aim should be to see how much ancient understanding of hallucinatory experiences evolved—or at least changed. Another aim should be to trace the connections and disconnections between co-existing ancient viewpoints, those of physicians versus those of lay-people, those of the educated versus those of the uneducated, those of the ultra-religious versus those of the more sceptical. An added dividend is that such an investigation will necessarily take us on a tour of some interestingly thorny historical problems such as Socrates' experience of a disembodied voice, and the resurrection of Jesus.

It may be too simple to suppose that the archaic Greeks considered all hallucinations to be the work of superhuman beings, but the central question is clearly when, why and how far 'secular' physiological/psychological understandings of hallucinations took over, and how long they persisted. Athenian tragedy shows us hallucinations of superhuman origin, but these hallucinations also, in all or most cases, make psychological sense. A philosophical tradition, especially visible in surviving texts of Aristotle and the Epicureans, expressed a purely human understanding of the phenomena. Hallucinations as medical symptoms were seen in a certain way by ordinary Greek and Roman physicians, but were not necessarily seen in the same way by everyone else. As for puzzling visions and voices experienced by apparently healthy people, they were often debated, and many will always have found superhuman agency of some kind the most likely explanation. The aim here is to disentangle these strands of thought, for Greek and Roman antiquity down to Augustine, who for these purposes may be considered the beginning of the Middle Ages.

Hallucinations are highly diverse, quite apart from the fact that they may or may not be symptoms of serious mental disorders. They may affect any sensory organ (though we shall be concerned here with visual and auditory sensations). They may be one-shot experiences or they may be recurrent. They may consist of seeing/hearing things when there is nothing to be seen or heard, or of more or less grossly misidentifying what is visible or audible. And there are borderline cases. Should we, for example, include sightings of ghosts (many intelligent Greeks and Romans believed in them)?[1] I would suppose that we should, even though ghosts as hallucinations are anomalous. For ghosts are often promiscuous, in the sense that they make themselves visible and audible to anyone (but not all ghosts do that). Another borderline case is the 'sensed presence', the experience that explorers and soldiers, in particular, sometimes seem to have that some supportive person is nearby though not actually visible or audible; this is a theme thoroughly explored in a new article by Gabriel Herman,[2] but since sensory error is not involved I shall say nothing about it in this paper.

More troublesome are sensory errors that are brief illusions rather than hallucinations. Cognitive psychologists like to dream up illusions, such as the Fraser spiral, in which the eye sees something which the brain insists on interpreting as something else; these are not hallucinations. Another situation: I think that I see a certain old friend at a party; I am wrong, but I am not hallucinating—it is someone like her, and I quickly and willingly admit that I was wrong. But if I persist in error, can I rightly be said to be hallucinating? My error may be an error of interpretation not perception. When, in a rather commonplace incident, a couple in Perth Amboy, New Jersey, said that a window in their apartment 'started creating an image of the Virgin', and convinced others that the image was there,[3] they were, if they were reporting their experience honestly, hallucinating—but perhaps not both of them and perhaps not in the central sense of the term. Later we shall consider the case of Pheidippides (p. 295), who encountered the god Pan in the mountains—was that perhaps just a misinterpretation, later elaborated, of a passing glimpse of a goaty man or a humanish goat? Here, however, the fact that Pan both appeared and spoke (see below) makes it reasonable to speak of a hallucination.

---

[1] For a convenient selection of sources on Greek and Roman ghosts see Ogden 2002, Chapter 8. He leaves out the discussion in Pliny, *Letters* 7.27. I cordially thank Maria Michela Sassi, Erin Roberts, Chiara Thumiger, and Glenn W. Most for their helpful criticisms of an earlier draft of this paper.

[2] Herman 2011. I thank Professor Herman for sending me his paper prior to its publication.

[3] This from the *New York Times* of October 1, 2000.

Then there is the problem of delirium—a fairly common feature of ancient medical reports. A desperately sick person talked nonsense, but was (s)he hallucinating? It may be impossible to tell.

In consequence of all this, definition is not easy. Here, however, is a definition adopted in a very useful recent work by two psychiatrists who thoroughly discuss the difficulties in earlier definitions (but in truth the concept is much as Esquirol defined it nearly two centuries ago).[4] A hallucination is, they say, 'a sensory experience which occurs [to a person who is awake] in the absence of corresponding external stimulation of the relevant sensory organ, has a sufficient sense of reality to resemble a veridical perception, [and] over which the subject does not feel s/he has direct and voluntary control'. (Thus this definition includes experiences that a person recognizes as hallucinations while they are going on, as in Charles Bonnet Syndrome).[5] That is all, of course, quite a long way from expressing the tiresome, alarming, indeed frightening quality that many hallucinations possess.

All the more frightening in modern times because a person who hallucinates is quite likely to be labelled a schizophrenic. Hallucinating can also be a symptom of, among a number of other serious conditions, *delirium tremens* and Parkinson's disease. The awkward fact is, however, that people who are suffering from no apparent mental disorder also sometimes hallucinate.[6] As far as I can tell, no one knows with any degree of precision how many such people there are; I have seen various estimates.[7] The recently bereaved are particularly likely to 'see' and/or 'hear' the person they have lost; this is not a fringe phenomenon, but something experienced by a large proportion of the human race.[8] There is a significant implication: just as it is fairly easy to identify people who (even without the help of LSD) have experienced hallucinations, it can be expected—though it cannot be proved— that many ancient people too, those of a certain age at least, learned from

---

[4] Aleman and Larøi 2008, 15, quoting David 2004, 108.

[5] On the latter see Plummer 2011.

[6] Aleman and Larøi 3, citing Johns and Van Os 2001. This fact is often emphasized in Payne 2011.

[7] 4 per cent of the population every year: Nayani and David 1996. Slade and Bentall 1988, 68–76, review a number of studies, most of which appear to show that between 10 % and 25 % of modern Anglophone populations hallucinate at least once in a lifetime. See further Johns and Van Os 2001. Methodological rigour has often been lacking (see David 2004, 111, for the softness of at least some of the data in question), but the article of Langer et al. 2011, which provides up-to-date bibliography, indicates that there has been some improvement in this respect.

[8] On evidence from Sweden see Grimby 1993, 1998. See further Aleman and Larøi 2008, 31, Casey 2010, 490–491.

their acquaintances what hallucinations were like even if they never hallucinated themselves. That may ease our task. On the other hand, any culture in which the notion is quite widespread that divine beings sometimes send waking visions will necessarily have a great deal invested in making sure that descriptions of such visions conform to its cultural norms (and we shall shortly see how this factor seems to have affected ancient descriptions of hallucinations).

Scholars exist, however, who think that we should not apply the term 'hallucination' to anything that occurred in antiquity, since there is no equivalent Greek or Latin term. Latin *alucinatio* usually meant 'mental wandering' in general, without any implication that sensory error was involved.[9] The Greek vocabulary for hallucinatory experiences is characteristically rich, especially in the matter of things seen: we meet *phantasmata*, but also *eidola* (images or spectres) and *doxai* ('appearances', as we might say); but there is no specific word for either visual or auditory hallucinations, and no single word that covers both.

Thus we shall be considering attitudes of the ancients towards phenomena that for them did not have a single identity—which should impose a certain caution. Yet although the ancients tended to keep auditory and visual hallucinations separate from each other, some of the more reflective among them knew that the two were inter-related. Thus when Socrates is discussing the unreliability of sense perceptions with Theaetetus and he brings in the perceptions of the insane, he speaks both of distorted hearing and of distorted seeing in parallel with each other.[10] Likewise, a speaker in Plutarch's dialogue *On the* daimonion *of Socrates* brings together the two main kinds of hallucination even as he contrasts them: 'he often heard Socrates express the view that people who claimed to have encountered some divine being visually were impostors, while he paid close attention to people who said that they had heard some kind of voice'.[11] The speaker drew the obvious

---

[9] However in the relatively late medical writer Caelius Aurelianus one has the impression that the word has a more precise meaning: *Acute Diseases* 2.166 and 167, 3.176. In the first and third of these passages I. Pape translated the term as 'Wahnvorstellungen', delusions. In the last one it is distinguished from *mentis alienatio*.

[10] Plato, *Theaetetus* 157e: 'The defect [in this argument] is found in connection with dreams and illnesses, especially madness [*mania*], and everything else that is said to cause errors of sight (*parhoran*) and hearing (*parakouein*) and the other senses (*paraisthanesthai*). For you know that in all these the theory we were just presenting [that the senses do not deceive] seems without doubt to be refuted'. Cf. Aristotle, *De insomniis* 1.458b31–32, Longus, *Daphnis and Chloe* 2.26.5.

[11] *On the* daimonion *of Socrates* 20 = *Moralia* 588c.

conclusion that Socrates' *daimonion* was 'the perception of a voice, or the mental apprehension of discourse that reached him in some strange way'.[12] And ancient hallucinations were sometimes both visual *and* auditory—less often, however, than we might have expected. This is probably the best way to take Herodotus' famous tale (6.105) about the Athenian runner Pheidippides (or Philippides), who, in the course of his two-day run to Sparta during the invasion crisis of 490, encountered the easily-recognized god Pan, at a lonely spot in the mountains: apparently Pan both looked the part, and spoke.[13] Similarly, the theatre-goer of Abydos or Argos who imagined dramatic performances in an empty theatre (and regretted being cured), was imagined as having both 'seen' and 'heard' them.[14] The physician Theophilus, in a case described by Galen as insanity (*paraphrosune*), suffered from the illusion that noisy flute-players had invaded his house and were playing there all day and all night; he both saw them and heard them.[15]

In *Dreams and Experience in Classical Antiquity* I argued that while at least one characteristic type of dream known in an antiquity is no longer experienced in the modern west (the 'epiphany dream'), the main features of dreaming are much the same now as they were then. As far as I can tell, there is no systematic difference between classical and modern hallucinations, but that is a quite provisional conclusion. It is an obvious possibility, for example, that the Greeks and Romans hallucinated divine figures more often than modern Europeans do. A culture that is deeply convinced of the existence of superhuman but anthropomorphic beings, whether it is the god Pan or the Virgin Mary, is probably more likely to hallucinate them. Saudi Arabian schizophrenics are reported to experience hallucinations with religious content more often than (presumptively less religious) British schizophrenics.[16]

---

[12] The term *daimonion* cannot be translated exactly: 'divinity' makes it too grand, 'spirit' not grand enough.

[13] There is no reason why we should consider this epiphany as 'auditory rather than visual' (Hornblower 2001, 143, following Versnel 1987, 49); Herodotus gives no hint of that—on the contrary, *prospiptei* and *phanenai* (ch. 106) indicate an (apparent) physical presence. See further Borgeaud 1988 [1979], 243 n. 3.

[14] Ps.-Aristotle, *De mirabilibus auscultationibus* 31 (specifying seeing), Horace, *Epistles* 2.2.128–140 (specifying hearing).

[15] *On the Differences of Symptoms* 3 = VII.60–61 K. Pigeaud 1988b, 163, has this wrong.

[16] Kent and Wahass 1996; Aleman and Larøi 2008, 28. *Plus ça change*: religiously-inspired group hallucinations seem to have been relatively common in sixteenth- and seventeenth-century England: Walsham 2010, 87–91.

In what follows I propose to deal first with what we can call, with all proper reservations, the fictional sources. To some readers that may seem a strange procedure. I follow it for two reasons, partly because some of the great imaginative stories—the story of Orestes above all—bulk large in modern thinking about mental disorders in antiquity, but more importantly because they bulked large in ancient thinking on the subject, so that the philosopher Chrysippus, for instance, when he is explaining visual hallucinations, turns at once to Euripides' Orestes.[17] Celsus and Tertullian, simply to mention two more examples, when they are discussing *insania* and the reliability of the senses respectively, naturally bring in Orestes too (and even Soranus did so on one occasion).[18] How did people—both those inside and those outside the various narratives concerned—respond to such phenomena?

When I have discussed fictional texts, I will turn to texts that claim to describe real events, such as those that describe the visions of Paul of Tarsus on the road to Damascus and of Brutus before the Battle of Philippi. And finally I shall turn to the medical and other analytic evidence.

The most recent publication that deals with this topic in any detail is *Ai confini dell'anima* by Giulio Guidorizzi (2010). This respected scholar asserts that the numerous divine epiphanies experienced by waking characters in the Homeric poems (there are by my count about forty in the *Iliad*, notably fewer in the *Odyssey*—but as B.C. Dietrich demonstrated it is often unclear what exactly was supposed to have been seen[19]) mean that having visions of the gods was for Homer's audience about 700 BC an everyday experience (a notion derived from the frankly absurd theory of Julian Jaynes[20]). He recognizes that when similar things happen in later epic poems such as the *Argonautica* and the *Aeneid*, they mean nothing of the kind, for Apollonius and Vergil used divine epiphanies as a conventional plot mechanism. Guidorizzi in effect makes the old error of supposing that Homer sprang fully formed from nowhere: he supposedly related to nothing except real life.

---

[17] *Stoicorum Veterum Fragmenta* II fr. 54. He also brings in Theoclymenos from the *Odyssey* (on whom see below). Orestes again, in a similar context: fr. 65. It hardly needs saying that stories about the heroes had a status quite different from that enjoyed in modern times by even the most iconic of literary heroes; though in fact one might turn to *Don Quixote*, for instance, to find out how hallucinations were regarded in its author's time and place.

[18] Celsus, *De medicina* 3.18.19; Tertullian, *De anima* 17.9. Caelius Aurelianus, *Acute Diseases* 1.122, brings Hercules and Orestes into his discussion of *phrenitis*, and this is a translation of Soranus.

[19] Dietrich 1983. The bibliography is extensive.

[20] *The Origin of Consciousness and the Breakdown of the Bicameral Mind* (Boston, 1976).

Here I leave aside the divine epiphanies that appear in Minoan and Mycenaean art (according to Burkert);[21] and I leave aside all problems about the composition of the Homeric poems; I merely observe, banally enough, that Homer was the heir of an already powerful and sophisticated tradition of oral poetry which had numerous conventions of its own.[22] When Homer's audience listened to his descriptions of divine epiphanies, all it needed was a ready acceptance of the idea that the gods, *at some time in the past* (epic poems are seldom set in an offensively realistic present), had been willing to visit the heroes (for they do not of course visit social riff-raff). It is, however, highly plausible to suppose that somewhere in the more or less remote background of the Homeric epiphanies there lie hallucinations, all the more so because they have some common features with hallucinations as we know them: (a) they are usually audible (and visible when they are visible) to a single individual only—if the bystanders see anything they 'mistakenly' think that it is a human being;[23] and (b) they often give instructions. It is scarcely necessary to say that this evidence tells us nothing whatsoever about the actual incidence or nature of hallucinations in seventh-century Greece.

The Homeric poems describe very few experiences that the poet himself regards as in any sense hallucinatory. The strange scene at the end of *Odyssey* Book 20 (lines 350–370) featuring the Suitors and the prophet Theoclymenos is in fact the only such case: in Odysseus' palace, the prophet sees the walls covered in blood and the court full of ghosts, *eidola*, and presumably he alone sees these things.[24] The scene is a fascinating and artful one: Athena has just plunged the suitors into a fit of insanity which apparently involves their not seeing what is in front of them, cooked meat also running with sinister blood (349) (but then their mood changes—why?). When Theoclymenos says what he can see, one of the suitors—unable to see the same things because he is out of his mind, or because they are only visible to Theoclymenos?—concludes from this (real or supposed) hallucination that the prophet is insane (*aphrainei*, 360), and in consequence should be turned

---

[21] Burkert 1985 [1977], 40.

[22] As to how Homer used divine epiphanies see esp. Dietrich 1983, 70.

[23] Thus in *Iliad* 2.279–282, for example, Athene seems to the Achaeans to be a herald (we are not told here that Odysseus recognizes her, but shortly before this he recognized her from her voice, 182). In 2.781–810 Iris, sent by Zeus, is apparently recognized by Hector as a goddess, but to the other Trojans she seems to be Priam's son Polites.

[24] Commentators give other examples of Greek visions of blood, such as the Delphic oracle in Herodotus 7.140.

out into the market-place. Visual hallucinations are thus proof of insanity, but failing to appreciate that they may be prophetic is also a mark of insanity.

This scene is a minor one. In Athenian tragedy, by contrast, hallucinations, mostly visual, are often at centre stage; that holds for the *Choephori*, the *Persae*, the *Ajax*, the *Orestes*, the *Hercules Furens*, and the *Bacchae*, and hallucinations also make appearances in the *Agamemnon*, in the *Prometheus Vinctus*, in *Iphigeneia in Tauris* and elsewhere.[25] A goodly proportion of the surviving plays.

These tragic hallucinations raise all sorts of questions, religious, dramaturgical, artistic, social and indeed political. I concentrate here on the poets' actual understanding of the phenomenon, as far as it can be discerned. Obviously we shall not expect the dramatists to medicalize visions seen and voices heard—though they do indeed 'show ... interest in the developing medical terminology and treatment' of Hippocratic times.[26] Right from the beginning, however, namely Aeschylus' *Persae*, madness is sometimes regarded as a sickness.[27] And hallucinatory visions are usually in tragedy signs of madness, in all the plays I mentioned with a single apparent exception, the *Persae*: whereas the Queen Atossa, at the time she sees the spectre or ghost (*eidolon*) of Darius, is on the edge of derangement (see lines 604–606; cf. 702),[28] the chorus of Persian elders, who are of sound mind, also see it (lines 694–696). Presumably that is possible because the Athenians by-and-large believed in ghosts, and put seeing ghosts in a different category from seeing other visions (it was not in itself a sign of mental illness).[29]

It is striking that the hallucinatory experiences we see on the Athenian stage, while they almost all have superhuman aspects to them, are also, in every instance, credible psychological case-histories on a purely human

---

[25] For the first six of these plays, see below. The other passages alluded to are *Agamemnon* (Cassandra) 1114–1129, 1214–1222, *PV* (Io) 566–588 (on this scene see S. Said's paper later in this volume), *IT* (Orestes) 267–300. In Euripides' *Helen*, a play teeming with error and deception, Menelaus seems to think for a time (557–604, esp. 575) that he is hallucinating. On the *Alcestis* see n. 28 below.

[26] Collinge 1962, Padel 1995, 159, Papadopoulou 2005, 59.

[27] Aristophanes fr. 322 Kassel and Austin (1984) shows that for the late-fifth century Athenians madness (*mainesthai*) was a sickness on a par with physical sicknesses.

[28] 604–606: 'before my eyes appears the enmity of the gods, and there roars in my ears a cry that is not of good cheer—such a blast of evils terrifies my mind' (not an easy passage to translate). H.D. Broadhead (1960, on 603–606) recognizes 'visual and aural hallucinations' here.

[29] The case of dying Alcestis is similar: when in Euripides, *Alc.* 252–263, she sees and hears Charon summoning her that may be taken as a poeticized version of normal experience.

level.[30] That obviously applies to the experience of Atossa. Even in the *Agamemnon*, where the person who sees the vision is Cassandra, the audience might, I suppose, think of her truth-telling madness as a result of her sufferings as well as of the power of Apollo. More clearly, in the *Choephori*, when Orestes begins to hallucinate the Furies (no one else can see them), they are both a superhuman external force and a result of his own intensifying madness; the human side of the story gains force from the delay that intervenes between the moment when he returns to the stage after murdering his mother (973), still sane but only just (*emphron*, 1026), and the moment when he catches sight of the Furies (1050). In Euripides' *Orestes*, what provokes the hero's on-stage hallucination of the Furies is, convincingly, the fact that Electra, after some forty lines of dialogue with him, suddenly mentions their murdered mother (*Orestes* 249–254).[31] Even in the (endlessly debated) *Ajax*, where Sophocles makes the hallucinatory madness of Ajax the result of the anger of Athena (*Ajax* 762–777), that anger is a consequence of an action—namely Ajax's arrogant refusal of the goddess's help—that reflects a character fault (it is *not* his anger over losing the arms of Achilles to Odysseus that drives him mad).[32]

A character fault also contributes to the hero's hallucinatory madness in another much-debated play, *Hercules Furens*. Heracles mistakes his own children for those of the hated Eurystheus, and kills them.[33] In fact his actual madness has as its sole cause Hera's old anger over the infidelity of Zeus in fathering Heracles in the first place,[34] and this is underlined by the fact that personified Lussa ('Madness') takes over the hero entirely because Hera has told her to. But the direct consequences of Heracles' madness arise from the extreme violence of his character. His murderous revenge against King Lycos, who was on the point of exterminating the hero's family, will have seemed entirely reasonable to the Athenian poet's audience, but the

---

[30] For the hypothetical role of anxiety in the production of hallucinations see al-Issa 1995, 368. The following remarks about tragedy necessarily omit many problems of interpretation. I leave aside the scene in Euripides' *Cyclops* 576–589, where the hallucinations are caused by drunkenness.

[31] 'ELECTRA: Conspicuous for infamy was the race of daughters that Tyndareus fathered—throughout Hellas their names are evil. ORESTES: Then be you different from those wicked ones. You can. And don't just say it, think it too. ELECTRA: Alas my brother, your eyes are wild. Quickly you've changed from good sense to insanity (*lussa*)'.

[32] See further Harris 2001, 174.

[33] Euripides, *HF* 936–1000.

[34] See among others Simon 1978, 135–136, Guardasole 2000, 201–203, Kosak 2004, 169–174, Papadopoulou 2005, esp. 81–83.

next step, murdering the supposed children of Eurystheus, is the act of an uncontrolled man of blood.[35]

Another case that has given rise to endless dispute is the *Bacchae*. My view is in effect that a large part of the play's dramatic brilliance consists in the poet's combination of divine punishment for impiety with a psychologically plausible account of the origins of that impiety. The play contains no fewer than four instances of fantastic hallucinations, three experienced by Pentheus, one by Agaue.[36] All this is embedded in a play that is shot through with Pentheus' other more or less wilful misunderstandings.[37] As for the murderous hallucination of Agaue, it is the culmination of her madness, which was of course wished on to her by Dionysus—not without reason, as we belatedly learn (1302–1303), since she was among those who had rejected him.[38]

In short, Athenian tragedy, taking most hallucinatory experiences as signs of insanity—but always temporary insanity—, combined in various ways both divine and human causation. We can presumably extend this attitude to most of the thinking members of the Athenian audience: in their imagination hallucinations were signs of ill health, which might stem from divine ill-well, but might also be prompted by the inner processes of humans themselves.[39]

An apparent hallucination in Menander's mostly lost play *Phasma* ('The Apparition') leads to a suggestion of quack medical treatment.[40] The unidentifiable New Comedy dramatist who wrote the play on which Plautus based the *Menaechmi* introduced a scene of feigned madness. The symptoms included the apparent sufferer's hearing the voice of Apollo (ordering him to commit murder) and his imagining that he is riding in a chariot. The response of the other characters to this madness is medical not religious.[41]

---

[35] To justify this problematical reading in full would require a disproportionate amount of space. Heracles' extreme violence, it may be noted, is already visible when he threatens a general massacre of ungrateful Thebans (ll. 568–573). For a fuller discussion see D. Konstan's paper later in this volume.

[36] 617–621, 630–631, 918–922 (Pentheus), 1114–1278 (Agaue).

[37] Cf. Leinieks 1996, chapter 10, not to be agreed with on all points.

[38] Thus while it is true in a sense that 'Agave's deranged act as a mad woman completely contravenes the behaviour we might expect of her character' (Thumiger 2007, 98), this discounts too much the seriousness of her 'offence'.

[39] Drabkin 1955, 224, detects a 'naturalistic' attitude towards insanity in *Orestes* and *Iphigeneia in Tauris*.

[40] At least this seems the best way of taking ll. 47–56 Sandbach = 22–31 Arnott.

[41] The hallucinations: *Menaechmi* 862–871; cf. 840–841, 849. The response: 872–875, 882–888.

(The doctor who is summoned makes a fool of himself, however).[42] Elsewhere in the play it is nonetheless assumed that madness can be treated by religious means.[43]

Let us turn now to texts that purport to describe actual real-world hallucinatory events. Our evidence is skewed towards miraculous epiphanies, often featuring gods or heroes. The earliest important case is Herodotus' story telling how the runner Pheidippides/Philippides encountered and was addressed by the god Pan, at a lonely spot in the mountains (6.105).[44] The historian emphasizes that the Athenians believed Pheidippides' account, which seems to hint that he, Herodotus, had some reservations about its truth.[45] A modern scholar is likely to say that either Pheidippides was lying, or he experienced a hallucination of the type that certain kinds of people ('primitives' in the older terminology) may quite easily encounter in lonely landscapes.[46] What would Herodotus have said if he had discussed the matter more fully? He might have said that the choice was between supposing that Pheidippides had lied or accepting that he had really seen the god Pan; but we cannot entirely exclude the possibility that he might have offered a purely psychological explanation such as Aristotle would have been capable of formulating (see below).

Divine epiphanies are of course innumerable in the ancient sources—even the catalogue of the gods who appeared during battles is a fairly long one.[47] None of them is known to us from eyewitness accounts and almost none even from contemporary sources: one such is commemorated by an Athenian inscription probably put up to honour the dead after the Battle of Koroneia in 447 BC, and it is remarkable because the demigod who appeared

---

[42] Stok 1996, 2291–2296. See also Most, this volume p. 396.

[43] *Menaechmi* 288–292, 310–315, with Stok 2303–2310.

[44] 'Pheidippides used to say, and he told the Athenians, that Pan came suddenly upon him [*prospiptei*] on Mount Parthenion above Tegea. Pan, he said, called out his name and told him to ask of the Athenians why they paid him no attention, in spite of his benevolence towards them and his often having been useful to them in the past, as he would be again in the future. When their affairs were once more in fair shape, the Athenians trusted that this story was true, and they built a shrine of Pan under the Acropolis, and ever since this message they court him with annual sacrifices and a torch-race'.

[45] One recalls the detachment with which Herodotus recounts the story that at the Battle of Marathon the Athenian Epizelos saw the *phasma* of a giant hoplite (6.117).

[46] If one wants to elaborate a rationalistic approach, it is worth recalling that Pheidippides was probably dehydrated and under great stress. Cf. n. 30. 'Food and water deprivation are also generally recognized as conducive to the experience of hallucination' (Slade and Bentall 1988, 32; for the effects of stress see ibid. 84–92).

[47] Pritchett 1979, 11–46.

helped the other side (the Boeotians) defeat the Athenians (which was of course a good excuse).[48] But the general pattern is intriguing: high classical writers tend to distance themselves from such stories with such formulae as 'they say that ...'; the exceptions are the relatively credulous Justin and Pausanias.[49] Some epiphanies are recorded in civic inscriptions.[50] Otherwise all unequivocal claims that gods had made appearances in war come from religious sources such as Delphi or the temple of Athena at Lindos.[51] Such stories were generally judged to be either true or false. Did anyone suppose that sometimes they were subjectively true but the product of fantasy or fear? Epicureans and philosophers of the New Academy must sometimes have come close to this position, but the tendency of sceptics, as far as I can tell, was rather to suppose that such stories were conscious human inventions.[52]

However the most famous of all real-life pre-Christian hallucinations, if that is what it was, must be Socrates' *daimonion*. For two generations now,[53] Socrates has been seen by many scholars as a mythical figure about whom rather little can be known, especially perhaps with regard to his religiosity; so both the facts and contemporary reactions are hard to recover. In Plato's later years, it was already part of the Socrates myth that he had special access to truth-telling dreams.[54] As for his *daimonion*, one may be puzzled by the fact that on one occasion (*Phaedrus* 242c),[55] Socrates is represented as saying that he 'seemed' to hear the voice (*edoxa*). However Plato's language is consistent with real hallucinations. The word *edoxa* should not worry us, since the noun *doxa*, as I noted earlier, is regularly used to refer to hallucinations that really were perceived. Plato is in fact reasonably clear when he says in *Apology* 31d that 'something divine and *daimonion* comes to me ... I have had this from my childhood; it is a voice of some sort or

---

[48] Pritchett 26. An important fifth-century case is the Stoa Poikile at Athens, where the paintings showed various figures who had appeared at the Battle of Marathon (large bibliography).

[49] When Dionysius of Halicarnassus (*Roman Antiquities* 2.68) protests against 'those who ridicule all the epiphanies of the gods which have taken place either among the Greeks or among the barbarians', he seems to feel outnumbered.

[50] Cf. Pritchett 1979, 44.

[51] For cases of the latter type see Pritchett 22, 29–30.

[52] Cf. again Dionysius of Halicarnassus, *Roman Antiquities* 2.68, where the key word is *alazoneiais*.

[53] Since Gigon 1947.

[54] Harris 2009, 25, 161.

[55] For a succinct account of Plato's and Xenophon's testimony on this topic see Guthrie 1969, 402–404. For a more detailed analysis see esp. Long 2005.

other (*phone tis*) that comes to me ...'.[56] And Xenophon too clearly thought (*Apologia* 12) that Socrates really did hear a voice. Both authors, and no doubt Socrates himself, must have thought that a superhuman being was somehow involved—a *daimon* in fact.[57] Socrates heard it often (*Apol.* 40ab, *Euthydemus* 272e). What is most interesting perhaps is that while Socrates' disciples evidently treated the phenomenon with respect, there seems to be no evidence that even his numerous contemporary detractors tried to use it as proof that he was mad.[58]

Plato also refers to a phenomenon well known to modern students of hallucinations, namely hallucinatory visions of the recently deceased.[59] In the *Phaedo* (81cd) Socrates tells us that 'we should suppose that the body is burdensome and heavy and earthly and visible. And such a soul [of a person who has been devoted to his body] is weighed down by this and is dragged back into the visible world, out of fear of the invisible and of Hades, and so, as they say, it flits about the monuments and tombs, where shadowy apparitions [*phantasmata*] of souls have been seen, images [*eidola*] of those souls that have not been completely released but partake of the visible and for that reason are seen'. For Plato, who also refers in the *Laws* (11.927a) to dead souls 'that concern themselves with human affairs', that is simply a natural fact, and not apparently one that reflects on the sanity of those who have seen such visions.[60] Given the religious and artistic background in Athens, that is just what we ought to have expected.[61]

In later times, educated persons often seem to have been ambivalent about stories that claimed to describe hallucinatory visions that were supposed to have taken place in historical time. This ambivalence is nicely dramatized by Plutarch in his life of Brutus: during the preparations for

---

[56] The word *tis* may refer to the voice's uncertain origin and is not evidence that what Socrates heard was only something like a voice.

[57] I see no reason at all, contrary to McPherran 2011, 125, to suppose that Socrates, or anyone else, thought that Apollo was 'behind' the *daimonion*.

[58] Unless Aristophanes, *Clouds* 357, contains an allusion, which I very much doubt. Gigon 1947, 166 and 175, argued that Plato was embarrassed by Socrates' *daimon*, and this view may be supported by Plato's use of the allusive phrase *daimonion semeion* (*Apol.* 40b and c, *Rep.* 6.496c, etc.). But Plato's stress on Socrates' heroic nature (as the recipient of veridical dreams, for example) suggests otherwise.

[59] See Aleman and Larøi 2008, 31, 67–68.

[60] Other authors who refer to visions of the recently deceased: Hippocrates, *On Diseases* 2.72 (below, p. 302), Lucretius 1.131–135 (below, p. 304), Augustine, *Epist.* 158.8.

[61] Figures who may have represented the dead appeared on the third day of the Anthesteria every spring (Burkert 1985, 237–242, etc.). Athenian funerary *lekythoi* often show a life-like *eidolon* of the dead person appearing to a survivor (Oakley 2004, esp. 165–168).

the Battle of Philippi, Brutus experienced a 'great sign' in the form of a 'monstrous and fearful shape' that visited him one night in his tent, and spoke to him.[62] His slaves neither heard nor saw anything. Cassius, however, being informed of this visitation, would have none of it, since he was notoriously an Epicurean: 'perception by the senses is a pliant and deceptive thing', he is made to say, and especially untrustworthy when one is physically exhausted.[63] Plutarch, for his part, seems to have been embarrassed by the tradition about Socrates' *daimonion*,[64] perhaps—though this is not at all clear—because 'hearing voices' had become, over the intervening 500 years, more of a symptom of mental disorder.[65] This embarrassment may re-appear when an authoritative speaker in *On the* daimonion *of Socrates* argues that 'what reached him [Socrates] was not, one would conjecture, spoken language (*phthongos*) but the words of a *daimon* making contact with his intelligence *without a voice* by the revelation of their sense alone'.[66]

What actually happened to Paul of Tarsus on the road to Damascus is wholly unrecoverable, but the story as told in Acts (three times, with variations) is nonetheless of interest here, because it shows that a story that has clear marks of describing a hallucination could readily be used, in the milieux in which Acts circulated and early Christian proselytization took place, as by no means a sign of mental disorder but, quite the contrary,

---

[62] *Brutus* 36: 'It was the middle of the night, his tent was dimly lit, and the whole camp was wrapped in silence. As he was thinking and reflecting, he thought he perceived (*aisthesthai*) someone coming into the tent. Turning his eyes towards the entrance he beheld a strange and dreadful apparition (*opsin*), consisting of a monstrous and fearful shape standing silently by his side. Summoning up the courage to question it, 'Who are you', he asked, 'man or god, and what do you want with me?'. The phantom (*phasma*) replied, 'Brutus, I am your evil spirit (*daimon*). You will see me at Philippi'. Brutus said calmly, 'I shall see you''. Plutarch also told this story in *Caesar* 69, drawing the conclusion that the assassination of Caesar had not pleased the gods.

[63] *Brutus* 37: 'This is our doctrine, that ... the intelligence (*dianoia*) is rather keen to alter and transform what is perceived from something that has no real existence into any shape it likes. ... the imagination (*to phantastikon*) is by nature in continual motion, and this motion is imagination (*phantasia*) or thought. In your case too the body is under stress, which naturally excites and deceives your mind. As for *daimones*, it is incredible that they exist, and if they do that they have the appearance or the speech of humans, or a power that extends to us ...'.

[64] *On the* daimonion *of Socrates* 11 = *Moralia* 581b and d.

[65] Cicero, *De divinatione* 1.122–124, avoids referring to the famous sign as a *vox*. According to Josephus (*Contra Apionem* 2.263), some people said that Socrates was joking; the notion evidently appealed to Josephus not because it would have saved Socrates from being thought insane, but from being thought blasphemous. Apuleius, however, in *De deo Socratis* expresses no embarrassment that Socrates should have heard a *daemon*, indeed he suggests (21) that Socrates probably saw the *daemon* too.

[66] *On the* daimonion *of Socrates* 20 = *Moralia* 588e.

as an unequivocal sign from God (though many contemporaries obviously rejected this view).[67] Seeing Apollo struck (some) Greeks and Romans as a sign of madness; seeing Jesus after his death would no doubt have struck some of them in the same way, but to some others it seemed an authentic epiphany.

We should probably also think that a few at least of the more than 1,300 *ex iussu* and similar inscriptions catalogued and analysed by Gil Renberg—inscriptions in honour of gods set up by diverse ordinary Greeks and Romans on the command of the god in question[68]—resulted from hallucinatory experiences. Yet the lack of explicit epigraphical testimony about appearances to individuals[69] suggests that such incidents will have been quite rare.

For those well-educated persons who, however, lacked deep knowledge of philosophy it was not easy to exclude the superhuman. Pliny junior (*Letters* 7.27) and Tacitus (*Annals* 11.21) both tell how Curtius Rufus, a man of undistinguished birth who was an assistant to the governor of the province of Africa Proconsularis (this will have been while Tiberius was emperor), 'was strolling alone at midday in a deserted colonnade' at Hadrumetum when a female figure of superhuman size appeared to him. (In ancient dreams, divine figures and divine messengers were commonly described as being of unusual height).[70] She announced that she was 'Africa' and that she had come to foretell Curtius' future: one day, he would return to this province as its governor, and die there. And sure enough, thanks to powerful patrons and his own energy, Curtius rose through the senatorial ranks to become governor of that province; and having seen the same figure on his return to Africa, he duly died there. Several observations are in order. One has to be that Curtius must originally have told the story about himself, and been believed, at least by many; presumably it helped him to gain

---

[67] Acts 9:3–19, 22:6–11, 26:12–16. It is interesting that the motif of the country road should recur. In chapter 9, Paul heard a voice and also apparently saw Jesus (v. 17; but 22.7 contradicts this) as well as a blinding light, but his companions, though they heard the voice 'saw no one'. In chapter 22 they do not even hear the voice. The core of the experience is in any case private and a set of commands. Paul alludes to the event in a very vague fashion in Galatians 1:16. There are of course a number of other visions in the NT: J.B.F. Miller 2007 provides bibliography.

[68] Renberg 2003. It is to be hoped that a revised version of this work will soon appear in print.

[69] Of all these texts only one, a Greek text of the second century AD from Rome (*Inscriptiones Graecae Urbis Romae* 184, Renberg no. 681), specifies that the author had encountered a god face to face)—and it was Pan. See further Renberg 2010, 48–49.

[70] For numerous examples see Pfister 1924, cols. 314–315.

high-level patronage. Pliny probably represents a widespread upper-class attitude when he says (7.27.1) that Curtius' story encouraged him (Pliny) to believe that *phantasmata*, ghostly figures, exist that possess *numen aliquod*, some sort of divine nature,—though he also holds that such visions may be caused by fear.[71] Tacitus, however, contents himself with the fact that Curtius saw and heard the female figure and later 'fulfilled the fateful omen'; for him it is a good story and that is enough.

Another good story, better-known, appears in Plutarch's essay *On the Obsolescence of Oracles* 17 (*Moralia* 419b–d). A merchant ship carrying many passengers sailed from Greece to Italy. One evening, the wind dropped and the ship drifted near the island of Paxos. While almost everyone on board was awake, there suddenly came from the island the voice of someone loudly calling one Thamus, which happened to be the name of the Egyptian who was the steersman. Twice Thamus was called and made no reply, but the third time he answered, and the caller, raising his voice, said, 'When you come opposite to Palodes, announce that 'Great Pan is dead''. Thamus did what he was told, and even before he had finished saying 'Great Pan is dead', there was a great cry of lamentation, not of one person but of many (the point of the story was to show that *daimones* such as Pan could die). As quite a number of people were on board, the story soon spread, and Thamus was sent for by the emperor Tiberius, who became thoroughly convinced that the story was true. Scholars have offered various interpretations of all this;[72] here it is enough to say, first, that while an hallucination may possibly have been at the root of this sequence of events, it was as a story quite *sui generis*;[73] secondly, while no one in Plutarch's dialogue expresses any surprise that the travellers believed that something supernatural had happened, the attitude of the author and his contemporaries remains undefined (there may be some implication that Tiberius was too credulous).

Both the status of the witness and the exact nature of the experience would of course influence how it was taken. When the controversialist Celsus wanted to discredit the supposed resurrection of Jesus, he pointed out that Mary Magdalen was (a) female and (b) insane;[74] thus she was

---

[71] For his continuing uncertainty see 7.27.15. Compare Lucan's comment, à propos of the macabre portents and omens he describes before and after the Battle of Pharsalus (many people saw Mount Pindus colliding with Olympus, and so on): 'one cannot know whether they believed because of prodigies sent by the gods or because of their excessive terror'.

[72] See Borgeaud 1983.

[73] Quite different from the stories in which people saw and/or heard Pan himself (see above and cf. Longus 2.26–29, where Pan produces diverse effects and appears in a dream).

[74] Origen, *Contra Celsum* 2.59, 60.

doubly untrustworthy as a witness in the eyes of any ancient male.[75] He further pointed out that many people had seen *phantasmata* of the dead among the tombs (and this was undoubtedly true—see above, p. 297): hence seeing Jesus alive after the crucifixion was nothing extraordinary.[76] The Magdalen's dubious status was probably what led to the early creation of other versions of the resurrection story that depended on her less or not at all.[77] Origen, however, reasons that the Magdalen can only have been deluded (hallucinating) if she had been one of those who are 'completely out of their minds and suffering from *phrenitis*'—which notwithstanding the gospels he denies (they of course attribute her condition to demons not sickness). But this will not mean that Origen held that hallucinatory experiences always had natural causes, as distinct from being the work of demons.

As noted earlier, our evidence is skewed towards hallucination narratives that feature epiphanies of one kind or another. What would the same writers have said about less dramatic and less intelligible hallucinations? Before answering let us consider what medical, naturalistic and philosophical writers have to say about such phenomena.

We can turn first to the Hippocratic texts, namely *Internal Affections* 48, together with *Prognostic* 4, *Diseases* 2.72, *Glands* 12, and *Diseases of Girls*. In *Internal Affections* 48 the patient who is suffering from such-and-such a complaint (it cannot be identified) thinks pieces of wool in his blanket are lice; and later 'there seem to appear before his eyes reptiles and every other sort of beast, and hoplites fighting, and he imagines himself to be fighting among them; he speaks out as if he is seeing such things .... When he ceases to be out of his mind, he immediately regains his senses .... This illness mostly befalls people when they are in other lands and if they are travelling a lonely road and fear seizes them because of an apparition ...'.[78] From

---

[75] Most 2005, 13, mentions in this context the 'uncontestedly low status [of women] as witnesses in first-century Palestine'.

[76] *Contra Celsum* 2.60.

[77] The versions that make the Magdalen the original witness are in Mark and John: Mk 16:9–11, 'from whom he had formerly cast out seven devils' (there is no need here to discuss the textual problem raised by this passage), Jn 20:10–18. In Lk 24:1–32 the first witnesses are men (cf. also I Cor. 15:5); in Mt 28:8–8 the Magdalen and 'the other Mary' are the first witnesses. In a Protestant work of reference Fuller 1993, 648, dodges all difficulties by saying that the resurrection was 'not historical in the sense that ordinary events are' (contrast I Cor. 15:14), a fine example of what Morton Smith used to call 'pseudo-orthodoxy'. Controversial writers on this topic sometimes debate whether a hallucination was in question.

[78] See Dodds 1951, 131 n. 90. But the words 'because of an apparition (*phasmatos*)' were an unwarranted addition by the editor Littré.

these passages it is clear that the Hippocratic doctors were familiar with visual hallucinations and regarded them as standard symptoms of various illnesses, such as *phrenitis*,[79] that ill-defined form of madness which figures so largely in ancient medical discussions of mental illness. In *Glands* 12 the author writes about a certain kind of brain illness that 'reason is disturbed and the victim goes about thinking and seeing alien things, bearing this type of disease with grinning laughter and grotesque visions [*phantasmasin*]'. *Diseases of Girls* refers twice in a few pages to visual hallucinations, without fitting them into a specific nosological framework.

One might ask whether the distrust of the senses that is a marked feature of Greek philosophy from an early date made it easier to fit hallucinations into a secular thought-world. The central pre-Aristotelian text here is the *Theaetetus*, since it has so much to say about sensation, and though it mentions misperceptions only in passing, it is evidently alluding to hallucinations (see above), and thus testifies to the fact that the high culture could treat them as part of the natural world. Unfortunately the topic is not pursued,[80] even though it could have helped Socrates to 'refute' the theory that knowledge is sensation.

As far as a naturalistic understanding of hallucinations is concerned, the next important text is a passage in Aristotle's treatise *On Dreams* (2.460b3–16):[81]

> [while awake], we are easily deceived with respect to our perceptions while we are in the grip of passion [*en tois pathesin*], different people being affected in different ways, a coward when he is afraid, a lustful person when he is excited. The former, on the basis of a slight resemblance, seems (*dokei*) to see his enemies, the latter his beloved. The more passionate he is, the slighter the resemblance that gives rise to these impressions. In the same way, everyone becomes prone to being deceived while they are dominated by anger or by any appetite .... That is why animals sometimes appear on the walls to people

---

[79] *Prognostic* 4: 'they hunt in the empty air ... snatch chaff from the walls—all these signs are bad and deathly'; *Diseases* 2.72: 'the [*phrenitis*] patient is afraid, and sees terrible things and frightening dreams and sometimes the dead'.

[80] Cf. Bostock 1988, 75.

[81] The claim is false that 'it was the early Christian writers who first systematically considered the nature of hallucinatory experiences' (Slade and Bentall 1988, 4–5, misled by Sarbin and Juhasz 1967). It is also incorrect to say that 'hallucination' first appears in English in a translation of Ludwig Lavater's *De spectris, lemuribus et magnis atque insolitis fragoribus* (Geneva, 1570) (*Of Ghostes and Spirites Walking by Nyght*, London, 1572) (Slade and Bentall 7, deceived once again by Sarbin and Juhasz 1967). The word was first used in a sense resembling its modern one by Sir Thomas Browne in 1646, who coined a number of other terms. By 1646 the text of Caelius Aurelianus (see above, n. 9) had been printed several times.

in a fever, from a slight resemblance in the combination of lines ... if they are not seriously ill, they are aware of the illusion (*pseudos*), whereas if their condition is more serious, they react by moving around ....[82]

In other words, visual hallucinations come not just to those who are physically ill but to those who are in certain psychological states, which Aristotle identifies, using the categories that were available to him, as more-or-less extreme passions or desires. Some interpreters appear to think that what Aristotle is discussing here is simply one-shot errors, such as mistaking the identity of someone on the other side of the street,[83] and 'everyone becomes prone to being deceived' supports such a view. But the reference to fever strongly suggests that Aristotle also has hallucinations in mind, even if he is not thinking of them exclusively. Not that Aristotle seems to have been much interested in hallucinations—there is little if anything about them in *On the Soul* or *On Sensation*. So we are left with more questions than answers (amid the huge scholarly literature that Aristotle's philosophy of mind has generated). Presumably he held that they were the work not of the senses but of what he calls *phantasia* (cf. *On the Soul* 3.3). The view that intense emotion was liable to produce hallucinations has no known Hippocratic antecedent, and one wonders what experience lay behind this opinion. It is in any case obvious that Aristotle's views about hallucinations, like his views about dreaming, will have been entirely naturalistic.

Stoics and Epicureans alike offered naturalistic explanations of visual hallucinatory experiences. Chrysippus (see above, n. 17) refers to visual hallucinations as *phantasmata*; they occur, he says to people who are suffering from *melancholia* or madness.[84] Lucretius deals with the subject briefly, promising at the beginning of his work that he will discuss the sources of the hallucinations of the dead that are experienced by the sick and by healthy people in dreams (1.131–135). In Book IV, however, he liquidates the subject in two lines with a mention of the *simulacra* that fly through the air and bring frightening images to people both waking and sleeping (4.26–44, esp. 33–34).[85] He may also allude to hallucinations later when he talks about our 'seeing' the dead (4.732–734), though it is the mind not the eyes that is doing the 'seeing'

---

[82] Freely translated, with an acknowledgement to the version by David Gallop (1991).

[83] Van Der Eijk 1994, 197, for instance, refers to the errors in question as 'Sinnestäuschungen'.

[84] Chrysippus also supposedly said that every inferior (*phaulos*) person was insane: *Stoicorum Veterum Fragmenta* III no. 663.

[85] Commentators have been concerned about the fact that the first passage but not the second refers to things seen by the sick.

there.[86] The *phasmata* and *phantasiai* referred to by Diogenes of Oenoanda fragment 10 are probably visually hallucinatory experiences,[87] but he simply expressed a normal Epicurean view about them.

In the first two centuries of our era, medical understandings of hallucinations continued of course to be naturalistic; that is what we find in Celsus, Aretaeus and Galen.[88] Celsus describes a form of fever-accompanied mental illness (*insania*) which he calls *phrenesis* (clearly the condition that others called *phrenitis*): if this grows intense, the patient 'receives certain unreal images' ('quasdam vanas imagines accipit') (3.18.3); when it is fully developed, 'the mind is completely subjected to those images'. (Various dreadful instructions follow about how such patients should be treated). Then there is a different kind of *insania*, in which the patients 'imaginibus, non mente falluntur', like Ajax and Orestes (3.18.19), which seems to mean that (visual) hallucinations are their principal or only symptom. To know how to treat such a patient, the most important thing is to see whether the patient is sad or cheerful.

Aretaeus is slightly more detailed: he describes both auditory and visual hallucinations as symptoms of mental illness,[89] while Galen expands on the passage in Hippocrates, *Prognostic* 4, that was mentioned earlier,[90] and elsewhere describes the case of Theophilus (also mentioned earlier), who imagined that flute-players were playing in his house all day and all night

----

[86] 'Many images [*simulacra*] of things are moving about in many ways and in all directions, very thin, which easily unite in the air when they meet, since they are like spiders' webs or leaf of gold. They are in fact much thinner in texture than those that take the eyes and assail the vision, since these penetrate through the interstices of the body, awake the thin substance of the mind within, and assail the sense of sight. Thus it is that we see Centaurs and the limbs of Scyllas and faces of Cerberus and images of those for whom death is past and their bones rest in the earth, since images of all kinds are being carried about everywhere, some that come into being spontaneously in the air itself, others that are thrown off from all sorts of things, and others again that are made of a combination of these shapes ...'.

[87] See M.F. Smith 1993.

[88] And that is clearly what we would have found in Soranus, to judge from the work of Caelius Aurelianus.

[89] *On the Causes and Signs of Chronic Diseases* 1.6: 'They [victims of *phrenitis*] misperceive things, and see things that are not present, and things that are invisible to others appear to them to be visible; those who are suffering from *mania* on the other hand see as they ought to ... [But as *mania* progresses] some experience ringings and rumblings in the ears which can even sound like trumpets and flutes ... If the illness turns towards *melancholia*, dark-blue or black images appear before their eyes, whereas those who are suffering from *mania* see red or purple images, which to many seem like lightning flashes ...'.

[90] *Commentary on Hippocrates' Prognosticon* 1.23 (VI.71–75 K): 'those who are suffering from acute fever, pneumonia, *phrenitis* or headache think that they see outside themselves things that are within their own eyes ...'; he explains this at some length.

(*On the Differences of Symptoms* 3 = VII.60–61 K)—'this was the form of his insanity (*paraphrosune*)'. None of these three authors makes any blanket statement about hallucinations, and it is worth remembering that Galen's views about dreams were by no means wholly rationalistic;[91] but it is highly unlikely that they left any room for hallucinations of supernatural origin.

Christians took various views. Tertullian's opinion—apart obviously from his belief in the resurrection of Jesus—conformed to what has emerged as the general view of educated Greeks and Romans of high classical times, namely that visual hallucinations were a natural phenomenon that accompanied more or less specific mental disorders. Defending the reliability of the senses, Tertullian (*De Anima* 17.9) attributes the famous hallucinations of Orestes, Ajax and Agaue to their *furiae*, but it is reasonably plain that he means by that not some demonic beings but their naturally occurring insanity (Furiae in the former sense had no part in the stories of Ajax or Agaue, as Tertullian knew).[92]

Early Christian thinking about the status of waking visions is too large a subject for this paper.[93] I note, however, that Augustine, while he is aware that the fever of *phrenetici* can lead to visual hallucinations, also holds that they may also be caused by the involvement of 'some other spirit, whether evil or good'[94] (all this in *De Genesi ad litteram* 12.12.25).[95] (He also thinks that they may result from 'nimia cogitationis intentione'—excessive mental concentration—, an idea for which I find no exact parallel in earlier texts). The effect of this is that a hallucinating person may see at the same time someone who is really present and someone who is not. He claims to have had personal contact with such persons, 'who talked with those who were not there'—that is to say experienced combined auditory and visual hallucinations—, and claims that when the experience is over some can describe it and others cannot.[96] What matters here, however, is the return to high intellectual respectability of the view that a hallucinatory experience may be caused by an external being.

---

[91] Harris 2009, 209–212.

[92] 'Those who are insane, such as Orestes ... Will you blame their eyes for these falsehoods, or their *furiae*? To those who suffer from jaundice through an excess of bile, all things are bitter ...'. For the *furiae* of Hercules see also *Ad Nationes* 2.14.8.

[93] On the connection between asceticism and hallucinations see esp. Dulaey 1973, 52–55, 95.

[94] 'conmixtione cuiusquam alterius spiritus seu mali seu boni'.

[95] Unfortunately the account of this text provided by Aleman and Larøi 2008, 10–11, is confused.

[96] I have found little about forgetting in the scientific literature on hallucinations.

What conclusions should we draw? First, there is in fact no readily detectable development in the understanding of hallucinatory experiences between the Hippocratics and the fourth century AD. It is certainly possible, however, that Athenians (and other Greeks) of the fifth century BC had a more vivid sense of the possibility of hallucinatory experiences caused by superhuman forces than anyone, any educated person at least, ever did again until the age of Augustine, whose allusion to the operation of good and evil spirits we have just noted. But this obviously does not mean that a rationalistic view reigned uncontested, even among the educated, in the intervening era: we have seen plenty of evidence to the contrary. As for interaction between the views of different kinds of people, it has to be admitted that popular views are largely unknowable. 'We observe the demon-possessed, the smelly and noisy from the arch point of view of upper-class writers of philosophy or fiction, but still have no idea what it felt like to be one of them', writes Dench,[97] with some understandable exaggeration.

Both medicine and philosophy most definitely led the lay-person towards a secular understanding of hallucinatory experiences—but who was willing to follow? Doctors seldom if ever wrote about Orestes, but for anyone else who had even a moderate education, he was real enough, and it was easy to think that his 'Furies' were outside him. No doubt, in the end, one's ideas about whether the ravings of an insane person were demon-inspired or a sad fact of natural life will have depended on vastly variable circumstances of culture and temperament.

---

[97] Dench 2011, 27.

CURE AND (IN)CURABILITY OF MENTAL DISORDERS IN ANCIENT MEDICAL AND PHILOSOPHICAL THOUGHT*

Philip van der Eijk

Introduction

How do accounts of mental disorders in Greek and Roman medical and philosophical texts address the question of the treatment of these conditions? Are such mental conditions deemed curable or not, and if not, for what reasons? What criteria are mentioned in the texts to distinguish between curable and incurable conditions? And, if cure is deemed possible, what does it look like?

A comprehensive discussion of these issues is obviously impossible within the limited scope of this paper; but I will try to summarise what I think is the broader picture, and illustrate these points with five examples, taken from different authors and time frames in the Graeco-Roman world.[1] First, we will consider the account of intelligence (*phronêsis*), lack of intelligence (*aphrosunê*) and various intermediate states, as well as the treatment

---

* I am grateful to William Harris for his invitation and for his generous patience, and to the participants at the conference for their comments. This paper has arisen from the research project 'Medicine of the Mind, Philosophy of the Body—Discourses of Health and Well Being in the Ancient World', based at the Humboldt University, Berlin, and supported by the Alexander von Humboldt Foundation.

[1] Even within the restrictions of this paper to medical and philosophical texts (thus excluding literary, historiographical, epigraphic and archaeological sources), no claim to comprehensiveness can be made. Much could be said on the ways in which medical authors such as Celsus, Aretaeus and Caelius Aurelianus conceptualise mental illness (cf. the discussion in Caelius Aurelianus, *Acute Affections* III.13.109–111, of the question whether *hydrophobia* is a mental or a physical illness) and address the treatment of mental disorders such as *phrenitis, lêthargos, apoplexia, mania*, or *melancholia*, including the use of light therapy (Aretaeus, Caelius Aurelianus) and music (Aretaeus); see the discussions by Drabkin 1955; Simon 1978; Gill 1985; Stok 1996 (with extensive bibliography), Pigeaud 1987, 2008a and 2008b; and McDonald 2009; and on the 'therapy of the word' in ancient medicine see Lain Entralgo 1970. Another area that would require a discussion in its own right is the whole discourse of Stoic and Epicurean philososophy as a 'medicine of the mind'; see Nussbaum 1994 and Gill 2010. For discussion of the theme 'incurability' in Hippocratic texts (though not focused on mental illnesses) see von Staden 1988.

recommended for these states, in the medical work *Regimen*, chs. 35–36; then we will turn to Plato's discussion of the two types of diseases of the soul (*nosoi peri psuchên*) and their treatment in the *Timaeus*, and to Aristotle's discussion of degrees of curability in his account of weakness of will (*akrasia*) in *Nicomachean Ethics* VII. We will then take a big chronological leap and move to the second century CE, to Galen's approach to mental illness and to the diagnosis and treatment of affections and errors of the soul, and to Ptolemy's account of affections of the soul and their varying modes of curability in the *Tetrabiblos*.

In doing so, we will find some fundamental issues recurring. The very concept of mental versus physical illness, how that distinction was made and defined, how it was applied in ancient medical and philosophical discourse and how it affected the question of treatment and cure, is of course deeply problematic. This question is discussed, at a much more fundamental level, elsewhere in this volume, but it cannot be entirely avoided here.

Yet it is not just the adjective mental that raises problems, but also the noun to which it is to be connected. For at least equally important is the question of what kind of states, or conditions, or characteristics, we are concerned with. In talking about the ancient material, we tend to use expressions such as mental illness, condition, disturbance, dysfunctioning, disorder, failure, deficiency or impairment, as if they were interchangeable and as if it were clear what they included or excluded. However, as we are acutely aware from today's medical discourse, such terms are not value-free, and one has to be extremely careful in their usage, as they have implications for the way people who are believed to be affected by such conditions are being perceived, labelled, categorised and indeed stigmatised by society, by policy makers and health insurance companies. The example of disability studies, and the historiography of disability, has shown how difficult it is here to develop a terminology that does not prejudge such issues of categorisation and at the same time takes due account of the problem of matching historical and contemporary terminology.

Furthermore, a term such as disorder would seem to exclude states that are considered not necessarily pathological but for which treatment is nevertheless available, in ancient texts as well as in modern society. For example, grief and bereavement in the ancient world were the subject of an extensive *consolatio* literature, and we may think of similar modes of counselling, coaching and guidance in today's world. Clearly, in antiquity, as today, one did not have to be ill in order to qualify for therapy, treatment or care of some sort or the other.

As far as the Graeco-Roman world is concerned, the texts present a great variety of states of mind (to use another expression that is meant to be neutral and descriptive, yet is already invested with a number of assumptions), ranging from what we would call clinical conditions to character flaws, cognitive as well as moral and behavioural failure. Sometimes, the conditions mentioned in the ancient texts are presented as acute mental disturbances, e.g. delirium, paralysis or stroke, offering little hope of cure and often resulting in death or permanent disability within a few days. Yet many of them are described in ways that would make us regard them as chronic conditions, long-term structural states that manifest themselves in periodic bouts or outbursts or in recurring erratic behaviour; here, treatment often does not seem to aim at cure but rather at making the situation manageable or bearable.

The fundamental question here is how to categorise these phenomena, whether they are clinical or moral, cognitive or behavioural. This has important implications for the question of responsibility and blame. To put it crudely, is the insane person responsible for his actions or is his illness to blame for his behaviour? How did he get mad in the first place? Is he to blame for this, or those responsible for his upbringing, or society at large? Or is his condition congenital, or perhaps the product of natural and environmental factors beyond human control?

These are not just modern questions, for ancient authors were well aware of these issues. They realised that attempts in early Greek medicine and natural philosophy to explain the extremes of human mental health or illness in natural terms came dangerously close to a reductionist view of mental life and a determinist, if not racial view of human psychological ability. When discussing outstanding intellectual achievement or error, creativity or stupidity, moral excellence or depravity, ecstatic joy or pathological despondency, the question arises whether this is all down to one's physiological temperament, one's *krasis*, the balance of humours and qualities in one's body—or, to mention a modern equivalent, is mental health, or the lack of it, all down to one's genes?

Philosophers like Plato and Aristotle were well aware of these issues. They refused to accept the materialist implications of some medical and naturalistic theories. Their position was that although the influence of the body on the soul can be very profound and extend even to cognitive faculties like memory and discursive thought, this does not mean that mental states and processes are necessarily *governed* by physical states. This, they argued, is only the case when something has gone wrong in the structure or management of the psycho-physical composite of the human organism, in the way it has come about and has been developed and maintained. By contrast, they argued, the combination of a frugal, healthy regimen with philosophy, as a kind of care for the soul, can enable people to resist the movements of the body and even impose their will on bodily states.

They also realised that these issues have implications for the question of curability, and the nature of the cure proposed. For ancient authors (medical as well as philosophical) argued that even if a particular mental condition may be natural or congenital, that does not mean that one cannot do anything about it. Hence they made distinctions between states or conditions that could be treated by means of dietetic and pharmacological means, those that require psychological and philosophical treatment, those that call for a combination of both, or those that admit of neither.

Finally, questions of treatment and cure inevitably also raised issues of expertise and authority. When people in the ancient world were confronted with mental disorder, for example in their family or in the community they were part of, what did they do? To whom did they turn for advice and treatment? Who were considered the experts in these matters? Who had the authority to determine, diagnostically, that someone was suffering from a mental illness and to decide, therapeutically, on the kind of treatment that was required? Was it the doctor, the philosopher, the priest, the gods—and any gods in particular? In the light of the increasing specialisation within ancient medicine (eye-doctors, midwives, surgeons), were there any specialists (human or divine) in the understanding and treatment of mental illnesses?[2]

These are important questions, but answers are not easily available, as the information is often scanty and scattered over a large variety of sources; and much work still needs to be done. What follows is inevitably selective, but I hope it will give some idea of the directions of further research in this area.

Medical Writers of the Late Fifth and Early Fourth Century BCE

It is generally agreed that Greek medical writers of the late fifth and early fourth century did not make a categorical distinction between mind and

---

[2] A case study by Chaniotis into propitiatory inscriptions of Lydia and Phrygia in the second and third century CE shows that some deities (Apollo Tarsios, Mes Axiottenos, Meter Tarsene) were approached for help in cases of mental insanity; yet the latter two are also invoked in cases of eye diseases, and Mes Axiottenos also in cases of diseases of the legs and the breast; see Chaniotis 1995, 338 and 342.

body, or between mental and physical illness. And while being innovative in many other ways, in this respect they adhered to existing patterns of thought as represented in Greek epic or tragedy, where no such distinction is made either. In the plays of Euripides and Sophocles, representations of madness are at least as frequent as accounts of physical illness, but there seems to be no categorical differentiation between the kind of mental frenzy that characterises Heracles, the mysterious chronic illness that affected Philoctetes or the lovesickness of Phaedra: they are all labelled *nosos*, 'disease', without explicit indication of the area affected. Moreover, they are all considered divine afflictions, attributed to the anger or wrath of a divine force;[3] and they manifest themselves in a combination of mental and physical symptoms. Cure, if at all possible, is something only the gods can effect; and when there is reference to herbal treatment (as in the case of Philoctetes), this is meant in terms of soothing and pain relief rather than cure.

In these two latter respects—causal explanation and treatment—the medical writers of the classical period do mark, of course, a striking innovation: they no longer assign these conditions to the influence of specific gods but to identifiable causes in the human body, the patient's personal history or lifestyle or environment, and they claim that these conditions can be treated, just as any other disease, by means of dietetic measures, drugs or surgery, or a combination of these.[4] They do not, however, distinguish mental illness as a separate category. It is rather that, in their discussions of disease, they frequently also discuss disturbances of the mental, cognitive, behavioural or motor functions of the body, but they present all these mental affections as being of a physical nature and having a bodily cause.[5] This, for instance, is the pattern that emerges from the ways in which the nosological treatises transmitted under the name of Hippocrates, such as *Affections, Internal Affections* and *Diseases* I, II and III, discuss *phrenitis* and

---

[3] There is no reason to believe that it was especially, or exclusively, mental diseases that were believed to be of divine origin. Epidemic disease, or various kinds of chronic disease, were also believed to be sent by the gods. See Kudlien 1968.

[4] On the question of the divine in medical texts of the classical period see van der Eijk 2005a, ch. 1. *Regimen* is the only text of this period that mentions prayer to the gods alongside dietetic measures; yet the context is prevention of illness, not treatment; see van der Eijk 2004.

[5] For general discussions see, e.g., Pigeaud 1980; Singer 1992; Bartos 2010; Gundert 2000; van der Eijk 2011. The picture becomes more complicated once we take other, non-Hippocratic medical texts into consideration: thus the fourth century medical writer Diocles of Carystus is credited with the notion of psychic pneuma (*psuchikon pneuma*) in his explanation of a number of diseases such as *errhipsis* ('lying prostrate'), *lêthargos, kephalaia* ('headache'), *spasmos, kunikos spasmos* ('dog's spasm'), and *melancholia*; see Diocles, frs. 77, 78, 80, 101, 107, 108 in van der Eijk 2000.

other diseases that, in later medical history, became the standard examples of mental illness, such as *mania, melancholia, lêthargos* and *kephalaia*. A further case in point is the author of *The Sacred Disease* who, in chapters 14–17, discusses a considerable number of what we could call mental or psychological activities, experiences as well as disturbances (thinking, feeling, perceiving, moving, derangement) without ever mentioning the word for soul, *psuchê*.

Even the author of *Regimen* (which is usually dated to the first half of the fourth century BCE), although he does speak about soul (*psuchê*) as distinct from the body (*sôma*), still conceives of the soul as something corporeal, whose workings and failings can be described in material terms and influenced, modified and treated by dietary measures.[6] In particular, chapters 35 and 36 of *Regimen* present what could be categorised as a materialist view on human intellectual activity, mental sanity and madness. These chapters are concerned with variations in mental or cognitive performance that are said to be due to specific fluctuations in the balance, or blend (*sunkrêsis*), of fire and water in the soul. These variations are presented under the rubric of *phronêsis*, and its negative counterpart *aphrosunê*, often translated as 'intelligence' (or, perhaps better, 'cognitive awareness') and 'lack of intelligence' (or, perhaps better, 'senselessness'). Yet translations for these, and related terms, are notoriously problematic. A better impression of what the author has in mind can be gained from his characterisations of the specific variations he goes on to describe. He distinguishes a number of types, differentiated according to their degree of intelligence, memory capacity, concentration power, swiftness or sharpness of thinking, and stablity of judgement.[7] While these differences in intellectual or cognitive ability still seem to be within the range of what is healthy, the author at some point comes to speak of people who, as a result of a specific blend of fire and water, are out of their mind (*embrontêtoi*) and suffer from insanity (*maniê*): they weep for no reason, fear what is not dreadful, are pained by what does not affect them,

---

[6] For a more extensive discussion of the psychological theory of *Regimen* see van der Eijk 2011. Parts of that discussion are summarised here.

[7] Apart from the adjective *phronimos* (and its counterpart *aphrôn*) being used in comparatives and superlatives, we also find references to varying degrees of memory (*mnêmonikôtatê*, 152,6 [VI.514 L.]), sharpness (*oxuteron*, 154,22 [VI.520 L.]) or dullness (*nôthroteron*, 152,11 [VI.514 L.]) quickness and slowness of mind (*tachutês, braduteros*, 154,25 [VI.520 L.]; 152,29 [VI.516 L.]), and degrees of concentration (*paramonimoi, hêsson monimon*, 152,11–12 [VI.514 L.]; 154,23 [VI.520 L.]). All references to *Regimen* follow the page and line numbers in the CMG edition by Joly and Byl 1984, followed by the volume and page number of the Littré edition (L.) in brackets.

and are oversensitive.[8] Likewise pathological seems the case of the people who, according to the author, are half insane (*hupomainesthai*), very close to insanity (*maniê*) and get out of their mind (*mainesthai*) at the wrong time.[9]

The explanation for these variations given by the author of *Regimen* is likewise given in terms indicating differences of degree. For example, the most intelligent soul with the best memory is correlated to a mixture of the moistest fire and the driest water. In this mixture both fire and water are called most self-sufficient (*autarkestaton*) in virtue of their mutual balance.[10] The author further distinguishes three types of soul in which fire dominates water, and three in which water dominates fire.[11] Thus the activities of the soul are closely linked to bodily states, conditions and processes; and the soul itself, too, is presented as something physical, a part of the body.[12]

As far as the treatment of these states is concerned, the author presents all these variations as capable of being corrected and manipulated by the doctor by means of dietetic measures and drugs. Carefully differentiating between the various conditions, he offers an extensive physical therapeutic regime including food, drink, exercise (walks and various types of running),

---

[8] CMG p. 154,9–10 (VI.518 L.).

[9] CMG p. 156,3–6 (VI.520 L.). The reference to 'dreaming' (*oneirôssein*) here is puzzling, especially in the light of what the author will say later on in Book 4 of the same work, where he presents a great variety of dream interpretations, some of which are given a favourable, others an unfavourable interpretation. It has been suggested that here in ch. 35 the author is thinking of hallucinations in the waking state, or of a specific type of dreams, such as nightmares (Joly translates 'cauchemars') or perhaps wet dreams (though wet dreams are usually indicated by *exoneirôssein*); Joly's interpretation receives some support from Book 4, p. 230,8 (VI.662 L.), where dreams (*enhupnia*) about the crossing of rivers, approaching warriors and bizarre shapes are said to be signs of insanity (*maniê*). Yet it remains somewhat curious that while in Book 4 the author makes a large number of distinctions between different kinds of dreams, here in ch. 35 he seems to present *oneirôssein* as one category *tout court* which is as a whole unhealthy.

[10] CMG p. 150,29–152,1 (VI.512–514 L.).

[11] The author further explains the mechanics of these mental states and processes in terms of movement and stability, with the former being characteristic of water, the latter of fire (152,4–5 [VI.514 L.]), in terms of passages (*poroi*) that may become too hollow (*koiloteroi*, 152,17), and in terms of exits (*diexodoi*, 152,21) that are emptied so that there is no blockage to the passages of the soul (*poroi tês psuchês*), by which the author presumably means the passages through which the soul moves. Cf. the reference to circuits (*periodoi*) in 152,30 (VI.516 L.): 'For as the circuit is slow, the sensations, being quick, impinge (on the soul) spasmodically, and their mixing (with the soul) is very partial owing to the slowness of the circuit. For the sensations of the soul that act through sight or hearing are quick, while those that act through touch are slower, and produce a deeper impression.' See Jouanna 2012.

[12] This would suggest that the author's view on the soul-body relationship is somewhat similar to that of the Epicureans, and the distinction between soul and body would have to be understood in terms of one special part of the body as distinct from the rest of the body.

wrestling, induced vomiting, baths, vapour and shower baths, massage, unc-
tion, fomentations, sexual intercourse, slimming down, dehydration, and,
in some cases, even aggressive drug treatment such as the purgative use of
hellebore.[13] While the treatment is adjusted according to each variation, it
is consistently motivated in terms of its impact on the physical condition
underlying the mental disturbance; and the suggestion clearly is that treatment can be successful in most cases. For example, the person in whom
there is a very pure mixture of fire and water but where the fire is slightly
dominated by the water, suffers from dullness of sensation, but if this condition is treated properly, he may become more intelligent than natural. He
should adopt the following regimen:

> Such a person is benefited by using a regimen inclining rather towards fire,
> with no surfeit either of food or of drinks. So he should take sharp runs, so
> that the body may be emptied of moisture and the moisture may be stayed
> sooner. But it is not beneficial for such a person to go wrestling, have massage
> or similar exercises, for fear lest, the passages becoming too hollow, they be
> filled with surfeit. For the motion of the soul is of necessity weighed down by
> such things. Walks, however, are beneficial, after dinner, in the early morning
> and after running; after dinner, that the soul may receive drier nourishment
> from the things that enter; in the early morning, that the exits may be emptied
> of moisture and the passages of the soul may not be obstructed; after exercise,
> in order that the secretion from running may not be left behind in the body
> to contaminate the soul, obstruct the exits and trouble the nourishment. It is
> beneficial also to use vomiting, so that the body may be cleansed of impurities
> left behind owing to any failure of exercise to purify, and after the vomiting
> gradually to increase the amount of food for more than four days at least.
> Unction is more beneficial to such persons than baths, and sexual intercourse
> should take place when the onsets of water occur, less, however, at the onsets
> of fire.[14]

Yet there are limits to the curability of mental states. For in chapter 36,
the author points out that whereas those mental conditions that are due
to the mixture of fire and water can be cured, this is not the case for some
other mental features, such as irascibility, indolence, craftiness, simplicity,
quarrelsomeness, and benevolence.[15] States like these, he argues, are caused
by the nature of the passages through which the soul moves or against which

---

[13] CMG p. 154,11 (VI.518 L.); 156,15 (VI.522 L.).

[14] CMG p. 152,13–28 (VI.514–516 L.), tr. W.H.S. Jones, slightly modified.

[15] CMG p. 156,23–24 (VI.522 L.): Τῶν δὲ τοιούτων οὐκ ἐστὶν ἡ σύγκρησις αἰτίη· οἷον ὀξύθυμος,
ῥᾴθυμος, δόλιος, ἁπλοῦς, δυσμενὴς, εὔνους· Note the use of οἷον, which indicates that this list is
not exhaustive.

it collides or with which it mixes.[16] And this, the author claims, is not possible to change through regimen, 'for it is impossible to change invisible nature'.[17]

For all the problems this passage raises,[18] it seems clear that the author is trying to make a categorical distinction between different mental states, some of which are curable, some incurable. From the examples given in the text, one may be inclined to think that the distinction is between cognitive capacities and defects and pathological cases of insanity on the one hand, and moral dispositions (or ethical character features) on the other. Yet the use of *phroneousin* in 156,27, if taken in the same sense as *phronêsis* at the beginning of chapter 35, hardly supports such a restriction of incurable states to the ethical sphere; and the words translated 'craftiness, simplicity' (*dolios* and *haplous* in 156,24) seem to have a cognitive side to them as well. A further problem is posed by the fact that the distinction the author makes is based on an alleged difference in underlying cause: mental states due to the mixture can be changed, mental states due to the nature of the passages cannot be cured. Yet it is not clear how, and on the strength of what criterion, the physician is to determine whether a particular mental state is caused by the mixture or by the nature of the passages. Nor does the reference to

---

[16] CMG p. 156,24–27: τῶν τοιούτων ἁπάντων ἡ φύσις τῶν πόρων δι' ὧν ἡ ψυχὴ πορεύεται, αἰτίη ἐστί. δι' ὁποίων γὰρ ἀγγείων ἀποχωρεῖ καὶ πρὸς ὁποῖά τινα προσπίπτει καὶ ὁποίοισι τισὶ καταμίσγεται, τοιαῦτα φρονέουσι. These passages (*poroi*) have been mentioned in the previous chapter (152,17 [VI.514 L.]). The idea seems to be that the soul is moving through these passages, and can thus be affected by their characteristics.

[17] CMG p. 156,27–28 (VI.524 L.): φύσιν γὰρ μεταπλάσαι ἀφανέα οὐχ οἷόν τε. This is an enigmatic explanation. The invisibility of the passages as such cannot be the problem, for earlier on in ch. 35, the author mentioned that one can influence the width of the passages by means of diet and life-style (CMG p. 152,17 and 21 [VI.514 L.]). Perhaps the point of the present passage is that it is not clear *how* the nature of these passages affects mind and character: even if we know that it does, the mechanism through which it does so remains obscure and hence is not accessible to dietetic treatment. Another possibility is that the author is thinking primarily, if not exclusively, of treatment by regimen: if you want to change someone's character or psychological disposition, diet will not be sufficient or suitable to change your passages: you may need more aggressive drugs, or perhaps even the surgeon's knife (or, alternatively, a philosopher or a psychotherapist).

[18] For a more extensive discussion see van der Eijk 2011. I have suggested there that one way of reading the text is that these psychological features or states not caused by the mixture of fire and water are somehow less closely associated with the body than others, and hence less, or even not at all, accessible to physical treatment. It seems that, in the author's thinking, there are different *modes*, or different *degrees* in the extent to which psychological states and processes are tied to the body and susceptible to manipulation by means of physical treatment. Even if, in the author's view, all psychological states and processes are, in the end, physical, it is still possible for some states or processes to be, so to speak, more physical or less physical than others.

the underlying cause itself explain the incurability, for the author goes on to draw an analogy with another state caused by the nature of the passages, i.e. the state of the voice: yet that state, he concedes, *can* be changed by 'making the passages smoother or rougher'.[19] Why it is possible to change the passages in this case, but not in the case of the mental states mentioned in 156,24, remains unclear.[20]

Plato's Category of 'Diseases of the Soul' and Their Treatment

References to madness and insanity are, of course, frequent in Plato's dialogues, and *mania* can take different forms, as we learn from the *Phaedrus*: some are divine, some natural, some are beneficial, some pathological.[21] For our purposes, the most relevant discussion can be found in the extensive theoretical account of the causes of disease in the *Timaeus* (81e7–90d7).[22] At some point, the text makes a categorical distinction between diseases (*nosê-mata*) in the region of the body (*peri to sôma*) and diseases in the region of the soul (*peri psuchên*), though with the specification that the latter, too, are due to a condition of the body (*dia sômatos hexin*, 86b1–2). As examples of these diseases of the soul, Timaeus first mentions *anoia* ('mindless-ness'), which he subdivides into two kinds: *mania* and *amathia* (86b3–4).[23] In the sequel, he lists the sufferings that these two kinds of disease give rise to: excessive pleasures and pains leading to obsessive, pleasure-seeking and paranoid, pain-avoiding behaviour, leading in turn to dysfunctioning of

---

[19] CMG p. p. 156,28–32 (VI.524 L.): 'Likewise, what kind of voice one has is caused by the passages of the breath; for the voice has to be of the nature of the vessels through which air moves and the things against which it collides. And this (the voice) one can make worse or better, since one can make the passages of breath smoother or rougher, but the above is impossible to change by regimen.' I take *keino* to refer to 'these things' (*ta toiauta*) in 156,27 or, more vaguely, to the fact of their being dependent on the nature of the passages. He does not tell us how one can change the nature of the passages in this case, presumably we have to think of voice exercises.

[20] Jones 1931, 295 n. 1, comments: 'We can change the *poroi* (throat, nose) that give characteristics to voice, but we cannot get at the internal *poroi* along which the *psuchê* travels.' But this does not answer the question *why* change (and cure) is possible in the one case but not in the other.

[21] *Phaedrus* 244A–250C.

[22] For a recent discussion see Grams 2009.

[23] Plato does not tell us what the difference between the two is. On the face of it, *mania* seems to refer to a state of excitement and passion, due to a slavish following of bodily pleasures and wrong ambitions; *amathia* rather seems to be a state of dullness of the mind or clinical stupidity (cf. 88b4–5).

vision and hearing, mental confusion and failure to reason properly; particular attention is given to lack of self-restraint in sexual matters (86c7–d5).
Further down, he mentions *duskolia* ('bad-temperedness') and *dusthumia*
('despondency'), *thrasutês* ('rashness') and *deilia* ('cowardice', 'phobia'?),
and *lêthê* ('forgetfulness') and *dusmathia* ('inability to learn') as examples
of the various kinds of diseases (*pantodapa nosêmata*) affecting the three
parts of the soul respectively (87a5–7). It is, again, impossible to find satisfactory translations for most of these terms, but they range from what we
would call the emotional domain through to behavioral dysfunctioning to
cognitive and learning disabilities.[24]

The causes for these conditions are divided between an inferior condition of the body (*ponêran hexin tou sômatos*) and uneducated nurturing
(*apaideuton trophên*, 86e2). As to the former, Timaeus mentions several
physiological states and processes, such as an abundance of sperma being
produced by the marrow (86c4) leading to excessive sexual desire, or a state
of width of the bones causing fluidity and moisture in the body (86d4), or
acid and salty phlegms and bitter and bilious humours wandering around in
the body without being able to be disposed of (86e5–6) and thus interfering
with the circular movement of the soul (*phora tês psuchês*). As to nurturing,
trophê is probably meant not only in the physical, corporeal sense but also
contains an element of upbringing, as becomes clear from the reference to
bad nurturing in 87b6–7 (*trephontes ... trophê*).

What is further striking is that there is a certain insistence in the text
on what we would call the clinical nature of the conditions: thus right at
the beginning (86b3), Timaeus says that one has to agree (*sunchôrêteon*)
that *anoia* is a disease of the soul (*noson tês psuchês*). And after making
the subdivision of *anoia* into the two kinds of *mania* and *amathia*, the text
goes on to explain that, indeed, one has to call (*prosrhêteon*) the sufferings
brought about by either of these conditions disease (*noson*, 86b5). This
insistence is taken up a few lines further down (86d1–5): The person who
is frantically pre-occupied (*emmanês*) with the satisfaction of his bodily
desires has a soul that is diseased and mindless (*nosousan kai aphrona*)
because of the body (*hupo tou sômatos*); and although his evil behaviour
might lead one to think that he is not clinically but willingly bad, the truth
of the matter is that lack of self-restraint in sexual matters is a disease of
the soul (*nosos tês psuchês*), because for the most part it is brought about

---

[24] For a discussion of these conditions see Tracy 1969, 125–136 and Gill 2000.

by the state of one substance (i.e. the seed) that is fluid and moisturising as a result of the porosity of the bones. It is therefore not correct, Timaeus goes on (86d6–7), to blame people who show lack of self-restraint in these matters as if they were willingly behaving like this: for no-one is willingly bad, the bad person becomes bad through causes beyond his control, viz. the inferior condition of the body and the uneducated nurturing we already mentioned.[25]

All this shows that Plato's references to diseases of the soul are not to be taken as metaphors for states of ignorance, as the allusion to the Socratic principle of 'no one does wrong knowingly' and the reference to the healing (*iatika*) power of intellectual study (87b3) might lead one to think. They are *genuine* diseases, caused no less by bodily states than by lack of education; and they are not moral dispositions, but pathological conditions. Their cure is likewise to be taken literally, as addressing both the underlying bodily condition and the state of the soul itself.

This becomes clear from the account of the treatment of these conditions in 87c1–89d2. The aim is first of all to bring about the right proportion (*summetria*) between soul and body, i.e. to restore the balance between the two.[26] For a soul that is too strong in relation to the body it belongs to, shakes it (*diaseiousa*) and fills it with diseases, causes it to become overheated (*diapuros*) and instable (*saleuein*) and brings about fluxes (*rheumata*, 88a1–2); and a body that is too strong for the soul causes the latter to become 'numb and unable to learn and unable to remember' (*kôphon kai dusmathes amnêmon te*), leading to the greatest of diseases, *amathia* (88b4–5). To address these kinds of imbalance therapeutically, a regime of physical and mental exercise (*gumnastikê*) is required, physical in the case of excessive mental activity, mental in the case of excessive physical activity. For even mental movements such as musical and mathematical training have a physical, corporeal impact: just as the circuit of the soul (*phora tês psuchês*, 87a1) can get mixed up with vaporous moisture arising from humours in the body,

---

25 ... νοσοῦσαν καὶ ἄφρονα ἴσχων ὑπὸ τοῦ σώματος τὴν ψυχήν, οὐχ ὡς νοσῶν ἀλλ᾽ ὡς ἑκὼν κακὸς δοξάζεται· τὸ δὲ ἀληθὲς ἡ περὶ τὰ ἀφροδίσια ἀκολασία κατὰ τὸ πολὺ μέρος διὰ τὴν ἑνὸς γένους ἕξιν ὑπὸ μανότητος ὀστῶν ἐν σώματι ῥυώδη καὶ ὑγραίνουσαν νόσος ψυχῆς γέγονεν. καὶ σχεδὸν δὴ πάντα ὁπόσα ἡδονῶν ἀκράτεια καὶ ὄνειδος ὡς ἑκόντων λέγεται τῶν κακῶν, οὐκ ὀρθῶς ὀνειδίζεται· κακὸς μὲν γὰρ ἑκὼν οὐδείς, διὰ δὲ πονηρὰν ἕξιν τινὰ τοῦ σώματος καὶ ἀπαίδευτον τροφὴν ὁ κακὸς γίγνεται κακός, παντὶ δὲ ταῦτα ἐχθρὰ καὶ ἄκοντι προσγίγνεται. Cf. also 87b4, where people are said to become bad in ways that are most against their will (*akousiôtata*).

26 87d1–3: 'In order to bring about health and disease, virtue and vice, no balanced proportion (*summetria*) or lack of proportion (*ametria*) is of greater importance than that of the soul itself in relation to the body itself'.

likewise healthy, corrective mental exercise can, in return, have a beneficial effect on the state of the body (88c4–7).[27]

The chief therapeutic principle is movement (*kinêsis*) (88b7), a gentle shaking of the body to enable a process of cleansing (*katharsis*) from harmful materials to take place and to allow the bodily parts and components to get settled (*sustasis*) into their orderly position (89a6). This is best done by physical exercise (*gumnasia*), or by the gentle motion brought about by sailing or travelling; thirdly, one may resort to the use of drugs (*pharmaka*), but only in very severe cases, for drugs are aggressive and destabilizing, and only to be used when more gentle, dietetic remedies are insufficient. Timaeus' insistence on the dangers of drugs in the treatment of mental illness in 89b3–d2 is remarkably emphatic, and paralleled by the reference to the treatment by drugs as 'problematic' or 'painful' (*chalepon*) in cases of physical illnesses such as *tetanos* and *opisthotonos* (84e10). It echoes similar cautions regarding the use of drugs in other medical texts of the time.[28] After this digression, Timaeus sums up his therapeutic regime in 90c: for every person and for every condition there is just one therapeutic principle, 'to provide the nurture (*trophai*) and the movements (*kinêseis*) appropriate to each individual'. These movements can be physical as well as mental; but then, in Plato's account here, even mental movements have a physical impact.

We may ask what makes all these conditions, for all their bodily aspects, 'belong to the soul' rather than to the body. Presumably, it is the fact that they manifest themselves predominantly in the psychic domain of emotions, feelings, and cognitive failure.[29] This probably explains Plato's

---

[27] Cf. 87b7–8: 'one should try to avoid evil both by upbringing and by intellectual pursuits'.

[28] On the special status of treatment by drugs in ancient therapeutics see van der Eijk 2005a, 112, with references to contemporaneous medical literature; cautions regarding the use of drugs are also found in Diocles, fr. 153 and 183a.

[29] Cf. the criteria mentioned by Caelius Aurelianus, *Acute Affections* III.13.109–111 on the question whether hydrophobia is a disease of the soul or of the body: 'Some say that it is a disease of the soul, on the ground that desire or longing is a function peculiar to the soul rather than the body ... And so, they say, hydrophobia, too, being the desire for drink, is a disease of the soul. Again, since fear, sadness, and anger are affections of the soul and those who have hydrophobia fear water, it must consequently be admitted that theirs is an affection of the soul.' Yet Caelius does not agree that these conditions apply, and he points out that desire and fear arise from the interaction between body and soul; that the diseases' antecedent cause (the bite by a dog) is physical; and that many symptoms of the disease are physical as well. He concludes: 'For affections of the soul, in the meaning of the philosophers, are affections of our judgement. But the disease of hydrophobia derives from a bodily force and is therefore a bodily disease, though it also attacks the psychic nature,

choice of examples, for in principle, his discussion does not seem to be restricted to *mania* and *amathia* or to the other conditions mentioned, as the use of *pantodapa* in 87a2 shows. Ancient medical texts recognised a great variety of mental disorders, such as *melancholia, phrenitis*, epilepsy, apoplexy, lethargy and *kephalaia*, and Plato must have been aware of at least some of these other disease names and with what they were believed to signify; but he does not, in the context of the *Timaeus*, mention them or tell us whether, and if so in what way, they are different from *mania* and *amathia*. The only exception is 'the sacred disease', which is mentioned in the context of diseases of the body (85b2), even though, as Roberto Lo Presti points out elsewhere in this volume, the cause Plato mentions for epilepsy is not very different from the humoural explanation given for some mental diseases in the later section. But the explanation probably is that epilepsy is, of course, a disease with strong, indeed striking bodily manifestations, and psychic problems are only part of the picture.

How are we to evaluate this discussion in the broader context of Plato's philosophy? Is Plato's *Timaeus* suggesting, for example, that *all* cases of lack of self-restraint (*akolasia, akrateia*) in sexual and other bodily desires are ultimately pathological? Or is it that only *some* are—the ones that he has been talking about here—and that these cases are to be treated physically as well as psychologically, whereas other cases of such behaviour arising from moral dispositions are vices (*kakiai*) for which the individual can be blamed and for which psychological or philosophical correction is the treatment called for? This is what the distinction in causes between 'an inferior condition of the body' (*ponêran hexin tou sômatos*) and 'uneducated nurturing' (*apaideuton trophên*) could be taken to imply—although nurturing and education are also mentioned in the therapeutic section dealing with the treatment of pathological cases. On this line of thought, Plato would regard genuine mental illness as due to bad management of the body, and mental health—in the clinical sense—a matter of keeping to a regimen in which the body and its influence on the soul through passion and desire is

---

as do mania and melancholy.' (tr. Drabkin 1950). A parallel case would be pleasures of the soul versus pleasures of the body. Cf. Aristotle, *Nicomachean Ethics* 1117b28, where ambition (*philotimia*) and love of learning (*philomatheia*) are given as examples of pleasures in which the body is not involved. On the pleasures derived from contemplation, i.e. theoretical study, see Aristotle, *Nicomachean Ethics* 1153a1, 1153a22, 1174b21. Cf. Nemesius, *Nature of Man* 18: 'Some pleasures are of the soul, some of the body. Those are of the soul which belong to it by itself, such as those involving study and contemplation, for these and similar pleasures belong to the soul alone.'

kept under strict regulation. Yet if this is Plato's view, the question arises—similar to the situation in *Regimen*—how and on the strength of what criteria pathological and moral cases are to be distinguished: is it a matter of degree of severity? Or is it a matter of differences in causation? Yet how are such differences determined?

Another possibility is that the account is, indeed, meant to be comprehensive and that Plato really wants to say that, *ultimately*, all immoderate behaviour is pathological—and, consequently, that cure should also address the physical side of things. In this way, Plato would be advocating a comprehensive regime—therapeutic as well as preventative—addressing all cases of sickness of the soul and consisting of physical as well as psychological or philosophical measures.

Once again, the distinction between clinical and moral states of mind is proving both problematic in theory and, if it is accepted, difficult to determine in practice. Likewise, the question of blame is raised, but it is not clear how exactly it is answered. Is the cause or origin of conditions such as *mania* and *amathia* within the individual's control? The *Timaeus* seems to deny this, and to shift the responsibility to those who are in charge of upbringing and education—parents, teachers, the society that, by means of education and training, should prevent these mental conditions from occurring or, once they have occurred, correct and address them by means of a therapeutic regime. Here, the question of curability comes in: the *Timaeus* is optimistic that these conditions can indeed be cured, although perhaps not all equally easily; there is no suggestion that any of these cases are incurable.

Aristotle's Analysis of Weakness of Character

Like Plato, Aristotle was clearly fascinated by forms and expressions of mental insanity and ecstatic states of the mind. Even though no dedicated systematic discussion has been preserved, references to people who are insane or possessed or beside themselves, or prone to such states, indicated with terms such as *manikos, ekstatikos, existamenos, emmanês, entheos, enthousiasmos*, are frequent in the surviving Aristotelian works.[30] Furthermore, as could be expected from the son of a court physician, Aristotle's work displays great interest in the physiology and pathology of mental states in general,

---

[30] See the discussion by Croissant 1932; Preus 1986; van der Eijk 1994, 321 and 330.

such as cognition and the emotions, as his famous theory of *katharsis* (which has strong medical overtones) and his account of emotions in book II of the *Rhetoric* testifies. Aristotle, more than Plato, acknowledges that emotions have their place within human nature, and that a regulated expression or even outpouring of these emotions can be conducive to health and mental stability. Mental health for Aristotle is a combination of natural and cultural factors, physical and environmental as well as psychological and moral; and on the basis of his definition of bodily health as a 'good balance', a *summetria* or *eukrasia*, between the constituent factors, he likewise understands mental health as being based on a balance, an *eukrasia*, between constituent factors such as the elementary qualities and the specific ratios between heat and cold.[31] Underlying this is the notion of *krasis*, the physical mixture or proportion of elementary qualities that Aristotle adopted from Greek medical theory and that we already encountered in the treatise *Regimen*.

Yet what happens when the *krasis* gets the upper hand? This is what seems to be the case in a group of people to whom Aristotle refers a number of times, calling them *hoi melancholikoi* ('melancholics').[32] This is a notion that Aristotle inherited from earlier medical texts, but which he modified and reformulated in the terms of his own physiology and anthropology. Piecing together the relevant remarks scattered over his writings, we get a more detailed picture of this type of people, who are characterised by a range of disturbances in the cognitive and ethical domain, such as being haunted by a multitude of images or appearances (*phantasmata*), which cause them to have poor recollective capacities and bizarre (though sometimes prophetic) dreams. They are intense, impetuous, capricious and obsessively pleasure-seeking in their behaviour, and let themselves be carried away by imagination and passion rather than guided by rational deliberation. One passage in particular speaks of their urge for satisfaction of bodily desires in terms that resemble our modern concepts of remedial pleasure and addiction: 'melancholics are by nature constantly in need of cure, for the mixture of their bodies keeps them in a constant state of irritation, and they are subject to intense desires all the time.'[33] All this is caused by their particular physiolog-

---

[31] See Tracy 1969.

[32] Again the translation is tentative and lays no claim to complete accuracy. For a reconstruction of Aristotle's concept of melancholy see van der Eijk 1990 (reprinted in van der Eijk 2005a, ch. 5).

[33] *Nicomachean Ethics* 1154b11–15: οἱ δὲ μελαγχολικοὶ τὴν φύσιν δέονται ἀεὶ ἰατρείας· καὶ γὰρ τὸ σῶμα δακνόμενον διατελεῖ διὰ τὴν κρᾶσιν, καὶ ἀεὶ ἐν ὀρέξει σφοδρᾷ εἰσίν· ἐξελαύνει δὲ ἡδονὴ λύπην ἥ τ' ἐναντία καὶ ἡ τυχοῦσα, ἐὰν ᾖ ἰσχυρά· καὶ διὰ ταῦτα ἀκόλαστοι καὶ φαῦλοι γίνονται.

ical constitution (*phusis*) or mixture (*krasis*), which is determined, *inter alia*, by a specific presence of black bile in their bodies.[34] Thus we are dealing not just with a temporary episode but with a long-lasting state, in some cases present from the moment of birth; and the melancholics can be regarded as chronically ill patients who are, as Aristotle puts it, in continuous need of cure (*iatreia*).[35]

Like Plato, Aristotle attributes failure to achieve or maintain mental health and moral excellence to a number of different causes, including the influence of disturbing physical, environmental and dietary factors. This becomes clear from his discussion of another intriguing mental state, *akrasia*, lack of moral self-restraint, in *Nicomachean Ethics* book VII. *Akrasia* is usually regarded in scholarship as an ethical state of weakness, and its treatment or correction is likewise believed to be of a moral, psychological nature rather than a matter of dietetics or drugs.[36] Yet there are good reasons to believe that Aristotle considered *akrasia*, at least in some of its manifestations, a medical, clinical condition rather than just a moral disposition.[37] This is indicated by the fact that for one of the two types of *akrasia* recognised by Aristotle (rashness, *propeteia*, versus weakness, *astheneia*),[38] the melancholics are the prototypical example: it is not just that akratic people are *compared* to melancholics, but rather that melancholics are a specific, indeed the most obvious *example* of the condition.[39] A further indication is that Aristotle's account of *akrasia*, and related forms of moral deficiency (such as profligacy, *akolasia*), is cast in strikingly medical terms that cannot be dismissed as being 'just' analogy.[40] Aristotle uses terms such as easily

---

[34] Black bile (*melaina cholê*) is mentioned as a characteristic of the melancholic nature in *Sleep and Waking* 457a31–33. For the physiological basis see van der Eijk 2005a, 152–155. The discussion of melancholy in *Probl.* XXX.1 is probably, at least in its present form, by a later Peripatetic, although it does contain a large number of genuine Aristotelian ideas and phrases; see van der Eijk 2005a, 155–167.

[35] 1154b11.

[36] See the recent collections of studies edited by Bobonich and Destrée 2007, and by Natali 2009.

[37] See Francis 2011.

[38] The word *astheneia* itself, too, may have medical overtones: it is often used in medical texts to refer to sickness in general.

[39] *NE* 1150b25–28, 1151a1–5 and 1152a17–20. See van der Eijk 2005a, 148–152.

[40] See the medical and physiological terminology in the following extracts: 'The profligate (*akolastos*) cannot be cured (*aniatos*), whereas the unrestrained man (*akratês*) can; for vice (*mochthêria*) resembles diseases (*nosêmatôn*) like dropsy and consumption (*huderôi kai phthisei*), whereas unrestraint is like epilepsy (*epilêptikois*), vice being a chronic (*sunechês*), unrestraint an intermittent (*ou sunechês*) evil. ... The unrestrained man is so constituted

cured (*euiatos*), difficult to cure (*dusiatos*) and incurable (*aniatos*); at one point, he says that *akrasia* is curable whereas *akolasia* (profligacy) is incurable, and he explains this by comparing the former to epilepsy, the latter to dropsy and consumption, the former being non-continuous (*ou sunechês*), the latter continuous (*sunechês*).[41] The whole discussion of *akrasia* in the *Nicomachean Ethics* strongly reminds us, as said, of addiction and other forms of neurotic behaviour; it is at any rate clear from Aristotle's discussion that he believes that these conditions have a physical side to them.[42]

This clinical nature becomes even more relevant when viewed against the background of the medical and Platonic evidence reviewed above. Plato had insisted that one cannot blame people whose lack of self-restraint in pleasures of the body is caused by a sickness of the soul (*nosos psuchês*) due to physical causes. There is no doubt that Aristotle was aware of this discussion in the *Timaeus*, and his own discussion of *akrasia* is to be seen against that background. Particularly striking in this regard is the similarity between Aristotle's division of *akrasia* into two types, rashness and weakness (*propeteia* and *astheneia*), and Plato's division of *anoia* into the more excitable *mania* and the more dull-witted *amathia*.

(*diakeitai*) as to pursue bodily pleasures that are excessive and contrary to the right principle without any belief he ought to do so, whereas the profligate, because he is so constituted as to pursue them, is convinced that he ought to pursue them. Therefore the former can easily be persuaded to change, but the latter cannot ... The unrestrained man knows the right in the sense not of one who consciously exercises his knowledge, but only as a man asleep or drunk can be said to know something. ... Cure is easier (*euiatotera*) in the case of unrestrained people of the melancholic type than in the case of people who deliberate as to what to do but fail to keep to their decision. And those who have become unrestrained by habit are more easily cured than those who are unrestrained by nature, since habit is easier to cure than nature. ... Bodily pleasures appear more desirable than others because pleasure drives out pain, and excessive pain leads men to seek excessive pleasure, and bodily pleasure generally, as a cure ... Bodily pleasures are sought because of their intensity, by people who are incapable of enjoying others ... many people being constituted in such a way that a neutral state of feeling is to them positively painful. Similarly the young are in a condition resembling intoxication, because they are growing; and youth is pleasant in itself. Melancholics are in constant need of such cure: their mixture (*krasis*) keeps their bodies in a constant state of irritation, and their appetites are continually active; hence any pleasure, if strong, drives out the pain.' (*Nicomachean Ethics* 1150b32–1154b18, excerpts, tr. Rackham). For discussion of the medical terminology and its Hippocratic background see Francis 2011, 164–170.

    41 *Nicomachean Ethics* 1150b32: ἀλλ᾿ ὃ μὲν ἀνίατος ὃ δ᾿ ἰατός· ἔοικε γὰρ ἡ μὲν μοχθηρία τῶν νοσημάτων οἷον ὑδέρῳ καὶ φθίσει, ἡ δ᾿ ἀκρασία τοῖς ἐπιληπτικοῖς· ἡ μὲν γὰρ συνεχὴς ἡ δ᾿ οὐ συνεχὴς πονηρία.

    42 See Francis 2011, 146–147 for interpretation of Aristotle's references to a 'natural' (*phusikos*) discussion of *akrasia* (1147a24) and to the views of the *phusiologoi* (1147b8, 1154b7) in his discussions of *akrasia* and of pleasure.

Yet, as is well known, Aristotle did not think the Socratic principle that no-one does wrong knowingly is sufficient to account for the complex phenomenon of *akrasia*. Nor did Aristotle think that *akrasia* itself was beyond human control. Natural *akrasia*, even if its cause is a congenital deficiency not of one's own making, may still be overcome by means of a corrective therapeutic regime, even though it may be more difficult to cure than acquired *akrasia*. As for acquired *akrasia* due to habituation, the ultimate cause lies within oneself (or those responsible for one's nurturing and education), and in a failure to manage one's bodily desires properly; this brings one in a state that makes one no longer capable of controlling oneself.[43] Again, the modern comparison with addiction is illuminating: someone who has ignored all advice and has given in to smoking or drinking brings his body in a condition in which he loses control over it and where his body starts to dominate him. And, like the case of smoking, the treatment (*iatreia, therapeia*) of *akrasia* will consist in a mixture of physical and psychological training. Although Aristotle does not tell us what the cure (*iatreia*) he refers to looks like, it may well be a similar combination of moral guidance, persuasion and counselling on the one hand,[44] and medical, dietetic and pharmacological measures on the other.[45]

Will such treatment be successful? What determines the degree of curability? Why are some states more easily cured than others? Why are some beyond cure? Aristotle does not answer these questions directly.[46] What is clear is that he regards states that are more deeply rooted in a person's nature as more difficult to cure, for as he says at some point, habit is easier to cure than nature.[47] On the other hand, he regards the kind of *akrasia* for which the melancholics are prototypical, i.e. the rash type of lack of self-control that does not deliberate at all, as more easily cured than the other kind, i.e. the weakness (*astheneia*) of those who lack self-control because they fail to stick to the decisions they had reached by rational deliberation.[48] Like the author of *Regimen*, Aristotle does not offer criteria on the strength of which the therapist can discern whether something is curable or incurable: is it the

---

[43] *NE* 1114a1–30.
[44] This is indicated by the use of *eumetapeistos* in 1151a14.
[45] See Demont 2005, 282–285.
[46] Some evidence may be gleaned from *NE* X.9, which discusses corrective physical, medical and educational arrangements in the polis.
[47] *NE* 1152a27–28.
[48] *NE* 1151a1–5. For an attempt to resolve the tension between these passages see van der Eijk 2005a, 150 and Francis 2011, 168–169.

nature or cause of the condition (but how is this determined?), the length
of time that has elapsed since it started, the willingness or unwillingness
of the patient to co-operate,[49] the physical condition of the patient?[50] Nor
does he go into the question of the kind of treatment that is to be followed
in individual cases. Perhaps he regarded these questions as too specific,
detailed and practical for the purposes of his general ethical theory, and
therefore left it to experts like doctors, trainers and teachers to deal with
the specifics.[51] Yet his remarks about the curability of human error in the
field of practical action anticipated the views of Stoics and Epicureans, who
presented their philosophies as 'medicines of the mind', authoritative guides
to health, mental as well as physical, and diagnostic as well as therapeutic;
and since they, like the author of *Regimen*, were materialists when it came
to their views of mental and psychological activities, one may assume that
physical therapy (dietetics, drugs) made up a significant component of their
therapeutic regime.[52]

---

[49] Cf. *NE* 1114a1–16, referring to a patient disobeying the doctor's instructions.

[50] Here it is relevant to bear in mind Aristotle's belief that health and disease are relative
notions that depend on the individual and on individual circumstances. Health is different
in people with excellent natural endowment from people born with various imperfections or
disability (*pêrôsis, pêrôma*); and likewise bringing about health is, for the doctor, a different
matter in those with excellent physical constitution and individuals (such as women and
slaves) of inferior constitution. Furthermore, even within one individual of excellent physical
condition, the perfection of health can only take place in adulthood. Cf. Tracy 1969, 318:
'The objective of the expert, then, like that of nature, is to bring the individual subject to
the highest perfection *of which it is capable*. Where the subject is richly endowed by nature
the expert may be able, through careful guidance, to bring it to the absolutely best form of
physical, moral, or political life. But in most cases, perhaps, the matter of potentiality of the
subject will be so imperfect that it cannot be made proportionate to the absolutely best form
by *any* effort of the expert over any period of time. ... the physician's task is not only to produce
the most perfect health, but his help is required perhaps even more to produce a relative
degree in persons of inferior constitution ... Because the patient is by nature imperfectly
constituted, the physician can never hope in this case to achieve the perfect *mesotês* of the
absolutely best condition. His objective, then, must be the relative *mesotês* possible to a
woman or old man, and to this particular patient wih her, or his, individual limitations. And,
as we have seen, the more precarious the state of the patient, the greater will be the skill and
care required of the physician (1320b34–39)'. And further down, Tracy 1969, 327–328: 'This
perfection of health can occur in human beings, however, only at the prime of life, when the
process of growth is complete and the process of decay not yet begun.'

[51] On the limits of Aristotle's interest in medical matters see Demont 2005, 283–284.

[52] See Tieleman 2003 on the medical nature of Stoic therapeutics; more sceptical is Gill
2010; see also the older study by Nussbaum 1994, who, like Gill, interprets most references to
treatment in the Hellenistic sources metaphorically.

Galen's Treatment of Mental Illnesses
and of the Affections and Errors of the Soul

Galen's approach to mental illness is in various ways indebted to the authors we have considered.[53] When it comes to the relationship between body and soul, Galen comes very close to the materialist position we found in *Regimen*; like this author, and like the Stoics and Epicureans, Galen argued in his influential treatise *That the Capacities of the Soul Follow the Mixtures of the Body* that even intellectual and cognitive performance can be enhanced or weakened by means of dietetic and pharmacological treatment; and in the course of his discussion, he gives several examples of mental dysfunctioning caused by physical causes.[54] The implication clearly is that psychological health and well being are the domain of the doctor as much as the philosopher.

In accordance with this principle, Galen's nosological accounts of various kinds of mental illness identify bodily causes and advocate treatment by medical means (dietetics, pharmacology, surgery).[55] These accounts are scattered over his immense œuvre, but one particularly informative discussion can be found in Book III of *Affected Parts*, where Galen deals with epilepsy, melancholia, lethargy and phrenitis and a number of other diseases manifesting themselves in disturbances of the cognitive and emotional domain. Thus his discussion of 'the melancholic humour' (*melancholikos chumos*) in *Affected Parts* III.9–10 explicitly addresses the question of the 'psychic' nature of the disease, with its characteristic manifestations in fear and despondency (*phobos* and *dusthumia*), even in cases where the disease does not arise in the brain but in the region of the stomach and causes damage to the mental faculties by means of co-affection (*sumpatheia*). As far as its treatment is concerned, Galen says that this is different depending on the cause and its localisation:

> For the treatment, this distinction is of no small importance: when the blood becomes melancholic throughout the whole body, it would be appropriate to start the treatment with venesection; but when only the brain is affected, the patient does not require venesection ... Your diagnosis should be based on this criterion: does the whole body have the melancholic humour in it, or is it just gathered around the brain?[56]

---

[53] For general discussion of Galen's views on mental illness see Pigeaud 2008b; McDonald 2009.

[54] See the discussion by Singer 2013 and Jouanna 2009.

[55] See McDonald 2009; Pigeaud 2008a.

[56] *Affected Parts* III.11 (VIII.182 K.); see the translation of the relevant sections by van der Eijk and Pormann 2008, 273–287.

Galen goes on to specify how one can apply this criterion in specific cases by means of a detailed physical examination of the patient's body and the kind of food he has taken, if necessary supplemented by information about his exercises, pain, sleeplessness and worries, as well as environmental factors such as season, place and age. As for treatment, apart from venesection, he mentions 'many baths and a moist, juicy diet, without any other remedy'; but he adds that, if the disease has become chronic, 'there is a need for remedies greater than the ones mentioned', presumably including more aggressive pharmacological treatment.[57]

However, this is only one side of the coin. For when we turn to Galen's work(s) devoted to the *Diagnosis and Treatment of Affections and Errors of the Soul*, we get a very different picture. The discussion there is moral rather than medical, and it deals with the development and management of character, and the correction of emotional and cognitive malfunctioning *(pathê* and *hamartêmata* respectively) such as anger and erroneous moral judgement in a manner strongly reminiscent of Stoic ethics. There is no explicit consideration of physiological aspects either in the domain of causal explanation or corrective treatment. As far as the causes for psychological affections and errors are concerned, we hear mainly about upbringing and education, and the therapeutic correction of moral flaws and the improvement of character are entrusted to teachers, guides and critical friends.[58]

How are these two sides to be squared, and what is the relationship of the one to the other? This has been the topic of considerable scholarly debate,[59] and explanations have varied, ranging from assumptions of a development in Galen's ideas to considerations of the genre, audience and rhetorical purposes of the works in question. A further suggestion has been that one should read the works as being complementary, and that physiological and psychological cure are to be applied side by side—bearing in mind that, as in the case of Stoicism, in Galen's view even intellectual teaching and persuasion ultimately impinge physically on the soul, which is itself physical too.[60]

While being sympathetic to this latter view, I would like to add one specification, derived from the title of two relevant Galenic treatises. Galen had argued that the capacities of the soul follow the *mixtures* of the body. This important qualification locates the determining influence not just in

---

[57] *Affected Parts* III.11 (VIII.192 K.); tr. van der Eijk and Pormann 2008, 287.
[58] See the discussion by Gill 2010; Singer 2013.
[59] See the summary in Singer 2013.
[60] See Hankinson 1993, esp. 220–222.

any part of the body but in the mixtures or *kraseis*—again, a notion familiar from earlier Hippocratic and Aristotelian discussions. What these mixtures are, we learn from another important Galenic work, the *Peri kraseôn* or *De temperamentis*. Briefly summarised, they are states of the body, and of parts of the body, constituted by the proportion between the four elementary qualities hot, cold, dry and wet. Thus what is 'mixed', i.e. related to each other in specific proportions, are the elementary qualities hot, cold, dry and wet. What is mixed is *not* the humours, although these can be characterised by the elementary qualities; and the term mixture (or temperament) is not a matter of humoural balance or imbalance, as is often thought, but refers to the relationship or proportion between the elementary qualities. In this regard, too, Galen follows Aristotle.[61] In total, he believes there are nine such mixtures, one good mixture or balanced state (*eukrasia*) and eight bad mixtures or states of imbalance (*duskrasiai*). In the good mixture, all qualities are present in the proportion that is right and appropriate for that particular genus or species of living beings. In the simple bad mixtures, there is one quality that predominates, i.e. it is present to a stronger degree than is the norm for that kind of living beings; and in the composite bad mixtures, both qualities are present to a stronger degree than is the norm for that kind of living beings. The use of expressions such as 'good mixture' and 'bad mixtures' does not mean that all human beings with a bad mixture are necessarily suffering from some kind of ill health, for health and disease admit of degrees, although one may presume that they are more susceptible to ill health and disease as a result of their constitution. There can further be variations between different genera or species; and there can be variations within one particular species (individual or sub-specific variations), such as the human species.

Galen refers to these mixtures as *hexeis*, states or dispositions.[62] Thus, while being subject to change by diet and drugs, they have a certain stability and are not just incidental, episodic physiological states that change all the time. There are congenital (*sumphutoi*) mixtures and those that have been acquired as a result of long term habituation.[63] There may be a hereditary side to the mixtures as well,[64] and climate, habitat and environment may

---

[61] See van der Eijk 2013a and 2013b; Tracy 1969; den Dulk 1934.
[62] *Mixtures* 31,20 (I.558 K.) and 60,10 (I.604 K.); references to *Mixtures* are to the page and line numbers in the Teubner edition by G. Helmreich, Leipzig 1914, followed by the volume and page number in the Kühn edition (K.).
[63] *Mixtures* 60,6–21 H. (I.604–605 K.).
[64] *Mixtures* 68,18–19 (I.618 K.); 67,27 (I.616 K.); 69,2 (I.618 K.).

further play a role.[65] Not only bodies as a whole, but also bodily parts have a mixture. And both kinds of mixture can be diagnostically determined by means of touch or vision, or a combination of sensation and reasoning.[66]

It is these mixtures, then, according to Galen, in which the close psychophysical correlation between the mental and the physical resides. Indeed, the perfect harmony between the two underlies Galen's picture of the ideal person that he sets out in a remarkable passage from *Mixtures*, Book II:

> Such, then, is the body of the most well-mixed man; his soul, similarly, will be precisely in the middle between boldness and cowardice, hesitancy and rashness, pity and envy. Such a person would be good-spirited, affectionate, generous, intelligent. It is from these things, then, that the most well-mixed person is recognised primarily and especially; but quite a few others are present in conjunction with them—things that follow from these necessarily. For such a person also eats and drinks in a well-proportioned way, and digests his food well, not just in his stomach but also in his veins, and throughout the whole condition of his body; and, to speak generally, all his natural (*phusikas*) and psychological (*psuchikas*) activities are faultless. For he is in the optimum state as regards perception and motion of the limbs; he also always has a good colour and good breathing; he is midway between somnolence and insomnia, smoothness and hairiness, and the black and white colour; as a child his hair will be more red than black, when he reaches his prime, the reverse.[67]

Furthermore, Galen's theory of mixtures explains how medical treatment of psychological states can be effective. The elementary qualities hot, cold, dry and wet and their varying proportions also constitute the domain in which treatment by means of dietetics and pharmacology is said to operate. This is set out in the third book of *Mixtures*, which is essentially devoted to pharmacology and where the basic outlines are given of Galen's therapeutics, which will be expounded in more detail in his grand *Therapeutic Method*, his work on drug treatment (*Simples*) and his account of dietetics in *The Properties of Foods*. We have to assume that all physical treatment—and hence also the psychological treatment it facilitates—works by its impact and interaction with the mixtures in the body: all substances (foods, drinks, drugs) that

---

[65] *Mixtures* 74,7–75,2 (I.628 K.).

[66] *Mixtures* 59,24–60,4 (I.603–604 K.).

[67] *Mixtures* 41,24–43,9 (I.575–577 K.), tr. Singer and van der Eijk 2014. For similar psychophysical correlations see 73,1 H. (I.625 K.): 'Rather, we should in this case conclude that there is a very high degree of heat in the heart, and therefore also that it he is spirited.', and 84,9–13 H. (I.643 K.): 'The bodily condition of one who was cold and dry from the beginning will be white, soft, bare, lacking in veins and in articulation, thin, and cold to the touch, while the character of his soul will be lacking in resolve, cowardly, easily dispirited.'

are administered to the body, their varying dosages and modes of preparation and application, and other therapeutic remedies such as massage and exercise, all work through the agency of the four elementary qualities interacting between the constitution of the therapeutic agent and the mixture of the human body. Galen describes their capacities (*dunameis*) and the conditions of their actualisation (*energeia*) in great detail in book III of *Mixtures*; and again, there is an optimistic tenor here suggesting that most states of the body—and, consequently, of the mind—are capable of being treated in this way.

Yet this is not the whole story. For at two points in the discussion of *Mixtures*, Galen makes it clear that not everything in the body is down to the mixtures. There are some features of the human body-soul composite that, so to speak, precede the mixtures in the order of their design. They are the result of 'craftmanship of nature', and this, Galen says at one point, 'shapes the parts of the body in a way which is in accordance with the character traits of the soul.'[68] Apparently, some natural, anatomical and physiological features of a human individual do not fall under the rubric of the mixtures, and any psychological features that are correlated to these features escape the determinism of the mixtures.

Furthermore, a passage in Galen's *Art of Medicine* points out that there are some characteristics of human bodies that are, so to speak, posterior to the mixtures. For while it is possible, to some extent, to relate a person's character traits to his physiological state and thus to diagnose, on the basis of these traits, what kind of mixture a person may have, there are exceptions to this:

> Whatever has been said on the subject of moral characteristics, here or in any other discussion, of diagnosis of the mixture, applies to innate characteristics, not to those—good or bad—which come about through philosophy.[69]

The context of this passage is the connection between physical states and character traits. And while, on the whole, and in keeping with *Mixtures*, Galen tends to explain the latter by reference to the former, he makes a distinction between innate characteristics and features that are the result of philosophical training, allowing the latter a state of relative independence that the former do not have. The implication clearly is that these characteristics produced by philosophy are not subject to treatment by means of

---

[68] *Mixtures* 79,22–23 (I.636 K.), tr. Singer and van der Eijk 2014.
[69] *Art of Medicine* 11, p. 309, 2–7 Boudon-Millot (I.336–337 K), tr. Singer 1997.

diet and drugs; presumably, we have to assume, they are to be corrected only by philosophical training, either good or bad. Which ones these are, Galen does not explain here, just as, somewhat disappointingly, he does not explain what the psychological features are that are due to the craftmanship of nature and that precede the determination by the mixtures. Yet it is clear that Galen does not believe that physical treatment is appropriate to all mental states and that there are some conditions that are beyond bodily influence and curable by means of psychological or spiritual means only. This, I suggest, is where the spiritual and moral regime of his other treatise, *Diagnosis and Treatment of the Affections and Errors of the Soul*, comes in, addressing anger, rage and other character flaws through an ethical rather than a medical mode of therapy.[70] And here, we do find explicit indications of the limits to curability: several times Galen cautions that cure may not always be possible, and in most cases this seems due to the time that has elapsed since the beginning of the condition.[71]

Galen is operating here on the by now familiar borderline between the pathological and the ethical, and the distinction is not always clear. Once again, *ultimately*, the impact of moral and spiritual guidance on an individual's soul and character is, itself, of a corporeal nature, since in Galen all psychic processes and states are, ultimately, corporeal. But on the surface, in mode of description and of course also in actual therapeutic practice, there is a distinction between an ethical regime and a treatment consisting of dietetic or pharmacological measures. Thus we see that, in Galen, once again the question of cure is different depending on the origin or cause of the features that are to be cured. The treatment is different whether we are dealing with features of the human psycho-physical composite that are due to the initial design: these, like the 'passages' of the soul mentioned by the author of *Regimen*, are the way they are and, one may assume, they are not accessible to treatment. Then there is the large area of features due to the mixtures, and these are all, in principle, open to treatment, unless there are supervening external features (*mêdenos exôthen empodizomenou*). Thirdly, there is the area of character traits that are the product of philosophy; and here, one may assume, the treatment will be different once again; and again, curability will depend on the specific circumstances.

---

[70] See, e.g. *Affections and Errors* 5, CMG p. 16 (De Boer) (V.22 K.), referring to irrational madness, rage and anger.

[71] Galen, *Affections and Errors of the Soul*, CMG p. 20,15–19 (V.29 K.), p. 25,9–11 (V.37 K.), p. 35,5–9 (V.52 K.).

Ptolemy's Affections of the Soul

We conclude with a little-known but most informative discussion of mental illness that can be found in a work by one of Galen's contemporaries, Ptolemy, in his *Tetrabiblos*, book III, ch. 15 (14).[72] And there are good reasons for this, for Ptolemy seems to be well aware of medical views, e.g. when he speaks of human mixture (*krasis*) in terms of proportions between the elementary qualities hot, cold, dry and wet,[73] when he speaks of the mixture of the soul (*psuchikê krasis*),[74] or when he refers to diseases caused by gatherings of the moistures (*hugrôn ochlêseis*);[75] and his account of bodily injuries and affections in III.13 (12) is rich in medical terminology.

The *Tetrabiblos* is, essentially, an astrological text making predictions about states, experiences and events that may happen to a person (both physically and psychologically), based on certain assumptions about the causal influence of the planets on human life, in particular that of the constellations or configurations of the planets at the time the person was conceived or born.[76] These astrological assumptions, which Ptolemy spells out elsewhere in his work,[77] need not concern us here too much. What is relevant for our purposes is that in chapter 15, mental affections (*pathê psuchika*) are distinguished as a separate category from bodily injuries and affections (*sinê kai pathê sômatika*), which are the subject of ch. 13;[78] and affections (*pathê*) of the soul are distinguished from qualities or features

---

[72] I have referred to the chapter, page and line numbers of the Teubner edition by F. Boll and A. Boer, Leipzig 1940, whose chapter division differs slightly from the Loeb edition by F.E. Robbins 1940 (R., mentioned in brackets). See also Cumont 1937, Geller 2010 and Tucker 1961. I am grateful to Henry Mendell for bringing this passage to my attention and for discussing it with me.

[73] Pp. 143,23; 144,3 f. 16 f.; 145,22 and 147,5 f. (pp. 308, 310, 312, 316 R.). I am aware that the term *krasis* is also used to refer to planetary relationships, e.g. 'the mixture of the different natures' mentioned at p. 120,1 f. (p. 248 R.), or the 'good mixture' of hot and cold (*to eukraton*) mentioned in p. 18,17 ff.; 19,4 (p. 36 R.); see also p. 32,18 ff. (p. 64 R.).

[74] P. 168, 13 (p. 360 R.).

[75] P. 118, 4 f. (p. 244 R.).

[76] P. 107,8–11 (p. 222 R.), distinguishing between *spora* and *kata tên apokuêsin ektropê*. See also p. 122,14 f. (p. 254 R.).

[77] E.g. in I.4–10, where he discusses the role of the elementary forces in the causative effect of the planets on life on earth; see also in III.1.

[78] The distinction between the two is defined on p. 148,25 ff. (p. 320 R.): 'an injury (*sinos*) affects the subject once for all and does not involve lasting pain, while disease (*pathê*) bears upon the patient either continuously or in sudden attacks.' Further down in the chapter, Ptolemy refers to blindness as impairment (*pêrôsis*, p. 149,9, p. 320 R.) and to deformations (*lôbêseis*, p. 151,13, p. 324 R.) such as hunchback, crookedness, lameness, or paralysis.

of the soul (*poiotêtes psuchikai* or *idiômata tês psuchês*); the latter are also
referred to as ethical (*êthikos*),[79] and they are the subject of ch. 14. In turn,
these features and qualities of the soul are distinguished from bodily form
and mixture (*morphê kai krasis sômatikê*), which are the subject of ch. 12.

Thus it seems that all the distinctions we have been discussing between
the mental and the physical, the moral and the pathological, have been
implemented here.[80] When we look at what Ptolemy has to say on these
affections of the soul,[81] it appears that they are not just excesses (*huperbal-
lonta*) or extremes (*akra*) of the vices and character flaws he has been discussing in the previous chapter. Those that Ptolemy is concerned with in this
chapter are utterly disproportionate (*ametria*), pathological (*nosêmatôdê*)
and they affect a person's whole nature (*holê phusis*), which includes both
the intelligent (*dianoêtikon*) and the affective (*pathêtikon*) part of the soul.[82]
As examples, Ptolemy mentions people suffering from epilepsy (*epilêpti-
koi*),[83] people suffering from mania (*maniôdeis*),[84] people struck by demons
(*daimonioplêktoi*) and people suffering from moisture in their heads (*hugro-
kephaloi*).[85]

The severity and (in)curability of these diseases, and indeed the mode of
their cure, is said to depend on the planetary constellation that causes them.
Thus we hear that

---

[79] P. 158,2 (p. 338 R.).

[80] In practice, though, there seems to be some overlap, as in the listings of people's
character features caused by certain planetary constellations in ch. 14 (13 R.), we do find
features very similar to some of the pathological features mentioned in ch. 15 (14 Robbins),
such as lasciviousness and sexual indulgence (cf. p. 165,1–9, p. 354 R. with p. 171,16–173,19,
pp. 368–370 R.). Yet Ptolemy seems to be aware of this when he says (p. 169,15–20, p. 362 R.)
that 'most of the moderate diseases have, in a way, already been distinguished in what has
been said about the character (*idiômata*) of the soul, and their increase can be discerned
from the excess of injurious influences; for one might now with propriety call 'diseases' those
extremes of character which either fall short of or exceed the mean (*tês mesotêtos*).' Yet
in the present chapter he is concerned with 'Those affections, however, which are utterly
disproportionate and as it were pathological ...' (p. 169,21f., p. 364 R.).

[81] According to the first paragraph, he only deals with a selection (*exaireta*); see previous
note.

[82] In contrast to *dianoêtikos*, 'affective' (or 'emotional') seems preferable for *pathêtikos*
to Robbins' 'passive'. Yet further down, (p. 171,16–19, p. 368 R.), the contrast is between
poiêtikos and *pathêtikos*. In ch. 14 (13) (p. 154,17–20 R. 332 R.), Ptolemy divides the soul into a
'rational and intellectual part' (*to logikon kai noeron meros*) and a 'sensitive and non-rational'
(*aisthêtikon kai alogon*) part.

[83] Note that epileptic seizures are also mentioned, together with 'falling fits' (*ptôma-
tismoi*), in the chapter on physical diseases, III.14 (13), p. 153,11ff., (p. 330 R.).

[84] Further down, *maniai kai ekstaseis* are mentioned in one breath (p. 171,5, p. 366 R.).

[85] P. 170,8 (p. 364 R.).

when the maleficent planets are by themselves and rule the configuration in the manner stated, the diseases of the rational part of the soul which we have mentioned as being caused by them are, to be sure, incurable, but latent and obscure. But if the beneficent planets Jupiter and Venus have some familiarity to them when they are themselves in the western parts and the beneficent planets are angular in the east, they make the diseases curable, but noticeable; if it be by Jupiter, curable by medical treatments, a diet, or drugs, if Venus, by oracles and the aid of the gods.[86]

Thus the (planetary) gods are not only the causes of diseases, in some cases they are also to be invoked for their treatment. Furthermore, some of these mental diseases, depending on their cause, become incurable, the subject of talk, and conspicuous. Thus Ptolemy goes on to say:

> in epilepsy (*epilêpsias*), they involve the victims in continuous attacks, notoriety, and deadly peril; in madness and seizures (*manias kai ekstaseis*), they cause instability, alienation of friends, tearing off clothes, abusive language, and the like; in demonic seizures (*daimonioplêxiais*), or gatherings of moistures (*hugrôn ochlêseis*), (they involve the victims in) possession (*enthousiasmois*), confession (*exagoriais*), torments (*aikiais*), and similar manifestations.[87]

Ptolemy then moves on to a discussion of pathological perversion affecting the other, affective (*pathêtikos*) part of the soul, again caused by planetary configurations at the time of conception or birth and depending in their details on more specific variations in constellation.[88] As in the case

---

[86] μόνοι μὲν οὖν οἱ κακοποιοὶ κατὰ τὸν προειρημένον τρόπον τὴν ἐπικράτησιν τοῦ σχήματος λαβόντες ἀνίατα μὲν ἀνεπίφαντα δὲ ὅμως καὶ ἀπαραδειγμάτιστα ποιοῦσι τὰ προκείμενα τοῦ διανοητικοῦ τῆς ψυχῆς νοσήματα· συνοικειωθέντων δὲ τῶν ἀγαθοποιῶν Διός τε καὶ Ἀφροδίτης ἐπὶ μὲν τῶν λιβικῶν μερῶν ὄντες αὐτοὶ τῶν ἀγαθοποιῶν ἐν τοῖς ἀπηλιωτικοῖς κεκεντρωμένων ἰάσιμα μὲν εὐπαραδειγμάτιστα δὲ ποιοῦσι τὰ πάθη. ἐπὶ μὲν τοῦ τοῦ Διὸς διὰ θεραπειῶν ἰατρικῶν καὶ ἤτοι διαιτητικῆς ἀγωγῆς ἢ φαρμακείας, ἐπὶ δὲ τοῦ τῆς Ἀφροδίτης διὰ χρησμῶν καὶ τῆς ἀπὸ θεῶν ἐπικουρίας. (p. 170,11–22, pp. 364–366 R.; tr. Robbins, slightly modified). Curability and incurability also figure in Ptolemy's account of physical injuries and diseases in III.13 (12); thus on p. 153,18–154,3 (p. 330 R.), the absence of the influence of beneficent planets causes injuries and diseases to be incurable and painful (*aniata kai epachthê*), whereas the presence of such influence makes them easy to remove (*euapallakta*). Furthermore, we find a similar distinction between medical and divine healing: Jupiter is said to 'cause the injuries to be concealed by human aid through riches or honours, and the diseases to be mitigated; and in company with Mercury he brings this about by drugs and the aid of good physicians' (*pharmakeiais ê iatrôn agathôn epikouriais*), while Venus is said to 'contrive that through pronouncements of the gods and oracles (*prophaseôs theôn kai chrêsmôn*) the blemishes shall be, in a way, comely and attractive, and that the diseases shall be readily moderated by divine healing (*tais apo theôn iatreiais euparêgorêta*).' (p. 154,3–9, pp. 330–332 R.).

[87] P. 171,2–9 (p. 366 R.; tr. Robbins, slightly modified).

[88] P. 171,19 ff. (p. 368 R.).

of affections of the active or rational part of the soul, he concentrates on
the extreme cases (*exaireta*), and these, he says, manifest themselves particularly in the domain of sexual aberrations from the natural, both on the
male and the female side, where natural and unnatural seem to refer to
active and passive positions in sexual intercourse. Thus on certain planetary configurations, men become 'addicted to natural sexual intercourse,
and are adulterous, insatiate, and ready on every occasion for base and lawless acts of sexual passion, while the females are lustful for unnatural con-
gresses, cast inviting glances of the eye, and are what we call *tribades*; for
they deal with females and perform the functions of males.'[89] On other configurations, he argues, it is the men who exceed in unnatural sexual activities, becoming soft and effeminate. Further manifestations of these kinds
of sexual behaviour are discussed, varying in degrees of secrecy, openness
and shamefulness. Yet again other constellations, especially the influence
of Jupiter, make for 'greater decorum, restraint, and modesty', while Mercury tends to increase notoriety, instability of the emotions, changeability
and foresight.[90]

Ptolemy's categorisation of these kinds of sexual activity as pathological and unnatural need not come to us as a surprise, as it reflects attitudes attested elsewhere, e.g. in Aristotle's notorious condemnation of male
homosexuality (*NE* 1148b27–34) or, almost a millennium later, in Caelius
Aurelianus' description of male homosexuality as a chronic disease (*Chronic
Affections* IV.9).[91] What is relevant for our purposes is, again, that affections of
the soul include not only states of mind but also tendencies and behaviour;
and that they are labelled as pathological (*nosêmatôdê*) and thus, at least
theoretically, distinguished from moral dispositions.

Thus we see that underlying Ptolemy's account is a categorical distinction between affections of the body (including injuries and diseases) and
affections of the soul; and the latter include what we would call character
flaws and moral weaknesses on the one hand and, again in our terminology,
clinical, psycho-pathological states, disorders, behavioral patterns on the
other. A further recurring characteristic in Ptolemy's account, mentioned
more prominently than in the other sources we have looked at, is the public
or private aspect of the conditions mentioned, whether they are latent or
conspicuous and, if the latter, to what extent they are much discussed and

---

[89] P. 172,5–14 (p. 368 R.).
[90] P. 173,16–19 (pp. 370–372 R.).
[91] See Keuls 1995, 264 and Schrijvers 1985.

much criticised.[92] Furthermore, we find statements about the treatment of the conditions mentioned, at least for the first group of conditions affecting the rational, active part of the soul. Some are said to be curable, others incurable, and curability and incurability are said to vary according to the cause of the disease;[93] likewise, the nature of the cure differs according to the cause. Yet, most remarkably, Ptolemy makes a further difference between treatment of affections of the active, rational part by medical means and treatment of the same group of affections by means of oracles and the aid of the gods.[94] The criterion for this distinction seems entirely a matter of whether the affection is caused by one planet or the other, not by any categorical difference in causation, symptoms or time that has elapsed since the beginning of the disease. What is further striking is that Ptolemy says nothing about any treatment of the affections of the affective part of the soul, the ones that manifest themselves in sexual aberrations: are we to infer from this that Ptolemy regarded them as incurable?

Conclusion

We have seen how ancient medical and philosophical authors, when confronted with manifestations of mental disorder, tried to make sense of these phenomena by making distinctions, sometimes implicitly, sometimes explicitly, and classifications: between conditions of the mind and conditions of the body; between conditions caused by psychological and cultural or by physical and environmental factors; between acute and chronic conditions; between clinical, pathological conditions and moral, ethical states

---

[92] Again, this point is also made in relation to physical diseases, e.g. p. 154,9–11 (pp. 330–332 R.): 'If, however, Saturn is by, the healing will be accompanied by exhibition and confession of the disease' (*meta paradeigmatismôn kai exagoriôn*, tr. Robbins). Public confession (*exagoria*) is also mentioned, but apparently as a symptom of disease rather than an accompanying phenomenon of the healing process, in p. 171,9–13 (p. 366 R.): 'Of the places that possess the configuration, those of the sun and Mars aid in causing madness, those of Jupiter and Mercury, epilepsy; those of Venus, divine possession and public confession' (*theophorias kai exagorias*, tr. Robbins).

[93] A further relevant passage in this connection can be found in book IV, ch. 9, where Ptolemy discusses various modes and causes of death. One category he mentions is death through disease, and here he distinguishes between diseases caused by Saturn, Jupiter, Mars, Venus and Mercury: the latter, he says, kills through 'madness, distraction, melancholy, the falling sickness, epilepsy (*maniôn kai ekstaseôn kai melancholiôn kai ptômatismôn kai epilêpseôn*), diseases accompanied by coughing and raising, and all such ailments as arise from the excess of deficiency of dryness' (p. 201,5–8, p. 430 R., tr. Robbins).

[94] On the role of the gods in earlier medical texts see van der Eijk 2004.

of mind; between cognitive, emotional and behavioural disorders; between congenital and acquired conditions; between conditions to be treated by means of dietetic and pharmacological means, those that need psychological treatment, those that allow a combination of both, and those for which one needs to take recourse to the gods through oracles and prayers; and between conditions that are curable, easily curable, difficult to cure, or incurable. We have further seen that these authors were mostly confident about the possibility of treating these conditions; at any rate there is no suggestion that they regarded any of these conditions as by definition beyond cure, or more difficult to cure than bodily conditions. And finally, we have seen that they tried to develop, with varying degrees of clarity, criteria in order to apply these distinctions to individual cases, though in the end leaving a great deal of room to the judgement of the therapist. Whatever one may think of the practicability of their endeavours, in doing so they raised questions about moral responsibility and medicalisation that are still facing us today.

PHILOSOPHICAL THERAPY AS
PREVENTIVE PSYCHOLOGICAL MEDICINE

Christopher Gill

What contribution was made to the treatment of mental illness in antiquity by philosophical essays on the therapy of emotions? To what extent can we—moderns—recognize in these essays a credible response to mental illness? In this discussion, I explore both these questions, in the belief that each of these lines of enquiry may illuminate each other. A key point, bearing on both questions, is the suggestion that the philosophical essays were intended to function as a psychological analogue for ancient medical regimen, or what we call 'life-style management' or 'preventive medicine'. I begin by developing this suggestion in general terms before relating this idea to the emergence of a distinct genre or body of writings on the therapy of the emotions in the Hellenistic and Roman Imperial periods. Next, I analyse the core strategy of this kind of philosophical therapy, identifying four key recurrent themes. I illustrate this schema, referring especially to Galen's newly found essay, *Avoiding Distress*, taken as representing a Platonic-Aristotelian approach, on the one hand, and to Seneca's *On Peace of Mind*, representing the Stoic approach, on the other. I then return to the idea that such works are designed to function as preventive psychological medicine, and ask whether they embody an approach to psychological health-care that we could find useful under modern conditions.

Ancient Philosophy as Preventive Medicine

First, I consider whether we can take seriously the thought that philosophical essays on the therapy of the emotions were seen in antiquity as a credible and potentially effective way of helping people cope with psychological illness or disorder. This is distinct from the question how far this ancient practice corresponds to modern methods of psychological care; but trying to correlate it with current methods may help us to make better sense of the function of these practices in their original setting. Some earlier scholarship has proposed that we should see the function of these ancient works as comparable with modern cognitive psychotherapy. The relevant point of comparison is that the patient is addressed as a responsible agent, capable in principle of understanding the causes of her own current distress and of relieving this by a deliberate programme of actions or thoughts.[1] This approach can be contrasted with psychoanalysis or other modern methods of psychotherapy which focus on trying to detect the unconscious roots of current disturbance, on the assumption that doing so, in itself, holds the prospect of psychological cure. Another relevant modern practice is counselling, which can be seen as a less technical version of cognitive therapy.[2] Although this comparison provides a starting-point for understanding the ancient genre, there are limitations to the analogy. For one thing, modern cognitive therapy and counselling are offered to people who already feel distressed and in need of some external support or guidance of this kind, whereas this is not necessarily the case with the ancient methods. Also, at least some ancient thinkers, certainly the Stoics and to some extent the Epicureans, characterize as mad or psychologically sick people who would not regard themselves in this way. These points of difference create what are, on the face of it, significant difficulties for the comparison between ancient philosophical therapy and modern cognitive therapy or counselling.[3]

However, I would like to offer a response to this problem, and one which also throws light on the function of this kind of writing in the ancient context. A first move is to explore the significance of the parallel with (body-based) medical treatment which is such a prominent feature of this ancient philosophical practice.[4] In the modern context, we tend to identify medical treatment with responses, through drugs or surgery, for instance, to illness or injury that has already occurred. These responses also correspond to well-marked branches of ancient medicine. But another, and very important, part of ancient medical practice was *diaita* or regimen, 'life-style management', as we might say, especially as regards diet, exercise, and choice of environment.[5] In fact, regimen or preventive medicine also plays a role in modern Western medical and socio-cultural practice (as it has in some non-Western medical traditions); and many people think it should be given

---

[1] See Sorabji 2000, 153–155.

[2] See Gill 2010a, 355–357.

[3] See Gill 1985, 321–322.

[4] On this analogy, see Pigeaud 1981 for a comprehensive treatment; also Gill 2010a, 295, 301–302.

[5] On this aspect of ancient medicine, see Jouanna 1974, 232–253, Wöhrle 1990, Nutton 2004, 96–97, 166–170, 240–242, van der Eijk 2008a, 297–300.

much greater weight and resources in medicine and society generally. The well-recognized importance of regimen in ancient practice helps to explain, I think, the readiness of ancient philosophers to characterize their ethical teachings as 'therapy' for the psyche.

The function of the ancient philosophical works on the therapy of emotions is much closer to regimen than to reactive treatment after the occurrence of disease. The main focus is on promoting a way of life and set of attitudes that will prevent distress and (what the theory presents as) psychological sickness. Put differently, the ancient philosophical essays set out to develop what we might call emotional resilience, that is, the ability to cope with—what are usually seen as—personal disasters or problems without loss of emotional stability or inner calm. The readiness of ancient philosophers to direct their therapy at people who are not (or not yet) distressed fits in with this preparatory or preventive approach. The tendency, in at least some theories, to extend the boundaries of what should count as psychological illness, can also be linked with this objective. The underlying assumption, as I bring out later, is that all or much human distress is produced by the beliefs held by the people concerned, and that changing these beliefs will help to pre-empt this distress. The preventive or preparatory function of the writings on the therapy of the emotions can be defined, to some extent at least, by contrast with the function of ancient consolatory writings. Consolatory writings are explicitly directed at people who are currently distressed, especially by the recent loss of a loved relative. Although this genre of writings draws on similar themes and ideas to those used in the therapy of emotions, the approach differs, at least in responding to distress already experienced; and this kind of writing can be more readily compared to medical treatment designed for those already ill. By the same token, this kind of writing is more obviously analogous with modern counselling or cognitive therapy.[6]

The prevalence of ancient writings on regimen and the therapy of emotions reflects a more general feature of Greek and Roman culture. This is the assumption that a standard part of the life of an adult free male (at least, an educated, reasonably well-resourced male) is to direct his life towards the achievement of certain recognized goods, typically including health and happiness. Michel Foucault stressed the importance of this aspect of ancient culture, which he characterized as 'the care of the self', suggesting that it was

---

[6] On consolatory writings, and parallels with modern counselling or psychotherapy, see Baltussen forthcoming.

a distinctive feature of Roman life in the first and second centuries AD.[7] But, arguably, it is widespread from a much earlier period, and certainly forms part of the background of Hellenistic medical and philosophical thinking. Writings on regimen form part of the Hippocratic corpus, dating from the late fifth century BC onwards. Both Plato and Aristotle, in their ethical writings, presuppose as rather common this goal-directed attitude to the shaping or management of one's life, with a view to gaining what is regarded as happiness (*eudaimonia*).[8] This prevalent social attitude has a special bearing on the kind of writings being considered here. Teaching and writings on the therapy of emotions, like those on the management of physical regimen, seem to have been regarded as part of a mainstream set of social practices, at least among wealthy educated males, even if some of the views presented under this heading may have seemed extreme or implausible. This feature of the social context of the therapy of emotions relates to the question how far this is a practice that we, moderns, should want to adopt, a question pursued in the last part of this essay.

Ancient Writings on the Therapy of Emotions

What ancient writings, exactly, should we consider as offering therapy of the emotions and how do they relate to other works that can be characterized as 'practical ethics' in antiquity? How does the analogy with medical writings arise and how far does this analogy encourage us to see a close link with ancient regimen? There are a number of overlapping groups of writings, surviving in whole or part or known about, which are relevant here. The linkage or analogy with medicine is explicit and recurrent in these writings; the connection with regimen specifically is less explicit, though I shall argue that it is one that makes sense.

   In identifying relevant works, and in considering where they fit in the larger map of ancient writings of this kind, it is useful to hold in view a three-fold distinction sometimes drawn in antiquity: between protreptic, therapy, and advice. In connection with philosophically informed practical ethics, these three activities are, typically, seen as having interrelated functions. Protreptic offers encouragement to undergo therapy: therapy removes false beliefs that produce psychological sicknesses; advice replaces the false

---

   [7] Foucault 1990, 41–50.
   [8] See e.g. Plato, *Symp.* 204e–205a, *Rep.* 360e–361d, 588b–592b, Aristotle *NE* 1.1–5, 10.7–8. On this strand in Aristotle and Hellenistic philosophy, see Annas 1993, 27–46.

beliefs with true, or at least better-grounded, ones. The three-fold set of activities, taken as a whole, is seen as helping to lead from psychological sickness to—or towards—health, though the linkage between medicine and philosophy is most strongly signalled in connection with therapy.[9] A group of writings running from Chrysippus' 'therapeutic book' (third century BC) to Galen's *Psychological Affections* (second century AD) present themselves as offering therapy for the emotions, at least for those emotions seen as diseased. But these writings also often have protreptic or advisory dimensions, which are more or less fully integrated with the therapeutic aspect.[10] Other writings in this period which are not specifically presented as therapeutic, such as Epictetus' *Discourses* and Marcus Aurelius' *Meditations*, also seem designed to integrate these functions in a broadly similar way to the therapeutic essays.[11] A related group of writings focus, rather, on consolation, especially for the recently bereaved. Cicero wrote one to himself, as well as reviewing consolatory strategies, and consolations survive by Seneca and Plutarch. The consolatory writings overlap in themes and approach with philosophical writings on therapy; indeed, grief or fear of death is one of the principal kinds of psychological 'sickness' addressed by therapeutic writings, especially by Epicureans. In this essay, my main focus is on the philosophical (or philosophically inspired) essays which announce their role as being the therapy of the emotions. But it is important to recognize that they form part of a broader spectrum of Hellenistic and Roman writings on practical ethics, in which the idea of protreptic, therapy, and advice, as interlocked functions, is pervasive.

The analogy with medicine is crucial for identifying these therapeutic essays and making sense of their programme. The idea that philosophers offer treatment for the psyche which parallels the therapy offered by doctors for the body figures prominently in Plato and is ascribed to the fifth-century sophist Antiphon.[12] But the systematic exploration of this idea belongs to Hellenistic thought, particularly to Stoicism and Epicureanism.[13] Especially

---

[9] For this three-fold typology, see Stobaeus, 2.39.20–41.25, referring to Philo of Larisa (158–184 BC); on Philo's use of this typology, see Brittain 2001, 277–280. On typologies of this kind in Hellenistic, especially Stoic, philosophy, see Gill 2003, 42–43.

[10] On these writings, see Gill 2010a, ch. 5; also below.

[11] On these writings, as forms of practical ethics, see Hadot 1995, ch. 6, Long 2002, Sellars 2003, 2007.

[12] See e.g. Democritus, DK 68 B 31, Plato, *Charm.* 155b–157d, *Gorg.* 475d, 505c, *Rep.* 444c–e, *Soph.* 227c–230e, *Tim.* 86d–90d. See further Laín Entralgo 1970, 97–98, Mackenzie 1981, chs. 10–11, Lloyd 2003, 208–212, 237–238.

[13] See Nussbaum 1994, Sorabji 2000, part 2.

important for promulgating this theme was the fourth book of Chrysippus' (lost) work *On Passions* (or *On Emotions, Peri Pathōn*), which seems to have been the first work of this kind explicitly characterized as 'therapeutic' in aim. The underlying assumption is that certain emotions are bad and constitute psychic illnesses, including emotions such as anger not conventionally regarded as inherently problematic. Chrysippus' book seems to have focused on promoting the idea that (most) emotions are psychological sicknesses and on systematic analysis of their nature and sub-types. In this respect, his work can be seen as protreptic, encouraging readers to see their emotions as needing therapy. However, promoting this understanding of emotions can also be seen as an integral part of the therapeutic process and as the beginning, at least, of acquiring a better and more 'healthy' belief-set. Chrysippus also addresses practical questions about the timing of effective therapy and about the best way to approach different types of people affected.[14] Seneca's *On Anger* is the one surviving Stoic work which falls squarely within the therapeutic category. Seneca's work, like that of Chrysippus, gives a prominent role to presenting most emotions as bad, and not just those normally seen as excessive or extreme. But Seneca also includes an extensive discussion of *remedia*, modes of treatment that one can and should apply to oneself. To this extent, this book also embraces advice, but of a type that is specifically linked with the conception of emotions as diseased and needing cure.[15]

Epicureanism also adopted from an early stage the analogy between the roles of philosophy and medicine and linked this motif with a radical critique of many emotions and desires not conventionally conceived as bad or as 'sick'.[16] However, Chrysippus' 'therapeutic book' seems to have been the first one which took this topic as its main theme and function. Although Chrysippus' approach to therapy is criticized by later Epicurean thinkers on this topic, his work may, none the less, have been influential in stimulating a series of Epicurean writings which also characterize as 'diseased'

---

[14] For reconstruction of this work and interpretation, see Tieleman 2003, chs. 4, 6 and Appendix (325–326); for analysis of its aims, see Gill 2010a, 280–295. For the medical-philosophical analogy in Stoicism, see e.g. Long and Sedley 1987 (= LS), refs. to LS normally to section and passage, LS 65 L, R, S; also Galen, *PHP* V.437 Kühn, 5.2.22–24, p. 298.28–38 De Lacy 2005, discussed in Gill 2010a, 309–310. (Kühn 1819–1833 is the 20-volume collection standardly used for references to Galen's works. References to Kühn are normally given in a combination of Roman and Arabic numerals, as here.)

[15] Seneca *Ira* 2.18–36, 3.5–43. For a synopsis of this work, see Cooper and Procopé 1995, xxxiii–xxxv; for analysis, Gill 2010a, 297–300.

[16] See e.g. LS, 25 C, J; Diogenes of Oenoanda fr. 2 Chilton 1971.

emotions not generally regarded in this way and which encourage their readers to attempt to cure them.[17] We have remains of, or know about, writings by Philodemus (first century BC) addressing anger and the fear of death. In the same period Book 3 of Lucretius' poem *The Nature of the Universe* can be seen as an extended treatment of the latter theme, designed to offer a set of philosophical arguments, embracing both 'physics' and ethics, against fear of death and thus offering 'cure' for those readers open to this form of treatment.[18] Although Stoics and Epicureans took the lead in this line of thought, the approach was taken up by other philosophical movements, sometimes with salient modifications. Cicero, for instance, whose main affiliation is with Academic Scepticism, offered an eclectic or independent version of therapeutic discourse, mainly directed at treating grief and fear of death, in his *Tusculan Disputations*.[19] Plutarch, whose typical stance is Platonic (or, in ethical psychology, Platonic-Aristotelian) wrote an essay on the management of anger in a style that is strongly influenced by Stoicism.[20] Essays on 'cheerfulness' (*euthumia*) or 'peace of mind' (*tranquillitas animi*) were composed by the Stoics Panaetius and Seneca and by Plutarch, writing in a more positive version of the therapeutic mode.[21] Galen, characteristically extending his scope from medicine into philosophy, composed a number of essays on practical ethics, of which two survive, both on the therapy of emotions. One is the newly discovered *Avoiding Distress*; the other is *On the Diagnosis and Cure of Psychological Affections*, the first half of a two-part work on emotions and errors.[22] Thus, we have a rather large body of works on the therapy of emotions, falling within what seems to be a continuous tradition, but written from different intellectual standpoints.

Why do we find the persistent use of the medical analogy in this type of writing? There are a number of reasons that plausibly explain this motif. One is that, from Plato onwards, the idea of medicine has connotations of authoritative expertise—despite the fact that the precise nature of medical

---

[17] Gill 2010a, 282 (referring to Philodemus *Ira* 1.10–20 Indelli 1988) and 295–297.

[18] See further Nussbaum 1994, chs. 4–7, Warren 2004, Tsouna 2009.

[19] See esp. *Tusc.* 1–2 and 5; see further Lévy 1992, 445–494, Erskine 1997.

[20] Becchi 1990, Waterfield and Kidd 1992, 168–175.

[21] See Gill 1994, Van Hoof 2010, ch. 4.

[22] The second work is referred to below as '*Psychological Affections*', and the standard Latin abbreviation is *Aff. Dig*; for translation of this work see Singer 1997, 100–127; for new translations of both works with introduction and commentary, see Singer forthcoming. For the Greek text of *Avoiding Distress* (Latin abbreviation, *Indol.*), see Boudon-Millot 2007 and Boudon-Millot et al. 2010.

expertise was a highly contested question in antiquity.[23] The adoption of
the medical stance is linked, especially in Stoic and Epicurean writings,
with the protreptic function of these writings. Health is generally, perhaps
even universally, seen as a human good; hence the offer to treat psychological sickness and provide a pathway towards psychological health constitutes a powerful encouragement to engage with the type of practices being
commended in this way.[24] The move by philosophers to undertake the role
of psychological doctor is also linked with the fact that ancient medicine
is predominantly focused on treatment of the body, or at least of the living person in her physical nature.[25] Hence, there was a substantial gap in
the scope of ancient medicine that philosophers were well placed to try
to fill. This move was reinforced by the fact that, on the more theoretical
aspects of medicine (physiology, for instance), there was substantial overlap
between ancient philosophy and medicine.[26] However, the ideas and methods advanced under the heading of psychological 'therapy' had their roots
elsewhere, especially in ancient ethical theory.

Was philosophical therapeutic discourse explicitly compared in antiquity with medical regimen, as distinct from the other branches of ancient
medicine? On the face of it, the answer is 'no'. Indeed, both Epicureans and
Stoics sometimes attempted to associate their psychological treatment with
the use of medical drugs or surgery.[27] However, it is evident that their use
of this kind of language was metaphorical. Even if ancient doctors tried to
treat mental illness, in part at least, by means of drugs or (much less commonly) surgery, these methods are not at all like the philosophical practices
characterized in analogous terms.[28] Ancient regimen, on the other hand, is
much more directly comparable with philosophical therapy. It constitutes
a programme of long-term management of the aspects of physical life that
are amenable to personal control, notably diet, exercise and related activi-

---

[23] On this point, see Lloyd 2003, 237–238.

[24] See further, in connection with Chrysippus, Gill 2010a, 285–288.

[25] See further Gill 2010a, 301–304.

[26] This is very clear in Galen's *QAM*, which cites medical and philosophical works equally
in support of the thesis that constitutes its title, *Psychological Faculties Depend on Bodily
Mixtures*, trans. in Singer 1997, 150–176, and forthcoming.

[27] The Stoic policy of 'extirpating' emotions, Cicero, *Tusc.* 3.13, 61, *Stoicorum Veterum
Fragmenta* (*SVF* = von Arnim 1903–1905) 3.443–444, 447, suggests surgery. The Epicurean idea
of philosophy as a 'four-fold remedy' (*tetrapharmakon*) (LS 25 J) suggests use of drugs. See
further Nussbaum 1994, 116–117, 389–340.

[28] For medical treatment of mental illness, see Pigeaud 1981, ch. 1, McDonald 2009 (on
phrenitis), and, on Galenic treatment, Nutton in this volume.

ties, and choice of environment.[29] State of mind or mood is also sometimes recognized as a factor that can affect physical health and that one should, accordingly, try to control.[30] In this respect, regimen is broadly similar, in the physical sphere, to the kind of advice offered by philosophers about the long-term management of emotions, along with related aspects of psychological life. It is an indication, perhaps, of the closeness of the two methods that we find attempts by practitioners of each method to appropriate the other sphere. For instance, Plutarch, author of a series of essays on practical ethics, including some on the therapy of emotions, also wrote a treatise on regimen, centred on combining management of health and a successful social life.[31] Galen, on the other hand, as well as writing on the therapy of emotions from a philosophical standpoint,[32] insists in one work that medicine, and specifically regimen, is more effective at making people psychologically better than philosophical guidance.[33] This suggests that ancient thinkers familiar with both modes of activity recognized them as having salient similarities.

Taken overall, one might offer this picture of the relationship between medical and philosophical approaches. Philosophers, notably Stoics and Epicureans, use the medical analogy, especially terms that evoke drugs and surgery, specifically to characterize the function of philosophical therapy (as distinct from protreptic and advice), namely to remove misguided beliefs that promote psychological sickness. However, there is a much closer, and non-metaphorical, relationship between regimen and philosophical discourse in this area. This is particularly true if we do not just focus on the 'therapy' dimension of philosophical discourse, but consider the overall aims of this kind of practice, integrating protreptic, therapy, and advice. Indeed, advice on the long-term management of one's life, with a view to physical or psychological health is the main common thread. The fact that regimen plays such a substantial role in ancient medicine may indeed have

---

[29] See Hippocrates, *Regimen*, Plutarch, *Precepts of Healthcare*, Galen, *On the Preservation of Health*; see further n. 5 above.

[30] See e.g. Galen, *The Art of Medicine* I.367 K (trans. in Singer 1997, 374), and commentary to Hippocrates, *Epidemics* VI (*CMG* 10,2,2), XVIIA 484.7–33, 485.17–19, 22–25, 487.18–23; see further García-Ballester 1988, 147–152, Gill 2010a, 318–319.

[31] Plutarch's *Moralia* ('Moral Essays') include *On Avoiding Anger and On Peace of Mind* (discussed below) as well as *Precepts of Health Care* (on the latter work, see Van Hoof 2010, ch. 8).

[32] See works cited in n. 22 above.

[33] *QAM* IV.768, 807–808 K, trans. in Singer 1997, 150, 169; see further Jouanna 2009, Gill 2010a, 319–321.

been one of the factors that made it plausible for philosophers to present their guidance as psychological medicine.

Core Strategy of Philosophical Therapy

I now consider the core strategy of these works of philosophical therapy. First, I outline this strategy in general terms, referring to the key themes in ancient philosophical theories that underpin this strategy. Subsequently, I illustrate features of this strategy, referring especially to Galen's *Avoiding Distress* and Seneca's *On Peace of Mind*, taken as exemplifying Platonic-Aristotelian and Stoic approaches respectively. Fundamental to this strategy is the aim of persuading people that all human beings, to some extent at least, have the ability and scope to achieve happiness or well-being by their own efforts. Distress or psychological disturbance is presented as being not—or largely not—the result of external circumstances, but as deriving from mistaken beliefs about what happiness requires and what constitutes happiness or the good life. Also crucial for the strategy is building on this recognition of what happiness requires. The method offers extensive advice on how to rebuild one's belief-set and thus to construct a framework of thinking (about actions, feelings, relationships, for instance) that provides a secure pathway to happiness. In terms of the three-fold distinction noted earlier, between protreptic, therapy, and advice, different aspects of this process can be correlated with one or other of these functions. From another standpoint, the process as a whole can be seen as therapeutic, in the sense that it tackles the roots of psychological sickness and helps people work towards health. It is important to note that the beliefs promoted in this way, and the component elements of the strategy, are taken to be objectively true and capable of being supported by well-grounded and systematic argument (though the therapeutic works do not set out to provide that argument). The beliefs promoted are not just advanced *in order to* alter the state of mind of the people offered this kind of treatment, or to *make them feel* less distressed—though this is claimed to be an outcome of a successful therapeutic process.[34]

I now consider more closely the key elements in this strategy. As will become clear, there are significant differences of view between ancient

---

[34] On this point, in Epicurean thinking, see Tsouna 263–265, challenging the views of Nussbaum 1994, ch. 4. Nussbaum 1994, 353–354, 491–492, herself accepts that this is true of Stoicism.

philosophical theories on how these elements should be conceived. However, there is also enough common ground for us to identify a single core strategy and set of key points. In bare outline, these four elements are: the conception of happiness involved, the psychological framework assumed, the formulation of the main therapeutic message, and advice about how to carry the therapeutic process forward. Although there are variations in the extent to which all four elements, especially the first two, are made explicit in any given example of therapeutic writing, the underlying presence of all four aspects is crucial for the credibility of the message and the effectiveness of the process.

The first element is the conception of happiness presupposed. A shared assumption of ancient philosophical theories is that happiness (in Greek, *eudaimonia*) is the natural target or goal of human aspiration, and also that this consists in an objective state, a condition of character and way of life, and not just a mood or set of moods (though its presence or absence affects one's moods).[35] A second shared assumption, and one fundamental for the therapeutic project, is that reaching happiness, or indeed making progress towards it, depends crucially on the person's own agency rather than on external factors. Within this common framework, there are significant differences of view, which form the basis for major, large-scale debates within theoretical works of ancient ethics in this period, such as Cicero's *On Ends*. Thus, for instance, the Stoics insist that, while virtue and happiness are not quite identical, virtue is the sole essential basis for happiness (it is both necessary and sufficient for happiness). On the other hand, in the Platonic-Aristotelian strand of thinking in this period, as adopted by Antiochus, for instance, some weight is given to 'external goods', that is, to factors such as health, the welfare of one's family or friends and material resources. More precisely, though it is recognized that the possession of virtue is the essential prerequisite for happiness, the achievement of the most complete kind of happiness is taken to depend on these further factors.[36] The Epicureans differ from the other theories in presenting pleasure, understood as absence of physical pain or psychological distress, as constitutive of happiness or the goal of life. However, the gap between the Epicurean and other theories is narrowed by the fact that they too see virtue as an essential basis for pleasure. The kind of pleasure that makes up happiness is regarded by

---

[35] See refs. in n. 8 above.
[36] The debate between these positions is played out at length in Cicero, *On Ends* 4–5, esp. 5.77–95 (see also 3.30–46). See further Annas 1993, chs. 19–21.

Epicureans as dependent on the kind of rational management of one's life that requires the proper exercise of the virtues (on an Epicurean understanding of what the virtues consist in).[37] Although the differences outlined here are intensely debated, they still allow the shared claim that the achievement of happiness depends crucially on one's own efforts as an agent, or that it is 'up to us', as Epictetus insistently puts it.[38] This claim is fundamental for all other aspects of the therapeutic strategy propagated by exponents of these theories, or by those, such as Galen, influenced by these theories.

The second element is an account of human psychology, one closely linked with a conception of ethical development (that is, development towards virtue and happiness, as understood by the theory). On this topic too, there are differences which give rise to intense, theoretical debate, but there is also a common core of ideas. The shared strand is the belief that all, or virtually all, adult human beings have some scope for exercising rational agency with a view to taking forward their development towards virtue and happiness, or towards a more complete form of these than they currently possess. The main topics of debate relevant for this element consist in the analysis of motivation, especially, how to understand the relationship between reason, emotion, and desire, and the prerequisites of ethical development. The Stoics, and to some extent the Epicureans, have a strongly unified view of human motivation, stressing that emotions and desires are shaped by beliefs and reasoning. In the Platonic-Aristotelian view, which is often pitted against the Stoic one in the first and second centuries AD, rational and non-rational aspects of motivation are seen as divergent in kind and potentially in conflict.[39] There is a related difference of view as regards the components of effective ethical development and their interrelationship. For the Platonic-Aristotelian approach, ethical development depends on the combination of a certain kind of inborn nature and habit-based upbringing in the right kind of family and community, and a form of rational education capable of enabling correct decision-making. For Stoics and also (though less emphatically) the Epicureans, the capacity of developing ethically is a property of all human beings as such, regardless of their specific inborn tendencies or upbringing. These two topics of debate are linked in that the greater scope seen for human development in the Stoic-Epicurean view is

---

[37] LS 21A–B, esp. B(6), M, O-P; also Cicero, *On Ends* 1.42–54. See further Annas 1993, ch. 16, Gill 1996, 395–397, Erler and Schofield 1999, 666.

[38] E.g. Epictetus, *Handbook* 1, *Discourses* 1.1.

[39] Key sources for this debate are Plutarch, *On Ethical Virtue*, and Galen *PHP* Books 4–5; see LS 65, also Gill 2006, ch. 4, 2010a, ch. 4.

connected with their belief that there is no fundamental cleavage between rational and non-rational parts of human psychology and so emotions and desires can be shaped or reshaped by changes of belief over a whole life-time by rational agency.[40] Despite intense arguments on these questions, both types of view allow some scope for adult human beings to play an active role within their own continuing ethical development, and thus to exercise the capacity to achieve happiness. This shared belief is, of course, closely linked with the shared assumption that happiness is the kind of state that depends crucially on the exercise of personal agency, rather than on external factors.

The third element in the process is the formulation of the central message of the therapeutic process (the scope for personal agency in working for happiness) in a form that engages effectively with the concerns of the person involved and his or her state of mind at the start of the therapy. Of course, we do not have independent access to actual discussions in antiquity and so we cannot tell exactly how, or how far, this kind of engagement occurred. But the writings we do have offer exemplary illustrations of this kind of dialogue, and sometimes adopt a literary form which seems designed to display the kind of engagement involved and the kind of therapeutic outcome intended.

The fourth element in the strategy is offering advice to the other person of a kind that is designed to enable him to rebuild his belief-set in a way that provides a secure basis for development away from the framework of beliefs that generates psychological sickness and towards well-being and happiness. The therapeutic writings offer a rich repertoire of such forms of advice, which can be supplemented by reference to related types of prac-tical ethics. Cicero, in his review of methods in *Tusculans* 3, highlights, for instance, preparation for (what are usually seen as) disasters, a technique shared by Cyrenaics and Stoics, and refocusing one's attention away from the causes of distress, a practice advocated by Epicureans.[41] Also relevant here are salient features of Stoic practical ethics, including Epictetus's advice to 'examine our impressions' before giving 'assent' to them, and Marcus' advo-cacy of 'stripping' situations to their moral essentials prior to responding to them.[42] In considering these methods, it is important to correlate them with the larger therapeutic strategy, and with the use to which this strategy is being put in any one context, as well as, in some cases at least, with the philosophical approach assumed.

---

[40] See Gill 2006, 130–138, 144–145, 178–182, 2010a, 201–208, 221–227.
[41] Cic. *Tusc.* 3.28–3, 33, 52; see further Sorabji 2000, chs. 15–16.
[42] See e.g. Epictetus, *Handbook* 1, *Discourses* 1.1.4–8. 1.27.1–13, 1.28.1–6, Marcus Aurelius, *Meditations* 3.11, 6.13, 12.2. See further Hadot 1995, 186–188, 193–199, Gill 2007, 179–180.

Examples of Philosophical Therapy: Galen and Seneca

I now illustrate this core strategy, with its four main elements, by reference to two works of philosophical, or philosophically informed, therapy: Galen's *Avoiding Distress* and Seneca's *On Peace of Mind*.[43] These two works are chosen for illustration because they are quite short and unified texts which exemplify the core strategy clearly, while also indicating the main differences between a Platonic-Aristotelian approach and a Stoic one. On some points, I refer to related works to illustrate the main elements and the way they are integrated with the strategy as a whole. The focus of the works differs, in that Galen's letter is centred on the question of how to withstand misfortune, whereas Seneca's dialogue addresses, initially at least, the problem of lack of a sense of purpose and consistency in one's life. However, both works include advice on confronting setbacks and have at their core ideas, of somewhat different kinds, about what is needed to provide the basis of emotional resilience and stability.

I begin with the third element, in the schema just outlined, the formulation of the central message, since this provides an overview of the shape of the two works.

Galen's *Avoiding Distress* takes the form of a letter to a young man wanting to know, for his own sake, how Galen has been able to cope with the loss of a huge number of his personal possessions (including many vital for his medical work) in the great fire of AD 192 at Rome, and has done so without loss of equanimity and emotional stability. This form enables Galen to use his own case as a paradigm and to deploy the first two key elements in the strategy (what is required for happiness and the psychological scope for agency that we have in seeking happiness) and to do so in a way that responds to the question posed by the addressee. Put more generally, the form allows him to show how the kind of thinking he is presenting, which is a non-technical version of the Platonic-Aristotelian approach, offers materials for enabling someone to strengthen his emotional resilience and the capacity to withstand what he sees as disasters.[44] Seneca's *On Peace of Mind* takes the form of a dialogue between Seneca himself and Serenus. The interlocutor presents himself as unable to maintain a consistent course of action

---

[43] On the Galen work, see n. 22 above. Seneca's work (*De Tranquillitate Animi*) is translated in the Loeb Classical Library (Basore, 1979, vol. 2) and The World's Classics (Davie and Reinhardt 2007).

[44] See introduction and notes to *Avoiding Distress* by Nutton in Singer forthcoming and Gill 2010a, 262–268.

and life and also incapable of sustaining stability in his character and state of mind. In response, Seneca offers a Stoic version of the ethical and psychological themes just outlined which shows how the interlocutor—or indeed, anyone—can chart and maintain a consistent and stable way of life and mode of character. Seneca also indicates how following this pathway can also enable someone to develop his capacity for withstanding disaster without loss of peace of mind, and in both respects to move towards happiness by his own efforts.[45] Thus, both these examples of the therapeutic genre formulate the core strategy outlined in a way that responds to the needs of the person concerned and offers a basis for relieving distress and lack of purpose in life and thus moving towards psychological well-being.

The importance of the first element in the core strategy is brought out very clearly in Galen's letter. In explaining to his addressee why he was not distressed by the loss of his possessions in the fire, Galen distinguishes his view from what he presents as the extreme position of the Stoics and Epicureans, that one can secure a kind of happiness that is invulnerable to *all* external circumstances. Towards the end of the essay, he says: 'Since you say that you have never seen me distressed, you may possibly imagine that I shall make the same pronouncement as some of the philosophers who promise that none of the wise will ever suffer distress' (70, cf. 48). He goes on to distance himself from both Stoic and Epicurean versions of this idea, associated with their respective ideals of *apatheia* (freedom from bad emotions) and *ataraxia* (freedom from distress). 'I make light of the loss of possessions without being quite deprived of them all and sent to a desert island, and [I make light] of bodily pain without [claiming that I am ready to be] placed in the bull of Phalaris' (71). Galen does not claim to have achieved the kind of complete or virtually complete invulnerability to external circumstances which is the goal of aspiration for both Stoicism and Epicureanism.[46] None the less, in specifying his positive ideal of happiness, he makes it clear that this ideal depends crucially on his own efforts.

> I am keenly aware that I depend on the quality of the state of both my body and my mind (*psuchē*), and so I would not like anything to arise from any external cause that could destroy my health or any disaster that could overpower my mind. Not that I neglect their welfare, but I always try, as far as

---

[45] Gill 1994, 4616–4624.

[46] Invulnerability to loss of possessions is presented here as a typical Stoic ideal and invulnerability to physical pain (feeling pleasure even if shut up in the bronze bull of the tyrant Phalaris over a fire) is presented as an Epicurean one. On these ideals, see further Gill 2006, 88–93, 102, 118–126; also e.g. LS 24 D and 63 L–M.

in my power, to endow them with sufficient strength to withstand whatever distresses them. Even if I do not expect my body to have the strength of Hercules or my mind to be like that they attribute to the sages, I think it better not to abandon deliberately any form of training.   (75–76)

Though presented as a purely personal ideal, this evokes the Platonic-Aristotelian ideal of happiness adopted by Antiochus, namely as a combination of psychic goods (virtue), some measure of bodily goods, such as health, and external goods, including material ones.[47] But, as Galen indicates here, both psychic and bodily aspects of this ideal require an ongoing programme of self-management (which is the fourth item in the core strategy).

There is less explicit focus on the conception of happiness in Seneca's *On Peace of Mind*. However, the Stoic approach is clearly implied. To achieve peace of mind, what is needed is not (as recommended by other thinkers) simply concentrating your activities or focusing on public—or private—life as such. What is required is a consistent matching of our own specific talents and inclinations to a way of life and set of projects that we can carry through consistently and unwaveringly in spite of setbacks and obstacles. What is also required is that we should conceive this process as part of a larger project of living a good human life, in other words, as the expression of virtue. It is thinking about our life in this way that enables us to achieve independence of fortune and external circumstances, which is linked with recognizing that this kind of success is up to us as agents. It is the consistent working out of this strategy, and only this, Seneca maintains, that will produce the peace of mind that Serenus is looking for.[48] At the centre of the work, Seneca places the Stoic ideal of the wise person (*sapiens*) who has achieved invulnerability to misfortune by following though this kind of life-plan and who thus shows that virtue is the only secure basis for happiness (11). This generalized ideal is supported by specific exemplars of the same principle (Socrates standing up to the 'thirty tyrants' in Athens and Julius Canus resisting the brutal Roman emperor Caligula, 5, 14). Although Seneca acknowledges the gap between these ideal figures and most people (11.1), fundamentally, the same conception of happiness applies to everyone.[49]

---

[47] See text to n. 36 above, and Gill 2010a, 264–266.

[48] See *On Peace of Mind* 2.3–5, 13, (referring to Democritus' approach to producing *euthumia*, 'cheerfulness'), 3–4, esp. 3.6 and 4.1, on the respective merits of public and private life and the importance of conceiving any way of life as a vehicle for the expression of virtue. On the background of Seneca's work, including Democritus DK 68 B3, see Gill 1994, 4609–4616; on Plutarch's alternative (though overlapping) strategy in *Peri Euthumias* (*On Contentment* or *On Feeling Good*), see Gill 1994, 4624–4631 and Van Hoof 2010, ch. 4.

[49] See further Gill 1994, 4615–4624.

As regards the second element in the core strategy, the psychological basis for exercising agency, both works refer to this element in a way that makes clear the different theoretical position underlying the therapeutic approach in each case. Galen's letter, like his related essay, *Psychological Affections*, stresses the contribution of his inborn nature and upbringing, especially the example of his father in providing the basis for emotional resilience in setbacks. His point is not that these factors ensure that Galen instinctively or automatically responds in this way. It is that his nature and upbringing have given him the capacity to use his education effectively and to build up, by his own efforts, the beliefs and attitudes that enable him to confront losses and disasters calmly.[50] In *Psychological Affections*, a similar view about ethical development is explicitly linked with a Platonic-Aristotelian account of psychological functions, as a combination of rational and non-rational 'parts' (or sources of motivation). The main conceptual link between these two points is that inborn nature and upbringing are seen as factors that shape our emotional (non-rational) character in a way that provides the basis for a rational response in framing our way of life and attitudes in adult life.[51] Thus, in Galen's case, and potentially for anyone with a similar nature or upbringing (or one that goes some way in the same direction), these factors give the foundation for the kind of measured and reflective response to material and personal losses that he recommends in both of his surviving therapeutic works.

Seneca's *On Peace of Mind* presupposes a competing Stoic view on development and on psychological functions, though one that is less explicit than in Galen's two therapeutic works. The Stoic position, outlined earlier, is that all human beings are constitutively capable of developing towards personal happiness (which depends on virtue), regardless of their specific inborn nature or upbringing. This is linked with a unified or holistic conception of psychological functions, according to which changes of belief at any stage of life will necessarily bring with them changes in emotional attitudes and desires.[52] In Cicero's *On Duties*, a work which is strongly influenced by the second-century BC Stoic Panaetius, these ideas underlie the theory of the

---

[50] See *Avoiding Distress* 58–62 and *Psychological Affections* ch. 8 (V.41–43 K), trans. in Singer 1997, 119–121.

[51] *Psychological Affections* ch. 6 (V.27–29 K), trans. in Singer 1997, 112–113, referring to the account of psychology in *Character Traits*, which survives in Arabic summary (included in Singer forthcoming). On the assumptions made by Galen about psychology and development, see Gill 2010a, 256–258.

[52] See Gill 2006, 132–134, 177–182.

four roles or *personae* which is presented there. According to this theory, while all of us (adult human beings) should aim to realize in our lives the virtues that form the basis for happiness, we should do so in a way that takes account of our specific natural inclinations, social background, and the kind of life-project we are capable of carrying through to the end.[53] Seneca's dialogue presupposes this set of Stoic assumptions. The therapeutic strategy assumes that we are naturally drawn towards different pathways in life. But it also assumes, in line with the four-*personae* theory, that, whatever our natural inclinations, we are capable of identifying a pathway that can serve as a vehicle for the expression of virtue. It also assumes that if we do this, we can withstand the setbacks and losses that potentially disrupt any given form of life, and can work consistently towards our overall goal (that of living a sage-like life of virtue) in a way that brings with it stability of purpose and emotional resilience. The pattern of ideas overlaps with the Platonic-Aristotelian ones underlying Galen's therapeutic works; but it also has some distinctive (Stoic) features which are underlined by Seneca's presentation.[54]

The fourth element in each case is offering advice or recommending practices which can enable the other person to move towards the desired goal. Here too, we can identify differences between the techniques advocated in each work. Although both works advocate cognitive or rational methods, the Galenic approach assumes that the effective deployment of these methods will require certain special preconditions (of inborn nature or upbringing) that do not depend solely on personal agency. The Galenic approach also assumes the effectiveness of habituation in modifying emotional attitudes over time, an idea linked with the idea that we have non-rational parts in our personality which need to be habituated rather than educated rationally.[55] Both these assumptions are absent from Seneca's Stoic version of therapy, as expressed in *On Peace of Mind*.[56] However, as regards the cognitive dimension of the techniques advocated, there is more similarity or

---

[53] Cicero, *On Duties* (*De Officiis*) 1.107–121; see also Gill 1988. The consistency of the Ciceronian approach here (following Panaetius) with standard Stoic thinking is stressed in Gill 2010b, 141–143.

[54] See further on the Panaetian background to Seneca's approach, Gill 1994, 4603–4624.

[55] See text to nn. 39–40 above. The importance of habituation is stressed esp. in *Psychological Affections*, ch. 4 (V.14–21), trans. Singer 1997, 106–109. The link between habituative treatment or 'correction' (*kolasis*), by contrast with rational education (*paideusis*), and Galen's Platonic-Aristotelian assumptions about psychology and development is brought out in ch. 6 (V.27–34 K), trans. Singer 1997, 112–116.

[56] Similarly, Seneca's *On Anger* (1. 2–21) rejects strongly the Aristotelian ideal of 'moderation of emotions', and, by implication, the ideas about psychology and development associated with this ideal.

overlap between the two works. For instance, in Galen's *Avoiding Distress*, we find advice designed to place what the other person sees as setbacks and disasters in a proper perspective by encouraging him to think about what really matters for human happiness and its opposite, avoiding a trivializing focus on relative differences between one's own situation and that of other people.[57] Crucial for Seneca's *On Peace of Mind*, on the other hand, is conceiving one's specific role in life as a vehicle for a larger project, that of living a certain kind of life, one centred on achieving happiness by the expression of virtue. Part of the intended effect of this move is to enable the person to place in a broader perspective the setbacks and (supposed) disasters that occur in the performance of one's chosen role, by re-conceiving that role as a vehicle for the larger project.[58] Underlying both these methods is the aim of drawing the other person away from the belief-set that sees happiness as dependent on external factors and towards one that recognizes one's own decisive role as agent in moving towards happiness.

Ancient Philosophical Therapy and Modern Practice

So far, I have mainly concentrated on analysing the role of ancient philosophical therapy in the ancient context. I now ask the more speculative—but also potentially practical—question, whether we moderns could usefully adopt this kind of therapy to enlarge our resources for confronting mental illness and emotional distress. In exploring this question, it is crucial to specify the area in which this kind of therapy might be useful. Like modern counselling or cognitive therapy, this kind of approach will not be useful in addressing people in acute states of mental illness (what are sometimes called schizophrenia or manic depression), where modern drugs are more likely to be useful in inducing some measure of emotional calm and self-control. The kind of cases where this question can usefully be raised are in what is sometimes called 'low-level' mental illness such as cases of long-term states of depression or anxiety or of situational distress, for instance, following bereavement.[59]

However, to pursue the question further, we need to acknowledge certain salient differences between the ancient methods and modern practices—differences which may prove to be an effective guide to what is potentially

---

[57] Galen, *Avoiding Distress* 39–47; here Galen draws on stock philosophical material also found in Diogenes Laertius 2.2 and Plutarch, *On Peace of Mind* 469 C–D.

[58] See text to nn. 52–54 above.

[59] Cf. Gill 2010a, 355–357.

most useful in the ancient approach. One difference derives from a feature that I have stressed throughout this discussion. This is the fact that the ancient writings on the therapy of emotion are best understood, on the analogy of ancient medical regimen, as preventive psychological therapy, designed to enable people to build up emotional resilience against setbacks and disasters before they have actually happened. This marks a clear point of difference from typical modern practices, in which counselling or therapy is applied to those who are already distressed and in need of guidance or treatment. A related difference is that the ancient writings, presumably reflecting normal practice in the culture, are directed at the patient or potential patient rather than the 'doctor' (meaning, in this case, the philosopher). Typically, I take it, modern texts on psychotherapy or counselling are addressed, primarily at least, to other practitioners or those training to practice, rather than the general public. A related difference is that, in antiquity, there is a rather prevalent assumption, at least among educated well-off adult men, that one can and should take care of one's psychological health and well-being and manage your life accordingly. A further differentiating feature is that this project of psychological self-care is usually framed in positive terms, those of the pursuit of happiness, for instance, and that it intersects with ethical reflection about the shaping and direction of one's life as a whole. Although these features can also be found in the lives of some individuals in contemporary Western culture, these are not standard features of modern social life.

These points of difference might lead one to conclude that this aspect of ancient culture is irrelevant to modern concerns, or, more broadly, that any given human culture evolves forms of psychotherapy that are appropriate to their own culture but not others. But another conclusion is possible. This is that these are all features of ancient culture that we moderns might usefully adopt, albeit perhaps with modifications. Indeed, these features overlap with some of the directions in which, according to some people, modern practice should be moving. In contemporary Western medicine, for instance, as noted earlier, there is a widespread view that we need to give greater weight to preventive medicine (by contrast with drugs, for instance) and that people can and should be expected to take responsibility for management of their own health. In the modern context, the focus has mainly been on the maintenance of one's bodily condition, for instance in avoiding obesity or alcoholism. But, since there is also an increasing recognition of the close interplay between bodily and mental aspects of health or sickness, it is clear that the same points could be made about psychological health. One might argue that ancient culture provides a paradigm we would do well to adopt, in which people can reasonably be expected to manage their lives in a way that promotes psychological well-being as well as a sound bodily condition.

A further line of argument might support this conclusion. Another feature of modern Western life is the widespread growth of 'self-help' or 'life-coach' manuals, which are now pervasive in bookshops and bookselling web-sites. The appeal of such books is, evidently, that they offer practical steps towards enabling people to address large questions such as the nature of human happiness or the meaning of life and to allow thought on these questions to inform the shaping of their lives. Of course, in modern (though not ancient) society, religion has been the traditional source of inspiration for this purpose, and this remains true for some people and some modern cultures or sub-cultures. But, for many people in modern Western society, the waning of religious practice has left a void in modes of discourse of this kind. The ancient works of philosophical therapy, if appropriately presented, could help to fill this gap in modern life. They offer a set of therapeutic approaches, directed at life-style management and the shaping of a life, which have a much firmer theoretical basis than many modern equivalents and which have been tested by sustained application over several centuries in antiquity. There are, of course, practical questions about what, or what more, needs to be done to make such works available and intelligible to modern readers who might want to use them in this way. But I think there is a strong prima facie case for thinking that the ancient therapeutic writings could play a valuable role of this kind in our society.

However, at this point a further objection to this line of argument looms. It might be argued that ancient ethical and psychological ideas are, quite simply, out of date, and cannot support a mode of therapeutic discourse that is meaningful for modern readers. But this objection is much less powerful, I think, than it might seem. Ancient ethical theories have, in recent decades, proved to be a powerful influence on modern virtue-ethics. Both in the revival of ethics based on the ideas of virtue and happiness and in the practical orientation of much ethical debate and inquiry, the current position in ethical philosophy is much closer to ancient thought than it was, for instance, in the early post-Second World War period.[60]

The question of the relationship between ancient and modern psychological ideas (which in both contexts are often linked with accounts of human physiology) is, of course, much more complex. Modern psychology

---

[60] See introduction to Gill 2005.

is, in its aspirations at least, a scientific, evidence-based, inquiry in a sense that is largely unknown in the ancient world. It might be concluded that this fact alone renders ancient philosophical therapy invalid for modern purposes. There are, however, a number of points to be made against this conclusion. As some recent discussions have brought out, there are strong analogies both between specific types of ancient and modern psychological theories and between the broader thrust of some areas of modern psychological debate. For instance, modern cognitive theories of emotion are anticipated by Stoicism. Also, recent debate based on research on the brain about how far human psychological functions are integrated or sub-divided has close analogies with Greco-Roman debate between Stoic and Platonic-Aristotelian approaches.[61] It is true that the ancient versions of these positions are not based on what we would regard as scientific investigation. But I think it is far from clear that the ancient theories (considered in their main claims and structure) have been invalidated by modern psychological research. Also, as the earlier discussion may have brought out, the ancient therapeutic works are informed by psychological theories at a rather general level. At this level, especially, I think it is unlikely that ancient claims about the scope for human agency and ethical development, in all, or at least many, people have been rendered obsolete by modern research.[62]

Obviously, these questions could be pursued much further than can be done here. But I think this discussion would support the following conclusion. The ancient works of philosophical therapy offer connected programmes, in different versions, for developing emotional resilience and a sense of purpose in life. The programmes are based on sophisticated philosophical ideas, worked out over several centuries, and they integrate ethical and psychological ideas in a way that is both theoretically strong and potentially effective for practical guidance. I hope this account has brought out both the rationale and role of these forms of discourse in ancient culture and has also indicated how they might be of substantive value and use in modern life and practice.[63]

---

[61] See Sorabji 2000, ch. 10, Nussbaum 2001, chs. 1–2, and Gill 2010a, 333–350.

[62] A distinct, but not irrelevant point, is that there appears to be a yawning and unresolved gap between current brain research and modern psychiatric categories for mental illness, according to the contribution by Roberto Lewis-Fernandez to the 2010 Columbia conference. This suggests that the contemporary position is far from settled or clear-cut and that there is scope for further reflective debate on how to analyse mental illness and cure which can be informed by ancient paradigms.

[63] I am grateful for the helpful comments on the oral version of this essay made at the Columbia conference in 2010 and also comments made on related papers given at Exeter.

PART V

FROM HOMER TO ATTIC TRAGEDY

FROM HOMERIC *ATE* TO TRAGIC MADNESS

Suzanne Saïd

It is agreed that 'madness' does not exist in the Homeric poems,[1] and is rather common or even central in Greek tragedy either as a metaphor or as frank clinical madness.[2] However, the vocabulary later appropriated by tragic madness—on the one hand ἄτη, *ἀάω, etc., and on the other μαίνο-μαι, μάργος, μαργαίνω and λύσσα[3]– already occurs in Homer.[4] But these two semantic fields never overlap and the only apparent exception (the story of Eurytion told in *Odyssey* 21.295–304) proves the rule. I propose in this paper to illuminate some distinctive features of tragic madness by looking at its prehistory and comparing it with its antecedents in Homeric poetry, pointing out both continuities and ruptures, instead of the usual comparison between tragedy and the Hippocratic writings.[5] The interest of such an approach, already suggested by B. Simon and R. Padel,[6] has been demonstrated for ancient epic by the book of D. Hershkowitz, who has shown how 'the words and deeds of Homeric characters can be appropriated by the representation of madness found in later epic tradition and transformed into images of madness'.[7] I shall focus mostly on Aeschylus, looking not only at descriptions of 'mad' characters but also at their presentation on stage, since tragic poets, as opposed to Homer, who only 'told in his myths the contests and battles of the demigods, rendered the myths in the form of contests and actions, so that they are presented not to our ears alone, but to our eyes as well', as Isocrates already said.[8] In the *Oresteia* this theatricalization of madness is pushed even further, since the audience is given with the *Eumenides*

---

[1] Simon 1978, 65–67; Padel 1995, 188, and Hershkowitz 1998, 126.

[2] Simon 1978, 67, 69–70, 89, and 100; Padel 1995, 167; Gill 1996, 257; Hartigan 1987, 126; and Guidorizzi 2010, 15.

[3] With the exception of νοῦσος, which is never applied to mental illness in Homer.

[4] See Simon 1978, 68, Padel 1995, 167, and Hershkowitz 1998, 159.

[5] See Dumortier 1935 and Ferrini 1978.

[6] Simon 1978, 68 and Padel 1995, 167.

[7] Hershkowitz 1998, 159.

[8] Isocrates *Ad Nicoclem* 49: Ὁ μὲν γὰρ [Homer] τοὺς ἀγῶνας καὶ τοὺς πολέμους τοὺς τῶν ἡμιθέων ἐμυθολόγησεν, οἱ δὲ [the tragic poets] τοὺς μύθους εἰς ἀγῶνας καὶ πράξεις κατέστησαν, ὥστε μὴ μόνον ἀκουστοὺς ἡμῖν ἀλλὰ καὶ θεατοὺς γενέσθαι.

an opportunity to share the true visions of Cassandra and Orestes. In order to better assess the originality of Aeschylean madness, I shall conclude with a comparison of his mad heroes to their Euripidean counterparts, Cassandra in *Troades* and Orestes in *Electra, Iphigenia in Tauris* and *Orestes*.

1. Homeric Madness?

Let us look first at Homer and the two semantic families of ἄτη and μαίνομαι and its associates λύσσα/μάργος/μαργαίνειν.

A. Ἄτη[9]

Rather than choosing between two interpretations of *ate*, 'damage of mind' and 'damage in life or fortune', let us attempt to establish its core meaning by looking at all its occurrences, as did R. Padel and D. Hershkowitz.[10]

Ate and cognate terms are applied to a wide range of behaviors that turn out to go against the best interests of the author. As D. Hershkowitz well said,[11] 'neither the state of mind of the actor nor some inherent quality of the action is at issue, but rather the subsequent reception of the action which then colors one's view of the actor's state of mind, as well as of the quality of the original action'. This is the reason why mistakes brought about by alluring promises of gods[12] or men,[13] actions of other men[14] or interventions of a god,[15] errors made out of carelessness,[16] intoxication[17] or stupidity[18] that

---

[9] On Homeric ἄτη see Dodds 1951, 2–27, Seiler 1954, Stallmach 1968, Saïd 1978, 75–83, Wyatt 1982, Padel 1995, 174–187 and Hershkowitz 1998, 125–160.

[10] Padel 1995, 174–187 and Hershkowitz 1998, 128–132.

[11] Hershkowitz 1998, 132.

[12] *Il.* 2. 111–115 = 9. 18–22, 8. 237: Agamemnon duped by Zeus who promised him he would return after sacking Troy.

[13] *Il.* 10. 391–399: Dolon who was lured into going by night to the Achaeans' ships by Hector who promised him the horses and the chariot of Achilles.

[14] *Od.* 10. 68, 12. 372: Odysseus victim of the behavior of his companions who opened the bag of the winds and killed the cattle of the Sun during his sleep.

[15] *Il.* 16. 805: Apollon stunning Patroclus.

[16] *Il.* 11. 340: Agastrophos forgot to bring his chariot close by and was killed by Diomedes; 16. 685–687: Patroclus disregarded the warning of Achilles and pursued the Trojans instead of returning after saving the ships.

[17] *Od.* 11. 6: Elpenor bewildered by drinking too much wine broke his neck by falling from the roof instead of using the ladder.

[18] *Od.* 15. 470: Eumaeus was kidnapped by Phoenicians because he stupidly followed his Phoenician nurse.

had fatal consequences for their author are *a posteriori* acknowledged as *ate* by their agent or by the narrator in the Homeric poems.

Even when *ate* is a crime or an offense to gods or men, emphasis is mostly put on the harm resulting from the action to its agent. In the *Iliad* the lack of consideration of Agamemnon for Achilles, which is the *ate par excellence* in the poem[19] is deemed as such by its victim, its witnesses and its actor only because Achilles is the best of the Achaeans and his anger has serious consequences for Agamemnon and the Greeks: deprived of their best warrior, they are unable to defeat the Trojans. In the same way, impiety is an *ate* because gods are always able to punish those who give offense to them. If behaviors such as those of Oineus, who forgot to give Artemis her due share of a sacrifice,[20] Paris,[21] who offended Athena and Hera by giving the prize of beauty to Aphrodite, or Ajax Oileus, who boasted that he escaped drowning 'despite the gods',[22] are labeled *ate*, it is only because their authors paid dearly for them, as emphasized by the context: Artemis sent into Oineus' orchards a boar who did much evil, Hera and Athena kept hating not only Paris, but also Priam, his people, and the sacred city of Troy, and Poseidon, after saving Ajax Oileus, killed him.[23] In the *Iliad*, murder is deemed an *ate* too, since it brings about exile for the murderer,[24] and in the *Odyssey* adultery or theft are branded as *ate* because of their fatal consequences for the agent, as demonstrated by the stories of Helen and Melampous.[25]

Because the gods, by definition immortal and blessed, are sheltered from fatal consequences of their mistakes, they ignore *ate*, and the exception proves the rule, for the story of Zeus' *ate*[26] explains why this phenomenon cannot any more happen among the gods. Once he has been deceived by Hera,[27] Zeus 'caught by the shining hair of her head the goddess *Ate* in the anger of his heart, and swore a strong oath, that never after this might *Ate*, who deludes all (ἣ πάντας ἀᾶται.), come back to Olympus and the starry sky. So speaking, he whirled her about in his hand and slung her out of the starry heaven and presently she came to men's establishments' (*Il.* 19.125–131).

---

[19] *Il.* 1. 412, 9. 116 and 119, 16. 274, and 19. 88, 91, 136, and 137.
[20] *Il.* 9. 537.
[21] *Il.* 6. 356 and 24. 28.
[22] *Od.* 4. 502–504.
[23] *Il.* 9. 533–536, 24. 27–28; *Od.* 4. 502–511.
[24] *Il.* 24. 480.
[25] *Od.* 4. 261–264, 23. 218–224: Helen; and 15. 231–234: Melampous.
[26] *Il.* 19. 95 and 113.
[27] *Il.* 19. 96–124.

Since the causes of *ate* matter less than its consequences for the reception of an action, they are often left unspecified through the use of the middle[28] or the passive[29] voice. Sometimes *Ate* herself is said to be the origin of delusion:[30] she 'harms' or 'damages' a man she 'follows', 'seizes' or 'ensnares',[31] and her victim can only 'endure'[32] her. At *Iliad* 9.505–507 and 19.91–94, she is even vividly personified.

When *ate* is given an explicit origin, it is always supposed to come from outside,[33] from an undefined god,[34] from Aphrodite,[35] from the Erinyes,[36] and, more often, from Zeus alone,[37] or associated with other supernatural powers such as other gods, fate and Erinyes.[38] Natural forces such as sleep or wine, alone or together with divine or human agents, may also explain the appearance of *ate*.[39]

But it is never the one who experiences the harmful consequences of an action who is presented as its subject, since no one willingly damages oneself. Retrospectively, the victim of *ate* cannot understand how he or she happened to behave in such a foolish way: such harmful behavior has to come from outside. The same idea is expressed in modern languages by expression such as the English 'what came over me?' or, even closer to the Greek, the French 'qu' est-ce qui m' a pris?'.

This explains why the first person singular ἀάω is never attested. The only occurrence of the third person singular in the active voice with a subject who experiences the ἄτη (*Od.* 21.297: ὁ δ' ἐπεὶ φρένας ἄασεν οἴνῳ, 'since he

---

[28] *Il.* 9. 116, 119, and 537, 11. 340, and 19. 137.

[29] *Il.* 16. 685 and 19. 113; *Od.* 5. 503 and 509, *and* 21. 301.

[30] *Il.* 16. 685, 19. 113 and 136 *Od.* 4. 503, 509, and 21. 301.

[31] 'harm': *Il.* 19. 128: Ἄτην, ἣ πάντας ἀᾶται, and 136 Ἄτης ἧ πρῶτον ἀάσθην; 'damage': 9.505–507 ἧ δ' ἄτη … βλάπτουσ' ἀνθρώπους, 513 βλαφθείς. 'follow': *Il.* 9. 513: τῷ ἄτην ἅμ' ἕπεσθαι; 'seize': *Il.* 16. 805: τὸν δ' ἄτη φρένας εἷλε, and 24. 480 ἄνδρ' ἄτη πυκινὴ λάβῃ; 'ensnare': *Il.* 19. 94: κατὰ δ' οὖν ἕτερόν γε πέδησε.

[32] *Od.* 21. 302: ἣν ἄτην ὀχέων ἀεσίφρονι θυμῷ.

[33] Simon 1978, 57 and Hershkowitz 1998, 131.

[34] *Od.* 23. 222–223.

[35] *Od.* 4. 261–262: ἄτην δὲ μετέστενον, ἣν Ἀφροδίτη / δῶχ', ὅτε μ' ἤγαγε κεῖσε φίλης ἀπὸ πατρίδος αἴης.

[36] *Od.* 15. 233–234.

[37] *Il.* 6. 356–357, 8.236–237, 19. 137, and 270–274.

[38] *Od.* 12. 371–372: Ζεῦ πάτερ ἠδ' ἄλλοι μάκαρες θεοὶ αἰὲν ἐόντες, / ἦ με μάλ' εἰς ἄτην κοιμήσατε νηλέϊ ὕπνῳ, and *Il.* 19. 87–88: ἀλλὰ Ζεὺς καὶ Μοῖρα καὶ ἠεροφοῖτις Ἐρινύς, / οἵ τέ μοι εἰν ἀγορῇ φρεσὶν ἔμβαλον ἄγριον ἄτην.

[39] 'Wine': *Od.*21. 293–296; Eurytion, 11. 61; Elpenor: ἆσέ με δαίμονος αἶσα κακὴ καὶ ἀθέσφατος οἶνος; 'sleep': *Od.* 10. 68–69: ἄασάν μ' ἕταροί τε κακοὶ πρὸς τοῖσί τε ὕπνος / σχέτλιος. See Padel 1995, 175–176.

damaged his wits through wine') is in fact a mere variation of the preceding line picturing the wine as the agent of the damage and the Centaur as its object (*Od.* 21. 295–296). This is echoed at l. 301 with a passive participle presenting the wits, *phrenes*, as the locus of ἄτη (ὁ δὲ φρεσὶν ᾗσιν ἀασθείς), which is followed at l. 302 by a participle picturing the ἄτη as a burden which the Centaur carries in his damaged *thumos* (ἣν ἄτην ὀχέων ἀεσίφρονι θυμῷ). The three other occurrences of ἄασεν or ἆσε singular, or ἄασαν plural always have as subject an agent external to the victim: in the *Iliad*, Zeus damaging through *ate* powerful kings (8.236–237 Ζεῦ πάτερ, ἦ ῥά τιν' ἤδη ὑπερμενέων βασιλήων / τῇδ' ἄτῃ ἄασας)[40] or, in the *Odyssey*, the wine associated with the fate apportioned by a god (11.61 ἆσέ με δαίμονος αἶσα κακὴ καὶ ἀθέσφατος οἶνος·) and the companions of Odysseus and wretched sleep (*Od.* 10.68–69 'ἄασάν μ' ἕταροί τε κακοὶ πρὸς τοῖσί τε ὕπνος / σχέτλιος.). If Helen put *ate* in her own *thumos*, it is only after a god's intervention.[41] Indeed in the Homeric poems the *thumos* and the *phrenes* are usually portrayed as a locus of *ate* or as an object affected by her.[42] The only exception occurs in *Iliad* 9.119, where Agamemnon explains the origin of his *ate* by the trust he put in his wretched spirit, ἀλλ' ἐπεὶ ἀασάμην φρεσὶ λευγαλέῃσι πιθήσας. Yet at 19.86–89 the same character denies any responsibility by saying that his *ate* was the consequence of an abnormal state of mind which had a supernatural explanation.

B. *Μαίνομαι and Cognate Terms*[43]

This verb, etymologically connected to μένος,[44] 'the most general Homeric word for vitality or energy',[45] is associated with it in the speech of Helenus and in the dialogue between Hera and Athena.[46] Yet in contrast to μένος, which has a positive value, μαίνομαι ('experience a heightened amount of μένος') 'marginalize[s] [its] subjects by placing them outside the boundaries

---

[40] See Padel 1995, 170.

[41] *Od.* 23. 222–224, Penelope speaking of Helen: τὴν δ' ἦ τοι ῥέξαι θεὸς ὤρορεν ἔργον ἀεικές· / τὴν δ' ἄτην οὐ πρόσθεν ἑῷ ἐγκάτθετο θυμῷ / λυγρήν.

[42] *thumos* as locus of *ate*: *Od.*23. 223; *phrenes* as locus of *ate*: *Il.* 19. 88; *Od.* 15. 233–234 and 21. 301; *phrenes* affected by *ate*: *Il.* 9. 377, 16. 805, and 19.137, *Od.* 21. 301, and the adjective ἀασίφρων 'à l'esprit égaré' (see Chantraine 2009, s.v. ἀάω): *Il.* 20. 183 and 23. 603; *Od.* 21. 302 and the noun ἀεσιφροσύνη 'égarement de l'esprit': *Od.* 15. 470.

[43] See Mauri 1990 and Heshkowitz 1998, 132–140.

[44] Chantraine 2009, s.v. μέμονα.

[45] Redfield 1975, 171 n. 17.

[46] *Il.* 6.100–101 (Helenus) and 8. 355–358 (Hector).

of mental normality'.[47] In the Homeric poems, it is mostly used in speeches as an insult (in the vocative[48] or second person singular or plural[49]) or for a pejorative purpose. In the *Iliad*, it is employed usually to condemn the raving fury of an enemy on the battlefield (it is applied to the Achaean Diomedes by the Trojans, Pandarus and Helenus,[50] and to the Trojan Hector by Odysseus and Hera, who sides with the Achaeans[51]), or more rarely to criticize immoral behavior such as the adulterous lust of Paris and Proitos' wife,[52] the disobedience of Hera and Athena to the orders of Zeus,[53] the refusal of Achilles to grant a proper burial to Hector,[54] the lack of gratitude of Zeus who thwarted Athena by helping the Trojans despite the help she gave to his son Heracles[55]), or an improper display of emotions (when the housekeeper compares Andromache to a mad woman[56]). In the *Odyssey*, where there are few battle-scenes, μαίνομαι is only once applied to the frenzy of the war-god Ares.[57] It is mostly used to criticize those who do not respect the laws of hospitality such as the Cyclops, the suitors, or the Centaur Eurytion.[58] Like *ate* and *menos*, which are often presented as gifts of the gods, *mania* is often associated with a divine intervention.[59]

In contrast with *ate, mania* is never acknowledged by its author or his allies. The few exceptions, when Diomedes alludes to the rage of his spear, or when Achilles evokes the rage of Patroclus' hands or the rage of Diomedes' spear, are only apparent. They are all, explicitly or implicitly, instances of embedded focalization and representations by the speaker of another character's perceptions.[60]

---

[47] Hershkowitz 1998, 142.

[48] *Il.* 3. 39 = 13. 769: γυναιμανές, 15. 128: μαινόμενε.

[49] *Od.* 9. 350 and 18. 406.

[50] *Il.* 5. 185 and 6. 101.

[51] *Il.* 8. 355 and 9. 238.

[52] *Il.* 3. 39 = 13. 769 and 6. 160.

[53] *Il.* 8. 413.

[54] *Il.* 24. 114: Zeus condemning the behavior of Achilles towards Hector's corpse and 24. 135: Thetis echoing the words of Zeus.

[55] *Il.* 8. 360.

[56] *Il.* 6. 389.

[57] *Od.* 11. 537.

[58] *Od.* 9. 350, 18. 406, and 21. 298.

[59] *Il.* 5. 184–187, 9. 239, and 15. 603–605.

[60] Explicit in the speech of Diomedes, *Il.* 8.110–111: ὄφρα καὶ Ἕκτωρ / εἴσεται εἰ καὶ ἐμὸν δόρυ μαίνεται ἐν παλάμῃσιν, and in the speech of Achilles, *Il.* 16.243–244: ὄφρα καὶ Ἕκτωρ/εἴσεται ... ἦ οἱ τότε χεῖρες ἄαπτοι μαίνονθ', implicit in the speech of Achilles who echoes Diomedes in *Il.* 16. 74–75.

Like *ate*, and for the same reasons, the occurrences of μαίνομαι in the narrative are rare. There are nevertheless two exceptions.[61] Yet one of them, the comparison of Andromache with a maenad in *Iliad* 22.460 is but a variation of the words of the housekeeper in book 6. In contrast to *ate*, it is also often applied to gods: it is once associated with Dionysos,[62] whose followers are later on called μαινάδες, and often characterizes the war-god Ares, who is the archetype of the frenzied warrior.[63] It is also used about gods such as Zeus, Hera and Athena.[64]

Whereas with *ate*, the stress is put on the harm done to oneself, with μαίνομαι the context explicitly emphasizes the harm done by enemies to friends.[65] Hence the two semantic fields never overlap. This is clearly demonstrated by the story of the Centaur Eurytion told by Antinoos to Odysseus in book 21 of the *Odyssey*. When Antinoos uses ἄτη, ἄασε, and ἀασθείς, the context always points out the damage done to the Centaur himself (295–302). By contrast, μαινόμενος is immediately followed with an allusion to the harm he did to others: in his frenzy he did much harm to the house of Peirithoös (μαινόμενος κάκ' ἔρεξε δόμον κάτα Πειριθόοιο, 298)

Λύσσα (3×), λυσσώδης (1×) and λυσσητήρ (1×), as well as μαργός (3×) and μαργαίνειν (1×), are rather rare in the Homeric poems. Λύσσα and its derivatives, like μαίνομαι, refer in the *Iliad* to the raving frenzy of the warrior and are applied in speeches to Hector,[66] but also once in the narrative to Achilles,[67] in contrast to μαίνομαι, which is never used for Achilles.[68] In the *Iliad*, μαργαίνειν occurs only once,[69] and like λύσσα and μαίνομαι, it is applied in a speech to the raving fury of Diomedes. In the *Odyssey*, μάργος is applied by Penelope to Antinoos who plotted Telemachus' murder and did not respect the suppliant beggar, and to Eurycleia who was driven mad by the gods when she gave her the news of Odysseus' return and the killing of the suitors.[70] It also occurs once in the narrative, applied to the beggar

---

[61] *Il.* 15. 605: Hector and 22. 460: Andromache.

[62] *Il.* 6. 132.

[63] *Il.* 5. 717 and 831, as well as 15. 128; *Od.* 11. 537.

[64] *Il.* 8. 360: applied to Zeus by Athena, and 413: applied to Hera and Athena by Zeus' messenger, Iris.

[65] Hera's speech, *Il. 8.356*: κακὰ πολλὰ ἔοργε: and Antinoos' speech, *Od. 21.298*: μαινόμενος κάκ' ἔρεξε.

[66] 4×: *Il.* 8.299, 9.239, 305, 13.53.

[67] *Il.* 21. 542.

[68] Hershkowitz 1998, 146.

[69] *Il.* 5. 882.

[70] *Od.* 16. 421–423, 23. 11–13.

Iros, 'famous for his ravenous belly and his constant appetite for eating and drinking' (μετὰ δ' ἔπρεπε γαστέρι μάργῃ / ἀζηχὲς φαγέμεν καὶ πιέμεν, 18. 2–3). Like ἄτη, warlike frenzy (μαίνεσθαι and μαργαίνειν) is often explained by divine interference[71] and is said to affect *phrenes*.[72] In contrast to ἄτη, it has physical effects such as pulsing heart, foaming mouth and fiery or glittering eyes.[73]

To complete this overview of the Homeric vocabulary, it is worth noting the occurrences of words expressing deprivation of wits such as ἄφρων, ἀφροσύνη, ἀφρονεῖν, and ἀφραίνειν. In the *Iliad*, with the exception of 4.104, where the poet points out the foolishness of Pandarus who listened to Athena and shot an arrow at Menelaus, they always occur in speeches, in order to denounce stupidity,[74] childish foolishness,[75] some crazy behavior of men or gods who oppose or want to confront a stronger character,[76] or criminal acts.[77] The verb ἀλύω, 'to be carried away', is used in narrative as well as in speeches to describe characters carried away by excessive physical pain or moral sorrow.[78]

Finally, one has also to take into account, in *Odyssey* 20.345–349, the descriptions of the laughter of the suitors an episode which is 'unexpected and surprising'.[79]

... μνηστῆρσι δὲ Παλλὰς Ἀθήνη
ἄσβεστον γέλω ὦρσε, παρέπλαγξεν δὲ νόημα.
οἱ δ' ἤδη γναθμοῖσι γελώων ἀλλοτρίοισιν,
αἱμοφόρυκτα δὲ δὴ κρέα ἤσθιον· ὄσσε δ' ἄρα σφέων
δακρυόφιν πίμπλαντο, γόον δ' ὠίετο θυμός.

---

[71] *Il.* 5. 185 and 881–882 (Diomedes), 9. 238 and 15. 603–605 (Hector); *Od.* 18. 406 (suitors), 23. 11 (Eurycleia).

[72] *Il.* 8. 360 and 413, 15. 128, as well as 24. 114 and 135.

[73] *Il.* 22. 460–461: pulsing heart; 15. 607–608: foaming mouth and glittering eyes, elsewhere assimilated to the eyes of the Gorgon (*Il.* 8. 348–349). This last symptom will become in Greek tragedy a distinctive sign of madness (see Theodorou 1993, 38 and Hershkowitz 1998, 134, n. 28).

[74] *Il.* 3. 220; *Od.* 6. 187, 17. 586, 20. 227 and 360, 21. 102 and 105.

[75] *Il.* 11. 389.

[76] *Il.* 2. 258: Thersites opposing Agamemnon; 7. 110: Menelaus wanting to confront Hector; 15.104: Olympians opposing Zeus; 16. 842: Patroclus fighting against Hector.

[77] *Il.* 5. 761 and 875, and 24. 157 = 186; *Od.* 8. 209, 16. 278, and 24. 457.

[78] *Il.* 5. 352 (narrative): Aphrodite carried away by excessive physical pain and 24. 12 (narrative): Achilles carried away by excessive moral sorrow; *Od.* 9. 398: the Cyclops carried away by excessive physical pain and 18. 333 and 393 (speech): Melantho and Eurymachus accusing the beggar Odysseus of being carried away by wine (speech).

[79] Guidorizzi 1997, 1.

In the suitors Pallas Athena stirred up uncontrollable laughter, and deviated their thinking. Now they laughed with jaws that were no longer their own. The meat they ate was a mess of blood, their eyes were bursting full of tears and their laughter sounded like lamentation.

Even if it does not include any of the words that will be used later on for madness, it is clear that this scene, which contains some exceptional expressions,[80] comes closer to the description of a fit of madness than any other passage in the Homeric poems. The intervention of the divinity causes a state of complete mental dissociation revealed in a series of precise symptoms (the deviation of the mind, the loss of control of the body, the association of laughter and tears) which are close to the manifestations of religious trance that took place in the Dionysiac and Corybantic cults. Here the rhapsode,

> having at his disposal in the compositional baggage of the epic neither the formulaic instruments nor the narrative models for describing such episodes ... has recourse analogically to a system of ideas which was foreign to his poetry but immediately recognizable by the audience inside its own culture ... in this perspective the reference to omophagy, decontextualized from Dionysiac ritual, confirms in the mind of the public the message that the rhapsode wants to transmit,

as G. Guidorizzi justly pointed out.[81]

To conclude, it is only on a first impression that madness is non-existent in the Homeric poems.[82] Forms of behavior branded as *ate, mania* or witlessness often come close to what we would call at least metaphorically 'madness'; and *Odyssey* 20.345–349 is truly a description of a fit of madness. Nevertheless, it is true that real madness is never distinguished by a special vocabulary from stupid or criminal behavior. In other words, 'the boundaries of what is considered normal behaviour—boundaries which define extremes and which are often defined by madness—appear to be much wider in Homeric than in Roman epic', as was well said by D. Hershkowitz.[83]

---

[80] Such as ἄσβεστον γέλω ὦρσε, παρέπλαγξεν which is used elsewhere for the material deviation of an arrow (*Il.* 15. 464) or a ship departing from its proper course (*Od.* 9. 81), αἱμοφόρυκτα (only occurrence in Homer).

[81] Guidorizzi 1997, 6–7 who refers to Jeanmaire 1951, 132–156.

[82] Theodorou 1993, 34, n. 4.

[83] Hershkowitz 1998, 153.

2. *Tragic Madness*

A. *Aeschylus*

In the complete tragedies of Aeschylus, the vocabulary of madness comes straight from Homer, with, on the one hand, ἄτη, ἀτηρός and, on the other, μανία, μαίνομαι, μάργος (10×), μαργάω (3×), μαργόομαι (1×), λύσσα (5×), ἀλύω (1×). But in contrast to Homer the two categories often overlap. The vocabulary of madness is also enriched by μῶρος (first occurrence in Simonides) and its derivatives μωρία (1×) and μωραίνω (1×), and the first occurrences of 'mental illness' (νόσος φρενῶν 1×), θυίας (3×) and βακχάω (1×). As in Homer, madness is always explained by a divine agency and affects the *phrenes*[84] or exceptionally the *noos*,[85] the *kradia*,[86] or the *thumos*.[87] Yet it is not only narrated in plays such as the *Persians*, the *Seven against Thebes* and the *Suppliants*, it is displayed on stage with Io in *Prometheus Bound*, Cassandra in the *Agamemnon* and Orestes at the end of the *Choephoroi*. In the *Eumenides* Aeschylus goes even further by making the vision of the mad man visible to the audience.

Ate is central in the first and most Homeric Aeschylean tragedy, The *Persians*, since the emphasis is put on the disaster brought upon the Persians by Xerxes. Sometimes *ate* clearly means the objective harm done by Xerxes to the Persians, when Darius reminds the audience that *hubris*, 'arrogance', blossoms and produces *ate*, 'disaster', whence one reaps a harvest of lamentation (821–822 ὕβρις γὰρ ἐξανθοῦσ' ἐκάρπωσεν στάχυν/ἄτης, ὅθεν πάγκλαυτον ἐξαμᾷ θέρος), or when the chorus evokes at l. 1037 'the calamities of our friends on the sea' (φίλων ἄταισι ποντίαισιν). It also refers to 'infatuation' at ll. 97–99 when the chorus fears a personified *Ate*, identified with the treacherous deception of the divinity (96 δολόμητιν δ' ἀπάταν θεοῦ) that fawns on man with friendly intent and misleads him into her nets[88] (98–99 φιλόφρων γὰρ ⟨ποτι⟩σαίνου-/σα τὸ πρῶτον παράγει/βροτὸν εἰς ἄρκυας Ἄτα). Yet, as in Homer, it is sometimes impossible to distinguish between the two sides of *ate*, objective damage or subjective harm caused by a delusion sent by the

---

[84] *Pe.* 750; *Sept.* 484, 757; *Ag.* 219, 1064, 1140, 1427; *Cho.* 1024, 1056; *Eum.* 330, 332; *PV.* 472, 673, 856, 878–879, 1054, and 1061.

[85] *Su.* 542.

[86] *Sept.* 781.

[87] *Sept.* 686–687.

[88] The metaphor of 'ensnaring' was already used by Homer 4×: *Il.* 9. 239, 305, 15.53, 19. 94 κατὰ δ' οὖν ἕτερόν γε πέδησε [Ἄτη l. 91].

gods, as at ll. 653–655, when the chorus opposes to the losses of Xerxes the successes of his father Darius who was 'a counselor equal to gods':

οὐδὲ γὰρ ἄνδρας ποτ' ἀπώλλυ
πολεμοφθόροισιν ἄταις,
θεομήστωρ δ' ἐκικλήσκετο Πέρσαις.

Here, one may translate πολεμοφθόροισιν ἄταις as 'in disasters that involved destructions of war', relying on the analogy with l. 1037, or as 'through infatuations that led to destruction in war' because of the parallel drawn between Xerxes and his father who was 'a counselor equal to gods'.[89] Again, at l. 1007 διαπρέπον οἷον δέδορκεν Ἄτα, A.F. Garvie[90] is not sure which translation to choose. 'How terrible is Disaster's (or perhaps 'Delusion's') gaze'.

Like Homer, the chorus attribute the responsibility for such an unexpected disaster to nameless divinities at ll. 1005–1106:

ἰὼ ἰώ, δαίμονες
ἔθεσθ' ἄελπτον κακόν.

But Darius wavers. Sometimes, he blames Xerxes himself for a decision he considers as madness at l. 719:

πεζὸς ἢ ναύτης δὲ πεῖραν τήνδ' ἐμώρανεν τάλας;

Did he undertook this foolish enterprise by land or by sea?

He denounces his 'mental illness' (an expression which is a clear departure from Homer) at ll. 750–751:

πῶς τάδ' οὐ νόσος φρενῶν
εἶχε παῖδ' ἐμόν;

Surely this was a mental illness that had my son in its grip,

and explains it by a combination of ignorance and youthful rashness[91] or by a lack of sound sense: Xerxes attempted the impossible, when he believed that he—a mere mortal—could prevail against all the gods and particularly Poseidon.[92] Yet, at ll. 724–725, Darius, like Atossa, clearly imputes this ill advised behavior to a god:

ATOSSA: γνώμης δέ πού τις δαιμόνων ξυνήψατο.
DARIUS: φεῦ, μέγας τις ἦλθε δαίμων, ὥστε μὴ φρονεῖν καλῶς

---

[89] Garvie 2009, 268.
[90] Garvie 2009, 359.
[91] *Pers.* 744: παῖς δ' ἐμὸς τάδ' οὐ κατειδὼς ἤνυσεν νέῳ θράσει.
[92] *Pers.* 749–750: θνητὸς ὢν θεῶν τε πάντων ᾤετ', οὐκ εὐβουλίᾳ,/ καὶ Ποσειδῶνος κρατήσειν.

ATOSSA: Some divinity has I think seized his mind
DARIUS: Indeed a mighty kind of daemon came upon him, so that he might lose
his mind.

If the *Persians* illustrates the continuity between Homeric and tragic *ate*,
the *Seven against Thebes*, where the war is seen from the point of view of
the besieged Thebans, can be used to demonstrate the close relationship
between Homeric and tragic *mania*. The Argive leaders are consistently
described with μαίνομαι, μαργάω, βαχχεύω, θυίας, employed for pejorative
purposes by their Theban adversaries. According to the chorus of Theban
women, they embody Ares' wild battle fury and the indifference to morality
characteristic of the war god:[93]

μαινόμενος δ' ἐπιπνεῖ λαοδάμας
μιαίνων εὐσέβειαν Ἄρης.

Furious Ares who subdues people and defiles piety is blustering. (343–344)

They 'boast loudly against the city with their frenzied mind' (ὑπέραυχα βά-
ζουσιν ἐπὶ πτόλει/μαινομένᾳ φρενί ll. 483–484). According to the messenger,
Tydaeus, 'ravening and eager for battle (μαργῶν καὶ μάχης λελιμμένος), cries
out like a snake in the midday heat and hurls abuses at the wise seer Amphia-
raus' (380–382). As for Homeric Andromache, a Dionysiac vocabulary is
also used to describe Hippomedon's frenzy. This warrior, 'possessed by Ares,
raves mightily in Bacchic frenzy like a maenad' (ἔνθεος δ' Ἄρει/βαχχᾷ πρὸς
ἀλκὴν θυιὰς ὥς, 498–499). The Seven are only once associated with *ate*, in a
context that first emphasizes the harm caused to its subject, when the chorus at ll. 312–316 asks the guardian gods of the city to cast upon those outside
the walls the cowardice that destroys men, the *ate* that makes them throw
away their arms and win glory for the citizens (312–316):

ὦ πολιοῦχοι/θεοί, τοῖσι μὲν ἔξω
πύργων ἀνδρολέτειραν
κάκαν, ῥίψοπλον ἄταν,
ἐμβαλόντες ἄροισθε
κῦδος τοῖσδε πολίταις.

Not only the Argives but also the Labdacids are portrayed as victims of a
personified *Ate* sent by the gods in the conclusion of the play, when the
chorus evokes successively the family turned in utter rout by the Curses,[94]

---

[93] see *Il.* 5. 761.
[94] *Sept.* 953–955: τελευταῖαι δ' ἐπηλάλαξαν/'Αραὶ τὸν ὀξὺν νόμον, τετραμμένου/παντρόπῳ φυγᾷ γένους.

the victory of *Ate* whose trophy is erected at the gate where the brothers were struck,[95] and the final triumph of the divinity over the two sons of Oedipus.[96] But, in contrast to Homer, *mania* and *margos* words are also used by 'friends', Eteocles and the Theban chorus, to characterizes the three generations of the Theban royal family, and the causation of this madness is simultaneously presented as human and divine and 'the attempt to determine how far necessity, on one hand, and Eteocles' own will, on the other, influence what he does seems dictated by modern ways of thinking'.[97]

At line 653–654, Eteocles himself, like Agamemnon in *Iliad* 19, suggests that his state of mind, which he acknowledges as madness, has some supernatural explanation: he belongs to a family that is 'maddened by the gods and greatly hated by them, the most miserable family of Oedipus' (ὦ θεομα-νές τε καὶ θεῶν μέγα στύγος,/ ὦ πανδάκρυτον ἁμὸν Οἰδίπου γένος· 653–654). He insists on the role of the gods,[98] and more particularly on the part played by Phoibos' hatred against Laios' family[99] and by Oedipus' curse.[100]

The chorus, after the death of the brothers, will also sing of the 'mad strife' (ἔριδι μαινομένᾳ, 935) which opposed them. But in contrast to Eteocles, they put the blame for the killing of a brother not only on an *ate* sent by the gods, but also on Eteocles' own misguided temper:

> τί μέμονας, τέκνον; μή τί σε θυμοπλη-
> θὴς δορίμαργος ἄτα φερέτω· κακοῦ δ'
> ἔκβαλ' ἔρωτος ἀρχάν.

> Why are you so eager, my son? Let no heart-consuming war-craving folly carry you away, expel this passion right from the beginning./ What are you set on, child? Do not let bursting passion and insane lust for battle carry you away. Expel right from the beginning the authority of harmful passion.[101]

(685–687)

They question his intent to 'cull his own brother's blood' (ἀλλ' αὐτάδελφον αἷμα δρέψασθαι θέλεις; 718) and condemn the impious mind that caused the death of the brothers (ὤλοντ' ἀσεβεῖ διανοίᾳ 831). But at the same time they stress the part played by the gods in the final disaster.[102] The impossibility of

---

95 *Sept.* 956–957: ἔστακε δ' Ἄτας τροπαῖον ἐν πύλαις,/ ἐν αἷς ἐθείνοντο.
96 *Sept.* 960: καὶ δυοῖν κρατήσας ἔληξε δαίμων.
97 Thalmann 1978, 148.
98 *Sept.* 689 and 719.
99 *Sept.* 691.
100 *Sept.* 70, 655, 695–697, and 709.
101 See also on Eteocles' passionate desire *Sept.* 692–694: ὠμοδακής σ' ἄγαν/ἵμερος ἐξοτρύνει πικρόκαρπον ἀνδροκτασίαν τελεῖν/αἵματος οὐ θεμιστοῦ.
102 *Sept.* 827, 832–833, 840–841, 885–886, 891, and 898–899.

distinguishing here between human will and divine intervention is clearly indicated by the use of the same verb to describe both the urge of Eteocles and the *eris* that fulfils Oedipus' curse.[103]

Oedipus himself, who is also given 'damaged wits' (Οἰδιπόδα βλαψίφρονος, 725) is explicitly called mad (alas in a passage manifestly corrupt!) when after the discovery of the incest 'in the madness of his heart (μαινομένα κραδίᾳ) he achieved two harms (δίδυμα κάκ᾽ ἐτέλεσεν)' (781–782), which must be the blinding of his eyes and the curse of his sons.[104]

So in *The Seven* madness becomes a recurrent phenomenon for the three generations of Labdacids. It is each time associated with passionate craving either for sex (Laios) or for blood (Eteocles), or with wrath (Oedipus),[105] and it is given at the same time and by the same speakers a divine and a human origin. This comes as no surprise after a reading of the *Iliad*, which juxtaposes in the same way the two strands of divine causation and human passion.

In the *Suppliants*, the vocabulary of madness is associated first with the Egyptians and second with Io. Like the Argive warriors in the *Seven*, the Egyptians in the *Suppliants* are seen through the eyes of their enemies, the chorus of Danaids and their father Danaus, and consistently described as mad in pejorative terms, with words belonging to the semantic fields of μαίνομαι and μάργος, but also with ἄτη, when the context emphasizes the harm caused by delusion to its victim, at lines 104–111:

> ἰδέσθω δ᾽ εἰς ὕβριν
> βρότειον, οἷος νεάζει,
> πυθμὴν δι᾽ ἁμὸν γάμον τεθαλὼς
> δυσπαραβούλοισι φρεσίν,
> καὶ διάνοιαν μαινόλιν
> κέντρον ἔχων ἄφυκτον, ἄ-
> τᾳ δ᾽ ἀπάταν μεταγνούς.[106]

Let ⟨Zeus⟩ look at the *hubris* of men, how it thrives, a stem sprouting at the prospect of marriage to me, its mind hard to dissuade—it has frenzied thoughts that goad it on, led by delusion to take up deceit.

---

[103] *Sept.* 698: ἀλλὰ σὺ μὴ 'ποτρύνου and 726 παιδολέτωρ δ᾽ ἔρις ἅδ᾽ ὀτρύνει.

[104] See Hutchinson 1985, XXV.

[105] *Sept.* 724–725: τὰς περιθύμους κατάρας 'his wrathful curses' echoed by 786 ἐπίχοτος τροφᾶς [Oedipus] 'angry at the origin of his sons'.

[106] There is a textual problem in this line, but it needs no discussion in the present context.

This madness is not only, as in *The Seven*, identified with 'arrogance' (ὕβριν, 104)[107] and wild fury (they are 'ravening and eager for battle').[108] It is also associated with lust (the origin of their excess and their mad intent is the prospect of marrying the Danaids). Again, as in *The Seven*, there is, with ἄτη, a close association between human motivation and divine interference (the delusion) and its result (the disaster).[109]

In the *Suppliants* there is also a descriptions of Io's madness through the evocations of the Chorus. This madness cannot be separated from the metamorphosis of Io turned into a cow by Hera.[110] She is repeatedly spoken of as a cow,[111] and once as a mixture of woman and cow[112] driven round and round by a gadfly dispatched by Hera.[113] Her many wanderings are real: she is kept continuously on the move by the gadfly and, propelled by it, flees among the tribes of men, cleaving the wavy strait separating Asia and Europe.[114] The madness and the wanderings of mind are relegated to the background, as M.G. Ciani well pointed out.[115] They are alluded to only at *Suppliants* 542 with the adjective ἁμαρτίνοος 542, 'erring in wits', and 562–564:

> μαινομένα πόνοις ἀτί-
> μοις ὀδύναις τε κεντροδα-
> λήτισι θυιὰς "Ηρας.

> frenzied by unworthy toils and pains inflicted by the gadfly's sting, a maenad possessed by Hera.

This is the same Bacchic vocabulary (θυιάς) as in the *Seven*. Again, as in the *Persians* and the *Seven*, the madness as well as its cure are explained by divine interventions: Hera was responsible for the metamorphosis, the wanderings and obviously the madness of Io (562–564), and it is Zeus who 'charmed away the pains of the wretched Io of many wanderings, driven

---

[107] See also *Su.* 30, 81, 426, 528, and 817: chorus, and 487: the king of Argos.

[108] *Su.* 741–742 μάργον Αἰγύπτου γένος/ μάχης τ' ἄπληστον· Compare with the description of Tydaeus in the *Seven* 380: Τυδεὺς δὲ μαργῶν καὶ μάχης λελιμμένος.

[109] See also at *Su.* 528–530 the same association between excess ὕβριν and black-benched ruin (μελανόζυγ' ἄταν) in the prayer of the chorus.

[110] *Su.* 299: βοῦν τὴν γυναῖκ' ἔθηκεν Ἀργεία θεός. see also 17, 44, 170, 275, 301, 303, 306: Io as a cow, and 568–570: Io as a mixture of woman and cow βοτὸν ἐσορῶντες δυσχερὲς μειξόμβροτον,/ τὰν μὲν βοός,/ τὰν δ' αὖ γυναικός.

[111] *Su.* 16, 45, 170, 275, 301, 303, and 306.

[112] *Su.* 568–570 βοτὸν ἐσορῶντες δυσχερὲς μειξόμβροτον,/ τὰν μὲν βοός,/ τὰν δ' αὖ γυναικός.

[113] *Su.* 16–17, 307–308, and 540–541.

[114] *Su.* 308, and 540–546.

[115] Ciani 1974, 70. On Io's madness see also Mattes 1970, 75–78.

round and round by the gadfly' (καὶ τότε δὴ τίς ἦν ὁ θέλξας πολύπλαγκτον ἀ-θλίαν οἰστροδόνητον Ἰώ, 571–573), and put an end to the treacherous illnesses plotted against her by Hera' (κατέπαυσεν Ἥρας νόσους ἐπιβούλους, 586–588).

In *Prometheus Bound*, Io's madness is staged and comes in the fore-ground.[116] Right from the beginning, it is obvious that Io in this tragedy is not any more a cow. Her self-introduction as 'a woman with cow-horns' (τὰς βούκερω παρθένου, 588) is in agreement with a description that closely as-sociates myth and psychology. Myth, with the evocation of the destruction or distortion of her former shape,[117] the mention of her horns (κεραστὶς δ᾽, ὡς ὁρᾷτ᾽, 674), the allusions to the stinging gadfly (ὀξυστόμῳ μύωπι χρισθεῖσ᾽, 674–675) and to the cowherd Argus (βουκόλος), the choice of σκίρημα, which is normally used for the leaps of young animals, for the description of her jumps,[118] her harassment by the gadly and the divine scourge (οἰστρο-πλὴξ δ᾽ ἐγὼ/μάστιγι θείᾳ γῆν πρὸ γῆς ἐλαύνομαι, 681–682) and the description of her many wanderings (ll. 700–735, 788–845).[119] Psychology, with allusions to 'the storm sent upon her by the gods' (θεόσσυτον χειμῶνα 643), which is a metaphor for madness, to her distorted *phrenes* (φρένες διάστροφοι, 673) and to her madness (ἐμμανεῖ σκιρτήματι 675).

Yet Io's madness is not only evoked through these brief allusions. Her hal-lucinations are also portrayed in her monody at ll. 566–583 and 593–608, which is, together with the *Oresteia*, the first representation of a fit of mad-ness on stage.[120] There, the gadfly that stings her is not any more a real one,[121] as in lines 674–675. It is confused with the *eidolon* of Argus the cowherd with countless eyes whom she sees and tries to keep away in panic:

χρίει τίς αὖ με τὰν τάλαιναν οἶστρος;
εἴδωλον Ἄργου γηγενοῦς·
ἄλευ᾽, ἆ δᾶ· φοβοῦμαι,
τὸν μυριωπὸν εἰσορῶσα βούταν.
ὁ δὲ πορεύεται δόλιον ὄμμ᾽ ἔχων,
ὃν οὐδὲ κατθανόντα γαῖα κεύθει.
ἀλλ᾽ ἐμὲ τὰν τάλαιναν
ἐξ ἐνέρων περῶν κυναγεῖ, πλανᾷ
τε νῆστιν ἀνὰ τὰν παραλίαν ψάμμον.

---

[116] Ciani 1974, 72–78.
[117] *PV.* 643–644: διαφθορὰν μορφῆς, 673 εὐθὺς δὲ μορφὴ καὶ φρένες διάστροφοι.
[118] *PV.* 599, and 675.
[119] *PV.* 565, 585, 608, 622, 784, 788, 820, and 829: πλανάω and its derivatives; 591, 838: δρόμος, 900: ἀλατεία.
[120] See Ciani 1974, 72.
[121] Contra Padel 1995, 79.

Wretched me, I am stung by a gadfly, the image of Argus, born from the earth. Alas! Move him away, I get frightened when I see the herdsman with countless eyes The Earth does not any more hide him. He marches against me with his deceitful eye. Coming from the dead he hunts me and drives me hungry along the sand of the sea-shore. (567–575)

This visual hallucination is followed by an auditory one, where the sound of the pipe which accompanies her lyrics is confused with the Pan-pipe of the cowherd: 'the shrill, wax-made pipe drones its soporific melody' (ὑπὸ δὲ κηρόπλαστος ὀτοβεῖ δόναξ/ἀχέτας ὑπνοδόταν νόμον·, 574–575). The sting of the gadfly again becomes a metaphor of the terror when she speaks to Zeus and asks him:

τί ποτέ μ', ὦ Κρόνιε παῖ, τί ποτε ταῖσδ'
ἐνέζευξας εὑρὼν ἁμαρτοῦσαν ἐν πημοναῖσιν,
    ἒ ἔ· οἰστρηλάτῳ δὲ δείματι δειλαίαν
παράκοπον ὧδε τείρεις;)

literally 'Having found me sinning in what respect ever, son of Kronos, did you yoke me in these sufferings and torment me, miserable and demented, by a terror driven by a gadfly?'. (577–582)

and in the conclusion of her lyrics, when she says to Prometheus

θεόσυτόν τε νόσον ὠνόμασας, ἃ
μαραίνει με χρίουσα κέντροισι φοιταλέοισιν;

You have rightly named the illness sent by the gods which withers me up, by stinging me with its wild roaming barbs (596–597)

madness, as in the *Persians*, becomes an illness sent by the gods;[122] the sting is again a metaphor describing the withering caused by physical pain; and the roaming can be an allusion to her physical wanderings or a metaphor for the distraction of her mind.[123]

Later on, before leaving the stage, Io gives the first description in tragedy of the physical manifestations of madness:

ἐλελεῦ, ἐλελεῦ,
ὑπό μ' αὖ σφάκελος καὶ φρενοπληγεῖς
μανίαι θάλπουσ', οἴστρου δ' ἄρδις
χρίει μ' ἄπυρος·
κραδία δὲ φόβῳ φρένα λακτίζει,

---

[122] As a matter of fact νόσος (596, 606, 632), and νοσέω (698) are often applied to Io's madness in the *Prometheus Bound*.
[123] See Griffith 1983 at l. 598.

τροχοδινεῖται δ' ὄμμαθ' ἑλίγδην,
ἔξω δὲ δρόμου φέρομαι λύσσης
πνεύματι μάργῳ, γλώσσης ἀκρατής·
θολεροὶ δὲ λόγοι παίουσ' εἰκῇ
στυγνῆς πρὸς κύμασιν ἄτης.

Alas, a spasm burns and madnesses that smite my wits inflame me, the
unforged spearhead of the gadfly stings me. My heart kicks my diaphragm
with panic. My eyes whirl, I am carried out of my track by the furious blast of
madness. I cannot control my tongue and my muddied words dash randomly
against the waves of loathsome ruin.   (877–886)

First the spasm: this is the first occurrence of σφάκελος, 'the spasm', which
will be found again in Euripides' *Hippolytus* to describe not the madness
but the acute pain of the dying hero,[124] and will become in the *Corpus
Hippocraticum* and Galen a technical term of debatable meaning.[125] The
metaphorical use of the gadfly again describes the acuteness of the pain.
There is also the violent move of the heart which kicks the diaphragm with
panic[126] and the rolling eyes, which will become later on a characteristic of
the madman,[127] both borrowed from Homeric descriptions of death.[128] The
disturbance of the mind is conveyed by a metaphor which combines chariot
racing (the uncontrollable chariot leaving the track) and nautical imagery
(madness is assimilated to a furious blast of wind). There is also the inability to control her tongue and inarticulate speech which are combined again
with a metaphor identifying madness as a storm provoked by *ate*. Thus in
Prometheus Bound, as in the *Persians* and the *Seven*, the Aeschylean vocabulary of madness does not separate *ate* and *lussa*. This description is so
vivid that some scholars have attempted to make a clinical or psychoanalytical diagnosis.[129] Yet, given the obvious echoes with Homeric vocabu-

---

[124] *Hipp.* 1351–1352: διά μου κεφαλῆς ἄισσουσ' ὀδύναι/κατά τ' ἐγκέφαλον πηδᾶι σφάκελος.

[125] See Galen, *De locis affectis* 2.92–93 and 8. 93.1.

[126] See also for Io's fear *P.V.* 567 and 580.

[127] Eur. *H.F. 868 and 932, Or.* 253, Bach. 1122–1123, 1166–1167, see Mattes 1970, 76.

[128] In the *Odyssey* λακτίζω describes the kicking of the feet of Iros struck by Odysseus (18.
99) and of the dying Antinoos (22. 88) and in the *Suppliants* 937 ἀπολακτισμοὶ βίου is used in
the same way to describe the 'kickings-off of life' and the convulsions of the dying warrior. In
the *Iliad* 16. 792, Patroclos slapped by Apollon rolls his eyes before dying (στρεφεδίνηθεν δέ οἱ
ὄσσε.).see Ciani 1974, 74.

[129] Kouretas 1930 concludes that Io was schizophrenic; Dumortier 1935, 5–6, 32, 70 and 74
that she was epileptic, given the similarities between the description of Io's madness and the
descriptions of epileptic maiden in the *Corpus hippocraticum*; Devereux 1976, 25–56, explains
it by Oedipal conflict, whereas D. and M. Gourevitch 1979 do not exclude any of these three
readings.

lary, it seems better to conclude, with M.G. Ciani,[130] that the Aeschylean description of madness is derived from Homeric descriptions of physical agony.

In *Prometheus Bound*, as in the *Suppliants*, Io is still driven mad by a divine agency which is either left vague, when Io speaks of an illness or a storm 'sent by the gods'[131] or imputed to Hera.[132] Yet because Io's episode contributes in this play to the portrayal of Zeus as a violent tyrant, it is Zeus who is more often said to be the cause of Io's madness.[133] But he will also be responsible for the cure: 'Zeus will restore you to your wits by touching you with a hand causing no fear and by touch alone' (ἐνταῦθα δή σε Ζεὺς τίθησιν ἔμφρονα/ἐπαφῶν ἀταρβεῖ χειρὶ καὶ θιγὼν μόνον, 848–849).

As in *The Persians*, the vocabulary of madness and mental illness is also metaphorically applied to Prometheus' inflexible attitude that goes against his best interests.[134] At the beginning of the play, Oceanos criticizes his 'foolish tongue' (γλώσσῃ ματαίᾳ, 329) and his 'sick temper' (ὀργῆς νοσούσης, 378). This criticism is echoed by the chorus and by Hermes: at ll. 472–474, the Oceanids portray him as deprived of wits, and wandering in his mind (ἀ-ποσφαλεὶς φρενῶν/πλάνῃ) and sick (ἐς νόσον/πεσὼν), a paradoxical behavior for a god who was able to render 'foolish' men (νηπίους ὄντας τὸ πρὶν, 443) 'capable of thought and possessed of intelligence' (ἔννους ἔθηκα καὶ φρε-νῶν ἐπηβόλους, 444), and demonstrated to them the mixtures of benevolent medicines through which they will repel all sicknesses (ἐγώ σφισιν/ἔδειξα κράσεις ἠπίων ἀκεσμάτων, / αἷς τὰς ἁπάσας ἐξαμύνονται νόσους, 481–483). At the end of the play, when Prometheus defies Zeus and refuses to tell him about his fatal marriage, Hermes, sent by Zeus as a warner as in *Odyssey* 1.35–43, again reproaches him for a defiant retort assimilated to madness and mental illness.[135] However, unlike Homeric *ate*, this 'madness' is not any more presented as an accident coming from outside. It is acknowledged by its author as a 'wilful mistake' with a first person active (ἑκὼν ἑκὼν ἥμαρτον, οὐκ ἀρνή-σομαι, 266).

---

[130] Ciani 1974, 73–74.
[131] θεόσσυτον: *P.V.* 596 and 643.
[132] *P.V.* 592, 600–601 and 703–704.
[133] *P.V.* 577–578, 736–738 and 759.
[134] See Ciani 1974, 75.
[135] *P.V.* 977: 977 κλύω σ᾽ ἐγὼ μεμηνότ᾽ οὐ σμικρὰν νόσον, 1054–1057: τοιάδε μέντοι τῶν φρενοπλή-κτων/βουλεύματ᾽ ἔπη τ᾽ ἔστιν ἀκοῦσαι. / τί γὰρ ἐλλείπει μὴ ⟨οὐ⟩ παραπαίειν/ἡ τοῦδ᾽ εὐχή; τί χαλᾷ μανιῶν;

In the *Agamemnon*, divine madness is staged again in the Cassandra scene.[136] The vocabulary of madness is first applied to her by Clytemnestra to convey an immediate evaluation of her refusal to answer her and obey her repeated injunctions to enter the palace,[137] although she is a slave: 'She is mad and listens to bad wits' (ἢ μαίνεταί γε καὶ κακῶν κλύει φρενῶν, 1064). Cassandra only breaks her silence after the departure of Clytemnestra, first with a lyric dialogue with the chorus (ll. 1073–1177), which opposes the supernatural vision of the prophetess inspired by Apollo to the limited vision of the old men of the chorus who criticize as inappropriate her associating Apollo with a cry of mourning[138] and are at first unable to understand the meaning of her prophecies.[139] What is for the chorus the palace of the Atreidai becomes a place haunted by gruesome crimes and murders both past and future. Her second sight enables her literally to see both past and future as if they were happening in the present[140] like the Homeric seer Calchas.[141] Her disconnected visions take the chorus and the audience both backwards, to the most distant past, the murder of the children of Thyestes[142] and the destruction of Troy,[143] and forward, to the immediate future with the murder of Agamemnon which is described realistically[144] as well as allegorically,[145] and her own death,[146] but also to a more distant future, seven years ahead, with the revenge of Orestes.[147] They also move in space from Argos and the palace of the Atreidai to Troy and the Underworld.

The accuracy of these hallucinations is soon to be proved. Her description of Thyestes' children's slaughter is endorsed by the chorus[148] and echoed, at the end of the *Agamemnon*, by Aegisthus.[149] In the following parts of the trilogy the audience will even become able to share her visions with their own eyes. At lines 980–982 of the *Choephoroi*, they are shown by Orestes,

---

[136]   see Leahy 1969; Lebeck 1971, 52–56; Taplin 1977, 316–322; Knox 1979, 42–55; Schein 1982; Effe 2000, 51–52.

[137]   *Ag.* 1039,1049, 1053–1054, 1059 and 1070–1071.

[138]   *Ag.*1074–1075 and 1078–1079.

[139]   *Ag.*1105 and 1112.

[140]   *Ag.* 1114 4 ἒ ἒ, παπαῖ παπαῖ, τί τόδε φαίνεται.

[141]   *Il.* 1.69–70.

[142]   *Ag.* 1096–1097 and 1217–1222.

[143]   *Ag.* 1156–1157 and 1167–1171.

[144]   *Ag.* 1100–1104, 1107–1111 and 1114–1118.

[145]   *Ag.* 1125–1129 and 1225–1235.

[146]   *Ag.* 1080–1082, 1100–1104, 1136–1139, 1160–1161, 1256–1263. 1275–1279, 1289–1294 and 1310–1317.

[147]   *Ag.* 1280–1291 and 1323–1326.

[148]   *Ag.* 1097–1098, 1106 and 1150–1155.

[149]   *Ag.* 1583–1597.

as a visible proof of the murder, 'the net of Hades' (δίκτυόν τί γ' "Αιδου, *Ag.* 1115)[150] seen by Cassandra, that is the robe in which Clytemnestra entangled Agamemnon. Again, her vision of the kindred Erinyes as a 'company' (στάσις 1117), a 'chorus singing together, not harmonious' (χορός/σύμφθογγος οὐκ εὔ- φωνος·1186–1187), or a 'band of revellers drunk with human blood' (πεπωκώς ...,βρότειον αἷμα κῶμος ... συγγόνων Ἐρινύων 1188–1190), and her perception of their song,[151] not only tally closely with their description in the *Choephoroi*, they are also an obvious anticipation of their apparition as a chorus in the *Eumenides*.[152] It is worth reading the Cassandra scene in conjunction with an episode that has no parallel in the epic tradition, the vision of the Apolline hereditary seer Theoclymenos in the *Odyssey*, following E.R. Dodds and G. Guidorizzi who well saw the similarities between the two episodes,[153] but emphasizing the differences more than they did.

> ἆ δειλοί, τί κακὸν τόδε πάσχετε; νυκτὶ μὲν ὑμέων
> εἰλύαται κεφαλαί τε πρόσωπά τε νέρθε τε γοῦνα,
> οἰμωγὴ δὲ δέδηε, δεδάκρυνται δὲ παρειαί,
> αἵματι δ' ἐρράδαται τοῖχοι καλαί τε μεσόδμαι·
> εἰδώλων δὲ πλέον πρόθυρον, πλείη δὲ καὶ αὐλή,
> ἱεμένων Ἔρεβόσδε ὑπὸ ζόφον· ἠέλιος δὲ
> οὐρανοῦ ἐξαπόλωλε, κακὴ δ' ἐπιδέδρομεν ἀχλύς.

Poor wretches, what evil has come on you? Your heads and faces, and the knees underneath you are shrouded in night and darkness; a sound of wailing has broken out, your cheeks are covered with tears, and the walls bleed, and the fine supporting pillars. All the forecourt is huddled with ghosts, the yard is full of them as they flock down to the underworld and the darkness. The sun has perished out of the sky, and a foul mist has come over. (20.351–357)

Like Cassandra, Theoclymenos sees in advance a murder to come and links the death of the suitors to their former crimes.[154] But he remains, like the Odyssean Proteus, who 'saw' (4.556) Odysseus crying in Calypso's island, an unconcerned observer, since his own death is not included in his prophecies, in contrast to Cassandra who is emotionally involved, tries to prevent what is coming,[155] and attempts to share her visions with the chorus.[156] Thus

---

[150] On the net and the bonds as a metaphor for the robe see *Ag.* 1127,1382–1383, Cho. 493, 981 and Lebeck 1971, 67–68.

[151] *Ag.* 1191–1192: ὑμνοῦσι δ' ὕμνον δώμασιν προσήμεναι/πρώταρχον ἄτης.

[152] See Padel 1995, 80.

[153] See Dodds 1951, 70 and Guidorizzi 2010, 108.

[154] *Od.* 20. 367–370.

[155] *Ag.* 1125–1126: ἆ ἆ, ἰδοὺ ἰδού· ἄπεχε τῆς βοὸς/τὸν ταῦρον·

[156] *Ag.* 1217–1218: ὁρᾶτε τούσδε τοὺς δόμοις ἐφημένους/νέους, ὀνείρων προσφερεῖς μορφώμασιν.

his prophetic ability, which also allows him to interpret omens, is a bless-
ing, whereas Cassandra's prophetic knowledge was turned by the wrath of
Apollo into a negative gift (she calls it an *ate* at line 1268) and a punishment
for breaking her agreement with him to have children.[157] Her prophecies
brought her only torments[158] and moral pains (her fellow citizens laughed
at her and called her 'beggar, poor wretch and starveling').[159] Moreover, they
include the knowledge of her own death, that is the only knowledge which
is useless (in *Prometheus Bound*, men were 'prevented from foreseeing their
death' by the Titan who 'planted in them blind hopes'[160]).

The motif of madness, first linked in the *parodos* to Agamemnon's decision to sacrifice his own daughter,[161] is also associated with Clytemnestra.
After the chorus have listened to the queen gloating about the murder of
her husband, they condemn her arrogant words,[162] explain them by a madness caused by bloodshed (φονολινεῖ τύχᾳ φρὴν ἐπτμαίνεται, *Ag*.1427), and
connect them with the stream of blood visible on her eyes, given that bloodshot eyes are a typical symptom of frenzy.[163] This madness is given a divine
origin first by the chorus and, later, by Clytemnestra herself. But Apollo is
replaced by the *daimon* of the race who falls upon the house, wields power
through women and fosters in their belly the lust of lapping blood.[164]

Orestes' frenzy is also linked to murder and explained, like all Aeschylean
madnesses, by a divine intervention. It comes, like the *ate* of Agamemnon and Melampous in Homer,[165] from the Erinyes, as suggested in the
Choephoroi by the vision of the Erinyes[166] and explicitly said in the *Eumenides*, where these 'mad'[167] goddesses sing a song synonymous with insanity
and derangement, ruining and binding the mind (τόδε μέλος, παρακοπά,/ πα-
ραφορὰ φρενοδαλής, ὕμνος ἐξ Ἐρινύων,/ δέσμιος φρενῶν (329–332). It will be
cured as well by a god.[168]

---

[157] *Ag*. 1203–1208.
[158] *Ag*. 1150–1151 and 1215–1216.
[159] *Ag*. 1270–1274.
[160] *P.V.* 248 and 250.
[161] *Ag*. 222–223: βροτοὺς θρασύνει γὰρ αἰσχρόμητις/τάλαινα παρακοπὰ πρωτοπήμων.
[162] *Ag*. 1399–1400 and 1426–1427.
[163] *Ag*. 1428: λίβος ἐπ' ὀμμάτων αἵματος ἐμπρέπει. About bloodshot eyes as symptom of
madness, see Eur. *H.F.* 933. This is also a characteristic of the Erinyes at *Andr*. 978 and *Or*.
256.
[164] *Ag*. 1468–1471 (chorus) and 1475–1480 (Clytemnestra).
[165] *Il*. 19. 87 and *Od*. 15. 234.
[166] *Cho*. 1048–1056.
[167] *Eum*. 67: τάσδε τὰς μάργους.
[168] *Cho*. 1059–1060 and *Eum*. 81–83, 232–234 and 282–283.

At the end of the *Choephoroi*, however, this frenzy is not first imputed to the murderer by an external witness, as in *Agamemnon*. It is Orestes himself who introduces the theme of madness with a simile describing himself as a charioteer driven off course and carried away by *phrenes* he cannot control;[169] then he mentions the fear ready to sing beside a heart ready to dance with the music of anger (πρὸς δὲ καρδίᾳ φόβος/ᾄδειν ἑτοῖμος ἠδ' ὑπορχεῖσθαι κότῳ,[170] 1024–1025). These physical symptoms are followed by hallucinations. The chorus considers them as 'mere fancies whirling him about' (τίνες σε δόξαι, φίλτατ' ἀνθρώπων πατρί, στροβοῦσιν;1051–1052), since they do not see them (ὑμεῖς μὲν οὐχ ὁρᾶτε τάσδ', 1061) and interpret them as a disturbance of his *phrenes* caused by the blood on his hands.[171] Yet these are true visions, as Orestes says at 1061: ἐγὼ δ' ὁρῶ, and his repeated use of deictics[172] also makes manifest the presence of the Erinyes. He does not content himself with identifying them, at ll. 1053–1054, as the fulfillment of the threat of Clytemnestra:[173] 'these are not for me fancies of troubles. They are clearly the angry hounds of my mother' (οὐκ εἰσὶ δόξαι τῶνδε πημάτων ἐμοί· / σαφῶς γὰρ αἵδε μητρὸς ἔγκοτοι κύνες, 1053), and he describes them precisely: these 'black-robed women' look like Gorgons wearing dark clothes and wreathed in snakes[174] (αἵδε, Γοργόνων δίκην,/ φαιοχίτωνες καὶ πεπλεκτανημέναι/πυκνοῖς δράκουσιν·, 1048–1050), 'they are coming in swarms and from their eyes they drip an unwelcome blood' (αἵδε πληθύουσι δή,/ κἀξ ὀμμάτων στάζουσι αἷμα δυσφιλές, 1057–1058) and they compel him to leave.[175]

B. *From Aeschylean to Euripidean Madness*

To assess the peculiarity of Aeschylean madness better, it is worth comparing it with the portraits of Cassandra's and Orestes' madness in the complete plays of Euripides which put these characters on stage, the *Trojan Women*, *Electra*, *Iphigenia in Tauris* and *Orestes* (there no allusion whatsoever to Orestes' madness at the end of Sophocles' *Electra*).

---

[169] *Cho*. 1022–1024: ὥσπερ ξὺν ἵπποις ἡνιοστροφῶ δρόμου/ἐξωτέρω· φέρουσι γὰρ νικώμενον/φρένες δύσαρκτοι. On this simile see also *P.V.* 883–884: ἔξω δὲ δρόμου φέρομαι λύσσης/πνεύματι μάργῳ.

[170] See *P.V.* 881: κραδία δὲ φόβῳ φρένα λακτίζει.

[171] *Cho*.1055–1056: ποταίνιον γὰρ αἷμά σοι χεροῖν ἔτι·/ἐκ τῶνδέ τοι ταραγμὸς ἐς φρένας πίτνει.

[172] *Cho*. 1048 and 1054: αἵδε; 1057: ἐκ τῶνδε; 1061: τάσδε.

[173] *Cho*. 924: ὅρα, φύλαξαι μητρὸς ἐγκότους κύνας.

[174] *Cho*. 529: the image of Orestes as a snake creates an analogy between the murderer and the goddesses who pursue him.

[175] *Cho*. 1050: οὐκέτ' ἂν μείναιμ' ἐγώ; 1062: ἐλαύνομαι δὲ κοὐκέτ' ἂν μείναιμ' ἐγώ.

In the *Trojan Women*, as in the *Agamemnon*, Cassandra appears on stage in one episode clearly divided by the meter into three parts, lyrics (308–340), iambic trimeters (353–443) and trochaic tetrameters (444–461). But Euripides substitutes the Dionysiac vocabulary of possession[176] for the μάντις terminology of Aeschylus,[177] though Cassandra is inspired by Apollo.[178] She was already portrayed as a Bacchic prophetess in the first part of Euripides' Trojan trilogy, *Alexandros* where she identified the victorious shepherd as the son of Priam and foresaw the disaster to come from him.[179]

Her lyrics are not any more a series of disconnected true visions ranging from distant past to near future. The hallucinations[180] she invites the chorus and Hecuba to share (ἰδού, ἰδού, 309) are clearly pathological. When she enters the stage, carrying a torch, she imagines that she is celebrating her wedding with Agamemnon. She believes that the *skene*, which was identified in the prologue as the barrack with the Trojan women still unallotted,[181] is a temple (τόδ'ἱερόν, 310); later she identifies it as 'the temple of Apollo crowned with bay leaves' (κατὰ σὸν ἐν δάφναισ ἀνάκτορον, 329–330), thus setting the whole marriage scene at Delphi, after having said that it was set in Argos (κατ' Ἄργος, 313). Her madness is also made manifest by her perversion of the wedding ritual—her carrying the torch normally carried by the bride's mother, her shouting a Bacchic cry (εὐὰν, εὐοῖ, 326), her invoking gods who had nothing to do with the wedding ceremony such as Hecate and Apollo,[182] and her frenzied rush that prevents her from carrying the torch straight.[183] Above all, she sings the 'bliss' of the bride and the groom and asks her mother to 'celebrate the bride with songs of bliss and acclamations',[184] a joyful song strikingly contrasting with the comments of Hecuba,[185] who laments and points out her madness:

[176] *Tr.* 170: ἐκβακχεύουσαν; 172: μαίναδ'; 307: μαινάς; 341: βακχεύουσαν; 367: Βακχευμάτων; 408: ἐξεβάκχευσεν; 415: μαινάδος, Id.Hec. 121. See Mason 1959, 89 and Papadopoulou 2000, 513 and 516–517.

[177] *Ag.* 1098, 1105, 1195, 1202, 1215, 1241 and 1275, see Mason 1959, 85 and Croally 1994, 229.

[178] *Tr.* 253–254, 408–409.

[179] Alexandros hypothesis P. Oxy 3650 col.i l. 27–28 and frgt 62 βακχεύει φρένα. See also *Andr.* 296–300.

[180] Well pointed out by Di Benedetto 1971, 55–56.

[181] *Tr.* 32–33: ὑπὸ στέγαισ/ταῖσδε.

[182] *Tr.* 322–323 and 329.

[183] *Tr.*348–349: οὐ γὰρ ὀρθὰ πυρφορεῖς μαινὰς θοάζουσ'.

[184] *Tr.* 311–312: μακάριος ὁ γαμέτας, / μακαρία δ' ἐγὼ βασιλικοῖς λέκτροις and 335–337 βόασον ὑμέναιον ὦ/μακαρίαις ἀοιδαῖς/ἰαχαῖς τε νύμφαν.

[185] *Tr.* 343–344: Ἥφαιστε, δαιδουχεῖς μὲν ἐν γάμοις βροτῶν, / ἀτὰρ λυγράν γε τήνδ' ἀναιθύσσεις φλόγα. On the contrast between Cassandra's exultation and Hecuba's lament, see Gregory 1991, 165.

O Hephaistus, you are the torch-bearer at people's weddings. But the torch you burn here is one of painful misery and a long way from what my high hopes were ... your plight has not given you sanity, my child (οὐδὲ σαῖς τύχαις, τέκνον, σεσωφρόνηκας), but you remain in the same state .... Let tears be exchanged for her wedding song.   (343–352)

Cassandra's spoken part also differs strikingly from that of her Aeschylean counterpart. It is not any more an elucidation of former cryptic visions expressed in a dense and obscure language. Indeed, at ll. 356–364, she does give a prophecy whose truth is vouched for by Apollo and clearly announces, as she did in *Agamemnon*, the death of the king and, in a paralepsis, her own death, Orestes' matricide and the overthrow of the House of Atreus. Later, explicitly relying again on Apollo's words communicated to her,[186] she predicts the death of Hecuba at Troy and the ordeals of Odysseus.[187] Yet these two predictions are only indirectly validated elsewhere, by the prophecy of Polymestor in Euripides *Hecuba*[188] and in the *Odyssey*.

A large part of her speech is devoted to a rational demonstration which has nothing to do with divine inspiration:

πόλιν δὲ δείξω τήνδε μακαριωτέραν
ἢ τοὺς Ἀχαιούς, ἔνθεος μέν, ἀλλ' ὅμως
τοσόνδε γ' ἔξω στήσομαι βακχευμάτων·

I shall show that this city of ours is more blessed than the Greeks are. I may be possessed by madness, but to this extent, I shall stand outside it.   (365–367)

Challenging the traditional celebration of the glory of the victor in an extraordinary example of sophistic rhetoric, she argues, from l. 368 to l. 402, that the Trojans are better off than the Greeks,[189] first disparaging the Greek victory (ll. ii. 368–385) and second celebrating the glory of the vanquished and eulogizing the Trojans (ii. 385–399).[190] How are we supposed to read this unsettling demonstration? The chorus points out the absurdity of such a song:

Χο. ὡς ἡδέως κακοῖσιν οἰκείοις γελᾶις
μέλπεις θ' ἃ μέλπουσ' οὐ σαφῆ δείξεις ἴσως.

You laugh with gladness at your own misfortunes and you sing things which perhaps you will show were not reliable/true when you sang them.
                                                                         (406–407)

---

[186] *Tr.* 428–429.
[187] *Tr.* 427–443.
[188] *Hec.* 1261–1273 and the *Odyssey*.
[189] Papadopoulou 2000, 523.
[190] On this speech see Di Benedetto 1971, 56–59, Croally 1994, 122–128 and Papadopoulou, 523–524.

The Greek herald Talthybius takes her words as a supplementary proof of Cassandra's madness:[191]

Τα. εἰ μή σ' 'Απόλλων ἐξεβάκχευσεν φρένας,
οὔ τὰν ἀμισθὶ τοὺς ἐμοὺς στρατηλάτας
τοιαῖσδε φήμαις ἐξέπεμπες ἂν χθονός.

Were it not Apollo who has driven wild your wits, you would have to pay for sending my commanders from this country with such ill-omened words.

(408–410)

Yet it seems better to dissent from them and acknowledge the truth of a demonstration indirectly corroborated in the prologue by the dialogue between Poseidon and Athena[192] announcing the tempest that will destroy the Greek ships on their way home.

In contrast to the *Choephoroi*, where it is staged, Orestes' madness caused by the Erinyes is only briefly referred to at the end of Euripides' *Electra* by Castor, who appears together with his brother:

δειναὶ δὲ Κῆρές ⟨σ'⟩ αἱ κυνώπιδες θεαὶ
τροχηλατήσουσ' ἐμμανῆ πλανώμενον.

The dreadful Keres, hound-faced goddesses will drive you wandering in frenzy.   (1252–1253)

In *Iphigenia in Tauris*, the intervention of the Erinyes also provides a mythical explanation for Orestes' madness and wanderings. As he says at ll. 81–86:

... διαδοχαῖς δ' 'Ερινύων
ἠλαυνόμεσθα φυγάδες ἔξεδροι χθονὸς
δρόμους τε πολλοὺς ἐξέπλησα καμπίμους·
ἐλθὼν δέ σ' ἠρώτησα πῶς τροχηλάτου
μανίας ἂν ἔλθοιμ' ἐς τέλος πόνων τ' ἐμῶν
οὓς ἐξεμόχθουν περιπολῶν καθ' Ἑλλάδα·

Then the Furies, taking turns, drove me away from home in exile; I roamed around across the land and came to ask you [Apollo] how I could put an end to the madness and the hardships I endured wandering through Greece.[193]

But the description of Orestes' fit of frenzy by a messenger at ll. 281–314, with its emphasis on physical symptoms (tossing of the head, moaning, shaking

191 See also *Tr.* 417–419.
192 *Tr.* 74–97.
193 See also *I.T.* 931–935, 941–942, and 1454–1456.

hands, shouting[194] and the allusion to the foaming mouth of Orestes at the end of the seizure[195])

ἔστη κάρα τε διετίναξ᾽ ἄνω κάτω
κἀνεστέναξεν ὠλένας τρέμων ἄκρας,
μανίαις ἀλαίνων, καὶ βοᾷ κυναγὸς ὥς·

He threw his head upwards and downwards, and trembling with his whole arms he started to shout, wandering about through his madness and shouted like a hunter. (282–284)

is unparalleled in Aeschylus and comes closer to the description of epilepsy in *The Sacred Disease*[196] than to the end of the *Choephoroi*.

These physical symptoms are accompanied by hallucinations that are first described in direct speech:

Πυλάδη, δέδορκας τήνδε; τήνδε δ᾽ οὐχ ὁρᾷς
"Ἀιδου δράκαιναν ὥς με βούλεται κτανεῖν
δειναῖς ἐχίδναις εἰς ἔμ᾽ ἐστομωμένη;
ἡ 'κ γειτόνων δὲ πῦρ πνέουσα καὶ φόνον
πτεροῖς ἐρέσσει, μητέρ᾽ ἀγκάλαις ἐμὴν
ἔχουσα, πέτρινον ἄχθος, ὡς ἐπεμβάληι.
οἴμοι, κτενεῖ με· ποῖ φύγω; ...

Pylades, don't you see how this hellish dragon fringed with terrible vipers tries to kill me? And, next to her, another, breathing fire and gore, flaps her wings and holds my mother in her arms, a mass of stone to hurl at me! Ah she will kill me! Where can I escape to? (285–291)

This hallucination is closely modeled on the Aeschylean description of the Erinyes at the end of the *Choephoroi*, where they are seen by Orestes, and in the *Eumenides*, when they appear on stage, with some significant changes. As in the *Choephoroi* their appearance provokes an impulse to flee:[197] instead of being wreathed with snakes (*Cho.* 1049–1050), they are throwing them at Orestes. In contrast to the *Eumenides* where they are explicitly said to differ from Harpies and have no wings,[198] they are flapping their wings as they usually do on Apulian vases in the second half of the fifth century.[199] Instead

[194] *I.T.* 282: κάρα τε διετίναξ᾽ ἄνω κάτω (see *H. F.* 867: τινάσσει κρᾶτα); 283: κἀνεστέναξεν ὠλένας τρέμων ἄκρας; 284: καὶ βοᾷ.

[195] *I.T.* 311: ἀφρόν see *Morb. Sacr.* 1.1. 362: Ἢν δὲ ἀφρὸν ἐκ τοῦ στόματος ἀφίη. See also 7.8.375.

[196] Ferrini 1978, 61–62 points out a parallel between *I.T.* 283: κἀνεστέναξεν ὠλένας τρέμων ἄκρας and *Morb. Sacr.* 7.1. 373: καὶ αἱ χεῖρες συσπῶνται.

[197] *Cho.* 1050 and 1062.

[198] *Eum.* 50–52.

[199] Giuliani 2001, 28: 'they are usually winged; the Berlin hydria, where they are wingless, is an exception.

of dripping gore from their eyes, as in the *Choephoroi*,²⁰⁰ they are breathing it on Orestes. The ghost of Clytemnestra who addressed, in a dream, the chorus of the Erinyes in the *Eumenides*²⁰¹ becomes a mass of stone hurled at Orestes.

But by contrast with the *Choephoroi*, Orestes' hallucinations are not any more true visions. They become empty fancies, as demonstrated by the comment of the messenger:

> παρῆν δ' ὁρᾶν
> οὐ ταῦτα μορφῆς σχήματ', ἀλλ' ἠλλάσσετο
> φθογγάς τε μόσχων καὶ κυνῶν ὑλάγματα,
> ἃς φᾶσ' Ἐρινῦς ἱέναι μιμήματα.

But none of these apparitions were there to see. He mistook the lowing of the cattle and the barking of the dogs, noises he claimed the Erinyes uttered as imitations.   (291–294)

Like the Sophoclean Ajax who confused the cattle with the Achaean leaders and killed them²⁰² or the Euripidean Agave who identified her son as a lion, the Euripidean Orestes mistook the cattle for the Erinyes:

> ὁ δὲ χερὶ σπάσας ξίφος,
> μόσχους ὀρούσας ἐς μέσας λέων ὅπως,
> παίει σιδήρωι λαγόνας ἐς πλευράς ⟨θ'⟩ ἱείς,
> δοκῶν Ἐρινῦς θεὰς ἀμύνεσθαι τάδε

Drawing his sword and rushing in the middle of the cattle like a lion, he thrust and stabbed their flanks and ribs, thinking that by so doing he was warding off the Erinyes.   (296–299)

In *Orestes* the fit of madness is not only reported by a witness as in *Ajax* and *Iphigenia in Tauris*, it is both reported by a witness (Electra) and presented on stage, as in the *Bacchae*.²⁰³ At the beginning of the play, where Orestes is said to be 'wasted with a savage sickness'²⁰⁴ and 'has taken to his bed' (34–35), the symptoms of his ailment are given an extensive description:²⁰⁵ general weakness,²⁰⁶ uncontrolled movements and jumps from his bed,²⁰⁷

---

²⁰⁰ *Cho.* 1058.

²⁰¹ *Eum.* 93–139.

²⁰² See Ciani 1974, 95.

²⁰³ *Bacch.* 1095–1136 (narrative) and 1169–1196 (staging).

²⁰⁴ The vocabulary of illness, which was never applied to Orestes' madness in the *Choephoroi* is often used in reference to it in *Orestes* (ll. 34, 43, 211, 227, 229, 232, 282, 314, 395, 407, 480, 792, 800, 881, 883 and 1016); see Smith 1967 and Theodorou 1993, 36–37.

²⁰⁵ See Ferrini 1978, 52–56.

²⁰⁶ *Or.* 227–228, 881, and 1016; *Morb. Sacr.* 1.3 354.

²⁰⁷ *Or.* 36–37, 44–45, 263, 278, and 326–327: λύσσας μανιάδος φοιταλέου. *Morb. Sacr.* 1.3 354, 1.11 362, 7.10 374.

refusal of food and bath,[208] filth,[209] dirty hair[210] (alluded to in the text and probably demonstrated by his mask: we know from Pollux, the existence of a young man mask called the squalid (πιναρός)[211]), panting,[212] disturbed and bloodshot eyes,[213] grim and unhealthy gaze,[214] foaming mouth,[215] fear[216] and shame.[217] These symptoms are so precise and so close to the descriptions of madness in Hippocratic writings that scholars have identified Orestes' illness either with delirium[218] or epilepsy.[219]

As in the *Choephoroi* and *Iphigenia in Tauris*, Orestes' fit of frenzy is accompanied by hallucinations. Immediately after the description of the first symptom of madness, the disturbance of the eyes,[220] the hallucinations begin:

> Op. ὦ μῆτερ, ἱκετεύω σε, μὴ 'πίσειέ μοι
> τὰς αἱματωποὺς καὶ δρακοντώδεις κόρας·
> αὗται γὰρ αὗται πλησίον θρώισκουσ' ἐμοῦ.

> Orestes: Mother, I beg you, don't threaten me with those blood-eyed, snaky maidens! For here they come, here they come, bounding up to me.

(255–257)

As in *Iphigenia in Tauris*, Orestes sees both his mother and the Erinyes. Yet, instead of Erinyes throwing Clytemnestra at him, it is Clytemnestra who is shaking Erinyes against him. In contrast to Orestes' visions, which were demonstrated to be true in *Eumenides*, in *Orestes* the ghost, the Erinyes as well as the bow he asks for from an imaginary attendant[221] are empty

---

[208] *Or.* 41–42, 189 and 226.

[209] *Or.* 226.

[210] *Or.* 223 and 225.

[211] Pollux 4. 137: ὁ δὲ πιναρὸς ὀγκώδης, ὑποπέλιδνος, κατηφής, δυσπινής, ξανθῇ κόμῃ ἐπικομῶν, see Donadi 1974, 114.

[212] *Or.* 84, 155 and 227.

[213] *Or.* 253: ὄμμα σὸν ταράσσεται and 836–837: φόνον δρομάσι δινεύων βλεφάροις; *Morb. Sacr.* 7.1 373 and 7.7 374: diverging eyes.

[214] *Or.* 389 and 479–480.

[215] *Or.* 219–220; cf. *Morb. Sacr.* 1.11 362, and 7.1 372.

[216] *Or.* 38, 269–270, 312 and 532; *Morb. Sacr.* 1.12 362, and 14.3 388.

[217] *Or.* 281–282; *Morb. Sacr.* 12.1 382.

[218] Theodorou 1993, 35 n. 16.

[219] Ferrini 1978, 50.

[220] *Or.* 253–254: Ηλ. οἴμοι, κασίγνητ', ὄμμα σὸν ταράσσεται, / ταχὺς δὲ μετέθου λύσσαν, ἄρτι σωφρονῶν.

[221] Many scholars (see Hartigan 1987, 134 n. 26) following the scholiast at 268 who says that the actors in his day imagine the bow, but thinks the original staging was otherwise posit that the bow was displayed on stage. Contra Di Benedetto ad loc. Smith 1967, 298. Donadi 1974, 118 and West 1987 at Or. 268, p. 200 and Willink 1986, at 268–274: 129–130.

imaginations, as pointed out first by Electra: 'you are not seeing any of the things you think you are sure of' (ὁρᾷς γὰρ οὐδὲν ὧν δοκεῖς σάφ' εἰδέναι, 259),[222] and second by Orestes when he says to Electra at l. 277: 'What am I doing, raving and out of breath?' (τί χρῆμ'; ἀλύω, πνεῦμ' ἀνεὶς ἐκ πλευμόνων, 277).

Like Heracles who 'thought' (δοκῶν, H.F.967) that his father Amphitryon was Eurystheus' father and kills his own sons, thinking that he was killing the children of Eurystheus, Orestes confuses friends with enemies: he takes Electra who attempts to restrain his unhappy jumping around[223] for an Erinys: 'Let go! You're one of my Erinyes, you're getting a grip on my waist for a throw into Tartarus' (μέθες· μί' οὖσα τῶν ἐμῶν Ἐρινύων / μέσον μ' ὀχμάζεις, ὡς βάλῃς ἐς Τάρταρον, 264–265).

Moreover—and this is may be the most innovative aspect of the play—Orestes' madness is not only explained by an external divine intervention. It is also given internal and psychological causes. Indeed, in *Orestes* the traditional notion of divine intervention still provides the explanation for the causation of madness: Electra (238), as well as the chorus (316–327, 365–369, 835), Menelaus (411, 423) and Tyndareos (531–532) attribute it to the Erinyes, some avenging spirit, or, more vaguely, to some god. They are echoed twice by Orestes, the first time during his fit of frenzy (260–270), the second time when he is worried that the goddesses may catch him with their frenzy (789–791) on his way to the assembly. At the very end of the play, in the speech of Apollo as *deus ex machina*, the announcement of the trial to come in Athens, where the Erinyes will act as plaintiffs (1648–1650), also reverts to the traditional view. But the play also questions this interpretation in the dialogue between Menelaus and Orestes:

Με. τί χρῆμα πάσχεις; τίς σ' ἀπόλλυσιν νόσος;
Ορ. ἡ σύνεσις, ὅτι σύνοιδα δείν' εἰργασμένος.
Με. πῶς φῄς; σοφόν τοι τὸ σαφές, οὐ τὸ μὴ σαφές.
Ορ. λύπη μάλιστά γ' ἡ διαφθείρουσά με ...
Με. δεινὴ γὰρ ἡ θεός, ἀλλ' ὅμως ἰάσιμος.
Ορ. μανίαι τε, μητρὸς αἵματος τιμωρίαν.

MEN.: What is wrong with you? What sickness is killing you?
OR.: My intellect—I am conscious of having done awful things.
MEN.: How do you mean? It's intelligent to be clear, not obscure.
OR.: It is grief in particular that is destroying me.
MEN.: Yes, this goddess is formidable, but still curable.
OR.: And frenzy-fits, retributions for my mother's blood.   (396–400)

---

[222] see also Or. 314–315: κἂν μὴ νοσῇ γὰρ ἀλλὰ δοξάζῃ νοσεῖν, / κάματος βροτοῖσιν ἀπορία τε γίγνεται.

[223] Or. 262–263.

The puzzlement of Menelaus at Orestes' answer clearly demonstrates the unusual character of an explanation that 'puts the emphasis on the effect of the crime on the mind (ἡ σύνεσις,) and emotions (λύπη) of the murderer'[224] and links Orestes' madness to a mental awareness and not the Erinyes.[225] However, it is worth pointing out that Euripides here chooses a purely psychological explanation and thus parts company with the author of *The Sacred Disease*, who attributed the cause of madness to the brain.[226]

Conclusion

In the Homeric poems, with the exception of *Odyssey* 20, there is no description of a fit of frenzy. The ἄτη words, always referring to some harm experienced by the subject and never associated with physical manifestations, are clearly distinguished from the μαίνομαι and λύσσα words always applied to some harm inflicted by the subject on others and often characterized by physical symptoms. Yet, both are equally explained by divine intervention. In Aeschylus the distinction between the two semantic families, both appropriated for the description of madness which is still caused by a god, tends to disappear. By contrast, in Euripides, vocabulary borrowed from Dionysiac madness becomes an integral part of the description of madness not only in the *Bacchae*, where the madness of Pentheus and Agave is explained by the intervention of Dionysos, but also in *Heracles* and the *Trojan Women*. Divine intervention is replaced by psychological explanation in *Orestes*, Physical symptoms receive more attention in all the tragedies that put madness on stage. If the three tragic poets put on stage the gods who caused the madness (the Erinyes in the *Eumenides*, Athena in Sophocles' *Ajax*, Lyssa ('Madness') in Euripides' *Heracles* and Dionysos in the *Bacchae*), it is only Aeschylus in the *Oresteia*, who makes visible for the audience the true visions of Cassandra and Orestes.

---

[224] Theodorou 1993, 40.
[225] Rodgers 1969, 254, and Theodorou 1993, 38.
[226] *Morb. Sacr.* 3.1 366: ἀλλὰ γὰρ αἴτιος ὁ ἐγκέφαλος τούτου τοῦ πάθεος ὥσπερ τῶν ἄλλων νοσημάτων τῶν μεγίστων.

THE MADNESS OF TRAGEDY

Glenn W. Most

> Non dimenticherò mai quella scena, di
> tutte le nostre facce mascherate, sguajate
> e stravolte, davanti a quella terribile ma-
> schera di lui, che non era più una ma-
> schera, ma la Follia!
>
> —Luigi Pirandello, *Enrico IV*

In Act II of Menander's *Aspis*, matters seem very bleak for young Chaireas. Cleostratus, the brother of the girl he loves, is thought to have died on a mercenary expedition abroad; now Cleostratus' greedy uncle Smicrines has announced that he will marry the sister, Cleostratus' heir, in order to inherit his booty. What to do? Chaireas and his stepfather Chairestratus can only tear their hair out and lament. But after all this is New Comedy: Daus, Cleostratus' loyal and resourceful slave, comes up, as comic slaves always do, with an ingenious plan. They will pretend that Chairestratus has gone mad and is dying of melancholy; after the old man's fake funeral, Smicrines will doubtless prefer to marry Chairestratus' extremely wealthy daughter rather than Cleostratus' only moderately wealthy sister and will be delighted to leave the latter for Chaireas.

Menander allows his characters, especially his stand-in Daus, to play knowledgeably, amusingly, and amusedly upon the contemporary technical vocabulary for madness and upon the experts who made good money out of diagnosing and, much more rarely, curing it. Already Chairestratus complains that he is doing terribly and has become melancholic because of the turn of events (Δᾶε παῖ, κακῶς ἔχω.| μελαγχολῶ τοῖς πράγμασιν 305–306); he has lost his self-control and almost gone mad (οὐκ εἴμ' ἐν ἐμαυτοῦ, μαίνομαι δ' ἀκαρὴς πάνυ 307). Then Daus takes over: Chairestratus must pretend to fall into a depression (ἀθυμίαν 331, ἀθυμοῦντ' 334)—after all, Daus opines sententiously, grief (λύπης 337) is the cause of most illnesses, and, he adds, with a pseudo-professional view to the specific circumstances of this particular patient, he knows that Chairestratus has a natural inclination to just such depressions (φύσει δέ σ' ὄντα πικρὸν εὖ οἶδα καὶ | μελαγχολικόν 338–339).

They will have to summon a doctor, a real intellectual (ἰατρός τις φιλοσοφῶν 340), who will diagnose pleurisy or phrenitis (πλευρῖτιν ... ἢ φρενῖτιν 341)—in any case, a disease sure to cause death quickly (342). He will have to be a foreigner, quick-witted and a bit of a braggart (374–375); in the absence of the real thing, Chaireas will fit out one of his friends with the necessary toupee, cloak, and walking-stick (377–378)—and, as we discover when the fake doctor enters, with a broad Doric accent as well (439–464). Daos provides Smicrines with his own quite professional sounding list of Chairestratus' symptoms, 'bile, some grief, loss of his mind, shortness of breath' (χολή, λύπη τις, ἔκστασις φρενῶν, | πνιγμός 422–423), and in a few moments his diagnosis will apparently be confirmed and further specified by the doctor (φ]ρενῖτιν 446, cf. 450–454).

Such scenes of intellectuals and professionals, fake and real, are common in Attic comedy; they permit us to estimate how far pseudo-scientific terminology had become diffused in various levels of contemporary Athenian society, just as in our own. The comic effect depends upon a shrewd interplay between familiarity and unintelligibility: to different degrees, different members of the audience must have heard such words, or ones much like them, and may well have even used them themselves, to describe themselves and others they knew, even if they were not always sure of just what they meant; seeing Smicrines being fooled will have reminded them how often they had wondered whether they were not being fooled themselves.

But if this scene in Menander tells us much about the dissemination of the technical discourse about insanity within the real language of his Athenian contemporaries, it also tells us much about the identification of the phenomenon of publicly staged insanity with the literary genre of Athenian tragedy. For Menander's comedies are full of clever stratagems like the one Daus proposes here. But this one, unlike all those others, turns out to have a manifest and significant relation with the genre of tragedy—as it were, it seems to be impossible for Menander to introduce a plot founded upon the appearance of madness without immediately and persistently invoking tragedy. When Chairestratus asks Daus what his plan is, the slave responds that they will have to stage an inauspicious kind of suffering, a real tragedy (δεῖ τραγῳδῆσαι πάθος | ἀλλοῖον ὑμᾶς 329–330). And when in Act III Daus' plan moves into the operational phase, Menander's text becomes adorned for almost thirty lines with the richest collection of tragic quotations in all his surviving oeuvre: an unidentified citation of the opening of Euripides' *Stheneboia* (407), an unidentified line from Chaeremon's *Achilles* (411), a line from Aeschylus' *Niobe* attributed explicitly to that playwright (412–413), an unidentified line (415), a line attributed explicitly to Carcinus (416), another unidentified line (417–418), one line attributed explicitly to Euripides from the beginning of his *Orestes* (424–425) and another one assigned explicitly to Chaeremon (425–426). Smicrines can protest all he wants to against Daus' gnomological rapture (414, 415, 425) but no power on earth, it seems, can stop him: for Daus, Menander, and Menander's audience, the connection between staged insanity and Attic tragedy is not only irresistibly funny in this comic context, it is also simply too strong to interrupt.[1]

This scene in Menander's *Aspis* is not only a remarkable document in the early history of gnomological collections of quotations from poets, organized thematically: surely many Athenians were likely to quote appositely in such situations, as Daus does, on the basis of just such handbooks; the comic effect here comes from the facts that it is a slave who is doing the quoting and that he just can't stop doing so. But this passage also reveals how great a fascination the madness of tragedy could still exert upon Athenian audiences, about a century after the deaths of Euripides and Sophocles. Not only, be it noted, the madness *in* tragedy, but also the madness *of* tragedy. For if the phrase 'madness *in* tragedy' denotes a limited group of certain definable scenes with an identifiable content to be found within the stable context of a given literary genre, the phrase 'madness *of* tragedy' also raises a question about that very context: just how stable is it? What is the relation between particular scenes of disorder and suffering, mental and physical, within tragedy, and the disorder and suffering that characterize in general terms tragedy itself? Indeed, can one entirely separate madness and tragedy from one another, or is it not rather the case that tragedy itself in a certain sense is a form of madness?

Greek tragedy, of course, contains many scenes of terrible suffering, what Aristotle indicated with the general term πάθος.[2] Suffering may be of at least two kinds, bodily and mental. Bodily suffering does indeed sometimes occur on the Greek tragic stage (think only of Heracles' torments in Sophocles' *Trachinian Women* and of Philoctetes' in *Philoctetes*); but a variety of considerations—theological, technical, psychological, and doubtless others—led the Greek tragedians to tend in general to remove most cases of physical torments from their spectators' direct inspection and to consign them instead to messengers' reports, offstage screams, and the audience's

---

[1] This passage is discussed by Paduano 1978 and more recently by Cusset 2003, 144–158 and Ingrosso's commentary on lines 408–443 (pp. 357–372). At line 330, ἀλλοῖον is Kassel's emendation of the papyrus' impossible ουκ'αλλοιον; another possible correction is Sisti's οὐκ ἄλλο γ'.

[2] Aristotle, *Poetics* 11.1452b11–13.

imaginations. The inevitable result was that, by a kind of compensation, it was psychological rather than bodily suffering that was most emphatically presented on stage. Adopting once again the terminology of Aristotle,[3] we might say that the tragic chorus and characters (and, too, the spectators) were exposed above all to two kinds of tragic emotions, fear and pity (of course other forms of pity and fear, and other emotions, were also involved): fear of physical and psychological suffering that had not happened yet but that seemed likely to be about to happen; and pity for physical and psychological suffering that had already happened or that was in the course of happening.

Among all the kinds of psychological suffering to be found in Greek tragedy, madness is the most extreme. We may define tragic madness as what happens when certain forms of psychological suffering—for example, love, grief, guilt, or anger—go beyond a certain limit and take on a unique and unmistakable degree of intensity. So if mental πάθος is one of the constitutive elements of tragedy, madness is the highest possible degree of that tragic mental πάθος. Dionysus is after all both the god of theater, including tragedy, and of intoxication verging on madness. We might say that, in a certain sense, a scene of madness is the very essence of Greek tragedy.[4]

The paradigmatic example of Greek tragic madness is Orestes; let us begin with his case, in order to establish the basic outlines of the ailment. Both Aeschylus and Euripides dedicate memorable and extended portrayals to the hero who, when he was relatively sane, committed the unspeakable crime of murdering his own mother, and later became a celebrated madman, pursued by the Erinyes who sought to punish him for that deed. Are the Erinyes real divine instances that exist independently of Orestes' mental state, or are they projections of his quite understandable feelings of remorse and anguish for what he has done, or in some way a mixture of both? In any case, Orestes is afflicted by bouts of recurrent insanity. In both Aeschylus and Euripides, his madness takes essentially the form of visual hallucinations. But there is a significant difference between the two tragedians' portrayals: in Aeschylus, Orestes sees things that are simply not there in the

---

[3] Aristotle, *Poetics* 6.1449b27, 14.1453b12; so already Gorgias B 11 (9) DK.

[4] The best study of this subject is Padel 1995. Somewhat less useful in the present context is Padel 1992. See also especially Schlesier 1985, and also Mattes 1970 and now Gerolemou 2011. It may well be of more than simply comparative interest that a whole genre of Japanese Noh dramas, the so-called Monogurui-mono, is focused on the madness of the (usually female) protagonist, who goes mad out of unrequited love, jealousy, or maternal love: see Bohner 1956 and now Savas 2008.

physical dimension to which he assigns them (they are real and present, of course, on a different, religious level, one to which he, gods, and divinely inspired figures have access, but not the chorus, other characters, or we spectators under normal circumstances); whereas in Euripides, Orestes sees figures that are really there physically but mistakes them as being other than they are. Aeschylus' Orestes commits a confusion about different ontological spheres; Euripides' commits one about different members of the same sphere.

As far as we can tell, it is the closing scene of Aeschylus' *Choephori* that introduces crazed Orestes onto the stage of world literature; and it does so in such a memorable way that many of the later dramatic versions of his insanity are best seen as direct responses to Aeschylus' text. At the end of the play, Orestes displays the corpses of Clytemnestra and Aegisthus, whom he has just murdered, and the net in which they had killed his father. Despite the horror of the sight of two dead bodies, and the greater horror of the fact that one of them is his own mother, whom he has slain, Orestes' speech accompanying this exhibition is lucid, balanced, lecture-like (*Choe.* 973–1006, 1010–1017)—until he suddenly states that he does not know how things will end and that, like a charioteer who has lost control of his horses,[5] he is being assailed by waves of fear and wrath (1021–1025). Yet by an effort of will he manages to dominate his growing anguish and pull himself together—but only briefly: at 1048 he cries out ἆ ἆ, and this *extra metrum* exclamation signals that he is passing into a phase of insanity. The unmistakable symptom of his madness is a visual hallucination: where the Chorus see only Orestes and the corpses, Orestes sees the Chorus and the corpses, but also Erinyes as well (1048–1062), and confusion falls upon his mind (ταραγμὸς ἐς φρένας πίτνει 1056). We might perhaps be tempted to think that what Orestes 'really' sees is the Chorus, a group of black-garbed women, whom he mistakes as being Erinyes; but this is impossible, for throughout these lines Orestes consistently uses the second person for the Chorus and the third person for the Erinyes, so he evidently has no difficulty in distinguishing the two groups and in recognizing that he is engaged with them in different ways, with the Chorus as his interlocutors and with the Erinyes as their victim. Repeatedly he designates the Erinyes with the deictic pronoun αἵδε (1048, 1054, 1057, 1061), normally reserved for indicating something near at hand and visible to all. But, despite his insistence, the Chorus cannot see

---

[5] Aeschylus' single but memorable charioteering simile may well have generated the false tale of Orestes' death in a charioteering accident in Sophocles' *Electra*.

them. In a certain sense, we have here a deliberate violation, on Aeschylus' part, of the grammar of such deictics: Orestes' persistence betrays his
recognition that the Chorus does not see what he sees (1061) and both establishes their difference from him and tries, fruitlessly, to draw them into his
madness. And what about us as spectators of this scene? What do we see?
Do we share the perspective of the Chorus, seeing nothing but the Chorus,
Orestes, and the corpses? Or do we share the perspective of Orestes, seeing
the Chorus, Orestes, the corpses, and the Erinyes? Aeschylus' text, of course,
is devoid of any stage directions that could clarify this question; and we cannot be certain how he staged it himself at the first production of the play
in Athens in 458 BCE. So what we spectators see depends upon what the
director of any given production chooses to make us see; and in fact different directors have made different choices in this regard. But it surely is
more effective dramatically for the director to make us see only what the
Chorus sees, thereby isolating Orestes even further within his incipient madness.

    This passage follows closely upon a series of lines, in Orestes' presentation
of the two corpses, that have emphasized vision and visibility (973, 980–981,
984–987, 1034–1035): after having insisted upon seeing what can be seen
by all, Aeschylus now has us see someone who sees what cannot be seen
except by himself. As it were, Aeschylus has trained his audience's sensitivity
towards the issue of vision and made it all the easier for us to be struck
by the visual element in Orestes' ailment. We have been brought into a
situation where we can easily recognize that Orestes sees something where
the Chorus see nothing. But this does not mean that Orestes sees something
that does not exist at all in any way whatsoever: instead, he sees something
that exists in a different way, in a different dimension, from what the Chorus
is capable of recognizing. After all, the Erinyes are real; they are not simply a
figment of Orestes' mind, any more than Apollo or Athena are; it is just that
they are not real in exactly the same way as the Chorus or Orestes is.

    It is precisely this difference that makes the beginning of the next and
final play of the trilogy, the *Eumenides*, so shocking: for here we come to
see exactly what, among humans, Orestes alone can see, humans but also
gods and Erinyes. In a certain sense, by being made to share his vision, we
are made to enter into his madness. At first we do not see the Erinyes ourselves, but only hear them described by a divinely inspired human being
who (unlike the Chorus of the *Choephori*) has been made able by a divine
instance to see them; in her description the Priestess repeats emphatically
words for vision in order to indicate how terrible these creatures are to see
(*Eum.* 34, 40, 49, 50, 51, 57). So at first we envision them only in our imagi-

nations, much as the Chorus of the *Choephori* supposed was the case with Orestes. But then Aeschylus allows, indeed requires us, together with Apollo and Orestes, to see them in person: when Apollo invites Orestes to see the sleep-struck Erinyes, the second person singular verb for seeing he uses (ὁρᾷς 67) is of course directed only to Orestes, but there can be little doubt that the hero's vision is supposed to be confirmed by our own as spectators. How exactly this was staged in 458 BCE is uncertain and controversial; the most economical hypothesis is that the σκήνη, a light wooden structure, was partly opened up in order to reveal the Erinyes sleeping at the Delphic *omphalos*. But however it was achieved, this *coup de théâtre* has an extraordinary psychological and theological impact. And it is not only a punctual, local dramatic effect of great theatrical sophistication and power, but also the culmination of a theme of madness and vision that Aeschylus has carefully constructed throughout the trilogy ever since the *Agamemnon*, where, just like mad Orestes, mad Cassandra (*Ag.* 1064, 1140) too had seen visions (*Ag.* 1114, 1125, 1217–1218), while that play's Chorus had seen nothing at all— or, to put it more precisely, where Cassandra had seen behind the σκήνη, within the royal palace, scenes of atrocious bloodshed and human suffering that had indeed happened already in the past or were about to happen in the imminent future, while the Chorus could not see, or refused to see, anything more than the present buildings and stone. Where ordinary people see only ordinary objects, both Cassandra and Orestes, in their madness, see extraordinary theological truths, in the form of terrifying visual hallucinations.

Euripides was one of Aeschylus' closest readers; and surely it is in large measure thanks to these scenes in the *Oresteia* that mad scenes involving Orestes become a stock feature of Euripides' theater. When, in *Iphigenia among the Taurians*, Iphigenia asks Orestes whether his madness on the beach had been due to the Furies, and he replies that this was not the first time that he had been seen to be so wretched (ὤφθημεν οὐ νῦν πρῶτον ὄντες ἄθλιοι 933), it is difficult not to read into his words, besides their obvious meaning, also a meta-theatrical acknowledgment that by this time such mad scenes of his had become conventional on the Athenian stage.

We can see how Euripides handles the same topic differently in two different plays, *Iphigenia among the Taurians* and *Orestes*. In the earlier play, the presentation of Orestes' madness is entrusted to a messenger's speech delivered by a Taurian cowherd (*IT* 281–307). At first, as in Aeschylus, the visual hallucinations of what are explicitly termed a madman (μανίαις ἀλαίνων 284) are set in contrast with an ordinary vision that sees nothing where, apparently, nothing at all is to be seen (285, 291–294[6]). But then the herdsman moves on to a second phase of his report, in which Euripides appears to innovate decisively with regard to his precursor: now Orestes really sees the same thing that the Taurians see, namely cattle, but he misinterprets them as though they were Erinyes and attacks them with his sword (296–300). Finally Orestes collapses, foaming at the mouth (307–308): the episode is over. In the *Orestes*, by contrast, Euripides dramatizes Orestes' bout of insanity by staging it before our eyes (253–277), rather than consigning it to the narrative report of a witness. Here too, however, Euripides structures the episode in precisely the same terms. Once again, insanity is named as such (μανίασιν λυσσήμασιν 270) and takes the form of visual hallucinations. And once again, Orestes begins by seeing something where there is nothing: he addresses his mother and asks her to keep the Furies away from him (255–257); it is in vain that Electra tells him that he in fact is seeing none of what he imagines to be seeing (259). But then, once again, Orestes moves from seeing something where there is nothing, to seeing some thing as though it were some other thing: he sees Electra, who is really there, but he mistakes her for a Fury (264–265). New is only that this time Orestes is made to suffer from haptic hallucinations as well: Electra really touches him, but he mistakes her embrace for an Erinye's. And finally, once again, Orestes recovers his senses, returns to himself, and asks what has happened (277): the episode, once again, is over.

We may summarize our clinical findings so far regarding the case of Orestes as follows. He is subject to recurrent bouts of insanity; each episode has a clearly marked beginning and ending; during his mad fits the same symptoms occur, and outside of them he seems to be fairly normal (if we can call a matricide normal). During these bouts, he is subject to extreme anxiety and terror and to hallucinations that are almost exclusively visual in nature. These latter consist either in his believing that he is seeing things when no one else is able to see them (Aeschylus, Euripides), or in his seeing some object x that others can see as well but in his mistaking this x as if it were some other object y (Euripides). Let us call the former kind of hallucination 'visions' as it involves believing that one sees something that belongs to quite a different ontological category from the rest of the world and the latter kind 'delusions' as it involves failing to distinguish between two differ-

---

[6] A difficult textual corruption mars this second passage and makes its exact meaning unclear; it is not entirely impossible that already here Orestes is shown to be responding erroneously to real stimuli, as he will certainly be doing shortly in any case.

ent objects that belong to the same ontological category. We might expect visions to be emphasized more, both because they have such interesting theological aspects and because, since they are premised upon the absence of any 'real' sensory stimulus, they might well be thought to be more terrifying. But, strikingly, it is the kind I have called delusions that seems, as far as we can tell, to have been added by Euripides (or by one of his lost post-Aeschylean predecessors), and this is certainly the one that he treats in such a way as to make it seem more climactic and more upsetting than visions. Why that should be the case is an interesting question. Perhaps he considered delusion to be more effective theatrically because it permitted spectators to see something that was really there and to recognize, without becoming confused, that Orestes was misrecognizing it. That is, the very simplicity of delusion (which after all reduces the mysteries of a divine second sight to a mere error in identification) might have made it, in Euripides' view, easier to manage in the theater—here too, as elsewhere, Euripides may be taking the opportunity to teach Aeschylus a brief lesson in proper dramaturgy. It is worth noting in this connection that Sextus Empiricus refers to Orestes' hallucinations a number of times as examples of epistemological error—and every time does so with reference not to his visions (which he never mentions) but to his delusions (which he has no difficulty in analyzing as mistaken interpretations of genuine sense impressions).[7]

Be that as it may, the central point I wish to stress is that Orestes' madness consists essentially in visual hallucinations. This may seem unsurprising to us; but it should not. Why should ancient tragic poets have chosen to emphasize in their depictions of mental disorder precisely visual hallucinations? Why do madmen on the tragic stage see visions and delusion so prevalently rather than experiencing other forms of sensory hallucinations, such as acoustic and olfactory ones, or other symptoms, like babbling or convulsions or depressions or paralysis or talking to themselves? We might perhaps be tempted to suppose that ancient Greeks tended to go mad in their own peculiarly Greek way: that is, we might wish to minimize the contradiction by historicizing it. This is not an entirely impossible way of trying to deal with this problem, but it is counter-intuitive to think that visual hallucinations were the only kind experienced by the ancient Greeks; and even if that were the case (which does not seem likely), this would require further explanation. Besides, ancient medicine focuses not only on visual hallucinations in its diagnosis of mental disorders, in this regard being not very

---

[7] Sextus Empiricus, *Against Logicians* 1.170,244, 249; 2.63, 67.

different from modern medicine;[8] so why should the tragedians do otherwise? So Orestes' problem is probably not just an ancient Greek problem. Alternatively, we might suppose that Orestes suffers from a very peculiar kind of madness, one found in him but otherwise, if indeed occasionally, only rarely: that is, we might try to reduce the scope of the problem by limiting it to the single case of Orestes. This strategy too is not quite impossible; but it must be pointed out that the ancients often discuss Orestes' madness without hinting in any way that it is anything but an entirely typical form of madness, and we would still wish to know why Orestes in particular suffers from just this type of malady. Moreover, we shall see later that other ancient tragic madmen are mad in exactly the same way that Orestes is. So Orestes' problem is probably not just Orestes' problem either.

Neither of these paths seems very promising: what are we to do? Instead, I would like to suggest a different approach to Orestes' peculiarly visual variety of madness, connecting it with the emphasis on vision in these scenes and in other scenes closely connected with them. My suggestion is that the depiction of tragic madness is being influenced by the essential visuality of the tragic medium itself. After all, the Greek theater was an essentially visual institution. Its very name, θεατρόν, proclaimed it as a place for 'seeing,' just as the spectator, θεατής, was someone who 'saw.' The architecture of the theater was designed so as to permit unimpeded sight lines for thousands of people who, whatever their differences in the rest of their lives, came together on the occasion of the dramatic festivals in order to sit together with their fellow citizens watching with them the very same spectacles.

My suggestion, then, is that one reason that the madness of a tragic hero like Orestes takes the form it does, above all that of visual hallucinations, is precisely because he is being presented on stage. Perhaps if the tragedian emphasizes the visual dimension of his hero's madness he does so because, in the context of the visual medium of theater, that is the aspect that can be staged most easily and the one that is likely to have the greatest effect upon the spectators. For it requires only a little reflection to realize that other forms of madness cannot easily be staged so effectively as visual hallucinations can. For example, how is a dramatic character supposed to convey to us that he is hearing voices? Either we will hear them too, in which case we shall not think he is mad; or we will not hear them, but at least some of us will wonder whether there really had been sounds that we ourselves

---

[8] See Jacques Jouanna (in the present volume) on the various kinds of mental disorders discussed by ancient medical treatises.

had missed. Visual hallucinations will inevitably be more striking than auditory ones, because we will generally be able to tell unambiguously that the objects the madman claims to see are not there at all, or are other than he supposes them to be. There are indeed several instances in Greek tragedy of what we would call auditory hallucinations, both staged (Dionysus' voice from the palace in the *Bacchae*) and reported (unidentified divine voices on the ship towards the end of *Iphigenia among the Taurians* and just before the disappearance of Oedipus in *Oedipus in Colonus*, and again the voice of Dionysus just before the murder of Pentheus in the *Bacchae*). But these are always considered to be episodes of genuine divine self-manifestation, never ones of human madness. As for gustatory, olfactory, or tactile hallucinations, these might well be very disturbing for the madman in question, but it would be difficult to convey them plausibly to the spectators sitting on the farthest benches. And what of depression? Probably, of all symptoms of mental disorder, this is the one that is hardest to envision as being dramatically effective—Euripides' Orestes may well suffer brief bouts of discouragement and depression, but just try to imagine a whole tragedy of Euripides devoted to Oblomov! So, put in these terms, it is not at all surprising that there is an emphasis upon visual hallucinations in this essentially visual medium.

But perhaps we can take another step and suggest a further theoretical implication of the visuality of tragic madness that might have been of interest for Euripides and for some of the more sophisticated members of his audience. On this reading, such scenes of visual hallucination are moments of self-reflection within the genre of tragedy, in which the spectators are implicitly reminded that they too are seeing what is not really there—both, seeing things that are not really there at all, and, especially, seeing one thing but taking it to be another than what it really is. For example, when the spectators, hearing the offstage screams of Agamemnon, imagine that Clytemnestra is murdering him, they are envisioning something that is not really there at all; but when they see an actor standing on the stage and dressed as a hero and they suppose that they are seeing Orestes, then they are seeing an object x (the actor) and mistaking it as the object y (Orestes). The kind of recognition that Aristotle assigns to the theatergoer, that of saying οὗτος ἐκεῖνος,[9] is not only a fairly low-level epistemological activity: it is also the basis of all dramatic illusion and may well be considered simply to be a cognitive mistake, though of course it is much more than that. But it is one thing to be momentarily in error about the identity of some person,

---

[9] Aristotle, *Poetics* 4.1448b17. Note the masculine gender.

imagining for a moment that an actor is in fact Orestes; it is a more serious, and more perplexing phenomenon, to suppose for the length of a whole
tragedy that what we are witnessing is not some costumed actors standing
in front of us and delivering their lines, but instead really Orestes and his relatives. In this sense, the staged madness of Orestes can be seen as a reminder
of the illusion that lies at the basis of all theatrical staging. Orestes, subject
to his visions, is not so very different from us spectators who envision him:
thereby our empathy for his predicament is enhanced, as is our perplexity
about our own predicaments.

These reflections may also cast further light on the development we noted
above, whereby the earlier, Aeschylean vision comes to be supplemented
later by the Euripidean delusion. For from the point of view of an implicit
theory of dramatic illusion, the case in which spectators imagine that there
is something when there is really nothing at all for them to observe is certainly rarer, and much less interesting, than the case in which the spectators
see an object x (for example, an actor or a painted wooden screen) and mistake it as an object y (for example, Orestes or the palace of Argos). For this
latter case is the fundamental premise of all dramatic illusion. After all, in
the theater we generally see something, which we take to be something else,
rather than seeing nothing at all. Even the happy madman of Argos about
whom Horace tells us[10] may well have spent his time sitting contentedly in
an empty theater—but it was a real, and really visible, theater that he was
sitting in. Had he imagined that he was sitting in the theater when he was
really sitting in his home, he would have been an ordinary and aesthetically
uninteresting madman; but his imagining that he was watching tragedies
when he was sitting in an empty theater made him just like the rest of the
tragic spectators, only more so.

Let us test these preliminary results by looking briefly at some of Orestes'
most notable mad colleagues: Ajax, Heracles, Pentheus and Agave (others
could easily be added, for example Phaedra). In Sophocles' *Ajax*, Athena at
first describes and narrates the hero's fit of violent insanity (μανιάσιν νόσοις,
Aj 59): like Euripides' Orestes, Ajax has been subject to delusions, seeing one
thing (cattle) and imagining he had been seeing something else (the Greek
commanders: 56–57, 64). But then Athena shifts from the narrative to the
dramatic mode: just as the *Eumenides* had first described the Erinyes and
then displayed them, Athena now shows mad Ajax to Odysseus, and to us,
as a play within the play, assigning to Odysseus the role of first spectator

---

[10] *Epist.* 2.2.128–140.

who will narrate what he has seen, in a further messenger's report, to the other Greeks (66–67). Euripides' *Heracles*, uniquely in our corpus, shows us a divinized figure of Madness herself, Lyssa, who will make Heracles insane in front of our eyes. She describes in clinical detail the external symptoms of the madness she is in the act of inspiring (*HF* 867–871); for the most part he too experiences delusions (865–866, 954–958, 962–971, 982, 989–990), but there is at least one passage which suggests he might also be subject to a vision (947–949). The passage is striking for its repeated references to the literary genre of comedy (935, 950–952): the interference between the genres of comedy and tragedy certainly heightens the horror of these events, but at the same time it makes even more explicit the meta-theatrical reflection involved in such a scene—the messenger watching Heracles' mad performance reminds us of ourselves watching him recounting it, his dramatized narration figures our own dramatic imagination. Heracles too, like Orestes, collapses at the end of his fit (1006–1008); but here too, just as the onset of his madness was assigned to divine intervention, so too its end is the work of a goddess, Athena (1002–1006). Finally, in Euripides' *Bacchae*, Pentheus, suffering from delusions under the influence of Dionysus, sees one thing (Thebes, the sun) as two things, and Dionysus as a bull (*Ba.* 918–922): his vision is due to a kind of quasi-alcoholic inebriation, and at the same time recognizes under the human mask of the god the bull as which he was also worshipped in the real world of Greek religion; yet at the same time his double vision has evident meta-theatrical connotations. Later in the play, Agave will become victim of far more terrible delusions, mistaking the object x (her own son Pentheus) for a different object y (a sacrificial animal: 1114–1142)—and yet, in a certain sense, she is right in her madness, and this is exactly what Pentheus is. Finally, there are manifest meta-theatrical implications in this scene, in which Pentheus is figured as a spectator who ends up becoming all too involved in the spectacle he is so anxious to observe.

It would doubtless be possible to extend this analysis of scenes of implicit self-reflection on the part of tragic texts by considering as well various non-tragic reflections about tragic madness and illusion in such authors as Gorgias,[11] Plato,[12] and Aristotle.[13] But to do so would trespass the limits of the present study and the objectives of the present volume. Instead, I shall close with a brief *amuse-oeil* on the depiction of tragic madness in

[11] Plutarch, *On the Fame of the Athenians* 348B–C = Gorgias B 23 DK.
[12] Above all the *Republic*, but also the *Ion* and other dialogues.
[13] Especially the *Poetics*.

the ancient visual arts. How did ancient painters depict Orestes' celebrated tragic madness? Of course, ancient visual artists, such as vase painters, were not obliged to even attempt to show madness, or any other object, of the same sort or in the same way as ancient verbal artists, such as tragic poets, did. But suppose the artists' choice of a story famous from dramatizations suggested to at least some of them that they might do well to try to show that story in a way reminiscent of what spectators had seen—or not seen—in the theater. This sounds easier than it would in fact have been. Depicting tragic madness poses very difficult problems for a painter. How can he show something that is invisible? How can he represent something visually that some people can see and others cannot? How can he depict an x that someone in the painting mistakes for a y? Modern artists like Henry Fuseli could rely on a repertoire of codified facial expressions that they could depict with precision and in detail. But most ancient vase painters at least were simply not up to this challenge. They often depict Orestes, but never do they make any attempt whatsoever to indicate that the Erinyes are less than fully visible, or are any less visible than Orestes is himself. It might be tempting to consider such depictions to be sophisticated attempts to place the viewer into the same position as Orestes occupies himself, so that we would share his hallucination and, like him, think the Erinyes no less real than he is. But surely this would be overly charitable: the artists in question presumably are not portraying the Erinyes as being just as real as Orestes is because they could have chosen to do otherwise but have preferred to enhance the terror of the scene by making them seem real, but instead they are portraying the Erinyes in this way precisely because they have no other way available to them to indicate their presence in any mode whatsoever.

The *Lexicon Iconographicum Mythologiae Classicae* lists several dozen Attic and South Italic vase paintings of Orestes and the Erinyes dating from the middle of the 5th century BCE to the second half of the 4th century BCE.[14] In the vast majority, Orestes is not represented as being manifestly insane: there is no visual token in such paintings to indicate unmistakably his madness (except, perhaps, for the very presence of the Erinyes, who are however themselves not indicated as being anything other than exactly as fully real as he himself is).[15] Only in a few cases does his bodily attitude—contorted,

---

[14] The relevant articles for the present discussion are the ones on Erinys (III.1.825–843, III.2.595–606) and Orestes (VII.1.68–76, VII.2.50–55). I refer henceforth to items in *LIMC* by their article and entry number.

[15] So Erinys 42 (Attic crater, 440–430; Paris), 45 (Attic pelike, 380–360; Perugia), 51 (Paestan amphora, 340; private collection), 55 (Apulian volute crater, 360–350; Bari), 60 (Apulian

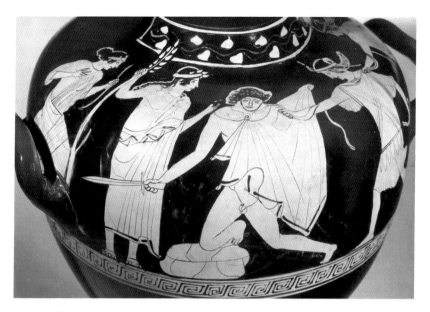

Illustration 1. Attic Hydria—Orestes in Delphi kneeling on a stone
altar. Findplace: Campania (?) Italy mid-5th century BCE.
Berlin, Antikensammlung, Staatliche Museen zu Berlin. Photo
(BW): Jutta Tietz-Glagow. © 2012. Photo Scala, Florence/BPK,
Bildagentur für Kunst, Kultur und Geschichte, Berlin.

spasmodic—or his facial expression—tormented, confused—suggest that
he might be in the grip of some terrible madness.[16] Among all the exemplars of this variously competent but basically quite conventional production, there is a single vase that stands out alone as a brilliant attempt to
convey Orestes' tragic madness in painterly terms. This is an Attic hydria
from about 450 BCE, conserved in Berlin (Illustration 1);[17] it is probably the

---

calyx crater, 350–330; Lecce), 64 (Paestan lecythos, 350–340; Paestum), 68 (Lucanian nestoris,
380–360; Naples); Orestes 16 (Apulian volute crater, 360–350; St. Petersburg), 17 (Apulian
volute crater, mid 4th century; Ruvo), 19 (Lucanian nestoris, ca. 330; Cambridge, MA), 20
(Apulian crater, 370–350; Bari), 24 (Apulian bell crater, ca. 360; Boston), 25 (Apulian oeno-
choe, ca. 350; Taranto), 31 (Apulian volute crater, 360–350; Ruvo).

[16] So Erinys 53 (Campanian bell crater, 360–350, Milan), 58 (Campanian hydria, 350–325,
Berlin), 46 (= Orestes 29; Apulian calyx crater, 360–350; St. Petersburg); Orestes 15 (Lucanian
calyx crater, second half of the 4th century; Copenhagen), 18 (Apulian volute crater, 360–350;
Berlin).

[17] It is Erinys 41, *LIMC* III.1.831–832, III.2.598. On this vase see especially Giuliani 2001,
particularly 27–28.

earliest extant vase painting of this episode and perhaps indicates an exceptional moment in the history of images of this scene before a relatively fixed
iconography had become established. It shows Orestes kneeling in exhaus-
tion and despair; on our left stand Artemis and Apollo who extends a helping
hand, while on our right two Erinyes run up, brandishing a snake in each
hand. The faces of all four figures are shown in profile—Orestes' too, as is
proven by his neck and hair. But the face of Orestes seems hardly like a face,
it looks more like an expressionless mask; and it has slipped around his head
and turned so that it is facing us.[18] The Erinyes have eyes only for him: they
are fully occupied by the dramatic situation in which they are engaged with
him. And it is towards them that Orestes' head is turned. But if his head is
in profile, his face is fully frontal; and what he sees is not the Erinyes—they
are too terrifying for him to endure to look upon them—but instead us, the
spectators, who are not in the scene at all but who are watching it from outside. By wearing something that looks like a mask, if it is really a mask that
it resembles, Orestes might be thought to be indicating to us that he is part
of a theatrical production. By completely rupturing the dramatic illusion in
a way that no tragic poet could possibly have done, he acts out for us his and
our awareness of its existence. By displaying to us his madness, he reminds
us of our own.

---

[18] The frontal view of a person's face is extremely rare in vase paintings of this period;
doubtless part (though probably not all) of the strangeness of the position of Orestes' head
and face on this particular vase is due to the technical difficulties entailed by the artist's
choice to depict Orestes in this posture. See in general Korshak 1987.

PART VI

MENTAL DISORDERS AND RESPONSIBILITY

MENTAL ILLNESS, MORAL ERROR,
AND RESPONSIBILITY IN LATE PLATO*

Maria Michela Sassi

The starting-point and pivot of my paper will be the much debated passage of the *Timaeus*, 86b–87b, where Plato gives a definition of mental disorder or, in his terms, 'disease of the soul' (*nosos ... psuches*), that is so broad as to include any immoral behavior resulting from psychic conflict. Plato also argues here that *all* psychic diseases are due to some defective condition of the body—according to the stronger reading, which I prefer, of the opening words, 86b2: *ta de peri psuchen dia somatos hexin teide*. One would have enough material for discussion on this point, except that Plato makes a further, unexpected step a few lines below, saying that 'no one is voluntarily wicked, but the wicked man becomes wicked by reason of some evil condition of body and unskilled nurture' (86d–e). This statement, besides being unique in explaining in purely physical terms the Socratic paradox that 'no one does wrong willingly', raises crucial questions about moral behavior and responsibility, not unlike Galen Strawson's famous argument, according to which we cannot be morally responsible for our actions in the way that is commonly supposed, because our actions are ultimately caused by the way we are, and the way we are is a result of heredity and early experience.[1]

The conception of immorality as a psychic disease is all but new in Plato's work. Ever since such earlier dialogues as the *Gorgias* and the *Republic*, as it is well known, he plays upon the analogy between medicine restoring physical health and justice bringing back the harmony among the different elements of the soul, whose 'internal war' (*stasis, Resp.* 440a) causes wrongdoing when the more irrational drives prevail over reason. One may even say that in elaborating this point Plato 'invented' the concept of mental health,[2] in spite of the problematic nature of the relationship (then and

---

* I am grateful to the participants in the conference whose questions and comments helped me significantly to reshape the earlier version of this paper. I feel especially indebted to Bennett Simon for his sensitive reading of the written draft and his invaluable suggestions.

[1] Cf. Strawson 1994.

[2] As Kenny 1969 put it. The most relevant passages are *Resp.* 409e–412a, 443b–445b; *Gorg.* 463a–466, 474c–479e. The complicated version of the standard analogy we find in *Soph.* 227c–

now) between the primarily moral meaning of this concept and the *medical* notion of mental health. Now, what Plato does in the *Timaeus* is exactly to provide a physiological basis to this complex of ideas, in that he assumes here not a mere analogy, but a strong interaction between body and soul. A crucial question about Plato's moral and political thought is whether and to what extent this move is going to support the elaborate theory of punishment that emerges from the *Laws*, where wrongdoing is considered as a 'sickness of the soul' that is to be cured with 'medical' methods—the point being whether the reference to medical therapy should be understood literally. Yet it seems appropriate to postpone this discussion and to give priority to a thorough analysis of our passage in the *Timaeus*, focusing first on another point of paramount interest, i. e., the fact that Plato is primarily committed in this context to defining a notion of 'mental illness' which is not necessarily tantamount to that of moral and intellectual error, although it largely overlaps with and has intriguing relations to it.

One should not forget that the medical section of the *Timaeus* opens at 81e6 with an extensive treatment of the diseases of the body, based on a humoral theory, which was considered well worthy of being mentioned at length in the medical doxography of the *Anonymus Londinensis* (cols. XIV.12-XVIII.8 Diels). That a philosopher might have some interesting things to say on medical matters was certainly not as surprising in an ancient context as it would be today, as Geoffrey Lloyd reminds us in remarking that 'the gap between the doctor and the lay person was, in any case, far narrower in the ancient world, where the former had no legally recognized qualifications they could cite to justify their right to practise'.[3] Although scholars on ancient medicine have taken Plato's theories seriously enough,[4] it seems to me that some work remains to be done for these to be positioned in the context of the Greek medical thought of the late fifth and early fourth centuries. With a view to this aim, I will proceed by subdividing the text in

---

229a is thoroughly examined by Balansard 2006. See also Simon 1973 for emphasis on Plato and Freud's sharing the vision of man as a 'creature in conflict', and Seeskin 2008 for a rich and up-to-date discussion of the Platonic background of the concept of mental health.

[3] Lloyd 2003, 153.

[4] See Pigeaud 1981, 52–53 and *passim* (on the contrary, Pigeaud 1987 neglects the passage); Nutton 2004, 117–118; last but not at all least, Jouanna and van der Eijk in this volume. Especially valuable are the philosophical analyses by Cornford 1937, 343–349; Tracy 1969, 123–136, Gill 2000; and the comments by Sorabji 2003, 152–155, and Gill 2006, 200–201. Schuhl 1968, 107–120 is appreciative, yet unfortunately hasty, whereas Joubaud 1991, 178–185 is rather confusing, particularly for introducing the notion of melancholy, which is not to be found in the *Timaeus*.

order to follow the argument step by step, not least in its zigzagging from the strictly medical to the moral perspective. The utmost attention is due to the beginning, partially quoted above (86b1–2):[5]

> Such is the manner in which diseases of the body come about; and those of the soul are due to the condition of the body in the following way.

As far as I know, no one, except Jouanna (this volume), has noted so far that Plato is the first in the Greek medical literature to conceptualize the notion of mental disease as such, i. e., as a disease that, while having organic causes, specifically affects one's cognitive capabilities and his or her relationship to the world. In fact, one would look in vain for any clear categorization of mental illness in the medical discourse of the time,[6] whereas— paradoxically enough—psychopathological manifestations, particularly of a manic kind, were not only easily recognized in the Greek society of the fifth and fourth centuries BC,[7] but also vividly represented on the tragic stage[8] and in mythological narratives,[9] that is, in contexts in which a belief in the supernatural origin of madness was prevalent. One might wonder if some 'hypercorrection' of the common belief was at work in the Hippocratic writers, in that they not only claimed a physical aetiology for such disturbances of the cognitive and behavioural functions as obsessive fears (*phoboi*), excitation (*manie*) and delirium with delusions (*paraphronein*), depression (*athumie* or *dusthumie*), and restlessness (*dusphorie*), but also tended to treat those disturbances as symptoms, not unlike others we would classify as physical (e.g. fevers, or the morbid quality of various discharges), within broader nosological pictures. Even *manie, phrenitis*, and *melancholia* oscillate between being identified as autonomous nosological entities and concomitant symptoms of some other categories of disease. Was it perhaps safer to look away from the 'dark' side of the patients' lives?

There are, it is true, some notable exceptions. For example, the short Hippocratic writing *Peri parthenion* (*Diseases of the Virgins*) provides a unique nosological framework of a particular kind of psychophysical imbalance

---

[5] I adopt the translation by Bury in the Loeb edition (1929), with some modifications.

[6] Among several authors making this point, cf. Drabkin 1955, Pigeaud 1980, Di Benedetto 1986, 35–69; Stok 1997; Andò 2007. Hankinson 1991 rightly points out that the physiological model of mind generally provided by the Greek doctors had Presocratic beginnings.

[7] Cf. Dover 1974, 126–129.

[8] Think, e. g., of Aeschylos, *Cho.* 1048–1062; Euripides, *Her.* 922–1015; *Iph. Taur.* 281–308; *Or.* 252–279.

[9] See, e.g., Marzari 2010 on the erotic madness of the Proetides.

affecting young girls. Although this disease has a clear physical cause, namely, the menstrual blood not finding a way out and thus pressing on the heart and diaphragm (*Virg.* 2.3), the symptoms recorded are mostly psychological—homicidal mania, terror of the dark, delirium, hallucinations leading to suicide (*Virg.* 3.1). Briefly, what is described is a general state of mental alienation, whose social origin is easily understood by the modern reader, if not by the ancient writer.[10] Even more significant is the conscious attempt to characterize epilepsy by the writer of *On the Sacred Disease*, who is also clear in distinguishing such states as fear and uneasiness (with loss of memory) from madness (*manie*), the former being caused by a *temporary* change (*metastasis*) effected by bile or phlegm on the temperature of the brain, the latter setting in if the same factors cause *continuous* damage (*diapthore*) of the brain (ch. 15).[11] Lastly, the author of *On Regimen*, Book 1, shows a similar awareness of there being cases in which the impairment of intelligence *is* the problem, famously describing in chapters 35–36 how intelligence (*phronesis*) may vary through different modes and degrees according to the balance of fire and water in the soul, with the possibility of people falling into depressive forms of *manie* if water prevails (*Vict.* I 35.7), or in delusional forms if fire does (*Vict.* I 35.11). Plato must have found food for thought both in *On the Sacred Disease* and in *On Regimen*,[12] and yet he seems to have 'digested' it while endorsing a model of mind that no medical writer ever had.

As noticed, no clear concept of the 'mental' is detectable in the Hippocratic writings, owing to the universal assumption of a 'monistic' concept of the body-soul complex, according to which mental activities, while having their own qualities, are totally grounded in the body.[13] To dwell on the trea-

---

[10] Cf. Andò 1990. I take the numbering of the chapters from the recent edition of Lami 2007.

[11] Cf. Lo Presti 2008, esp. 187–188.

[12] Jouanna 2007a has brilliantly shown that *On Regimen* has been influential for Plato's account of perception and knowledge in the *Timaeus*, and van der Eijk 2011 makes a point of the modes and degrees of mental performances being discussed in *Vict.* I 35–36 (see also their comments in this volume). See also Byl 2002, detecting a number of echoes of *Vict.* I 35 in *Alc. II*, 140c–e (which is, however, pseudo-Platonic).

[13] The fact that mental functions were commonly recognized to have some distinctive qualities actually undermines any qualification of the Hippocratic theories as 'monistic'. Although I here bypass the question by putting the word in quotation marks, I think that it is time to overcome the traditional dichotomy monism-dualism in looking at ancient medical models of mind. A new direction is suggested in this volume by Roberto Lo Presti, tracing in the classical medical accounts of epilepsy (including that of Plato) a concept of mind as an emergent property of the body.

tises whose possible influence on Plato I have supposed, it is notable that the word *psuche* is not to be found in *On the Sacred Disease*, where the mental functions and dysfunctions are traced to some part of the body such as the brain. As for *On Regimen*, suffice it to mention that intelligence is here a property of the *psuche*, yet this is a 'part of the body' (*moira somatos anthropou*, *Vict.* I 7.1) whose blending changes along with the changes occurring in the body as a whole. On the contrary, Plato sticks in the *Timaeus* to the 'dualistic' view that is the core of his psychology since the *Phaedo*, and has been refined in the theory of the three 'parts' of the soul in the *Republic*. Now we are told by Timaeus that the immortal, rational principle of the human soul has been created by the divine Demiurge with the same (non-material) stuff of which the cosmic soul is made. Then the Demiurge's assistants, the 'lesser gods', implant this principle in the physical body, and specifically in the head, whose shape has been intended as the most convenient for the circular movements of the rational soul to remain regular. At this very moment the 'mortal' kind of the soul is born in its two elements, the passionate or irascible one, associated with the heart, and the desiring and appetitive one, located in the liver (*Tim.* 40d–44c).[14]

The notion of psychic motions is crucial here because if we take it literally, as Thomas Johansen pointed out, it follows, importantly enough, that the soul, even if immaterial, does possess spatial *extension*. Therefore the soul-body dualism as conceived in the *Timaeus*, which does not assume soul and body to be ontologically different after all, is not of the Cartesian type, and Plato's theory escapes at least the main difficulty inherent in that of Descartes, that is, how to explain the interaction between soul and body. According to Plato, the body influences the soul thanks to the motions of both of them falling—in Johansen's words—'under a general mechanics explaining the motions of extended figures (whether two- or three-dimensional) in space'.[15] Therefore I think that the particular form of connection between soul and body that Plato endorses in the *Timaeus* is exactly what allows him to focus in this dialogue on the concept of mental illness, this being classified according to the specific entity it affects, i.e. the soul (it is significant that in the *Phaedrus*, where a different relationship between body and soul is envisaged, Plato's approach to the definition of mental illness is correspondingly different). Plato clearly diverges from the Hippocratic model on this point also in his tracing of epilepsy to a morbid

---

[14] Cf. Pradeau 1998; Fronterotta 2006.
[15] Johansen 2004, 142.

blending of white phlegm and black bile spreading over the head and shaking the circular motions (*periodoi*) of the rational *soul* (nevertheless, this account is included, curiously enough, in the section on the diseases of the body, 85a1–b2).

It should not surprise us, after what we have said, that a definition covering the whole range from the mildest psychic conflict to 'technical' insanity follows the initial statement on the diseases of the soul (86b2–c3).

> We must agree that mindlessness (*anoia*) is a disease (*nosos*) of the soul; and of mindlessness there are two kinds, the one of which is madness (*mania*), the other ignorance (*amathia*). Whatever affection a man suffers from, if it involves either of these conditions it must be termed 'disease'; and we must maintain that pleasures and pains in excess are the greatest of the soul's diseases. For when a man is overjoyed or contrariwise suffering excessively from pain, being in haste to seize on the one and avoid the other beyond measure, he is unable either to see or to hear anything correctly, and he is at such a time distraught and wholly incapable of exercising reason.

The word *anoia* properly means 'mindlessness', namely, a condition of general inability of reason to control the rest of the soul, dominated by desire for pleasures and fear of pains. We are reminded that for Plato every newborn baby suffers from *anoia*, a direct effect of the embodiment of the rational soul, whose revolutions get distorted both by bodily motions and by the assaults of the outside world (*Tim.* 43a–44d). A remedy for this universal condition comes when the psychic circuits gradually regain their original proportions thanks to one's developing since youth the natural potential for knowledge with the help of right upbringing, so as to escape the 'most grave disease' (*ten megisten ... noson*, 44c1–2) and return sound to Hades at the end of his or her life. However, this process being neither homogeneous nor uniform, *anoia* may always be there, in varied modes and degrees.

As for *mania* and *amathia*, they are both disturbances of one's relation to pleasures and pains, yet they are two opposite states of mind, respectively characterised by frantic excitement and dullness. While *amathia* belongs to Plato's moral vocabulary, and easily suggests a general defect in respect of knowledge and wisdom, the meaning of *mania* is more difficult to unpack, in that the word covers a large spectrum of behavioral disorders, from the more ordinary ones, in some way connected, in Platonic terms, to the ignorance of the real end of the action, to the most extreme and disturbed. This may be a recurrent question with the vocabulary of madness, and the categorization of it. As for the modern habit, just think of the title of a celebrated TV series, *Mad Men*. These are not people secluded in an asylum, but men of success, just frantically pursuing money, power, and sex in the world of the commercials of the Sixties in America. Their ordinary rash behavior, far from excluding them from society, is essential for them to integrate in it. Defining them 'mad' implies a more or less mild moral judgment, not a social stigma, and even less a medical diagnosis.

I suggest that things were not that different in Athens between the fifth and fourth centuries BC. According to Xenophon, Socrates was already well aware of what was at stake. He was apparently the first to explore the relation of ignorance of what is good, leading to immoral if not criminal conduct, to 'technical' madness. He seems also to have anticipated Plato in stating that the delinquents have to be cured of their ignorance rather than put in jail, whereas imprisonment is necessary for the 'madmen' who are really dangerous (*Mem.* I.2.50).[16]

> In reality Socrates held that, if you clap fetters on a man for his ignorance, you deserve to be kept in jail yourself by those whose knowledge is greater than your own: and such reasoning led him frequently to consider the difference between madness and ignorance (*ti diapherei manias amathiai*). That madmen (*tous mainomenous*) should be kept in prison was expedient, he thought, both for themselves and for their friends: but those who are ignorant of what they ought to know deserve to learn from those who know it (*tous de me epistamenous ta deonta dikaios an manthanein para ton epistamenon*).

In a later chapter Xenophon mentions a lucid definition Socrates gave of ignorance and madness as the two poles of a spectrum of graduated deviations from the normal behavior (*Mem.* III 9.6–7):

> Madness, again, according to him, was the opposite of wisdom, nevertheless he did not identify ignorance with madness (*manian ge men enantion men ephe einai sophiai, ou mentoi ge ten anepistemosunen manian enomize*). But not to know yourself, and to assume and think that you know what you do not, he put next to madness (*engutato manias*). 'Most men, however,' he declared, 'do not call those mad who err in matters that lie outside the knowledge of ordinary people: madness is the name they give to errors in matters of common knowledge'. For instance, if a man imagines himself to be so tall as to stoop when he goes through the gateways in the wall, or so strong as to try to lift houses or to perform any other feat that everybody knows to be impossible, they say he's mad. Most men don't think that people committing slight errors (*tous mikron diamartanontas*) are mad, but just as they call strong desire love, so they name a great delusion (*megalen paranoian*) madness.

---

[16] I adopt Marchant's translation of the *Memorabilia*, with slight changes.

Accepting Xenophon's testimony, usually neglected in Plato scholarship, should commit us to ask how many of Plato's ideas on punishment and/or cure of wrongdoing actually came from Socrates. I do not intend to discuss this problem thoroughly here, but at least one significant point should be noted. In the passage above, 'ignorance' refers to 'matters of common knowledge' (including the goals of moral action), whereas 'madness' is restricted to cases of the individual's total incapability to cope both with external reality and with himself.[17] On the contrary, Plato's assumption in the *Republic* that the individual's psychic balance is consubstantial with that of the city commits him to cataloguing *all* kinds of imbalance as pathological, in that they are disruptive of the social harmony—the obvious reference is to the *mania* of the tyrannical man (*Resp.* 573a–c, 577e–578a). In other words, Plato seems to think that *every* psychic conflict is a more or less serious form of madness, thus endorsing a view which is diametrically opposite to that of Thomas S. Szasz, the psychiatrist who famously claimed that mental illness just does not exist, because it is a 'convenient myth', that is to say, a construction depending upon the (illusory) assumption that social intercourse is 'inherently harmonious'.[18]

The fact remains that Plato's construction of *mania* is also well supported by a remarkable sensitivity to the 'most' pathological manifestations of it. In this regard the list of the symptoms of *mania* in the *Theaetetus* (157e) is to be mentioned, because of its including illusions of sight and hearing and of the other senses (*parakouein … paroran … paraisthanesthai*). Coming back to our passage in the *Timaeus*, we find right in the next section a description of erotic *mania* suggesting that Plato is drawing on some experience he must have of a pathological phenomenology (86c3–d1).

> And whenever a man's seed grows to abundant volume in his marrow, as it were a tree that is overladen beyond measure with fruit, he brings on himself time after time many pangs and many pleasures owing to his desires and the issue thereof, and comes to be in a state of madness *for the most part of his life* because of those greatest of pleasures and pains, and keeps his soul diseased and senseless by reason of the action of his body.

I think this passage allows us to make an exception to the principle of caution to be used in comparing ancient nosological frames to modern ones. In fact, I see no reason to deny that there might be in the ancient world

---

[17] In a similar vein, Aristotle would say in the *Nicomachaean Ethics*, III 2, 1105–1110, that only if one were *mainomenos* could one be ignorant (*agnoeseien*) of every contextual aspects of one's action, let alone of *oneself*.

[18] Szasz 1960.

a fair number of recognizable cases of what is currently defined today as Hypersexual Disorder, namely, a 'sexual drive disorder with an impulsivity component', that it is recommended as the diagnose when the condition *durationally* causes problems for the persons affected or those associated with them.[19]

One might ask why Plato does not mention female 'hypersexuality'—a concept replacing the older one of nymphomania. Male anxiety about female sexuality produced ambivalent effects in the Greek culture. On the one hand, it generated in literary representations a number of images of female lasciviousness (just remember the 'torrid' landscape described by Alcaeus, frg. 347 Lobel-Page). On the other hand, for reasons not entirely clear (yet close, I suspect, to those I hazarded above for the prejudice of Greek doctors against the more irrational aspects of human psychology) the scientific discourse tends rather to remove the fact that women have their own sexual appetites—we can even find such champion of heterosexuality as Aristotle stating in an ethical writing, amazingly, that it is inappropriate to say that women are incapable of controlling their desires, because 'they are passive, not active, in sexual intercourse' (*NE* VII 6, 1148b31).[20]

Be that as it may, it is noteworthy that in Timaeus' tale erotic *mania* is determined by the marrow's producing sperma in excess.[21] As this aetiological model shows up again in a 'norm-directed' version a little later in the dialogue, where the marrow's urging in the male genital organ is said to explain the basic desire for generation (*Tim.* 91b1–d5),[22] one can guess that acquaintance with cases of 'abnormal' sexual behavior may have inspired Plato's medical approach to the general issue of sexual desire.

More important for our discussion is the claim that abnormal sexual behavior, being physically determined, escapes moral judgment (86d1–5):

> ... his soul [*is*] diseased and senseless by reason of the action of his body (*nosousan kai aphrona ischon hupo tou somatos ten psuchen*), yet such a man is reputed to be voluntarily wicked and not diseased; although, in truth, this sexual incontinence, which is due for the most part to the abundance and fluidity of one substance because of the porosity of the bones, constitutes a disease of the soul.

---

[19] Cf. Kafka 2009.

[20] See Sassi 2001, esp. 82–139, for the approach of ancient science to the issue of female difference.

[21] It is to be noted that according to Plato the marrow (on whose role in the physiology of the *Timaeus* see Pradeau 1998) comes from the brain (cf. *Tim.* 82d–e, 91a–b).

[22] In the same passage, by the way, the reciprocal impulse in women is de-sexualized by confining the 'wildness' of desire to the reproductive organ, i.e., the wandering womb. See H. King 1998, 205–273, on the historical construction of hysteria.

This is in fact the claim that triggers the generalisation that follows, saying that *all* wicked behaviors are involuntary, given the assumption that states of mind always depend upon the physical conditions, and these are determined both by nature *and* lack of education (a point I shall consider later; 86d5–e2).

> And indeed almost all those affections which are called by way of reproach 'incontinence in pleasure', as though the wicked acted voluntarily, are wrongly so reproached; for no one is voluntarily wicked, but the wicked man becomes wicked by reason of some evil condition of body and unskilled nurture, and these are experiences which are hateful to everyone and involuntary.

Having insisted so far on situations of overwhelming pleasures, Plato goes on to consider some more-or-less pathological manifestations of psychic pain. Bile and phlegm, previously mentioned as the cause of epilepsy, come back as responsible for various forms of mental distress that are classified according to the part of the body where they accumulate and to the kind of the soul whose motions the vapor arising from them is going to upset (86e3–87a7).

> And again, in respect of pains likewise the soul acquires much evil because of the body (*dia soma pollen ischei kakian*). For whenever the humors which arise from acid and saline phlegms, and all humors that are bitter and bilious wander through the body and find no external vent but are confined within, and mingle their vapor with the movement of the soul and are blended therewith, they implant diseases of the soul of all kinds, varying in intensity and in quantity (*pantodapa nosemata psuches empoiousi mallon kai hetton kai elatto kai pleio*); and as these humors penetrate to the three regions of the soul, according to the region which they severally attack, they give rise to all varieties of irritability (*duskolias*) and depression (*dusthumias*), and they give rise to all manner of rashness (*thrasutetos*) and cowardice (*deilias*), and of forgetfulness (*lethes*) also, as well as of stupidity (*dusmathias*).

Forgetfulness and stupidity are affections of the rational soul, as rashness and cowardice are of the spirited one, and irritability and depression of the appetitive one. Interestingly, the aetiology of depression becomes clearer by looking at Plato's treatment of the liver, in whose surroundings the lower part of the soul is located (*Tim.* 70d7–72d2). In fact, the liver works as a mirror reflecting images of the commands coming from the rational soul so as to frighten the irrational one, and the bilious humors that are involved in the process produce pains and nausea, whereas, if sweeter images are sent by the reason, the bitterness of the liver calms down and the soul can be cheerful, sleep, and practise divination (71c–d). It is tempting to see here the picture of a sort of bipolar disorder, which makes a person alternate depression with euphoria. In any case, Plato's description acutely picks out the main remedy ancient societies had for containing this kind of disorder, namely, exploiting them creatively as experiences of religious ecstasis.[23] Most importantly, Plato provides here a physiological reduction of the divinatory phenomenon, which was identified in the *Phaedrus* as one of the forms of *mania* to be traced to divine possession.[24]

As for the ailments mentioned in this section, only irritability and depression correspond to nosological categories (the word *dusthumia* often also occurs in Hippocratic contexts as a technical word for despondency), whereas this is only partially the case for such broader states as forgetfulness and stupidity, even though possibly including amnesia and idiocy, respectively, and it is not at all so for such qualities as rashness and cowardice, where the usual assimilation of moral defects to mental illness emerges again.[25] We might even see the last pair, rashness and cowardice, as anticipating the equivalent one in Aristotle's theory of moral vices, where they are explained as extremes with respect to a virtuous *mesotes*, that is, in our case, courage. Yet in the *Nicomachaean Ethics* Aristotle differs from Plato, while at the same time staying close to Xenophon's Socrates, in explicitly limiting the field of mental illness to those cases of extreme deviance that are caused by certain diseases, physical damage, or mere bestiality (most frequent among barbarians), and thus do not allow moral judgment because, unlike virtues and vices, they are unnatural, if not inhuman, habits (*NE* VII 5.1149a5–18).[26]

> Indeed folly, cowardice, profligacy, and ill-temper, whenever they run to excess, are either bestial or morbid conditions (*hai men theriodeis, hai de nosematodeis eisin*). One so constituted by nature as to be frightened by everything, even the sound of a mouse, shows the cowardice of a lower animal; the man who was afraid of a weasel was a case of disease. So with thoughtlessness: people irrational by nature and living solely by sensation, like certain remote tribes of barbarians, belong to the bestial class; those who lose their reason owing to some disease, such as epilepsy, or through insanity, are morbid … vice that is natural to man is called simply vice, whereas the other

---

[23] The obvious reference here is to Dodds 1951. Add now Guidorizzi 2010.

[24] Brisson 1974, acutely, was the first to make this point. See, moreover, Dixsaut 2003; Rotondaro 1997 and Barker 2000 on the workings of the liver in the *Timaeus*; Linforth 1946 and Panno 2007, 93–100, on the process of rationalization cum physicalization of *mania* going on in the *Laws*.

[25] Tracy 1969, 125–136, is a thorough analysis of this section, and supplies a rich harvest of parallels to be found both in Plato (especially the *Laws*) and in the Hippocratic literature.

[26] Soardi 2010 and Darbo-Peschanski 2011/2012 are useful discussions on the topic emerging in *NE* VII: see also 1145a30–32, 1147a14–20, 1149b25–35. Of course, as Haksar 1964 remarks, Aristotle thinks that all except those who are (technically) madmen are responsible for acting wrongfully.

kind is termed not simply vice, but vice with the qualifying epithet bestial or morbid.[27]

Plato prefers continuity to differentiation, as he makes clear by insisting on the diseases of the soul being 'of all kinds, varying in intensity and in quantity' (*Tim.* 87a2), according to the size of the deviation from an ideal state of mental balance and the number of cases in which this is more or less temporarily disturbed owing to the individual combination of inborn constitution with the development of rational ways for controlling the faults in it. Family surroundings and the frame of the community are fundamental to steering each individual into a virtuous life, yet one's natural endowment seems to be of major weight in determining his or her capacity and will to pursue the good and happiness (87a7–b9):

> Furthermore, when, with men in such an evil condition, the political admin-istration also is evil, and the speech in the cities, both public and private, is evil; and when, moreover, no lessons that would cure these evils are anywhere learnt from childhood,—thus it comes to pass that all of us who are wicked become wicked owing to two quite involuntary causes. And for these we must always blame the begetters more than the begotten, and the nurses more than the nurslings; yet each man must endeavor, as best he can, by means of nur-ture and by his pursuits and studies to flee the evil and to pursue the good. This, however, forms a separate subject of discussion.

The last words are plainly rhetorical, as education is *not* a separate subject of discussion in the second part of the *Timaeus*, nor in the project of this writing as a whole. At the end of the nosological account Timaeus focuses on the issue of therapy, starting with equating health to beauty, and beauty to the right proportion (*summetria*) between the movements of soul and body (87c–d). While drugs are put in last place because they might even irritate if applied to weak forms of disease (*sic*! 89b2–3), gymnastics on the one hand and a combination of philosophy and music on the other are the right way to restore the regularity of the bodily and psychic movements, respectively, and thus the harmony between physical vigor and intellectual energy (87e–88c). There clearly reemerges here the role of gymnastics and music in education that was already outlined in the *Republic*, and it is here increased by founding it on the assumption that there is a strong interdependence between the movements of the soul and the body.[28]

---

[27] Rackham's translation, with slight modifications.
[28] Cf. esp. *Resp.* III, 405b–408b. The topic of childhood education is discussed in this volume by Katja Vogt.

We can at last raise the question of whether the *Timaeus'* particular version of the concept of mental illness, saying that injustice is literally a sickness, may have influenced Plato's theory of wrongdoing and punishment in his latest, political treatise. The answer is yes. As a matter of fact, the construction of the *Timaeus* seems to be aimed as a whole to providing a physical frame for the project of the *Laws*, by showing that both the world and the human being have been organised by the benevolent Demiurge in the best way he could, except for some unavoidable failings in human nature that it is the duty of the legislator to correct. That is why, as Richard Stalley was right to note, the idea that vice is a disease depending on bodily conditions is central to the legislation of Magnesia. However, Stalley was also right in refusing to take the *Timaeus'* account as a denial of the individual responsibility.[29] As Plato clearly says at *Tim.* 87a–b, human beings are responsible, if not for the way they were born, for accepting the direction of reason in the course of their lives, and thus taking care of their souls. This point is also crucial in the *Laws*, with the only difference that the educational process, which is described in the *Timaeus* as the parents' and nurses' job, is entrusted to the laws themselves. Therefore it is no wonder that these are to supervise, among other things, gymnastics and musical performances.[30] And when education turns out not to be effective enough to prevent the worst from happening, the penal code is there to administer a wide range of punishments going from pecuniary sanctions to humiliations, from mere talking to forced teaching in the notorious *Sophronisterion*, to persuade people to love justice and hate injustice. Only the incurable criminals, being dangerous for the city, must be eliminated by exile or death.[31]

To conclude, notwithstanding the likely influence of such models of mind as the elaborate distinction of degrees and modes of intelligence to be found in the Hippocratic treatise *On Regimen*, the general theory of human behavior emerging from the *Timaeus* is largely due to Plato's own work, functional as it is to his concern for social cohesion and the

---

[29] See, besides Stalley 1996, Saunders 1991 (whose assumption of a 'medical penology' of the *Laws* is, however, rightly criticised by Stalley), and Roberts 1987 (whose focus is on the issue of voluntariness in wrongdoing). Berges 2012 has recently made the good point that Plato regards a cure as a 'last resort', to be resorted to only if the individual's responsible development of his or her healthy soul through prevention and regular check-ups (according to the medical model) has failed.

[30] See Pelosi 2010 on the development of Plato's thought on the psychological effects of music from the *Republic* to the *Laws*, crucially elaborated in the *Timaeus*; Sassi 2008 on emotions and education in the psychology of the *Laws*.

[31] Cf. *Leg.* 735e, 862e–863a, 909a5.

psychological basis for it. Finally I suggest that Plato's admittedly broad model of mental disease is meant to answer questions about defining the boundaries between mental health and insanity that are still central to moral philosophy *and* to psychiatry.

THE RHETORIC OF THE INSANITY PLEA

David Konstan

1. *Agamemnon's Apology Revisited*

In his popular survey, *Wild Beasts and Idle Humours: The Insanity Defense from Antiquity to the Present*, Daniel Robinson writes: 'Surely one of the earliest recorded insanity defenses is to be found in Book XIX of the *Iliad* when Achilles and Agamemnon are at last reconciled'.[1] Robinson observes that, 'far from explaining his offending actions', Agamemnon 'disowns them'. The reference is to Agamemnon's claim: 'I am not responsible [*aitios*], but rather Zeus and Fate and the Fury that strolls through the air, who cast this violent madness upon my wits in the assembly, on that day when I myself took away Achilles' prize' (19.86–90).[2] Agamemnon launches on a lengthy narrative about Atê or 'madness', and concludes: 'Since I was mad and Zeus stole my wits away, I wish to please [Achilles] once more and give him numberless gifts' (137–138). In his review of Robinson's book, Kevin Crotty remarks that Robinson's argument 'is misleading, for, as Dodds long ago pointed out, Agamemnon is not attempting to exculpate himself'.[3] Crotty adds that 'the view of self reflected in Agamemnon's apology is subtly different from modern views, and, in particular, views the self as far more 'permeable'—more open to outside influences—without any sense, however, that this permeability exonerates the one who has injured another'.

Crotty's account of the difference between the archaic Greek and the modern sense of self invokes the notion of 'psychic intervention' proposed by Dodds.[4] Dodds writes in the chapter entitled 'Agamemnon's Apology': 'To ask whether Homer's people are determinists or libertarians is a fantastic anachronism: the question has never occurred to them, and if it were put to them it would be very difficult to make them understand what it

---

[1] Robinson 1996, 8.
[2] Translations are mine unless otherwise indicated.
[3] Crotty 1997; the reference is to Dodds 1951.
[4] Dodds 1951, 5.

meant. What they do recognize is the distinction between normal actions and actions performed in a state of *atê*.[5] Dodds sums up his argument by noting that 'all departures from normal human behavior whose causes are not immediately perceived ... are ascribed to a supernatural agency', and he adds: 'This finding will not surprise the non-classical anthropologist: he will at once produce copious parallels from Borneo or Central Africa'.[6] Dodds explains that the notion of *atê* served to enable Homeric man 'in all good faith to project on to an external power his unbearable feelings of shame'—shame, rather than guilt, since Homeric heroes, according to Dodds, are motivated not by the moral imperative of a quiet conscience but by 'the enjoyment of *timê*, public esteem'.[7]

Dodds' analysis has been highly influential, though there have been dissenting voices; but it is not, I think, necessary to account for Agamemnon's way of excusing his behavior—and he is indeed attempting to exculpate himself. Agamemnon clearly recognizes that he has treated Achilles unfairly, and so he properly offers compensation. This gesture is compatible with his claim that he was temporarily beside himself, and so not wholly responsible for his words and actions. Centuries later, Plato affirms in his treatise, *The Laws* (864D–E), that a person who commits an offense while mad or in the grip of illness or extreme old age must pay for the damage that he has done, even though he is acquitted of other penalties (unless his hands have been polluted by murder, in which case he must go into temporary exile). But the reason why Agamemnon appeals to *atê* or madness as the cause of his conduct, thereby transferring the blame to an external agency, is not, I think, that he has a more permeable self than later Greeks (or than we ourselves do for that matter), or that he and other Homeric characters automatically ascribe what they perceive as a departure from their usual behavior to supernatural agencies (whatever the case with cultures described by modern anthropologists). Nor is it that Homer's characters lack a sense of autonomous self or a fully realized understanding of responsibility.[8] After all, when Poseidon earlier seeks to encourage the Achaeans to fight more resolutely, he reminds them of the shame of defeat and adds: 'But if the

---

[5] Dodds 7.
[6] Dodds 13.
[7] Dodds 17.
[8] The idea that Homer lacked a vocabulary, and indeed a concept, of the self was given most forceful expression by Bruno Snell (1953); scholars have since criticized Snell's arguments, but the notion that Homeric heroes did not have a wholly autonomous self is still widespread (see Farenga 2006 for a sophisticated defense of the idea).

heroic son of Atreus, wide-ruling Agamemnon, was in truth wholly responsible [*aitios*], in that he dishonored the swift-footed son of Peleus, there is
nevertheless no way that we can relax from battle' (13.111–114): it is clear that,
in the eyes of Poseidon, Agamemnon bears full responsibility for the offense
to Achilles and the reversals suffered by the Achaeans, or at the very least
that Poseidon can, in these circumstances, make the claim and expect the
Achaean warriors to understand it.

Why then does Agamemnon himself accuse Atê and the Furies, rather
than take full responsibility for what he has done? The answer is to be
sought, I believe, not in an archaic conception of the self in Homeric epic but
in the norms that governed reconciliation and the appeasement of anger in
the classical world. The strategy of exonerating oneself by shifting the blame
to an outside agency or cause was, as we shall see, the principal technique
recommended in Greek and Roman rhetorical handbooks for placating a
person one had offended. Whether or not Agamemnon recognizes that he
was at personally fault is not the point, since the best way to assuage Achilles'
wrath and restore the relationship between them is to deny it. In other
words, Agamemnon is not seeking forgiveness.

The ancient Greek term that is most commonly translated as 'forgiveness'
is *sungnômê*. In fact, however, the Greek idea differs in fundamental respects
from the modern concept. In brief, we normally suppose that we grant forgiveness to someone who has wronged us, and done so deliberately; it would
be odd to forgive someone who has never done us any harm. What is more,
we are disposed to forgive those who are sorry for what they have done; that
is, we expect an apology and other manifestations of sincere remorse. This is
why many readers are dissatisfied with Agamemnon's defense: it seems shal-
low as an apology, which we expect to include a frank confession of one's
fault. But this pattern of confession and repentance is foreign to classical
practices for placating anger and achieving reconciliation.[9]

Aristotle discusses *sungnômê* briefly in the *Nicomachean Ethics*, but the
significant point is that he does so in the course of his account of involuntary behavior: thus, he observes that it is appropriate to grant *sungnômê*
when people have acted either under external compulsion or else in excusable ignorance of the circumstances (1109b18–1111a2). As he puts it: 'since
virtue concerns emotions and actions, and praise and blame are due in the
case of voluntary acts, whereas *sungnômê*, and sometimes pity [*eleos*], are
due in the case of involuntary acts, it is obligatory for those investigating

---

[9] The following argument is based largely on Konstan 2010a.

virtue to define what is voluntary and what is involuntary' (1109b30–34),
and he adds at once that 'it is believed that involuntary acts are those that
occur either by force or through ignorance'. Both actions performed under
compulsion and those done in ignorance admit of various descriptions, and
Aristotle addresses these complexities. Thus, if one's ship is driven astray in
a storm, or pirates take over the vessel, no one would accuse a passenger
of voluntarily changing course, for she or he has not contributed anything
at all to the result, whether actively or passively. But in situations in which
one acts out of fear, as when a tyrant who has power over one's parents and
children orders one to commit a shameful deed, there is some ambiguity as
to whether the act is voluntary or not. Aristotle says that 'such actions are
mixed, but they rather resemble voluntary ones' (1110a11–12). He then notes
that 'in some cases, praise is not given, but *sungnômê* may be, when someone does things one ought not to do on account of circumstances that are
beyond human nature and which no one could endure' (3.1, 1110a23–26).

Aristotle's discussion of involuntary action in the case of ignorance is
equally nuanced. For example, if one commits a wrong in ignorance, but
later feels no regret (*en metameleiâi*), then the act hardly counts as unwilling, since one would have done it even had one been fully aware; Aristotle
labels such an act, accordingly, 'not voluntary', as opposed to 'involuntary'
(1110b18–23). So too, wrongs done when one is drunk or in a rage are in
some sense done unawares, but are not genuinely involuntary. As opposed
to such character-based or generalized ignorance, Aristotle specifies that
what renders an act involuntary is a lack of knowledge of particulars, and
this is the kind of situation in which pity and *sungnômê* are appropriate
(1110b33–1111a2). One might, for example, mistake one's son for an enemy,
or mistakenly strike someone with a deadly weapon when one had reason to suppose that it was harmless, and such cases will naturally give rise
to regret once the facts are known. Aristotle gives as an example Oedipus'
misrecognition of his father, and indeed Oedipus himself makes the same
point in *Oedipus at Colonus*, where he insists, in his reply to Creon's allega-
tions, that he murdered his father and married his mother unwillingly (*akôn*,
964), since he did not know what he had done or to whom (976–977; cf. 983,
986–987).

Given this account of *sungnômê*, it is clearly incumbent on a person who
seeks pardon for an offense to plead either ignorance or some kind of external compulsion, and the tactic of shifting the blame to some other cause
or agent was recognized in the rhetorical literature and given the technical
name of *metastasis* or, in Latin, *transferentia*. There was, to be sure, some
variation in terminology. The rhetorician Hermogenes (2nd century AD),

for example, reports that 'some have divided off *sungnômê* from *metastasis* not on the basis of responsibility and non-responsibility (*tôi aneuthunôi kai hupeuthonôi*), but have simply called all those things that transfer the crime to something coming from without 'transferences' [*metastatika*], whether it is a storm and torture and any other such thing, and define only those things that transfer to some private passion of the soul [*idion ti pathos psukhês*] as pertaining to *sungnômê*, for instance pity or sleep or anything of this sort' (6.69–81). Hermogenes comments that this may not be wrong, for 'the former differ in nothing but name from *sungnômê*'. Apsines (3rd century) records a similar distinction, including among the reasons for *sungnômê* drunkenness and madness (276.3–7). Finally, Porphyry (3rd century AD) proposed to distinguish simply between crimes that are avoidable, which he listed under *metastasis*, and those that are not, and which fall under *sungnômê*, for example the case of the ten generals at Arginusae who were absolutely prevented by the storm from retrieving the bodies of the soldiers who had drowned in the famous sea battle fought there. It is evident that *sungnômê*, whether it includes such external pressures as storms and tortures, or is restricted to internal factors such as drunkenness, passion, or insanity, has nothing to do with asking forgiveness for a confessed wrong, but rather looks to denying or evading responsibility for an action by ascribing the cause to circumstances—whether internal or external—that are beyond the agent's control. Thus Malcolm Heath, in his translation of Hermogenes' treatise on issues, renders *sungnômê* as 'mitigation', and explains that it is invoked when 'an acknowledged *prima facie* wrong is excused as due to factors outside the defendant's control'.[10] Michel Patillon, in turn, in his French translation of the works ascribed to Hermogenes, renders *sungnômê* as 'excuse', which comes closer to the mark, since it is not a matter of diminishing or extenuating responsibility but of seeking exoneration by virtue of non-responsibility.[11]

We should not be surprised, then, that Agamemnon seeks to shift the blame for his mistreatment of Achilles; this is standard operating procedure in ancient Greece, where the modern habit of confessing one's guilt and pleading for forgiveness on the basis of sincere contrition and a change of heart was not part of the repertoire of strategies for reconciliation. Insanity in this regard is no different from pleading the excuse of drunkenness or passion or love or rage or youth or any other factor that explains away the act

---

[10] Heath 1995, 256, in the 'Glossary'.
[11] Patillon 1997.

and exonerates the offender. Thus Demeas, in Menander's *Samia*, seeking to excuse his earlier suspicions of his son (he believed that he had slept with his concubine), exclaims: 'I accused you unjustly: I was deluded, wrong, out of my mind' (*êgnoês, hêmarton, emanên*, 702–703). Like Agamemnon, Demeas acknowledges his error even as he disclaims full responsibility for it.

2. *The Madness of Ajax and Heracles*

If we continue to feel uncomfortable with Agamemnon's appeal to Atê as a way of evading blame, it may be because it seems entirely ad hoc: the only indication of insanity is his uncharacteristically poor judgment in insulting Achilles. To support the claim of diminished responsibility, we might have expected independent evidence of madness at the time of the offense. Had Agamemnon, for example, failed to recognize Achilles and attacked him because he believed he was a Trojan warrior who had entered the Greek camp, we would very likely agree that he was *ouk aitios* and acting in excusable ignorance of the particulars, as Aristotle puts it (caused by madness in this instance). In Sophocles' *Ajax*, Athena steals away the wits of Ajax and causes him, in his desire to avenge himself on the Greek princes for granting Achilles' arms to Odysseus rather than to himself, to mistake sheep for his enemies, and so to torture and kill them instead of Agamemnon, Menelaus, and Odysseus. Obviously, Ajax is not in his right mind, and his condition evokes the pity of Odysseus himself. In this case, however, his delusion does not exonerate him of the crime he had intended to commit, for madness was not the cause of his desire to murder the Greek leaders, which he does not renounce on recovering his sanity, but simply of his killing innocent animals in their stead.[12] Ajax's misrecognition, while testifying to his altered mental state, is incidental to the intended offense.

At the beginning of Euripides' *Heracles*, Amphitryon explains that he, his daughter-in-law Megara, and the children she has had with Heracles are to be killed by Lycus, the tyrant who has usurped power in Thebes. Lycus' motive is to destroy all the relatives of the former king so as to eliminate potential rivals for the throne. Heracles cannot help his family, since he

---

[12] Cf. Celsus, *De medicina* 3.18.19: 'tertium genus insaniae est ex his longissimum [longest-lasting or simply furthest from?], adeo ut vitam ipsam non impediat; quod robusti corporis esse consuevit. Huius autem ipsius duae species sunt: nam quidam imaginibus, non mente falluntur, quales Aiacem vel Orestem percepisse poetae ferunt; quidam [that is, others] animo desipiunt.' On images, cf. Aretaeus, *On the Treatment of Acute Diseases* 5.1.3 (92.3–7 Hude).

has gone to Hades to capture Cerberus, the hound of hell. Just when the situation seems hopeless, Heracles appears, and when Lycus returns to kill his family, he slays Lycus instead. At this juncture, Iris, the messenger of the gods, and Lyssa, that is, 'Madness' personified, descend and announce that, at Hera's orders, they are going to drive Heracles mad. The results are instantaneous: Heracles begins foaming at the mouth, and imagines that he has driven in a chariot to Argos, where he will take vengeance on Eurystheus, the king who obliged him to undertake his many labors. Heracles' father asks in alarm: 'My son, what is happening to you ...? Is the slaughter of the corpses whom you just now killed making you frenzied?' (965–967). Under the impression, however, that he is in Eurystheus' palace and that his father and children are those of Eurystheus, he kills his three sons and Megara as well, collapsing just before he manages to add his father Amphitryon to the carnage. When Heracles awakens and becomes aware of what he has done, he contemplates committing suicide—he is, in Aristotle's phrase, *en metameleiâi*—but at this point Theseus, whom Heracles had rescued from Hades, arrives with troops from Athens, with the intention of driving out the tyrant Lycus. Heracles accepts Theseus' offer of refuge, and departs with him for Athens.

In his deluded condition, Heracles unintentionally slays the very people whom Lycus had sought to destroy. There is no question but that the madness induced in him at Hera's behest absolves Heracles of the murder of his kin: he did not, in his frenzy, know who they were, any more than Oedipus was aware that the man he slew and the woman he married were his biological father and mother. We might wish to inquire whether the vengeance that Heracles proposed to take against Eurystheus—slaying his entire family— was also a symptom of his altered state of mind, or did his madness reside solely in his confusion over the identity of his victims? If the latter, then his behavior in attacking the presumably innocent children and wife of his enemy does not appear to be different, in principle, from that of Lycus in regard to Heracles' own family, and the moral distinction between Heracles and Lycus is blurred if not altogether eradicated.

The tragedy itself passes over in silence the analogy between Heracles' intention to kill Eurystheus' children and Lycus' plan, and critics are divided over its significance. Ever since Wilamowitz, some have seen Heracles' madness as a consequence of his own nature or actions; most recently, for example, Robert Emmet Meagher states that 'Lyssa is merely a prop, an empty mask, as it were. Herakles' madness neither required then nor requires now any elaborate explanation for those who have taken part in the insane rampage of war'; his domestic violence is simply an extension of his martial savagery, and he is best understood as a 'trauma victim'.[13] If this is the case, then Heracles may seem to bear at least a very large measure of responsibility for the murders. Kathleen Riley, after surveying earlier views, arrives at the opposite conclusion: 'There is nothing in Euripides' portrait of the sane hero to suggest that killing is attractive to him or that his normal use of violence is excessive',[14] and she takes the cause of his madness to be wholly external, that is, induced by Lyssa at Hera's behest. On this view, brutality in the home and violence at war are neatly quarantined, with no suggestion that the two might be connected. But Riley also notes that 'The madness of Herakles … is dramatized, paradoxically, in an extremely well-reasoned and orderly manner', and that 'Herakles' hallucinatory exploits, which appear to the bystanders as crazed and haphazard, are, in his mind, one continuous and logical sequence of events'.[15] This reason within madness is understandable if the essential feature of Herakles' condition is his mistaken identification of his family with that of Eurystheus and his fantasy that he has travelled to Eurystheus' palace, rather than his decision to slay the tyrant and his kin.

If it is plausible, as I think it is, to understand Heracles' madness as residing in the same kind of error or confusion as Ajax's when he mistakes sheep for the Achaean leaders, then both tragedies are predicated on a similar effect: madness causes one to be ignorant of the particulars, and hence excuses the immediate action but has no bearing on the larger intention, that is, killing Agamemnon and the rest or, in Heracles' case, Eurystheus and his wife and children.[16] To put it another way, it is not their moral reasoning that is damaged by the bout of insanity, but their perceptive faculties, which are subject to hallucination. In this respect, the effect of madness on them is the opposite of that which Agamemnon alleges in his defense. If his behavior was in some sense involuntary, it is as a result of compulsion rather than ignorance, to use Aristotle's distinction.

3. *Cicero's Distinction*

In Xenophon's *Memorabilia* (3.9.6–7), Socrates explains that madness consists in making errors in regard to matters that everyone knows to be true,

---

[13] Meagher 2006, 48, 50.

[14] Riley 2008, 37.

[15] Riley, 34.

[16] Plato, *Timaeus* 86B, distinguishes between two ailments of the mind, the one being madness (*mania*), the other ignorance (*amathia*), these being subclasses of *anoia*; both arise principally from excessive pleasures and pains.

for example, a person who imagines that he is too tall to pass through the gates of the city, or that he is able to lift a house. A particularly famous case was that of Menecrates, who styled himself as Zeus and went so far as to offer to help out Philip II of Macedon; Philip is said to have replied: 'Philip to Menecrates: get well' (*hugiainein*), instead of 'be well' (*khairein*, Hegesander *FHG* fr. 5, from Athenaeus 7.33–34). But among the most common symptoms of insanity was a loss of control over one's emotions, above all in respect to anger, and surely this is what Agamemnon is relying on as evidence of his irrational behavior, and which he explains by reference to the intervention of Atê. In overreacting as he did to the demand that he return his war prize and insulting Achilles for backing it up, Agamemnon caused harm to the entire army. His disproportionate rage amounted to a form of insanity.

Extreme rage might be deemed a form of insanity, as in Horace's dictum, 'anger is a brief madness' (*ira furor brevis est: animum rege, qui, nisi paret,/ imperat*, *Epistles* 1.2.62; cf. Philemon fr. 156: 'We're all insane when we're angry').[17] William Harris gives several illustrations of the connection between anger and madness, and points out that Homer himself characterizes Agamemnon's fury at Achilles as an incapacity to think (*oude ti oide noêsai*, 1.343).[18] But the equation of anger with madness was not sufficient to excuse any and all outbursts of rage on the grounds of diminished responsibility. For even if full-blown anger was at times tantamount to madness, the onset of anger could be deemed to be within a normal person's control. Thus, Seneca writes that there is no more direct route to madness than anger (*On Anger* 4.36.5: *nulla celerior ad insaniam uia est*), and cites Ajax as a prime example of the maxim: 'Madness drove Ajax to death, but anger drove him to madness' (*Aiacem in mortem egit furor, in furorem ira*). The case of anger would thus be analogous to that of drunkenness: true, a drunken individual is not fully conscious, and hence not responsible for his or her actions, but he or she does have the prior obligation not to become inebriated to the extent of losing all control.

The problem is treated with particular clarity by Cicero in his *Tusculan Disputations*. In the third book Cicero enters upon a discussion of the emotions by inquiring whether the sage is subject to distress (*aegritudo*) and other disturbances of the mind, such as fears, passionate desires, and bouts of anger (*formidines, libidines, iracundiae*, 3.7). Cicero affirms that these feelings, along with pity, envy, and the like, are called *pathê* in Greek, which, he

---

[17] Philemon fr. 156 Kassel and Austin 1989.
[18] Harris 2001, 63–64, 344–345.

says, would be literally rendered as *morbi* or 'sicknesses' in Latin, as being movements of the mind that do not heed reasoned arguments; but because calling the passions 'sicknesses' sounds odd in Latin, he prefers *perturbationes*. But Cicero immediately proceeds to dub such sentiments a form of madness (*insania*, 3.8), which, being no less rare a usage, provokes an expression of surprise on the part of his interlocutor. Cicero explains that *insania* basically signifies a lack of *sanitas* or health in the mind, just as *morbus* indicates the absence of health in the body; the emotions deprive us of tranquility of spirit, and this is just what mental illness is. Since wisdom is the health of the mind, it is incompatible with the passions. Thus, ancient Latin usage (as Cicero interprets it) confirms the Stoic claim that all emotions are a form of madness or mental instability (3.9–10).

Cicero concludes that Latin is indeed more precise than Greek in this respect, since it separates out the mental and the physical. He goes on to explain that in Latin one says that people are 'out of control' (*ex potestate*) when they are carried away by desire or anger, 'although anger itself is a part of desire; for the definition runs: anger is a desire for revenge' (3.11)—a point on which the Stoics were in agreement with Aristotle. Cicero now professes to be puzzled as to why the Greeks should call a condition such as anger *mania* ('madness'), and claims that Latin speakers do better in distinguishing between *insania*, which involves a lack of wisdom, and *furor*, or real craziness. The Greeks too, he says, mean to say something of the sort, but they miss the mark by employing the term *melankholia* for the latter condition, as though it were merely a matter of bile and not often a consequence of intense anger, fear, or grief, as happened, for example, to Ajax and Orestes. Someone afflicted by *insania*, according to Cicero, can still manage his own life, more or less—as indeed a person subject to ordinary anger can; but a person in the grip of *furor* is prohibited from doing so by law. *Furor* is thus a greater thing (*maius*) than *insania*, and yet, Cicero says, the sage is susceptible to it, though not to *insania*. This is in line with the Stoic view that even sages may suffer a physiological or physical trauma which would rob them of their mental faculties,[19] but of course they would not, like Ajax, arrive at such a state as a result of an excess of passion (for the distinction between madness as a result of physical illness, and madness as a consequence of poor character or upbringing, cf. Plato *Laws* 934D–E).

Cicero, then, distinguishes among three categories—physical sickness (*morbus*) and two types of mental disorder, which we might render as loss

---

[19] Cf. Graver 2002, 83.

of control or hysteria (*insania*) and wholly delusional or raving psychosis of the sort that leaves a person unable to function (*furor*). Anger is an instance of *insania*, and may in extreme cases lead to *furor*, though *furor* may also be produced in other, more organic ways—and with regard to these, not even the sage is invulnerable.[20]

The distinction is important to Cicero, precisely because if anger is equated with madness in the strict sense of *furor*, which had legal recognition as a cause of diminished responsibility, then no one who acted in a fit of rage, or who was subject to extreme anger, could be held accountable for his or her actions.[21] Interestingly enough, Donatus, in his commentary on Virgil's *Aeneid*, worries about just such a form of exculpation in the case of the brutal tyrant Mezentius. Donatus explains (ad *Aen.* 1.347–348) that in cases in which *furor*, that is, love or madness (*insania*) or mental sickness (*animi dolor*), drives people to commit grave crimes, they may be pardoned for the deed (*possunt habere veniam facti*), since such a person has sinned not voluntarily but on account of psychosis (*non vuluntate sed furore peccavit*.[22] Since Mezentius is described as mad (*Aeneid* 8.489), Donatus worries that he may be let off the hook for his unspeakable atrocities on an insanity plea.[23]

4. Conclusion: The Rhetoric of Madness

In the end, the decision to accept an excuse based on madness is a rhetorical matter. Was Agamemnon really out of his wits? He had affirmed as much to

---

[20] Cf. Stok 1996, 2360.

[21] Cf. Cicero, *De officiis* 1.27: 'Sed in omni iniustitia permultum interest, utrum perturbatione aliqua animi, quae plerumque brevis est et ad tempus, an consulto et cogitata fiat iniuria. Leviora enim sunt ea, quae repentino aliquo motu accidunt, quam ea, quae meditata et praeparata inferuntur'; Dyck 1996, 121–122; the argument may well be original with Cicero, since it is absent earlier Stoic sources. On *furor* in the Digest, see esp. 21.1.1.8 ff., where madness counts as a motive for reclaiming payment made on a slave if it is induced by fever or other physical cause, but not if it results from habitual irregular behavior caused by frequenting ecstatic cults and the like (cited in Toohey, this volume); this recalls Cicero's distinction between two causes of *furor*, but I would imagine that the type caused by self-induced frenzies is excluded because the master ought to have exerted better control of his slave. That a person cannot be accounted guilty if he is not *suae mentis*, see 29.7.2.3; for comparison of a madman with a child, 9.2.5.2; for madness as sufficient punishment on its own, 1.18.13–14 (all cited by Toohey). For a madman assigned to the care of a guardian, cf. Horace, *Epist.* 1.1.101–105.

[22] On Donatus' treatment of the *status venialis* or defense on the basis of non-responsibility, see the excellent account in Pirovano 2006, 93–146.

[23] Further discussion in Konstan 2010b.

Nestor, even before he sent Odysseus, Ajax, and Phoenix on the failed mission to appease Achilles with numberless gifts—though Odysseus did not see fit to repeat the precise words of Agamemnon's confession to Achilles at the time (9.115–120).[24] They would surely have been wasted on him, for Achilles was in no mood to hear excuses. Only after he had decided to return to battle in order to avenge Patroclus was he prepared to be reconciled with Agamemnon, and Agamemnon reached for the best defense available: acknowledge the impropriety of his rage, but pass off the blame—by *metastasis*—and thereby win pardon for having acted in some sense involuntarily, under the influence of extreme anger which is akin to madness. Since no one objected to the description, it served to acquit Agamemnon of full responsibility for the quarrel.

---

[24] Cf. Konstan 2010, 61–63.

PART VII

A ROMAN CODA

MADNESS IN THE *DIGEST*

Peter Toohey

Not a great deal has been published concerning madness in the *Digest*.[1] Despite the impression created by this neglect—that little is to be garnered from its apparently infrequent references to madness—there in fact exists a considerable amount of unambiguous allusion to mental disorder in this legal text. The *Digest* contains more on the subject than most other ancient works, even the literary and the medical. In fact it contains far more allusion to madness than could be covered in the space of a short essay. Because this abundant material is less well known, I have attempted to provide at least a representative sampling of some of the more intriguing commentaries within the *Digest* on madness. What emerges is a vivid and accurate picture of what it could be like to be mad in one pre-modern society. I say 'accurate' with deliberation, for there can be little doubt that what is termed madness in the *Digest* is madness. It is my opinion that the *Digest* provides the most illuminating portrait of madness that is preserved from the Greco-Roman world. And it is an accurate one.

The word 'portrait' is used with due circumspection. The term implies that the *Digest* is capable of presenting a unitary vision of madness. This is

---

[1] Margaret Trenchard-Smith's excellent and very thorough 'Insanity, exculpation and disempowerment in Byzantine law', (2010), came out after I had composed this article. It covers all of the data, and some more, that I do. But I have her article now, so I might point out the differences between my essay and hers. It is my intention to foreground the unexpected importance of Roman law as the major source for the understanding of madness at Rome in the classical period and indeed the most significant means by which we can avoid retrospective diagnosis. Trenchard-Smith wisely eschews such grandiose claims. Her essay, then, looks forward and indeed looks to comparisons with Byzantine law. Mine looks backwards, hoping to use the *Digest* to elucidate 'classical' Roman attitudes towards madness, especially those to be seen in medicine. Trenchard-Smith, given her 'medieval' remit and Byzantine interests, is also and understandably less concerned to emphasize the importance of law for an understanding of Roman social history—hence we stress different of the implications of the juridical evidence. Notable also are Nardi 1983 (which discusses most of the passages I touch upon), Diliberto '1984, and P. King 2000. There is a long examination of the madman in Roman law in Semelaigne 1869, 215–228. (also covered is 'Hippocratic medicine', Erasistratus, Asclepiades, Celsus, Aretaeus, Caelius Aurelianus, and Galen). There is not a great deal of guidance to be gained on the status of the *furiosus* to be gained from standard handbooks such as those of Buckland (2007) or Kaser (1989).

what I believe it does, for, as far as I can see, the *Digest* offers a strikingly consistent picture of the mad in the Roman empire. It does this despite the text's representing a compilation of the work of many jurists and a compilation that was drawn from a broad chronological base.[2] What then provides this unity, if it is not authorial nor chronological? I presume that this is produced because, when the *Digest* contemplates and meditates on madness, it is reflecting on real-life situations that are of a common and limited type and that persist through time. Furthermore it is reflecting on conditions with which the jurists and the readers of the *Digest* would have been quite familiar from their daily lives.

Retrospective Diagnosis

> quo tempore, ut Marcus Brutus refert, Octauius etiam quidam ualitudine mentis liberius dicax conuentu maximo, cum Pompeium regem appellasset, ipsum reginam salutauit.   (Suetonius, *Divine Julius* 49)

> At this same time, so Marcus Brutus declares, one Octavius, a man whose disordered mind made him somewhat free with his tongue, after saluting Pompey as 'king' in a crowded assembly, greeted Caesar as 'queen'.

What is the matter with Octavius? He sounds quite mad (not just of 'disordered mind') to have been bold enough to have made sarcastic comments in front of such powerful individuals as Pompey and Caesar, referring more or less openly to Caesar's alleged sexual relations with King Nicomedes of Bithynia. It would be easy to assert of a passage like this that it shows that Octavius was mad, or at least that Suetonius thought that he was mad. But of course we can never be sure, neither whether Suetonius thought that he was mad, nor whether he was in reality mentally unbalanced. To assert Octavius' madness is to assert what is usually termed a retrospective diagnosis. Retrospective diagnosis, however, is most successful where there are actual remains, such as mummified or frozen bodies. So, retrospective diag-

---

[2] Did the legal views on madness evolve and change during the reporting period covered by the *Digest*? Logically they must have. Yet the impression of this reader, at least in the case of the *furiosi*, is that there is a sameness to the way that the mad are characterized and to a degree legislated on. I presume that this is the result in the sameness of the way that madness was viewed by society at large—in which no great changes seem to occur until the influence of Christianity and its views on possession took root. Certainly there is no great change in the characterization of madness in the historical literature. But perhaps the one area where evolution is more obviously possible is in the application of curatorships. Johnston 1999, 41–42, is very helpful on this matter.

nosis may be helpful in ascertaining the cause of death for example of a King Tutankamen—a badly broken femur. His body survives and it can be subjected to scanning with an MRI, the DNA can be examined, and pathogens can be pored over. But retrospective diagnosis does not seem to help much where there is no body. So it is that the problems relating to retrospective diagnosis become especially prominent when it comes to the understanding of ancient madness, as we may encounter in the case of Octavius. What makes retrospective diagnosis of mental illness so perilous an enterprise is that a clear-cut expression for madness is usually lacking in passages such as the one that has just been quoted. The phrase which Suetonius uses, *valetudo mentis*, could apply to any one of a number of neurological conditions.

In the *Digest* madness is always named, clearly and unequivocally. Retrospective diagnosis therefore does not come into play, unless you believe that the ancients were incapable of recognizing madness. There are approximately two hundred and fifty passages in which madness is alluded to and, at lesser or greater length, discussed. There are therefore a very large number of passages in which some confidence can be felt that retrospective diagnosis is not required. In the case of the Roman legal code as it is preserved in the *Digest* the problem of retrospectivity therefore is not at issue. This is because of the variety of clear-cut terms that are used for or relating to madness. These are all expressions that seem to make reasonable sense as descriptors of insanity. The terms for madness or its absence in the *Digest* which I have noticed are: *aegritudo, amentia, demens, dementia, fanaticus, fatuus, furens, furiosus, furor, furere, furoris infortunium, gaudens simplicitate, imbecillus, insanus, languor animi, vitium animi, lunaticus, melancholicus, morio, non compos mentis, non suae mentis, captus mente, integritas mentis, resipiscens, sanitas, vecors,* and *vesanus.*[3] I do not believe that it is necessary to

---

[3] Nardi (1983, 18–45) has an extensive discussion of this topic. Trenchard-Smith (2010, 42) concludes of some of the terms: '*Furor* was understood to range in severity ... *Demens, amens,* and *mente captus* occasionally replace *furiosus* in legal texts; where their force is specific, *demens* designates a person in a delusional or senile state and *mente captus* someone who is mentally impaired. *Fatuus* and *morus* expressly convey mental deficiency; although the terms may vary in meaning from *furiosus,* in legal practice they were indistinct ...'. It would be, however, a confident person indeed who would be able to distinguish many of these terms, for the difficulties are not confined to the *Digest*. There are an array of seemingly different terms used by historical and other writers for madness—and some writers do seem to have their favorite words—which highlight the difficulties facing anyone wishing to differentiate them. So, for example and at random, we find, seemingly used interchangeably, *valetudo mentis* (Suetonius *Jul.* 49), *mente lapsus* (Suetonius *Aug.* 48), *insania* (Suetonius *Claud.* 55),

attempt to adjudicate on the applicability of these terms as descriptors for mental derangement. Nor do I believe that it is profitable to attempt to distinguish the overtones of these terms. Except in the most obvious of senses (*fatuus, morio,* or *gaudens simplicitate,* for example), they seem to be used more or less interchangeably (as can be seen, for example, with *furiosus* and *dementia: Dig.* 24.2.4 *Ulpianus 26 ad sab. Iulianus libro octavo decimo digestorum quaerit, an furiosa repudium mittere vel repudiari possit. et scribit furiosam repudiari posse, quia ignorantis loco habetur: repudiare autem non posse neque ipsam propter dementiam neque curatorem eius, patrem tamen eius nuntium mittere posse.* 'Julian asks in the eighteenth book of his *Digest* whether an insane woman [*furiosa*] can repudiate her husband or be repudiated by him. He writes that an insane woman [*furiosam*] can be repudiated, because she is in the same position as a person who does not know of the repudiation. But she could not repudiate her husband because of her madness (*dementiam*), and her curator cannot do this either, but her father can repudiate for her.').[4] In all of these instances the condition is described plainly as madness. The Roman law compendium, therefore, may well offer some of the most explicit evidence that there is for the description of the social experience of madness in antiquity.

Criminal Actions

The best English term for insanity as it is to be seen in the *Digest* is madness. This is because the most commonly used of all of the expressions for insanity is the adjective, used nominally, *furiosus*. It is of course linked to anger and it is close to the ambiguous English expression, 'being mad'.[5] And it is for this reason that the most representative English term for rendering mental illness as we encounter it in the *Digest* is madness. This stands to reason in a legal text. The *Digest* is concerned with madness when it interferes with the normal course of events. Hence passive conditions, such as a profound depression, are less of a problem for the legislators than are conditions of madness that are to be associated with violence and anger. The mad as they

---

amens (Suetonius *Claud.* 15), *demens* (Seneca *Con.* 2.3.3—Seneca rather favors this term), *dementia* (Tacitus *Ann.* 11.16), and so on. Perhaps easier to distinguish are *fatalis vaecordia* (of Messalina's lover, Gaius Silius—Tacitus *Ann.* 11.16) and *imminuta mens* (of Claudius—Tacitus *Ann.* 6.46).

   [4] Translations are taken from Watson 1998.

   [5] The confusion, as it relates the noun *furor,* is noted by Harris 2001, 64.

are depicted in the *Digest* can carry out some pretty terrible actions. Perhaps the following passage offers one of the most vivid instances (*Dig.* 1.18.14):

> Macer, *Criminal Trials book 2*: The deified Marcus and Commodus issued a rescript to Scapula Tertullus in the following terms: 'If you have clearly ascertained that Aelius Priscus is in such a state of insanity (*furore*) that he lacks all understanding through the continuous alienation of his mental faculties (*ut continua mentis alienatione omni intellectu careat*), and if there remains no suspicion that his mother was murdered by him under pretence of madness (*dementia*); then you can abandon consideration of the measure of his punishment, since he is being punished enough by his very madness (*furore*). And yet it will be necessary for him to be all too closely guarded, and, if you think it advisable, even bound in chains, this being a matter of not so much punishing as protecting him and of the safety of his neighbors. If, however, as very often happens, he has intermittent periods of relative sanity (*intervallis quibusdam sensu saniore*), you shall diligently explore the question whether in one such moment he committed the crime, and whether no indulgence is due to his illness (*morbo*). If you ascertain any such thing, you shall consult us, that we may consider whether the enormity of his crime (in the event of his having committed it when he could be held to have been fully aware) merits the infliction of extreme punishment'.

This remarkable passage provides a clear sense of what sort of excessive behavior could constitute madness in the eyes of the jurists. Aelius Priscus' plight is also very similar to that of Orestes, who was a genuine victim of intermittent insanity.

Characteristics of Madness[6]

The jurists in the *Digest* are understandably little concerned with the aetiology of madness. In one of the rare instances of aetiological information Labeo states (*Dig.* 47.10.15 pr.) that 'if a person derange another person's mind by a drug or some other means (*si quis mentem alicuius medicamento aliove quo alienaverit*), the action for insult lies against him.' And elsewhere (*Dig.* 21.1.1.9) Vivianus is quoted as stating that 'it does happen that a physical defect affects the mind also and makes the slave thereby defective; it can happen that he becomes mentally deranged (*frenetico*) by reason of a fever from which he suffers'. Drugs and fevers, notwithstanding, provide slim evidence for aetiologies.

---

[6] Peter King (2000, 17–43) has a discussion of this topic in which he attempts to place the characteristics of madness in the *Digest* within the broader field of Roman literature.

More clues, however, may be found that indicate how a mad person might characteristically act. Although the main concern of the *Digest* is to legislate rather than to diagnose, there are a certain few passages in which mad activity is described. Thus it is for the jurist Ulpian that madness could entail making a bizarre claim in one's will. He suggests that 'if someone should bequeath the gardens of Sallust, which are the emperor's, or the Alban estate, which is for imperial use, the addition of such legacies would be the act of a lunatic (*furiosi*)' (*Dig.* 30.39.8). For Modestinus madness can be evident in a desire for a bizarre burial: He tells us (*Dig.* 28.7.27 pr.) that:

> A certain man appointed an heir in his will under a condition, such as, 'if he throws my remains into the sea'; the question was asked, when the instituted heir had not met the condition, whether he should be expelled from the inheritance. Modestinus replied: The heir is to be praised rather than accused for not throwing the testator's remains into the sea according to his wishes but delivering them for burial, as a reminder of the condition of men. But this point must first be investigated, whether the man who imposed such a condition was even not of sound mind (*compos mentis*).

And for Paul madness can entail the extravagant mistreatment of one's children in a will (*Dig.* 5.2.19):

> A mother on her deathbed appointed an outsider as heir to three quarters of her estate, one daughter as heir to one quarter and passed over the other. The latter successfully bought a complaint of undutiful will ... [the mother's] last judgment is condemned as that of a lunatic (*furiosae*).

The next rather long passage illustrates what the jurists considered to be real mental failings in slaves that were for sale (*Dig.* 21.1.1.8–21.1.4.1):

> So if there be any defect (*vitium*) or disease (*morbus*) which impairs the usefulness and serviceability of the slave, that is ground for rescission ... 9. The question is raised in Vivianus whether a slave who, from time to time, associates with religious fanatics (*fanaticos*) and joins in their utterances is, nonetheless, to be regarded as healthy (*sanus*). Vivianus says that he is; for he says that we should still regard as sane those with minor mental defects (*animi vitia*) ... 10. Vivianus says further that although, at some time in the past, a slave indulged in Bacchanalian revels around the shrines and uttered responses in consonance therewith, it is still the case that if he does it no longer, there is no defect in him and there will be no more liability in respect of him than if he once had a fever; but if he persists still in that bad habit, cavorting around the shrines and uttering virtually demented ravings (*ut circa fana bacchari soleret et quasi demens responsa daret*), even though this be the consequence of excess and thus a defect, it is a still a mental, not a physical, defect, and so constitutes no ground for a rescission ... 4.1 But if a physical affliction should have mental consequences, say that the slave raves in consequence of his fever or wanders through the city quarters, talking nonsense in the manner of the

insane, there is, in such cases, a mental defect flowing from a physical one, and consequently, rescission will be possible. (*Sed si vitium corporis usque ad animum penetrat, forte si propter febrem loquantur aliena vel qui per vicos more insanorum deridenda loquantur, in quos id animi vitium ex corporis vitio accidit, redhiberi posse.*)[7]

Madness in this instructive passage is, it seems, particularly though not necessarily to be linked with the regular association with religious fanatics, or with Bacchanalians, or with those who cavorted round shrines and raved. Excess in behavior and perhaps an excess that runs counter to normally accepted behavior may point to madness. But actions such as raving in public throughout the city were the clearest signs of madness. It appears from the tone of this passage, furthermore, that such behavior was not at all uncommon.

There are other striking symptoms. Pomponius speaks of runaway or wandering slaves, whom he thought could be also mad (*Dig.* 21.1.4.3).[8] In a longish discussion of the grounds according to which a the sale of a slave could be judged as invalid he notes:

> Generally, the rule which we appear to observe is that the expression 'defect and disease' (*vitii morbique*) applies only in respect of physical defects; a vendor is liable in respect of a defect of the mind (*animi vitium*), only if he undertake liability for it, otherwise not. Hence, the express reservation of the wandering or runaway slave; for their defects are of the mind, not of physical (*hoc enim animi vitium est, non corporis*).

It was not just in raving, in wills, or in wandering that madness could be expressed. It seems that the mad, in the eyes of the jurists, may have been given to unintentionally hiding themselves away. Thus Ulpian, arguing in reverse mode, suggests that a person who willingly hides himself away cannot be said to be mad, but that by implication one that does not do this intentionally is mad (*Dig.* 42.4.7.9):

> So far does hiding (*latitatio*) require the intent and design (*animum et affectum*) of the person who conceals himself that it is rightly said that a lunatic

---

[7] Parlamento 2001, 1–20, expands on the notion of *vitium animi* and aims to show that the puzzling figure of the 'melancholic slave' in the lines to follow this passage should be understood in terms of Hippocratic (and Galenic) medicine and Cicero's *Tusculans* 3.5.11 as the victim of a *vitium animi* rather than a *vitium corporis* (something that might also have appealed to Seneca), hence offering grounds for rescission.

[8] Drapetomania, in the terminology of the awful 19th century physician Samuel A. Cartwright. This was a form of mental disorder that caused black slaves to attempt to escape captivity, he alleged (1851, 691–715). 'Hacking 1999, 57, explains this view.

(*furiosum*) cannot be subjected to a sale on this score; for a person who does not have control of himself (*suus non est*) does not go into hiding.

Hiding, it seems, requires volition. The madman, therefore, may openly flaunt his unusual predilections because he is not in control of himself (*suus non est*) and in this case may sequester himself without any conscious volition.

The mental defects of slaves can extend beyond such actions as wandering or running away. Venuleius at *Dig.* 21.1.65 pr. highlights as *vitia mentis* such unexpected activities as being 'addicted to watching the games or studying works of art or lying' (*si ludos adsidue velit spectare aut tabulas pictas studiose intueatur, sive etiam mendax ... teneatur*). While such *vitia* may not have quite constituted full blown madness, they do seem to partake of the condition, for the term *vitium animi* can be used elsewhere of those who are unquestionably *furiosi*.

What sort of a picture do these few passages provide of the madman in the *Digest* and no doubt in Rome? Behavior that was excessive and that defied societal norms, such as raving in public, participating in strange religious cults, wishing your body to be buried in unacceptably peculiar places such as at sea, and the making of wills that call upon the wealth of others or misapply your own, all seem to be associated with madness. It is possible too that wandering or running away in slaves also pointed to madness as did involuntary hiding. Such then are a few of the glimpses that may be gained of the characteristic behavior of the madman according to the *Digest*. One also has the impression that such individuals were reasonably common in Roman cities and that their movements were not necessarily constrained. How many of them were there? There can be no answer to this question from the *Digest*. And from what did they suffer? We cannot know from this legal text, for the *Digest* is not interested in nicety of diagnosis. Why should it? Its task was to settle on the proper treatment of the mad.

Understanding Madness

How did the Romans of the periods when the *Digest's* constituent elements were composed understand madness? Some assistance with this query is provided, for example, by the comments of Ulpian on the *lex Aquilia*, a law that covers damages. The question being discussed is this: what legal liability is incurred when a madman causes damages (*Dig.* 9.2.5.2)? Here is Ulpian's adjudication:

And accordingly, the question is asked whether there is an action under the *lex Aquilia* if a lunatic (*furiosus*) causes damage. Pegasus says there is not; for he asks how there can be an accountable fault in him who is out of his mind (*cum suae mentis non sit*) ... Therefore the Aquilian action will fail in such a case, just as it fails if an animal (*quadrupes*) has caused damage or if a tile has fallen (*si tegula ceciderit*); and the same must be said if an infant (*infans*) has caused damage ...

What is the common denominator that links madmen, tiles, animals and children under the age of seven (*infantes*)? A partial clarification is provided in *Dig.* 9.1.1.3: 'an animal is incapable of committing a legal wrong because it is devoid of reason (*nec enim potest animal iniuriam fecisse, quod sensu caret*)'. It is easy to see how this description of the mental capacity of an animal might be transferred to a *tegula*—it certainly lacks any form of *sensus*. But what of an *infans* and a madman, do they too lack *sensus*? The jurist Modestinus, helpfully, renders the link implicit in Ulpian's comment more comprehensible when he makes a link between the relative guilt for murder under the *lex Cornelia* of a child under the age of seven and a madman (*Dig.* 48.8.12—compare *Dig.* 6.1.60):

An infant (*infans*) or a madman (*furiosus*) who kills a man is not liable under the *Lex Cornelia*, the one being protected by innocence of intent (*innocentia consilii*), the other excused by the misfortune of his condition (*fati infelicitas*).

It seems as if both are ultimately let off the hook because they have no sense (no capacity for *consilium*) of what they are doing. This is made quite explicit in the case of the *infans* and by implication with the *furiosus*. What else does his *fati infelicitas* imply but being as devoid of sense as an animal or a falling tile?

The mad are frequently associated with children within the *Digest*. The link warrants further attention. The following technical passage also links up small children and the mad and may make this point more apparent. Their incapacity to offer assent is presumably the result of their being devoid of reason (*Dig.* 8.2.5):

In connection with servitudes [rights exercised over property belonging to another], when something is done against a man's wishes (*invitum*), we must not take this to mean that he openly objects, but that he does not give his consent. Thus, Pomponius asserts in his fortieth book that something can properly be said to be done against the wishes of an infant (*infantem*) or a lunatic (*furiosum*).

Infants and lunatics, lacking *sensus*, are, in other words, incapable of providing assent. As a parting point to this matter it deserves emphasis that the link between children and madmen is made, not because the *furiosi* are to be seen as childish, but rather, because children, like the mad, are devoid of reason. The same point could be made of the link between animals, tiles, and the insane: the latter are not animal-like but rather are devoid of reason.

There are other ways of understanding the mad which can be seen within the *Digest*. In one of the most beautiful of these Julian likens a madman to someone who is either absent (*absens*) or asleep (*quiescens*). Here is the context in which this is stated (*Dig.* 29.7.2.3):

> A lunatic (*furiosus*) is not understood to make a codicil, because he is not understood to perform any other legal act, as in all circumstances and in every respect he is treated like someone absent or asleep. (*Furiosus non intellegitur codicillos facere, quia nec aliud quicquam agere intellegitur, cum per omnia et in omnibus absentis vel quiescentis loco habetur.*)

It would probably be an exaggeration to suggest, on the basis of this characterization of the madman as someone *absens vel quiescens*, that the Roman attitude to the mad was a sympathetic one. This is because the *absentia* of the *furiosus* in this passage is perhaps better understood as being like that of, for example, a soldier on duty overseas and whose affairs need to be managed by another person. Paulus provides what is perhaps the most straightforward explanation for this use of *absens* (*Dig.* 50.17.124):

> Where presence, and not simply verbal assent, is necessary, a mute, provided that he has his wits, can be regarded as replying. Likewise, with someone who is deaf, he also can reply. 1. Someone who is mad (*furiosus*) is in the same position as someone who is absent, as Pomponius writes in the first book of his *Letters*. (*Furiosus absentis loco est et ita pomponius libro primo epistularum scribit.*)

Someone who is absent cannot speak for themselves nor can the madman. His psychological 'absence' is presumably based on the understanding of his being devoid of reason (*caret sensu*) and hence volitionally absent from those legal circumstances in which he or she finds themselves. There are, in addition to this passage from Paulus, a certain number of others which also pair the madman, in a legal setting, with an individual who is literally *absens*, sometimes one who has been taken captive by the enemy. Here is an example of this simple pairing (*Dig.* 23.4.8):

> When a son marries where his father is insane (*furens*) or has been captured by the enemy (*ab hostibus capto*) or where a daughter does so, there is no alternative to entering into a pact on the dowry with these people themselves.

This excerpt does not state that both parties are *absentes*, but the pairing implies that the mad father is subject to the same constraints as one who is captured by the enemy, being psychologically absent that is, and hence in no position to make decisions. Following is a second passage which makes much the same point and doubtless is based on the same notion of absence, real or psychological. It is surely significant that in this instance *infantes* are also included (*Dig.* 40.5.36 pr.):

> *Infantes*, lunatics (*furiosi*), captives of the enemy, and persons whose delay [in granting freedom [to a slave]] is due to religious scruple or a very honorable reason or some calamity or a very great risk to estate, civic status or reputation or sort some like cause, are not within the scope of the *senatus consultum* Rubrianum [which provides a magistrate with the right of offering liberty in those cases where the inheritor is unwilling]

There is, curiously, an even more natural link between being *absens*, captured by the enemy, and madness that is demonstrated by the next passage. The period of captivity for the Roman prisoner might render him literally insane. So we read (*Dig.* 49.15.26):

> It is of no concern in what manner a captive has returned, whether he was set free or whether he escaped from the power of the enemy by force or trickery, provided that he comes back with the intention of not returning thither; for it is not enough for a person to have returned home in body, if the spirit is elsewhere [*mente alienus*—in other words returned as a madman and incapable of *voluntas*]. But those who are rescued on the defeat of the enemy are reckoned as having returned with *postliminium* [regaining of public and private law rights on return from capture by the enemy]

It is clear from this passage that, sometimes at least, those who had been captured by the enemy returned *mente alienus*, rendered mad by the experience in other words. (The phrase *alienatio mentis* is used of madness in *Dig.* 1.18.14). The matter of fact manner in which Florentinus announces this possibility makes one wonder whether this was in fact a common occurrence. Florentinus may therefore provide an even more unexpected link between being mad and being captured by the enemy.

The other term, apart from *absens*, that was used to describe the madman was being asleep, or *quiescens*. It is easy to guess how this expression might characterize a madman, but it is worthwhile to hear this in the *Digest*'s own words (*Dig.* 41.2.1.3). Once again *voluntas* is at issue:

> A madman (*furiosus*), however, and a *pupillus* acting without his tutor's authority cannot begin to possess because they do not have the intention to hold, whatever their physical contact with the thing, as when one places something in the hand of a sleeping man (*sicuti si quis dormienti aliquid in manu ponat*).

Or (*Dig.* 41.3.31.3):

> If my slave or son holds anything by way of *peculium* or in my name, I possess
> it or even usucapt it through him, although I am unaware of it; and if he
> should go mad (*si is furere coeperit*), then, so long as the thing remains in
> the same condition, it is to be understood that possession remains in me and
> usucapion continues to run, just as would be the case if such a person was
> asleep (*dormientem*).

Let us attempt to sum up the results to this point of this brief survey of
some of the modes by which madness seems to be understood within the
Digest. The absent cannot speak for themselves—so captives, madmen, and
children (but not the mute who can physically indicate assent)—are subject
to a psychological 'absence'. But the mad and children (and animals and
falling tiles) also exhibit an absence of volition—they cannot choose to do
anything because *carent sensu*.

Understanding Madness's Appearances

Thus far I have been speaking of the understanding of madness in a more
intellectual sense. Another way of putting this might be to say that we have
been looking at how madmen were conceptualized in the *Digest*. On a more
practical or observational level the Romans of the *Digest* certainly understood that individuals could, during a normal life-span, become mad, they
could cease to be mad, they could cycle in and out of madness, and they
could stay mad. The jurists are quite matter of fact about this. Their understanding that madness could occur in interludes within an individual's life
was significant. For the jurist these interludes were vital, for the law needed
to understand whether a criminal action took place during an interval of
madness or of sanity (it is possible that the term *lunaticus* may imply someone who is subject to such periods of unreason—*Dig.* 21.1.43.6). This, one
could guess, was important not just as it would relate to punishment, but
also to legal liability in, for example, damage cases. So we read that (*Dig.*
14.4.4):

> liability ... attaches to a *pupillus* who acts fraudulently after reaching puberty
> ... and to a madman who acts fraudulently in a lucid interval (*furiosus sanae
> mentis dolum admittant*).

Or, more alarmingly (*Dig.* 48.9.9.1):

> Those who kill persons other than their mother, father, grandfather or grand-
> mother ... shall be punished capitally or put to the extreme penalty. Truly, if
> anyone kills a parent in a fit of madness (*per furorem*), he shall not be pun-
> ished, as the deified brothers wrote in a rescript in the case of a man who had

killed his mother in a fit of madness; for it was enough for him to be punished by the madness itself, and he must be guarded the more carefully, or even confined with chains.

And madmen could easily appear so sane that you might contract business with them. They also understood that not all mental problems were equal (*Dig.* 22.3.25.1):

> But if the person who claims to have paid money not due is a ward, *minor*, woman or man of full age who is a soldier, farmer, or a person inexpert in court matters, simple minded (*alias gaudens simplicitate*) or slothful, then the recipient must show that the money paid was properly received and owing to him.

But perhaps most interesting of all was their realization that madness could be feigned as a means for getting out of criminal actions, such as in the following (*Dig.* 27.10.6):

> The praetor must be careful not to appoint a curator [person who had, amongst other things, power of attorney over the madman] for someone rashly without the fullest investigation; for many feign madness or mental illness (*plerique furorem vel dementiam fingunt*) so as to escape their legal obligations by receiving a curator.

Infants and Madness

Despite the frequent pairing of the mad with children (Gaius, *Inst.* 3.109 suggests that 'an *infans* and one who is close to an *infans* in age does not differ much from a madman [*furioso*], because *pupilli* of this age have little intellect [*intellectum*]'), the *Digest* has very little to say of madness in the young. One intriguing excerpt asks of a mother (*Dig.* 38.17.2.31):

> What if she has not applied for a tutor or a curator for an insane (*furioso*) child? The more reasonable view is that she incurs [the penalty of the *senatus consultum*].

But I know of no other comparable passages. The *Digest's* longest discussion touching on madness in children has as its focus their legal care. Its suggestion is that, should a child in tutelage or liable for tutelage become mad, tutelage rather than curatorship ('care' in this passage) should be continued or applied to the child's protection. The passage goes on to propose that age rather than health (madness that is) is the issue in these matters and should also be the decider in the case of those whom we might term youths. Exposition of these views is provided by the following passage (*Dig.* 26.1.3):

If a person who has a tutor, whether *pupillus* or *pupilla*, becomes a lunatic (*si furere coeperint*), he is in a position where he, nonetheless, should remain in tutelage; this was the opinion of Quintus Mucius and approved by Julian, and we follow the principle that curatorship is redundant if the age of the person concerned requires tutelage. Therefore, if they have tutors, they are not admitted into care on account of their lunacy (*per furorem*), but if they do not have them and become lunatics (*furor eis accesserit*), nonetheless they are able to receive tutors, since the *Law of the Twelve Tables*, is understood not to apply to *pupilli* or *pupillae*. 1. Thus, because we do not allow agnates to be curators over the persons of *pupilli*, for that reason I also think that if someone under twenty-five becomes a lunatic (*furiosus*), he should be given a curator, not as a lunatic (*furioso*), but as an *adulescens*, as though the difficulty were one of age. Thus, we shall explain that where a person's age subjects him to care or tutelage, it is not necessary to find him a curator, as for a madman (*dementi*), and the Emperor Antoninus issued a rescript to this effect, since for the meantime one must give thought more to his age than to his insanity (*dementiae*).

For me and, I believe, for those interested in modern understandings of madness, what is striking is the nonchalance—if I can use this word—with which it is indicated that madness is possible in young children. It might have been expected that the condition, which normally becomes evident in later teens, might have been attributed to other causes.

Caring for the Mad: Curators

The use of the curator, from a modern standpoint, is one of the most unexpected of the modes by which the Roman madman could be cared for. It is, from our point of view, singular, although comparable procedures existed in ancient Greece (such was the purport of the *dike paranoias*)[9] and in classical Arabic law, according to Michael Dols in his great book, *Majnun: The Madman in Medieval Islamic Society*.[10] The distinction between Greece and Rome seems to have resided in the fact that for the Roman the appointment of a curator was a legal right. The concept of curatorship was a remarkable one, even if it practice may not have always lived up to the idea.

---

[9] The most helpful survey of madness in Greek culture with which I am familiar is Clark 1993. She discusses Greek law and madness as well as the *graphe paranoias* on 156–174. There is also Carr Vaughan 1919, which looks at Greek law on 59–72.

[10] Dols 1992 also discusses Roman law in this context (428–430). I have been helped by his summary. On the links between curatorships and madness there is also assistance to be derived from Tristán 2000 and Pulitano 2002. Trenchard-Smith cites Sesto 1956).

A curator was appointed for an individual over the age of 25 and that person was expected to manage the affairs of the *furiosus*—property, finance, as well as their physical well being. The curator was appointed by a legal magistrate, a praetor—it was a duty that could not be shirked and it could be expensive. So do we learn in *Dig.* 27.1.2.9:

> Moreover, those who are already administering three tutelages or three curatorships or three tutorships and curatorships all told, which are still in existence, that is, where the *pupilli* are not yet of age, are exempt from a forth tutelage or curatorship. Indeed, a curator of a lunatic (*furiosi*) rather than of a minor can count this last among the number of curatorships ...

And it was a duty that could have serious legal ramifications (*Dig.* 26.9.5):

> After the death of a lunatic (*furiosus*), an action on a judgment will not be granted against the curator who managed his affairs, any more than it will be granted against tutors, as long as it is certain that no renewal of debts was made with his consent after he had resigned his office, and that no obligation was transferred to the curator or tutor.

A curator could be a member of the family, a son, for example, but it was usually not. A husband, for example, could not act for his mentally impaired wife. It is also worth noting that a curator could be appointed for a *prodigus*, a *fatuus*, and individual who had been captured by the enemy, or a soldier on campaign. (It may or may not be significant that physicians, soldiers, and rhetoricians were excused from duty as a curator.) If an individual was under the age of 25 and did not have a parent, then the praetor could appoint a tutor whose responsibilities match those of a curator. A tutor, if the circumstances required it, could be appointed for an unborn child.

The reality of the exercising of the curatorship may have fallen short of the ideal, however. It has been suggested that there is always the possibility—though evidence is lacking—that 'the power to have someone confined as insane would have been abused.'[11] This might have been particularly acute in cases of intermittent insanity, where the accurate diagnosis of the appearance and disappearance of the condition might have presented a real diagnostic challenge. Might not the period of dependence be unnecessarily extended to an agnate curator's advantage? There is certainly evidence pointing to the problematic nature of intermittent insanity.[12]

---

[11] Johnston 1999, 41.
[12] The anonymous reviewer of this paper points to two Justinian enactments, *C.* 5.70.6–7, reporting on earlier juristic disputes about intermittent insanity.

How Were the Mad Looked After?

The task of care, even for the criminally insane like the parricide of *Dig.* 48.9.9.1 (mentioned above), belonged in the first instance to the family. It was only if this failed that the praetor or the provincial governor would step in. So we learn in *Dig.* 1.18.13.1–14 that:

> In the case of madmen whom their relatives cannot keep under control, there is a remedy to which the governor must resort, namely, that of confining them in prison. So held the deified Pius in a rescript … 14 'But since we have learned from your letter that his [the same individual referred to in *Dig.* 48.9.9.1] position and rank are such that he is in the custody of his own people or even in his own house, it seems to us that you will act rightly if you summon those by whom at the material time he was being looked after, and if you make inquiry into the cause of so neglectful an act, and if you make a decision against each one of them according as you find his culpability lesser or greater.
>
> For those who have custody of the insane are not responsible only for seeing that they do not do themselves too much harm but also for seeing that they do not bring destruction on others. But if that should happen, it may deservedly be imputed to the fault of those who were too neglectful in performing their duties.'

So it is that the madman is looked after at home by his relatives in the first instance. But if they are unable to do this, then the praetor steps in both to prosecute the family for any failings that their care may have resulted in, and to imprison the madman. Where this prison may have been is difficult to imagine, however, for in most periods of Roman society there were no such institutions.[13] Perhaps the rescript is referring to those temporary holding cells used to house prisoners awaiting further punishment, which did exist. And there were, of course, no hospitals for the criminally insane.[14] It must

---

[13] On prisons in Rome there is Krause 1996. Semelaigne (1869, 216–217) maintains that the lower class mad, if they were dangerous, were imprisoned. Were that true, it would be of interest for the case made by Foucault, cited below.

[14] The medical writer and adapter of Soranus, Caelius Aurelianus (*Chronic Diseases* 1.5, 172 Drabkin) speaks disparagingly of those physicians who prescribe that victims of mania (one version of *furor*), be constrained in bonds' 'physicians also prescribe indiscriminately that patients be kept in bonds (*vinculis aegrotantes coerci*) … [but] it is easier to restrain patients by having servants use their hands (*facilius aegros ministrantium minibus … retinere*) than by applying crude bonds (*inertis vinculis*)'. I deduce from the reference to the *ministrantes* that Caelius and Soranus have a home scene in mind. That offers one more piece of evidence as to how the *furiosi* in some circumstances and some periods were dealt with. Caelius (active in the fifth century in North Africa) also claims (*Chronic Diseases* 1.5, 179 Drabkin) that Titus, a pupil of Asclepiades (died come time in the first century BCE), 'prescribes that a patient

have been a different case for the poor whose lodgings and family situation would not have allowed them to look after the mad. The *Digest* tells us nothing about what must have happened to those unfortunate individuals.

More context, if not more detail, is provided by long passage that discusses the effects of madness within a marriage.[15] ('Within' must be stressed, for diagnosable madness prevented a marriage from taking place. So *Dig.* 23.1.8: 'It must be obvious that insanity (*furor*) is an impediment to betrothal, but if it arises afterward, it will not invalidate it.') The passage I have just referred to provides advice and rulings on the rights within marriage of a wife or a husband who has succumbed to insanity (*Dig.* 24.3.22.7):

> Let us see what is to be done if a husband or a wife becomes insane (*furere*) within a marriage. There can be no doubt that the person in the grip of insanity (*furore detenta est*) cannot repudiate the marriage, because that person is not in their senses. What if a woman is repudiated in these circumstances? If there were lucid intervals during the madness (*intervallum furor habeat*) or the disease is permanent but bearable for those connected with her, then the marriage ought not to be dissolved at all. Where a person who is aware of the situation and is of sound mind repudiates the other person who is insane (*furenti*) in the way we described above, that person will be to blame for the dissolution of the marriage. For what could be more generous than a husband and wife sharing in each other's misfortunes (*quid enim tam humanum est, quam ut fortuitis casibus mulieris maritum vel uxorem viri participem esse*)?

There are, however, grounds for a husband's seeking a divorce. These are directly related to the level of violence to which the madwoman is prone. So we hear (*Dig.* 24.3.22.7):

> But if the insane person is so violent, savage and dangerous (*propter saevitiam furoris*) that there is no hope of recovery and it is terrible for her attendants and if the other party fears for his safety and is tempted by the desire to have children because he has none, this person will be allowed, if of sane mind, to repudiate the other party who is insane (*furenti*), so that the marriage will be ended without blame attaching to anyone and neither of them will suffer damage.

In some instances, however, the husband may be unwilling to seek a divorce even in an intolerable situation. This may be because he has designs on the misuse of her dowry. In a case such as this recourse should be had to

---

be taken from his usual pursuits and put in bonds (*vinculis constringi*).' Thus the practice of constraining some *furiosi* by the use of *vincula* was acknowledged over a five-century period. (See also Celsus below.)

[15] Evans Grubbs (2002, 190) looks at issues related to these matters.

the curator or to other family members, such as the woman's father who can attempt to recover he dowry either for himself or for the daughter (*Dig.* 24.3.22.8–9):

> But suppose the woman has the most savage form of insanity (*in saevissimo furore muliere constituta*) and the husband does not want to end the marriage because he is too cunning for this, but treats his wife's misfortune with scorn and shows her no sympathy but clearly does not give her proper care, but misuses her dowry. Here the insane woman's curator or her relatives can go to court, to force the husband to give all this sort of support to the woman, to provide for her, to give her medicines, and to omit nothing a husband should do for his wife as far as the amount of the dowry allows. But if it is clear that he is about to squander the dowry and not enjoy it as a man should, the dowry should be sequestered, and the wife should have enough for the maintaining of herself and her household. All dotal pacts which the parties entered into at the time of marriage action must continue in their former condition and are dependent on the recovery of the health of the wife. Again, the father of the insane woman (*furiosae*) can legally bring an action to recover the dowry himself or for his daughter. For although the insane woman cannot repudiate, her father can certainly do so.

The passage finishes with a bizarre twist. What if the daughter's father himself goes mad after a divorce has taken place? I am not sure whether the advice here is an example of willful speculation, or whether it offers some sort of evidence that madness ran in some Roman families. At any rate, here is the jurists' advice (*Dig.* 24.3.22.10–11):

> If after the marriage has been dissolved the father becomes insane (*furiosus*), his curator can bring an action to recover the dowry with his daughter's consent, or where there is no curator the daughter can bring it, but she must give security that her act will be ratified. It has also been decided where a father is captured by the enemy (*ab hostibus captus sit*), an action to recover the dowry should be granted to the daughter.

Death and Suicide

The *Digest* does not have a lot to say about how the mad perish. There is one intriguing reference to suicide and madness, but, as far as I can see, this is all. It ought to be of considerable to those who link suicide to mental disorder rather than to difficulties in coping with life's challenges. It comes from *Book 3* of Arrius Menander's *Military Law* (*Dig.* 49.16.6.7):

> If a man has wounded himself or has attempted suicide in some other way, the Emperor Hadrian wrote in a rescript that the circumstances of the matter should be established, so that, if he had preferred to die out of inability to

bear pain, or *taedium vitae*, or disease, or madness, or shame (*si impatientia doloris aut taedio vitae aut morbo aut furore aut pudore mori maluit*), the death penalty should not be inflicted on him, but he should receive a dishonourable discharge

Suicide amongst the insane is forgivable. The link is something that could be deflected back to a character such as the Ajax of Sophocles.

Conclusion

Some forms of mental instability seem to fall outside the remit of the *Digest*—these are perhaps the ones that nowadays interest many people most, such as depression, melancholy, ennui, chronic boredom, all conditions that are of themselves harmful enough to individuals, but not necessarily harmful to society. The *Digest* was understandably not concerned with this type of problem. For the Romans of the centuries that are dealt with by the *Digest* madness seems to have been primarily a legal problem. A contrast could be made to the nineteenth, twentieth, and twenty-first centuries where madness is, I think it is fair to say, primarily seen as a medical problem—while perhaps for the seventeenth and eighteenth centuries madness was viewed a social problem.[16] Perhaps medicine mattered less as a solution in antiquity because, as we can see from Galen or Aretaeus or Caelius Aurelianus, there was very little that could be done by physicians to cure or even to mitigate mental disorder.[17] And very little could be done from a social point of view either when there were no hospitals, no prisons to speak of, and, effectively, no police force. But there was a highly articulated legal code whose role was the resolution, not the control, of difficult social issues. There was a code that could deal with such problems as might arise from insanity: those relating to marriage, inheritance, slave ownership, property and personal damages, and so forth.

The impression of the Romans that is left with a modern reader by the discussions of madness in the *Digest* is of a very practical people. Their practicality, though perhaps not always sufficient to the task at hand, was tempered by considerable compassion and even respect for those blighted

---

[16] The consideration of the historical periodization of madness begins with Michel Foucault. The complete version of his first book, which was on this topic, or at least the 1972 version, has now been published in full in English as *History of Madness* (Foucault, 2006).

[17] An overview of the history of madness which I have found useful is Leibbrand and Wettley 1961. It focuses on the medical sources and has no discussion of the legal sources.

by mental disorder.[18] I would like to finish with an excerpt that well captures this benign respect (*Dig.* 1.5.20):

> A person who has become insane is held to retain his previous status and dignity, and also his position as a magistrate and his power, just as he retains ownership of his property.

> Qui furere coepit, et statum et dignitatem in qua fuit et magistratum et potestatem videtur retinere, sicut rei suae dominium retinet.[19]

---

[18] They were not perfect. Celsus suggests that refractory *furiosi* might be beaten by physicians (*De Medicina* 3.18.21): 'If, however, it is the mind that deceives the madman (*insanientem*), he is best treated by certain tortures (*tormentis*). When he says or does anything wrong, he is to be coerced by starvation, fetters and flogging (*fame, vinculis, plagis*).' Caelius Aurelianus reports, but without support, on similar practices (*Chronic Diseases* I.5, 178–179): 'under the influence of Asclepiades' account, his pupil Titus, in Book II of his work *On the Psyche*, holds that flogging should be employed.' Titus, it seems, has a lot to answer for.

[19] My thanks to William Harris for asking me to deliver an oral version of this paper to *Mental Disorders in Classical Antiquity* conference at Columbia University in April, 2010, to the participants at that event, and to the anonymous reviewer of my paper. Different versions of this paper were read to the History of Neurology Interest Group (December 2009) and to the Mental Health Awareness Group (December 2010) in the Faculty of Medicine at the University of Calgary (many thanks to Dr's Frank Stahnisch, Andrew Bulloch and Scott Patten).

THE PSYCHOLOGICAL IMPACT OF
DISASTERS IN THE AGE OF JUSTINIAN

Jerry Toner

The year 560 CE saw the start of some very strange behaviour in the city of Amida on the upper reaches of the River Tigris: people began to 'bark like dogs, bleat like goats, meow like cats, cuckoo like cocks, and imitate the voices of all dumb animals'.[1] Not only that, but, according to John of Ephesus's account, groups of deranged sufferers 'gathered in groups, confused, troubled, disturbed, causing confusion', and they staggered about in the night on their way to the cemetery. They sang and raged in public and they bit each other; they uttered sounds 'as if with horns and trumpets', and used vulgar language 'as if from devils in person'. They would explode with laughter, and even utter 'immodest talk and evil blasphemy'. The disorder took on a physical expression, with the afflicted jumping about and climbing walls, 'hanging themselves upside-down, falling and rolling down while naked'. So extreme was their confusion that none 'knew either his house or home'.[2]

This bizarre group behaviour did not just erupt of its own accord. The fortress city of Amida, where John had been born, lay strategically on the river Tigris, in the border area with the Persian empire. Periodic warfare between the two great regional rivals made it an inherently unstable place. But the sixth century had seen the city struck by repeated hammer blows of misfortune. In 502 CE it had suffered a three month long siege at the hands of the Persians, and after it fell 80,000 of its inhabitants were slaughtered. The next two years saw vigorous Roman counter-offensives under the emperor

---

[1] An analysis of the psychological impact of disasters in the wider Roman world can be found in my forthcoming *Roman Disasters*. On mental health in ancient Rome, see the second chapter of Toner 2009.

[2] For a detailed analysis of John of Ephesus, see Harvey 1990, esp. 57–75, on the madness of Amida. John's account was originally contained in Part II of his *Ecclesiastical History* but survives primarily in Part III of the Chronicle of Zuqnīn, previously ascribed to pseudo-Dionysius. The two later major accounts of the Amidan episode draw on this source for their information: Michael the Syrian, *Chronique*, 9.32; and *Chronicon anonymum* 1234, LXII. See Harvey, 1990, 64 n. 44. All translations are from Harrak's version of *The Chronicle of Zuqnīn* 1999.

Anastasius. For the city dwellers inside the walls, these Roman sieges caused them to suffer even more greatly than the Persian defenders. The men were imprisoned, the women were sexually abused, and food became so scarce that people resorted to acts of cannibalism. Being returned to Rome under a settlement in 505 CE did not bring the population security. The largely Monophysite city was to suffer vigorous religious persecution at the hands of one of Justin I's orthodox henchmen, Bishop Abraham bar Kaili, a man of whom it was said that he employed a band of lepers to infect his Monophysite prisoners and pollute their property. He retained his bishopric for some thirty years. Then in 543 CE the Great Plague struck. John tells us that the city and its environs lost 30,000 dead in just three months. The shock of the plague brought the economy to its knees and famine ensued. Finally in 560 CE, following this great series of disasters, people were panicked by rumours of another Persian invasion. It was said that the false reports were spread by a band of 'rebellious demons' appearing in the guise of refugees fleeing from the supposed attack. Alarm spread and the people of the region 'migrated all at once, and great confusion and losses occurred everywhere for many days'. It was the final straw. The fear of renewed siege seems to have tipped some sections of society over the edge: 'It was rage, madness, frenzy', explains John. And so the city suffered a collective mental breakdown, which saw all the normal conventions of social behaviour overturned.

I want to start by examining this group behaviour in the light of what modern mental-health research can tell us about the psychological impact of disasters, before considering some of these findings in relation to the Late Roman world to see what light they can help shed on the mental health of the ancient population. For if there is one thing that anyone familiar with the history and literature of antiquity will know, it is that disasters are a recurrent feature of ancient sources. Whether natural disasters, such as earthquakes, volcanic eruptions, floods and droughts, biological calamities such as plagues and epidemics, man-made catastrophes, like wars, or disasters which cannot so easily be compartmentalized, like famines and shipwrecks, disasters were a hard fact of the harsh reality of Roman life.

Disasters were an in-built part of ordinary life in the Roman world. This is not to say that everyone suffered repeated catastrophe, simply that extreme trauma can be expected to have occurred with a certain degree of periodic regularity given the structural deficiencies of a pre-industrial society. Food crises were common, wars depressingly inevitable, and floods frequent. And as well as the headline-grabbing disasters of Pompeii or the defeat at Cannae, small scale, local disasters also brought widespread distress. Frequent shipwrecks that left communities shattered, isolated plagues of locusts and mice that left villages starving, and terrifying outbreaks of disease made disaster a permanent feature on the social horizon. Long drawn-out disasters such as war or famine probably hit the poor hardest. The most vulnerable in society were placed in a situation where they were exposed to extreme levels of mental stress when they were lacking any adequate resources to help them cope with them. The fact that Roman society assigned much of what can be termed 'emotion work' to women also meant that disasters placed them under particular pressure. Death in the family, household break-up, and inability to care for their children adequately all placed an extra burden on women. So too did the likelihood that during the recovery period there was a greater reliance on their role as caregivers and providers of emotional support at a time when mothering itself was probably made more difficult by the traumatic incidents that had affected the family.[3]

The Great Plague, which first arrived in the empire in 541 and spread to Constantinople the following year, raised the concept of disaster to a new level.[4] The calamity had been prefigured, we are told by John, by the appearance of terrifying phantoms at sea. Numerous spectres of boats of copper were seen, in which what looked like headless black people were sitting. But this was much more than a normal epidemic. When it reached Constantinople, it started with vigour first 'with the masses of poor people'. Sometimes, we are told, as many as 16,000 among them died each day. At first, people not only counted them but they also buried them 'with great diligence' and gave them proper funeral rites. But total disorder soon took hold. The plague struck down the wealthy and the powerful. All ages were humbled and crushed in what John describes as a 'wine press of wrath' in which 'all ranks were pressed on the top of each other'. People forgot about money and wills and possessions. Even 'selling and buying itself ceased'. A complete social dystopia had come about, where the catastrophe was so powerful that all forms of hierarchy had been destroyed.

Modern disaster research suggests that the psychological impact of such intensely stressful events would have been significant.[5] A large body of research has examined the link between the extreme stresses which deeply traumatic events exert upon individuals and their subsequent development of mental disorders.[6] Disasters are a world where 'un-ness' rules: the

---

[3] On gender and disaster, see Rodríguez et al. 2007, 130–146.
[4] On the plague in Constantinople, see Evagrius, *HE* 4.29; Procopius, *Wars* 2.22–23.
[5] For an overview of modern disaster research, see Rodríguez et al. 2007.
[6] On disasters and mental health, see López-Ibor et al. 2005, Neria et al. 2009, and Norris et al. 2002.

unexpected, the unmanageable and the uncertain take over and impose considerable psychological pressure on the individuals exposed to them.[7] In the immediate aftermath, individuals can display what is known as 'disaster syndrome'. They appear docile, stunned, shocked, and dazed, with an absence of emotion. They fail to respond to stimulus and shy away from any outward activity. These initial responses can last for a matter of hours or a few days at most. The most common longer-term mental disorders suffered by individuals in the aftermath of a disaster are post-traumatic stress disorder (PTSD), depression, anxiety and panic. PTSD is a relatively newly diagnosed disorder, first appearing in the third edition of the *Diagnostic and Statistical Manual of Mental Disorders*, published in 1980, before being revised in the fourth edition of 1994. It describes the development of a range of symptoms following exposure to an extremely traumatic stressor, either personally or as a witness, usually involving threat to the individual's life or serious injury. An essential element is that the individual must have experienced 'intense fear, helplessness, or horror'. The symptoms include the persistent re-living of the traumatic event in the form of recurrent dreams or intrusive flashback, feelings of detachment and withdrawal from society, apathy, and reduced emotional response. The lifetime prevalence rate among US citizens is between 1 and 14 per cent. In the wake of the 2001 attacks on New York, 7.5 per cent of a random group of adults living south of 110th Street in Manhattan exhibited the symptoms of PTSD. Most symptoms of mental disorder appear immediately following the disaster event and 70 per cent improve naturally with time. The prevalence rate among the group of New Yorkers fell from 7.5 per cent one month after the attacks to 1.7 per cent after four months and just 0.6 per cent after six. The severity and number of stressors that an individual suffers seem to be the most important factors in predicting the severity of mental health problems he or she will subsequently encounter. To use New York again as an example, the percentage of people suffering from PTSD one month after the attacks rose from 7.5 per cent to 20 per cent when the sample was taken from adults living south of Canal Street and hence much closer to the World Trade Center. The percentage increased to as many as 30 per cent when looking at those who were injured and 37 per cent among those who escaped from the Twin Towers themselves. In the most extreme situations, such as the Armenian earthquake of 1998 where high mortality was combined with numerous injuries,

---

[7] See Rodríguez et al. 2007, 42.

little rescue effort and prolonged homelessness, as many as two thirds of people showed the symptoms of PTSD.[8]

As indicated, PTSD is not the only response to trauma: depression, anxiety, somatic problems, poor sleep and alcohol abuse are other common symptoms, and there is high co-morbidity with other mental disorders. The considerable range of possible responses to disasters shows that no simple cause and effect can be established. This is partly the result of the fact that no two disasters are alike. Factors that act as buffers against the psychological stress that disasters induce include family and social support networks. One of the problems with many disasters is that family and social networks tend be disrupted, if not outright destroyed, and that daily life becomes that much more difficult because of various knock-on effects of the disruption. Additional stress factors can include the need to relocate, the overcrowding this usually results in, frightened children, a loss of a sense of security, and a loss of trust in those in authority. Factors that have been shown to help with recovery include having a purpose, social attachment, prayer, a sense of humour, acceptance of the situation without giving in to its difficulties, adaptiveness, and a general will-to-survive. Managing to find some kind of meaning to the disaster aids recovery, as does finding someone to blame for it, both of which can be neatly achieved by attributing it to God's will.

Disasters are inherently social events. It is, after all, only the fact that a human population is adversely affected by such things as earthquakes that makes them disasters at all. Disasters are also of sociological interest because the effects of most disastrous events are related to socio-economic status. Those at the bottom of the social pile tend to be more vulnerable to the negative effects of most extreme events, whether it is food shortages, flood or war. A disaster can be thought of, therefore, as an expression of social vulnerabilities which result from the underlying societal ordering. It is, for example, the fact that the poor of Bangladesh can only afford to live in areas liable to floods that makes them so susceptible to them when they happen. It is a social crisis generated from within. This is particularly important with respect to the psychological morbidity associated with disasters, because mental health problems are also related to socio-economic status. The poorest in society tend to be exposed to a wider variety and greater depth of social stressors in their everyday lives, meaning that they tend to experience higher levels of mental disorder. At any one time, therefore, a

---

[8] On PTSD see esp. Neria et al. 2009.

sizeable minority of the overall populace will already be suffering from mental health problems before a disaster strikes, and a disproportionate number will be from those of lower socio-economic status. Not only are the poor, therefore, more likely to suffer from mental disorders, they are more likely to be negatively affected by the consequences of a disaster, at the same time as having less access to resources to help them cope.

How much of this modern theory is applicable to the ancient world? To begin with, three caveats need to be stressed. The first is that most modern research of the mental health impact of disasters has concentrated on American examples. It is highly unlikely that these findings can simply be applied to Roman examples and expected to produce similar results. The second is that even in modern disasters, or even different analyses of the same disaster, the range of results concerning levels of mental disorders varies considerably. We must be careful, therefore, not to treat the figures quoted above as anything more than indicative, if informed, guesses. Thirdly, levels of reported mental disorder following modern disasters vary considerably from society to society. Cultural attitudes towards fear, resilience, and self have significant roles in affecting the reported level of mental health. These considerations suggest that the problems involved in applying such concepts to the ancient world mean that we should not imagine that we can use modern evidence to predict the degree nor the forms that such mental ill-health would have taken in antiquity. Each period of history attacks its inhabitants' mental health in its own particular way and in doing so generates its own unique form of mental disorder. Moreover, the mind is never purely a personal phenomenon. It is both individually and socially created and experienced, and is affected by broader societal processes. Conceptions about the relationship between disasters and individual psychiatric suffering will always be linked to wider social attitudes towards suffering, blame, and disorder. The best we can probably hope to achieve, therefore, is to explain something about how a certain style of psychiatric expression has emerged from a specific social and cultural context.

Religious ideas dominated most Roman explanations of disaster. They were primarily seen as acts of gods. Propitiatory attempts to placate the gods were therefore common and widely believed to be effective. Aristeides felt convinced that it was his sacrifice which had stopped the tremors of an earthquake.[9] The occurrence of disasters presents problems for reli-

---

[9] Aristeides, *Or.* 49.38–40.

gions in that, as well as requiring some level of justification, they disrupt the normal relationship between the natural and divine worlds.[10] Roman responses normally centred around rituals which declared that communal unity had survived the shock of the disaster and remained the basis for continuity. Such responses could take a range of forms, such as consultations with oracles, public prayer, communal processions, and ritual fasting. But scepticism towards the divine could also be an understandable response to the apparent injustices thrown up by a disaster and the clear failure of the gods to protect their devoted worshippers. Thucydides famously noted that the Athenians lost their faith in the gods during the plague at the beginning of the Peloponnesian War. That this was, perhaps, a fairly common response in the Roman world is suggested by Artemidorus' interpretation of dreams involving the desecration of religious sites: he says, 'to commit any sacrilegious act in a temple is inauspicious for all men and portends great crises. For men who are in great distress also abandon their reverence towards the gods'.[11]

Christians saw disasters more as an inbuilt, if mysterious, part of the divine plan for the universe. As such, disasters were simply something to be, at the very least, patiently endured, if not positively welcomed. The advent of a calamitous event represented a God-given opportunity for the individual and the community to repent and reform before the coming of judgement day made it too late. Disasters could also be interpreted within this framework as being a divine punishment for sin. The victims themselves were stigmatized and the blame attached to them. Disaster was seen as being caused by a moral impurity, one which the power of temptation could make highly contagious. Pseudo-Joshua the Stylite's chronicle covers what he calls the 'period of distress' lasting from 494–506 CE, and is replete with severe disasters. In fact, these serve as the 'ideological backbone' of the text, since they support both a moralistic interpretation of the terrible events which occur and also to highlight that this period should be seen as the run-up to that ultimate of all destructive events, the apocalypse.[12] In his view, it was the sins of the townspeople of Edessa which had brought a famine justly upon themselves. They had begun celebrations in the theatre a full seven days before the festival should properly have started, a festival, moreover, where lascivious mimes were enacted. For Joshua, it was no

---

[10] Garnsey 1990, 143.
[11] Artemidorus, *The Interpretation of Dreams* 2.33 trans. White 1975.
[12] Stathakopoulos 2004, 255.

coincidence that when the mimes were banned by the emperor Anastasius in 502 CE the famine eased within thirty days.[13]

That such powerfully moralistic views of disasters were problematic was implicitly recognised by widespread explanations which attributed them to external demons. In the *Life of St Simeon the Stylite*, a large ship is sailing to Syria when a dreadful storm arises. The passengers 'cried out and were distressed and supplicated with tears and groans', as 'they felt sure that they should never see dry land again, especially because they saw a man who was black and looked like an Indian [which probably means like an Ethiopian or a black African], who came and stood on the top of the mast'. This was a demon of whom it was said that 'every time he was seen in a ship he sank her'.[14] Materialistically conceived demons of this type were also blamed for loving to spread rumours about imminent disasters, often falsely. As Athanasius says in his *Life of Antony*, demons 'sometimes talk nonsense in regard to the water of the Nile'. For when 'seeing heavy rains falling in the regions of Ethiopia and knowing that the flooding of the River originates there, they run ahead and tell it before the water reaches Egypt'. Athanasius complains that it is no use to people to find out from demons what is going to happen days in advance; knowledge is not the basis of salvation but keeping the faith and the commandments.[15] Written as part of a long section against the popular use of oracles, what these passages tell us is that people did not automatically accept the Christian doctrine that their own moral failings were themselves responsible for their suffering. They preferred to see wicked supernatural agents as the problem.

Demons made excellent explanatory agents for disasters because of what Brown calls their 'anomalous' nature.[16] Demons were held responsible for all kinds of confusion in human social relations and so it made sense to attribute to them the great chaos and disorder of disasters. Mental disorder was also believed to be caused by demons. It is important to emphasise that demons were a complex phenomenon that cannot simply be approached from a comparative mental health standpoint; the role of demons in Roman society had social, political and, not least, theological aspects. But a society which placed great emphasis on the correct order of things found all kinds of disorder, including mental, deeply problematic and found it easy and natural to associate it with the demonic.

---

[13] *The Chronicle of Pseudo-Joshua the Stylite* ch. 30.
[14] *Life of Simeon the Stylite* in Lent 1915, 172–173.
[15] Athanasius, *The Life of Saint Antony*, ch. 32 & 33.
[16] Brown 1978, 20.

For it was the disordering effects of disasters that seem to have generated the greatest distress in Late Roman society. Disasters brought out into the open the conflicts and schisms which threatened to destabilize the Late Antique world. John of Ephesus, in his account of the flood that afflicted Edessa in 525 CE, explains the disaster as a punishment for the wicked behaviour of the orthodox bishop of the city, Asclepius. The bishop had tortured ten monks who shared John's Monophysite faith in order to make them submit to his Chalcedonian communion, and when they did not comply he imprisoned them, threatening to resume the torture on the next day. The same night, John writes, 'the flood occurred in such a way that it seemed to everyone that God had grown angry at the bishop and at the city on account of the torment of these blessed ones'. Understandably the populace reacted by trying to stone him to death.

The Chinese symbol for disaster is a combination of two different characters, one symbolising danger the other opportunity.[17] And as the previous example makes clear, disasters could also be seen as opportunities for competing groups to benefit at others' expense. Disasters smashed holes in the iron curtain of the social hierarchy, giving people an opportunity to escape from the stifling constraints of their social ties. For disasters were never only about death and destruction. They were also about recovery and regeneration. In the same way that a disaster, by damaging the social system, could create chances for members of the elite to establish and reaffirm patronage relationships between themselves and their suffering people, so too did it provide the Church with a compelling opportunity to display Christian leadership and thereby add momentum to the drive towards a deeper Christianization of Roman society. It was a way of converting people's sense of post-disaster disorientation into a clearly focused form. By stressing the decadence and immorality of the populace, Christian disaster accounts could hope to promote aggressively a purer world view, a world where higher standards of public behaviour would be driven forward by the example of moral Christian leadership.

In the same way that the disorder thrown up by disasters could be socially useful, so too could mental disorders play a beneficial role at times of social stress. The association of demonic interference with the occurrence of disasters allowed Roman society both to accept and to channel the disruptive influences unleashed by calamity. To focus simply on the negative mental health implications of disasters would be to overlook the very positive

---

[17] See Rodríguez et al. 2007.

functions such disorder could perform in a rigid society. People often needed change and the chaotic environments which disasters could so easily create gave a rare glimpse of alternative social orderings, however discomforting they might have been. It was, perhaps, the holy man who best embodied this imaginative release. Here was a man who through his own personal struggle was immune to the dangers of disasters. Here was a man who, through his proximity to God, had control and expertise over the forces of nature and their effects on man. A man who could drive away locusts and summon down the rains. A symbolic equivalence was established between the ascetic and the common man, which urged the individual to direct his personal stress through him towards the greater glory of God. When it was revealed to Daniel the Stylite that God's wrath was about to fall upon the city of Constantinople in the autumn of 465, he alerted the relevant authorities, both the archbishop and the emperor, 'begging them to order rites of intercession'. Unwilling to interrupt a forthcoming feast, they ignored the holy man's warnings. As a result, when the fire struck, 'all the inhabitants were in great distress and the majority had to flee from the city. They made their way to the holy man and each of them implored him to placate God's anger so that the fire should cease'. Interestingly, we are told that they would 'relate to him the personal misfortunes they had suffered'. One says, 'I have been stripped bare of great possessions'; another complains that, 'I ran away from that terrible danger only to suffer shipwreck of my scanty belongings'. The holy man's response was to weep with them and to emphasise that they had only themselves to blame: 'you should have importuned God and escaped his terrible wrath'. He also spoke 'many other words of counsel' to them and thereby 'turned their hopelessness into hopefulness'.[18] In this dramatic scene, not only can we see the holy man acting as a focus for communal stress, a figure who can help survivors adjust to their new reality of loss, but we also see him turning a dreadful happening into a shining opportunity for positive regeneration and optimism for the future. It was a dramatization used to express, in the deliberately exaggerated form of a disaster context, the emotional structure of a perfect society, one in which no personal suffering could be tolerated by wider society and each individual was held in the comforting embrace of the Church.

We can see all these various interrelated notions of disaster, mental disorder and the demonic at work in John of Ephesus' account of the effects of the Great plague and the mental breakdown of Amida. In the wake of

---

[18] *Life of St Daniel the Stylite* ch. 41 & 45 in Baynes and Dawes 1948.

the plague's first descent on Constantinople, the survivors were profoundly shocked. How, asks John, could 'the heart of the witness of these things not melt inside him'. How could his limbs not dissolve in pain while looking at white-haired old men whose hair has been 'soiled by the putrefaction of their heirs' and 'beautiful girls and virgins', who were 'looking forward to their bridal feasts', but instead are 'discarded, exposed, and soiled by the filth of the other dead'. But in the face of such overwhelming distress, there was 'neither crying nor mourning but only people shocked ... speechless like those drowsy from wine'. The plague seemed to leave their senses incapable of functioning normally. Everyone 'talked to his companion like men drunk with strong beer, baffled and confused. People were easily driven to insanity by the intoxicating plague'. In such a state of mental disarray, people were vulnerable to all kinds of demonic deception. Demons sought to 'mislead people and ridicule their madness', so they made a survivor state that if earthenware pots were thrown from the windows of upper stories the plague would leave the city. John records how 'foolish women ... set their minds to this madness'.

In John's account, the plague created a kind of negative carnival, a time when the normal rules of society were turned upside down.[19] The narrative emphasises how the great disaster created a Christian dystopia, where the extremes of plagues contrasted with the moderation of the good life. Everything is portrayed as the inverted image of what it should be. Plague meant a breakdown in social and moral order that reflected the dreadful nature of the sins that had caused it. Here was, in all its gruesome detail, a shocking foretaste of the eternal punishment that awaited those who did not take note and repent.

In Amida, the plague was but the latest in a long line of disastrous events to afflict the city. As we have seen, the culmination of this perfect storm of disasters was an attack on the mind. It was natural for the sane to try to treat this mental disorder by means of religion. They tried to cure the victims with religious ritual, by gathering them in churches. But even in such places where they should have been on their best behaviour, they continued to look and act differently: 'some were raging and foaming, while others were raving and uttering vulgar words as if from devils in person'. Such disorder lasted for a year and longer in Amida. Susan Harvey rightly points out that it was significant that holy men in the region remained within the city because it was simply too dangerous to live out in the bandit country

---

[19] An idea suggested by C. Jones 1996 concerning the plague in Early Modern France.

surrounding it.[20] This meant that they too were caught up in the plight of the city and so were unable to perform their usual role as a focus for psychological concern. John himself has no idea what caused the outbreak of what DSM IV would probably term 'shared psychotic disorder': 'only god knows,' he explains, 'for what reason and because of what sin this divine abandonment occurred ... that vicious demons might greatly control the youth to the extent of entrapping them in committing filthy debauchery among themselves inside the churches'. We can speculate that the enormous pressure which the threat of military invasion, in the aftermath of repeated disasters, generated an outbreak of mental disorder. But that would not do justice to the range of uses to which mental phenomena could be put in Late Roman society. Disordered, incomprehensible behaviour can also be seen as an oblique but critical reflection by the weak on their powerlessness in society. It represented a safe way to register discontent and perhaps even express defiance. The dangers involved in outright rebellion meant that misery found its expression in a language of mental disorder, a language whose grammar was inversion. It allowed a suffering population, and a disaffected youth, an idiom through which they could say something about the abnormally extreme psychological stress that their social environment was exerting upon them. The Roman world was a highly regimented society which had always made the expression of alternative ideas about society a dangerous business. Deploying the mind avoided the full force of official repression by the state. Psychiatric expression, therefore, became a vehicle for articulating a variety of societal tensions and frustrations in a safe and potentially positive way.

John's disaster narrative created a social dystopia to reflect a deep desire for the ideal society which was its mirror. His account of the many disasters, culminating in the coming of the great plague and the collective madness of Amida, used shocking stories to advertise the perfect Christian society it inverted. The quest for recovery in Amida involved a search for renewed social and religious harmony through rituals, penitence, vows, and processions. Slowly, the treatment began to work: 'one by one and little by little,' John tells us, 'they started to come to their senses. They grieved, wept, groaned and kept busy in prayer and in painful supplication at all time'. Through the medium of religion, the victims were able to be readmitted into normal life in a way that allowed them to avow publicly their renewed enthusiasm for society's ideals. Hence groups of those who had regained

---

[20] Harvey 1990, 57–75.

their senses 'went to Jerusalem and to other holy places for prayers, sorrow-ful, clad in black, making supplication, praying and weeping'. Social values were reasserted. Respect for God, His Church and the community were re-established, and through rituals of prayer and pilgrimage the community was able to state publicly its renewed mental vigour and integrity.

BIBLIOGRAPHY

Most editions of classical authors are omitted.

Adams, F., *The Genuine Works of Hippocrates* (London, 1849).

Adamson, P., *The Arabic Plotinus: a Philosophical Study of the 'Theology of Aristotle'* (London, 2002).

—— 'Miskawayh's Psychology', in P. Adamson (ed.), *Classical Arabic Philosophy: Sources and Reception* (London, 2008), 39–54.

Adamson, P., and Pormann, P.E., *The Philosophical Works of al-Kindî* (Karachi, 2012). (Adamson and Pormann 2012a)

Adamson, P., and Pormann, P.E., 'More than Heat and Light: Miskawayh's *Epistle on Soul and Intellect*', in A. Shihadeh, *On the Ontology of the Soul in Medieval Arabic Thought*, special issue of *The Muslim World* 102 (2012), 478–524. (Adamson and Pormann 2012b)

Aleman, A., and Larøi, F., *Hallucinations: the Science of Idiosyncratic Perception* (Washington, DC, 2008).

American Psychiatric Association, *Diagnostic and Statistical Manual of Mental Disorders, Fourth Edition Text Revision* (DSM-IV-TR) (Washington DC, 2000).

American Psychiatric Association DSM-5 Development, available at: http://www .dsm5.org/Pages/Default.aspx.

Anastassiou, A., 'Zum Enkephalos-Abschnitt der hippokratischen Schriften *De Morbo Sacro*', in Boudon-Millot et al. 2007, 35–40.

Andò, V., 'La verginità come follia: il *Peri parthenion* ippocratico', *Quaderni storici* n. s. 75 (1990), 715–737.

—— '*Psyche* e malattie psichiche nella prima medicina greca', in R. Bruschi (ed.), *Gli irraggiungibili confini. Percorsi della psiche nell'età della Grecia classica* (Pisa, 2007), 103–129.

Angelino, C., and Salvaneschi, E., *Aristotele: La 'melanconia' dell' uomo di genio* (Genova, 1981).

Annas, J., *The Morality of Happiness* (Oxford, 1993).

Arkoun, M., 'Deux épîtres de Miskawayh', *Bulletin d'Études Orientales* 17 (1961/2), 7–74.

Arseneault, L., Cannon, M., Fisher, H.L., Polanczyk, G., Moffitt, T.E., and Caspi, A., 'Childhood Trauma and Children's Emerging Psychotic Symptoms: A Genetically Sensitive Longitudinal Cohort Study', *AJPsy* 168 (2011), 65–72.

Asmis, E., 'Plato on Poetic Creativity,' in Kraut 1992, 338–364.

Asper, M., *Griechische Wissenschaftstexte. Formen, Funktionen, Differenzierungsgeschichten* (Stuttgart, 2007).

Assael, J., 'ΣΥΝΕΣΙΣ dans *Oreste* d'Euripide', *L'Antiquité Classique* 65 (1996), 53–69.

Atlan, H., *L'organisation biologique et la théorie de l'information* (Paris, 1972).

Ayache, L., 'Est-il vraiment question d'art médical dans le *Timée*?', in Calvo and Brisson 1997, 55–63.

Badawî, A., *Dirâsât wa-nuṣûṣ fî l-falsafa wa-l-ʿulûm ʿinda l-ʿArab* [Studies and Texts on Philosophy and Science among the Arabs] (Beirut, 1981).

Baker, G.A., 'The Psychosocial Burden of Epilepsy', *Epilepsia* 43 (2002), 26–30.

—— Jacoby, A., Buck, D., Stagis, C., and Monnet, D., 'Quality of Life of People with Epilepsy: a European Study', *Epilepsia* 38 (1997), 353–362.

Bakker, E.J. (ed.), *A Companion to the Ancient Greek Language* (Oxford, 2010).

—— 'Pragmatics: speech and text', in Bakker 2010, 151–178.

Balansard, A., 'Maladie et laideur de l' âme: la gymnastique comme thérapie chez Platon', in P. Boulhol, F. Gaide, and M. Loubet (eds.), *Guérisons du corps et de l'âme: approches pluridisciplinaires* (Aix-en-Provence, 2006), 29–42.

Baltussen, H. (ed.), *Acts of Consolation: Approaches to Loss and Sorrow from Sophocles to Shakespeare* (Cambridge, forthcoming).

Barker, A., 'Timaeus on Music and the Liver', in Wright 2000, 85–99.

—— 'Transforming the Nightingale: Aspects of Athenian Musical Discourse in the Late Fifth Century', in Murray and Wilson 2004, 185–204.

Barnes, J. (ed.), *The Complete Works of Aristotle: The Revised Oxford Translation* (Princeton, 1984).

—— 'Roman Aristotle', in J. Barnes and M. Griffin (eds.), *Philosophia Togata II: Plato and Aristotle at Rome* (Oxford, 1997), 1–69.

Barton, T.S., *Power and Knowledge: Astrology, Physiognomics, and Medicine under the Roman Empire* (Ann Arbor, 1994).

Bartos, H., 'Varieties of the Ancient Greek Body-soul Distinction', *Rhizai* 3 (2006), 59–78.

Bateson, G., *Steps to an Ecology of Mind: Collected Essays in Anthropology, Psychiatry, Evolution, and Epistemology* (London, 1972).

—— *Mind and Nature: A Necessary Unity* (New York, 1979).

Battezzato, L., *Linguistica e retorica della tragedia greca* (Rome, 2008).

Baynes, N.H., and Dawes, E., *Three Byzantine Saints: Contemporary Biographies* (Oxford, 1948).

Beard, M., 'Cicero and Divination', *JRS* 76 (1986), 33–46.

Becchi, F., 'La nozione di *orgē* e di *aorgēsia* in Aristotele e in Plutarco', *Prometheus* 4 (1978), 65–87.

Benveniste, E., 'La frase nominale', in *Problemi di linguistica generale* (trans. M.V. Giuliani, Milan, 2010), 179–199 (original ed.: *Problèmes de linguistique générale*, Paris, 1966).

Berges, S., 'Virtue as Mental Health: A Platonic Defence of the Medical Model in Ethics', *Journal of Ancient Philosophy* (on-line) 6, 2012, Issue I.

Berrettoni, P., 'Il lessico tecnico del I e III libro delle Epidemie ippocratiche. Contributo alla storia della formazione della terminologia medica greca', *Annali della Scuola Normale Superiore di Pisa* 39 (1970), 27–106 and 217–311.

Berthoz, A., *Le sens du mouvement* (Paris, 1997).

—— and Petit, J.-L., *Physiologie de l'action et Phénoménologie* (Paris, 2006).

Black, J.A., *The Four Elements in Plato's Timaeus* (Lewiston, NY, 2000).

Bleuler, E., *Dementia praecox, oder Gruppe der Schizophrenien* (Leipzig, 1911) (trans. J. Zinkin as *Dementia Praecox, or the Group of Schizophrenias*, New York, 1950).

Bobonich, C., and Destrée, P. (eds.), *Akrasia in Greek Philosophy. From Socrates to Plotinus* (Leiden, 2007).

Bohner, H., *Nô. Die Einzelnen Nô*. Mitteilungen der Deutschen Gesellschaft für Natur- und Völkerkunde Ostasiens, Supplementband 22 (Tokyo and Wiesbaden, 1956).

Bonanno, M., *L'allusione necessaria: ricerche intertestuali sulla poesia greca e latina* (Rome, 1990).

Bordt, M., *Platons Theologie* (Freiburg, 2006).

Borgeaud, P., 'The Death of the Great Pan: the Problem of Interpretation', *History of Religions* 22 (1983), 254–283.

—— *The Cult of Pan in Ancient Greece* (trans. K. Atlass and J. Redfield, Chicago, 1988) (original ed.: *Recherches sur le dieu Pan*, Rome, 1979).

Borges, J.L., *Other Inquisitions, 1937–1952* (trans. R. Simms, Austin, TX, 1964) (original ed.: *Otros inquisiciones*, Buenos Aires, 1952).

Bortolotti, L., *Delusions and Other Irrational Beliefs* (Oxford, 2010).

Bostock, D., *Plato's* Theaetetus (Oxford, 1988).

—— *Space, Time, Matter and Form: Essays on Aristotle's Physics* (Oxford, 2006).

Boudon-Millot, V., 'Un traité miraculeusement retrouvé, Sur *l'inutilité de se chagriner*: texte grec et traduction française', in Boudon-Millot et al. 2007, 73–124.

—— 'De Pythagore à Maxime Planude en passant par Galien: la fortune exceptionnelle de l'adage médicophilosophique ὡς μήτε πεινῆν μήτε ῥιγοῦν μήτε διψῆν', in Perilli et al. 2011, 3–27.

—— Guardasole, A., and Magdelaine, C. (eds.), *La science médicale antique. Nouveaux regards. Études réunies en l'honneur de Jacques Jouanna* (Paris, 2007).

—— Jouanna, J., and Pietrobelli, A. (eds.), *Galien: Ne pas se chagriner* (Paris, 2010).

—— and Pietrobelli, A., 'Galien ressusicité: Édition princeps du texte grec du *De propriis placitis*', *Revue des Etudes Grecques* 118 (2005), 168–213.

Bowie, E., '*Miles ludens*? The Problem of Martial Exhortation in Early Greek Elegy', in Murray 1990, 221–229.

Boyer, P. *Religion Explained: the Evolutionary Origins of Religious Thought* (New York, 2001).

Breslau, J., 'Introduction: Cultures of Trauma: Anthropological Views of Posttraumatic Stress Disorder in International Health', *Culture, Medicine, Psychiatry* 28 (2004), 113–126.

—— 'Response to "Commentary: Deconstructing Critiques on the Internationalization of PTSD"', *Culture, Medicine, Psychiatry* 29 (2005), 371–376.

Brillante, C., 'Il sogno nella riflessione dei presocratici', *Materiali e Discussioni per l'analisi dei testi antichi* 16 (1986), 9–53.

Brisson, L., 'Du bon usage du dérèglement', in J.-P. Vernant (ed.), *Divination et rationalité* (Paris, 1974), 220–248.

Brittain, C., *Philo of Larissa: The Last of the Academic Sceptics* (Oxford, 2001).

Brown, P., *The Making of Late Antiquity* (Cambridge, MA, 1978).

Buckland, W.W., *A Text-book of Roman Law from Augustus to Justinian* (3rd ed., rev. P. Stein) (Cambridge, 2007).

Bundrick, S.D., *Music and Image in Classical Athens* (Cambridge, 2005).

Burkert, W., *Greek Religion: Archaic and Classical* (trans. J. Raffan, Oxford, 1985) (original ed.: *Griechische Religion der archaischen und klassischen Epoche*, Stuttgart, 1977).

—— *Creation of the Sacred: Tracks of Biology in Early Religions* (Cambridge, Mass., 1996).

Burnyeat, M.F., *Culture and Society in Plato's Republic* (Salt Lake City, 1997).

—— 'Plato on Why Mathematics is Good for the Soul', *Proceedings of the British Academy* 103 (2000), 1–81.

Burton, T., *The Anatomy of Melancholy* (1621), ed. T.C. Faulkner, N.K. Kiessling and R.L. Blair (Oxford, 1989) (based on the 1632 edition).

Byl, S., 'Le vocabulaire de l'intelligence dans le chapitre 35 du livre I du traité du *Régime*', *Revue de philologie, de littérature et d'histoire anciennes* 76 (2002), 217–224.

—— 'Le délire hippocratique dans son contexte', *Revue Belge de Philologie et d'Histoire* 84 (2006), 5–24.

Calvo, T., and Brisson, L. (eds.), *Interpreting the* Timaeus—Critias. *Proceedings of the IV Symposium Platonicum* (Sankt Augustin, 1997),

Cambiano, G., 'Une interprétation 'matérialiste' des rêves: *Du Régime* IV', in Grmek 1980, 87–96.

Carr Vaughan, A., *Madness in Greek Thought and Custom* (Baltimore, 1919).

Cartwright, S.A., 'Diseases and Peculiarities of the Negro Race', *New Orleans Medical and Surgical Journal* (1851), 691–715.

Casey, M., *Jesus of Nazareth: an Independent Historian's Account of his Life and Thinking* (London, 2010).

Cellucci, C., 'Mente incarnata e conoscenza', in E. Canone (ed.), *Per una storia del concetto di mente* (Florence, 2005), 383–410.

Centrone, B., Μελαγχολικός in Aristotele e il *Problema* XXX 1', in B. Centrone (ed.), *Studi sui Problemata Physica aristotelici* (Naples, 2011), 309–339.

Chaniotis, A., 'Illness and Cures in the Greek Propitiatory Inscriptions and Dedications of Lydia and Phrygia', in van der Eijk et al. 1995, II, 323–344.

Chantraine, P., *Dictionnaire étymologique de la langue grecque. Histoire des mots* (Paris, 2009). (*DELG*)

Ciani, M.G., 'Lessico e funzione della follia nella tragedia greca', *Bollettino dell'Istituto di Filologia Greca dell'Università di Padova* 1 (1974), 70–111.

—— *Psicosi e creatività nella scienza antica* (Venice, 1983).

Clark, A., and Chalmers, D.J., 'The Extended Mind', *Analysis* 58 (1998), 10–23.

Clark, P.A., *The Balance of the Mind: The Experience and Perception of Mental Illness in Antiquity* (unpublished diss., University of Washington, 1993).

Clarke, E., 'Apoplexy in the Hippocratic Writings', *Bulletin of the History of Medicine* 37 (1963), 301–314.

Classen, C.J., 'Die Peripatetiker in Cicero's *Tuskulanen*', in Fortenbaugh and Steinmetz 1989, 186–200.

Classen, J., *Beobachtungen über den Homerischen Sprachgebrauch* (Frankfurt, 1879).

Clifton, F., *Hippocrates upon Air, Water, and Situation; upon Epidemical Diseases; and upon Prognosticks, in Acute Cases especially* (London, 1734).

Cohen, D., *Law, Violence and Community in Classical Athens* (Cambridge, 1995).

Collinge, N., 'Medical Terms and Clinical Attitudes in the Tragedians', *Bulletin of the Institute of Classical Studies* 9 (1962), 43–55.

Cooper, J.E., Kendell, R.E., Gurland, B.J., Sartorius, N., and Farkas, T., 'Cross-national

Study of Diagnosis of the Mental Disorders: some Results from the First Comparative Investigation', *AJPsy* 125 (1969), Supplement, 21–29.

Cooper, J.M., *Reason and Emotion. Essays on Ancient Moral Psychology and Ethical Theory* (Princeton, 1999).

Cooper, R., 'What is Wrong with the DSM?', *History of Psychiatry* 15 (2004), 5–24.

Corvisier, J.-N., *Santé et société en Grèce ancienne* (Paris, 1985).

Croally, N.T., *Euripidean Polemic. The Trojan Women and the Function of Tragedy* (Cambridge, 1994).

Croissant, J., *Aristote et les mystères* (Liège and Paris, 1932).

Crotty, K., rev. of Robinson 1996, *Bryn Mawr Classical Review* 10.14 (1997).

Cumont, F., *L'Égypte des Astrologues* (Brussels, 1937).

Cusset, C., *Ménandre ou la comédie tragique* (Paris, 2003).

Daly, D.D., 'Reflections on the Concept of Petit Mal', *Epilepsia* 9 (1968), 175–178.

Damasio, A.R., *Descartes' Error: Emotion, Reason, and the Human Brain* (New York, 1994).

―――― *The Feeling of What Happens: Body and Emotion in the Making of Consciousness* (New York, 1999).

D'Ancona, C., *Recherches sur le Liber de Causis* (Paris, 1995).

Dandrey, P. (ed.), *Anthologie de l'humeur noire: Écrits sur la mélancholie d'Hippocrate à l'Encyclopédie* (Paris, 2005).

Darbo-Peschanski, C., 'L'âme d'un fou à travers son acte dans Aristote, *Éthique à Nicomaque*', *Chora* 9/10 (2011/2012), 243–257.

Davey, G.C.L. (ed.), *Phobias. A Handbook of Theory, Research and Treatment* (Chichester, 1997).

David, A.S., 'The Cognitive Neuropsychiatry of Auditory Verbal Hallucinations: An Overview', *Cognitive Neuropsychiatry* 9 (2004), 107–124.

Davidson, H.A., *Alfarabi, Avicenna, and Averroes, on Intellect: Their Cosmologies, Theories of the Active Intellect, and Theories of Human Intellect* (New York and Oxford, 1992).

Davidson, J., *Courtesans and Fishcakes: the Consuming Passions of Classical Athens* (London, 1997).

De Boer, H., Mula, M., and Sander, J.W., 'The Global Burden and Stigma of Epilepsy', *Epilepsy and Behaviour* 12 (2008), 540–546.

Debru, A., 'L'épilepsie dans le *De somno* d'Aristote', in G. Sabbah (ed.), *Médecins et médecine dans l'antiquité* (Saint-Etienne, 1982), 25–41.

―――― 'Les démonstrations médicales à Rome au temps de Galien', in van der Eijk et al. 1995, I, 69–81.

Degen, R., and Niedermeyer, E. (eds.), *Epilepsy, Sleep, and Sleep Deprivation* (Amsterdam and New York, 1984).

de Jong, J.T.V.M., 'Commentary: Deconstructing Critiques on the Internationalization of PTSD', *Culture, Medicine, Psychiatry* 29 (2005), 361–370.

De Lacy, P., 'Galen's Platonism', *American Journal of Philology* 93 (1972), 27–39.

―――― 'Galen's Concept of Continuity', *Greek, Roman, and Byzantine Studies* 20 (1979), 355–369.

―――― 'The Third Part of the Soul', in Manuli and Vegetti 1988, 43–63.

Delatte, A., 'Les conceptions de l'enthousiasme chez les philosophes présocratiques', *L'Antiquite Classique* 3 (1934), 5–79.

Demont, P., 'Observations sur le champ sémantique du changement dans la Collection hippocratique', in López Férez 1992, 305–317.

――― 'About Philosophy and Humoural Medicine', in van der Eijk 2005b, 271–286.

Dench, E., rev. of Toner, *Popular Culture in Ancient Rome, London Review of Books*, 17 February 2011, 27–28.

den Dulk, W.J. (ed.), *Krasis. Bijdrage tot de Grieksche Lexicographie* (Leiden, 1934).

Denyer, N., 'The Case against Divination. An Examination of Cicero's De divinatione', *Proceedings of the Cambridge Philological Society* 31 (1985), 1–10.

De Sousa, R., *The Rationality of Emotion* (Cambridge, MA, 1991).

Devereux, G., 'The Nature of Sappho's Seizure in fr. 31 LP as Evidence of her Inversion', *CQ* 20 (1970), 17–31.

Devereux, G., *Dreams in Greek Tragedy: an Ethno-psycho-analytic Study* (Berkeley, 1976).

Diagnostic and Statistical Manual of Mental Disorders: see American Psychiatric Association.

Di Benedetto, V., *Euripide: teatro e società* (Turin, 1971).

――― *Il medico e la malattia. La scienza di Ippocrate* (Turin, 1986).

Dietrich, B.C., 'Divine Epiphanies in Homer', *Numen* 30 (1983), 53–79.

Diliberto, O., *Studi sulle origini della 'cura furiosi'* (Naples, 1984).

Dillon, J., 'How Does the Soul Direct the Body, After All? Traces of a Dispute on Mind-Body Relations in the Old Academy', in D. Frede and B. Reis (eds), *Body and Soul in Ancient Philosophy* (Berlin, 2009), 349–356.

Dixsaut, M., 'Divination et prophétie (*Timée* 71a–72d)', in C. Natali and S. Maso (eds.), Plato physicus. *Cosmologia e antropologia nel* Timeo (Amsterdam, 2003), 275–291.

Doctor, R.M., Kahn, A.P., and Adamec, C., *The Encyclopedia of Phobias, Fears and Anxieties* (third edition, New York, 2008).

Dodds, E.R., *The Greeks and the Irrational* (Berkeley and Los Angeles, 1951).

――― *The Ancient Concept of Progress and other Essays on Greek Literature and Belief* (Oxford, 1973).

Dols, M.W., *Majnūn: the Madman in Medieval Islamic Society* (Oxford, 1992).

Donadi, F., 'In margine alla follia di Oreste', *Bollettino dell'Istituto di Filologia Greca dell'Università di Padova* 1 (1974), 11–27.

Donini, P., 'Psychology', in Hankinson 2008, 184–209.

Dover, K.J., *Greek Popular Morality in the Time of Plato and Aristotle* (Oxford, 1974).

Draaisma, D., *Disturbances of the Mind* (trans. B. Fasting) (Cambridge, 2009).

Drabkin, I.E., *Caelius Aurelianus: On Acute and On Chronic Diseases* (Chicago, 1950).

――― 'Remarks on Ancient Psychopathology', *Isis* 46 (1955), 223–234.

Dulaey, M., *Le rêve dans la vie et la pensée de Saint-Augustin* (Paris, 1973).

Dumortier, J., *Le vocabulaire médical d'Eschyle et les écrits hippocratiques* (Paris, 1935).

Duminil, M.-P., *Le sang, les vaisseaux, le cœur dans la collection hippocratique* (Paris, 1983).

Eadie, M.J., 'Louis François Bravais and Jacksonian Epilepsy', *Epilepsia* 51 (2010), 1–6.

――― and Bladin, P.F., *A Disease Once Sacred: a History of the Medical Understanding of Epilepsy* (Eastleigh, Hampshire, 2001).

Eckert, M., *Theories of Mind. An Introductory Reader* (Lanham, MD, 2006)

Edelman, G.M., *Neural Darwinism: The Theory of Neuronal Group Selection* (New York, 1987).

—— *Bright Air, Brilliant Fire. On the Matter of the Mind* (New York, 1992).

—— *Second Nature. Brain Science and Human Knowledge* (New York, 2006).

Effe, B., 'Tragischer Wahnsinn: ein Motiv der attischen Tragödie und seine Funktionalisierung', in B. Effe and R.F. Glei (eds), *Genie und Wahnsinn: Konzepte psychischer 'Normalität' und 'Abnormität' im Altertum* (Trier, 2000), 45–62.

Elder, R., Evans, K., and Nizette, D., *Psychiatric and Mental Health Nursing* (second ed., Chatswood, NSW, 2009).

El-Hai, J., *The Lobotomist: A Maverick Medical Genius and His Tragic Quest to Rid the World of Mental Illness* (Hoboken, NJ, 2005).

Enders, H., *Schlaf und Traum bei Aristoteles* (Würzburg, 1923).

Enge, M., *Psychische Erkrankungen bei Hippokrates, Celsus und Aretaius* (Frankfurt, 1991).

Erler, M., and Schofield, M., 'Epicurean Ethics', in K. Algra, J. Barnes, J. Mansfeld, and M. Schofield (eds.), *The Cambridge History of Hellenistic Philosophy* (Cambridge, 1999), 642–674.

Errera, P., 'Some Historical Aspects of the Concept Phobia', *Psychiatric Quarterly* 36 (1962), 325–336.

Erskine, A., 'Cicero and the Expression of Grief', in S.M. Braund and C. Gill (eds.), *The Passions in Roman Thought and Literature* (Cambridge, 1997), 36–48.

Esquirol, J.-E., *Mental Maladies. A Treatise on Insanity* (trans. E.K. Hunt, Philadelphia, 1845) (original ed.: *Des Maladies mentales considérées sous les rapports médical, hygiénique et médico-légal*, Paris, 1838).

Evans, M., 'Plato and the Meaning of Pain', *Apeiron* 40 (2004), 71–93.

Evans Grubbs, J., *Women and the Law in the Roman Empire: A Sourcebook on Marriage, Divorce, and Widowhood* (London and New York, 2002).

Everson, S., 'The *De somno* and Aristotle's Explanation of Sleep', *CQ* 57 (2007), 502–520.

Farenga, V., *Citizen and Self in Ancient Greece: Individuals Performing Justice and the Law* (Cambridge, 2006).

Farr, S., *The History of Epidemics, by Hippocrates* (London, 1780).

Fehr, B., 'Entertainers at the *symposion*: the *akletoi* in the Archaic Period', in Murray 1990, 185–195.

Féré, C., *Les épilepsies et les épileptiques* (Paris, 1890).

Ferrini, F., 'Tragedia e patologia: lessico ippocratico in Euripide', *QUCC* 29 (1978), 49–62.

Fischer, K.-D., 'De fragmentis Herae Cappadocis atque Rufi Ephesii hactenus ignotis', *Galenos* 4 (2010), 173–183.

—— '*Ex occidente lux*: Greek Medical Works as Represented in Pre-Salernitan Latin Translations', in Perilli et al. 2011, 29–55.

Flashar, H., 'Die medizinischen Grundlagen der Lehre von der Wirkung der Dichtung in der griechischen Poetik', *Hermes* 84 (1956), 12–48.

—— (ed.), *Aristoteles*: Problemata Physica (Berlin, 1962).

—— *Melancholie und Melancholiker in den medizinischen Theorien der Antike* (Berlin, 1966).

Flemming, R., *Medicine and the Making of Roman Women. Gender, Nature, and Authority from Celsus to Galen* (Oxford, 2000).

—— 'Commentary', in Hankinson 2008, 323–354.

Fodor, J.A., 'The Mind-Body Problem', in Eckert 2006, 81–95.

Foës, Anuce, *Hippocratis Opera Omnia* (Frankfurt am Main, 1595).

Ford, A., 'Catharsis: the Power of Music in Aristotle's *Politics*', in Murray and Wilson 2004, 309–336.

Forschner, M., *Die Stoische Ethik* (Stuttgart, 1981).

Fortenbaugh, W.W., and Steinmetz, P. (eds.), *Cicero's Knowledge of the Peripatos* (New Brunswick, 1989).

Foucault, M., *The Care of the Self* (trans. R. Hurley, London, 1990) (original ed.: *Histoire de la sexualité* III, Paris, 1984).

—— *History of Madness* (trans. J. Murphy and J. Khalfa, London and New York, 2006) (original ed.: *Histoire de la folie à l'âge classique*, Paris, 1972).

Frances, A., 'A Warning Sign on the Road to *DSM-V*: Beware of its Unintended Consequences', *Psychiatric Times* (26th June 2009); available at: www.psychiatrictimes .com/display/article/10168/1425378 [accessed 14th December 2010].

—— 'DSM in Philosophyland: Curiouser and Curiouser', *Association for the Advancement of Philosophy and Psychiatry, Bulletin* 17 (2010), 2–5.

—— 'Good Grief', *The New York Times* (14 August 2010).

—— 'The Uses and Misuses of Psychiatric Diagnosis', Paper delivered at the conference 'Situating Mental Illness', ICI Kultur Labor Berlin, 28–29 April (2011).

Francis, S.R., 'Under the Influence—the Physiology and Therapeutics of *akrasia* in Aristotle's Ethics', *CQ* 61 (2011), 143–171.

Frede, D., 'Disintegration and Restoration: Pleasure and Pain in Plato's *Philebus*', in Kraut 1992, 425–463.

Frede, M., 'The Method of the so-called Methodical School of Medicine', in J. Barnes, J. Brunschwig, M. Burnyeat, and M. Schofield (eds.), *Science and Speculation: Studies in Hellenistic Theory and Practice* (Cambridge, 1982), 1–23.

—— 'The Stoic Doctrine of the Affections of the Soul', in M. Schofield and G. Striker (eds.), *The Norms of Nature: Studies in Hellenistic Ethics* (Cambridge, 1986), 93–110.

Freeman, W.J., 'Abstracts from Current Literature: The Neurology of Hippocrates', *Archives of Neurology and Psychiatry* 34 (1935), 654–658.

Freud, S., *Studies on Hysteria* (trans. J. Strachey, London, 1955) (original ed.: J. Breuer and S. Freud, *Studien über Hysterie*, Leipzig and Vienna, 1895).

Friedlander, W.J., *The History of Modern Epilepsy: the Beginning, 1865–1914* (Westport, CT, 2001).

Fronterotta, F., 'Anima e corpo: immortalità, organicismo e psico-fisiologia nel *Timeo* platonico', *Études platoniciennes* 2 (2006), 141–154.

Frontisi-Ducroux, F., and Lissarague, F., 'From Ambiguity to Ambivalence: a Dionysiac Excursion through the 'Anakreontic' Vases', in D. Halperin (ed.), *Before Sexuality: the Construction of Erotic Experience in the Ancient Greek World* (Princeton, 1990), 211–256.

Fuchs, R., 'Anecdota medica Graeca', *Rheinisches Museum für Philologie* 50 (1895), 576–599.

Fulford, K.W.M., *Moral Theory and Medical Practice* (Cambridge, 1989).

——, Thornton, T., and Graham, G., *Oxford Textbook of Philosophy and Psychiatry* (Oxford, 2006).

Fuller, R.H., 'Resurrection of Christ', in B.M. Metzger and M.D. Coogan (eds.), *The Oxford Companion to the Bible* (New York, 1993), 647–649.

Gallop, D., *Aristotle: On Sleep and Dreams* (Warminster, 1996).

García-Ballester, L., *Alma y enfermedad en la obra de Galeno* (Valencia and Granada, 1972).

—— 'Soul and Body. Disease of the Soul and Disease of the Body in Galen's Medical Thought', in Manuli and Vegetti 1988, 117–152.

Garcia Gual, C., 'Del melancolico como atrabilario. Segun las antiguas ideas griecas sobre la enfermedad de la melancholia', *Faventia* 6 (1984), 41–50.

Garnsey, P., 'Responses to Food Crisis in the Ancient Mediterranean World', in L.F. Newman (ed.), *Hunger in History: Food Shortage, Poverty, and Deprivation* (Oxford, 1990), 126–146.

Garofalo, I., 'La traduzione araba del *de sectis* e il *sommario degli Alessandrini*', *Galenos* 1 (2007), 191–210.

Garvie A.F., *Aeschylus' Persae, with Introduction and Commentary* (Oxford, 2009).

Geller, M., 'Look to the Stars: Babylonian medicine, Magic, Astrology and *melothesia*', Max Planck Institut für Wissenschaftsgeschichte, Preprint 401 (Berlin, 2010).

Gentili, B., and Luisi, F., 'La *Pitica* 12 di Pindaro e l'aulo di Mida', *QUCC* 49 (1995), 7–31.

Gerolemou, M., *Bad Women, Mad Women. Gender und Wahnsinn in der griechischen Tragödie* (Tübingen, 2011).

Ghaemi, N., 'DSM-IV, Hippocrates, and Pragmatism: What Might Have Been', *Association for the Advancement of Philosophy and Psychiatry, Bulletin* 17 (2010), 33–35.

Gigon, O., *Sokrates: sein Bild in Dichtung und Geschichte* (Bern, 1947).

—— 'Cicero und Aristoteles', *Hermes* 87 (1959), 143–162.

Gill, C., 'Ancient Psychotherapy', *Journal of the History of Ideas* 46 (1985), 307–325.

—— 'Personhood and Personality: The Four-*Personae* Theory in Cicero, *De Officiis* 1', *OSAP* 6 (1988), 169–199.

—— 'Peace of Mind and Being Yourself: Panaetius to Plutarch', in *ANRW* II.36.7 (Berlin, 1994), 4599–640.

—— 'Mind and Madness', *Apeiron* 29 (1996), 249–268.

—— *Personality in Greek Epic, Tragedy, and Philosophy: The Self in Dialogue* (Oxford, 1996).

—— 'The Body's Fault? Plato's *Timaeus* on Psychic Illness', in Wright 2000, 59–84.

—— 'The School in the Roman Imperial Period', in Inwood 2003, 33–58.

—— (ed.), *Virtue, Norms, and Objectivity: Issues in Ancient and Modern Ethics* (Oxford, 2005).

—— 'Psychophysical Holism in Stoicism and Epicureanism', in R.A.H. King 2006, 209–231. (Gill 2006a).

—— *The Structured Self in Hellenistic and Roman Thought* (Oxford, 2006). (Gill 2006b).

—— 'Galen and the Stoics: Mortal Enemies or Blood Brothers?', *Phronesis* 52 (2007), 88–120. (Gill 2007a).

—— 'Marcus Aurelius', in Sorabji and Sharples 2007, I, 175–187. (Gill 2007b).

—— *Naturalistic Psychology in Galen and Stoicism* (Oxford, 2010). (Gill 2010a).

—— 'Particulars, Selves and Individuals in Stoic Philosophy', in R.W. Sharples (ed.), *Particulars in Greek Philosophy* (Leiden, 2010), 127–147. (Gill 2010b).

——, Whitmarsh, T., and Wilkins, J. (eds.), *Galen and the World of Knowledge* (Cambridge, 2009).

Giuliani, L., 'Sleeping Furies: Allegory, Narration and the Impact of Texts in Apulian Vase-Painting', *Scripta Classica Israelica* 20 (2001), 17–38.

Gleason, M., 'Shock and Awe: The Performance Dimension of Galen's Anatomy Demonstrations', in Gill et al. 2009, 85–114.

Godderis, J., *Antieke geneeskunde over lichaamskwalen en psychische stoornissen van de oude dag. Peri Geros* (Leuven, 1989).

Görler, W., 'Cicero und die 'Schule des Aristoteles'', in Fortenbaugh and Steinmetz 1989, 246–263.

Gottschalk, H., 'Aristotelian Philosophy in the Roman World from the Time of Cicero to the End of the Second Century A.D.', *ANRW* II.36.2 (Berlin, 1987), 1079–1174.

Gourevitch, D., 'Asclépiade de Bithynie dans Pline: problèmes de chronologie', in J. Pigeaud and J. Oroz-Reta (eds.), *Pline l'Ancien: Témoin de son temps* (Salamanca and Nantes, 1987), 67–81.

—— 'La pratique méthodique: définition de la maladie, indication et traitement', in Mudry and Pigeaud 1991, 51–81.

Gourevitch, D. and Gourevitch, M., 'Histoire d'Io', *L'Évolution psychiatrique* 2 (1979), 263–279.

—— 'Phobies', *L'Évolution psychiatrique* 47 (1982), 888–899.

Gourinat, J.-B., 'La «prohairesis» chez Épictète: décision, volonté, ou «personne morale»?', *Philosophie Antique* 5 (2005), 93–134.

Gowers, W.R., *Epilepsy and Other Chronic Convulsive Diseases* (London, 1885).

Grams, L., 'Medical Theory in Plato's *Timaeus*', *Rhizai* 6 (2009), 161–192.

Graumann, L.A., *Die Krankengeschichten der Epidemienbücher des Corpus Hippocraticum. Medizinhistorische Bedeutung und Möglichkeiten der retrospektiven Diagnose* (Aachen, 2000).

Gravel, P., 'Aristote: sur le vin, le sexe, la folie, le génie. Mélancolie', *Études Françaises* 18 (1982), 129–145.

Graver, M.R. (tr.), *Cicero on the Emotions: Tusculan Disputations 3 and 4* (Chicago, 2002).

—— 'Mania and Melancholy: Some Stoic Texts on Insanity', in J. Sickinger and G. Bakewell (eds.), *Gestures: Essays on Ancient Greek History, Literature, and Philosophy in Honor of Alan Boegehold* (Oxford, 2003), 40–54.

—— *Stoicism and Emotion* (Chicago, 2007).

Gregory, J., *Euripides and the Instruction of the Athenians* (Ann Arbor, 1991).

Grieve, J. (trans.), *Aulus Cornelius Celsus, Of Medicine in Eight Books* (Edinburgh, 1814).

Griffith M., *Aeschylus, Prometheus Bound* (Cambridge, 1983).

Grimby, A., 'Bereavement among Elderly People: Grief Reactions, Post-Bereavement Hallucinations and Quality of Life', *Acta Psychiatrica Scandinavica* 87 (1993), 72–80.

—— 'Hallucinations Following the Loss of a Spouse: Common and Normal Events among the Elderly', *Journal of Geropsychology* 4 (1998), 65–74.

Grmek, M.D. (ed.), *Hippocratica: actes du Colloque hippocratique de Paris, 4–9 septembre 1978* (Paris, 1980).

—— *Les maladies à l'aube de la civilisation occidentale* (Paris, 1983).

—— 'Le diagnostic rétrospectif des cas décrits dans le livre V des *Epidémies* hippocratiques', in López Férez 1992, 187–200.

Guardasole, A., *Tragedia e medicina nell'Atene del V secolo a. C.* (Naples, 2000).

Guidorizzi, G., 'The Laughter of the Suitors: a Case of Collective Madness in the *Odyssey*', in L. Edmunds and R.W. Wallace (eds.), *Poet, Public and Performance* (Baltimore, 1997), 1–7.

—— *Ai confini dell'anima: i Greci e la follia.* (Milan, 2010).

Gundert, B., 'Parts and their Roles in Hippocratic Medicine', *Isis* 83 (1992), 453–465.

—— 'Soma and Psyche in Hippocratic Medicine', in Wright and Potter 2000, 13–35.

Guthrie, W.K.C. *A History of Greek Philosophy* III (Cambridge, 1969).

Hacking, I., *Mad Travellers: Reflections on the Reality of Transient Mental Illness* (London, 1999).

Hadot. P., *Philosophy as a Way of Life* (trans. M. Chase, Oxford, 1995) (original ed.: *Exercices spirituels et philosophie antique*, Paris, 1981).

Hagel, S., 'Calculating *auloi*—the Louvre *aulos* Scale', in E. Hickmann and R. Eichmann (eds.), *Studien zur Musikarchäologie* 4 (2004), 373–390.

——, *Ancient Greek Music. A New Technical History* (Cambridge, 2010).

Haksar, V., 'Aristotle and the Punishment of Psychopaths', *Philosophy* 39 (1964), 323–340.

Halliday, M.A.K., *The Language of Science* (London, 2004).

Hankinson, R.J., 'Galen's Anatomy of the Soul', *Phronesis* 36 (1991), 197–233. (Hankinson 1991a).

—— 'Greek Medical Models of Mind', in S. Everson (ed.), *Companions to ancient thought 2. Psychology* (Cambridge, 1991), 194–217. (Hankinson 1991b).

—— 'Actions and Passions: Affection, Emotion and Moral Self-management in Galen's Philosophical Psychology', in J. Brunschwig and M. Nussbaum (eds.), *Passions and Perceptions. Studies in Hellenistic Philosophy of Mind* (Cambridge, 1993), 184–222.

—— 'Body and Soul in Galen', in R.A.H. King 2006, 232–258.

—— (ed.), *The Cambridge Companion to Galen* (Cambridge, 2008).

Hanson, A.E., and Green, M.H., 'Soranus of Ephesus: *Methodicorum Princeps*', *ANRW* II.37.2 (Berlin, 1994), 968–1075.

Hardie, A., 'Music and Mysteries', in Murray and Wilson 2004, 11–38.

Harig, G., and Kollesch, J., 'Galen und Hippokrates', in *La collection hippocratique et son rôle dans l'histoire de la médecine* (Leiden, 1975), 257–274.

Harika, V., *Miskawayh: De l'âme et de l'intellect. Présentation, traduction critique et notes* (undergraduate thesis: Louvain-la-Neuve, 1993).

Harris, C.R.S., *The Heart and the Vascular System in Ancient Greek Medicine, from Alcmaeon to Galen* (Oxford, 1973).

Harris, W.V., *Restraining Rage: The Ideology of Anger Control in Classical Antiquity* (Cambridge, MA, 2001).

—— 'The Rage of Women', in S. Braund and G.W. Most (eds.), *Ancient Anger: Perspectives from Homer to Galen* (Cambridge, 2003), 121–143.

—— *Dreams and Experience in Classical Antiquity* (Cambridge, MA, 2009).

Hartigan, K.V., 'Euripidean Madness: Herakles and Orestes', *Greece & Rome* 34 (1987), 126–135.

Harvey, S.A., *Asceticism and Society in Crisis: John of Ephesus and the Lives of the Eastern Saints* (Berkeley, 1990).

Heath, M., *Hermogenes on Issues: Strategies of Argument in Later Greek Rhetoricians* (Oxford, 1995).

Heckelman, L.R., and Schneier, F.R., 'Diagnostic Issues', in R.G. Heimberg, M.R. Liebowitz, D.A. Hope, and F.R. Schneier (eds.), *Social Phobia. Diagnosis, Assessment and Treatment* (New York and London, 1995), 3–20.

Heiberg, J.L., 'Geisteskrankheiten im klassischen Altertum', *Allgemeine Zeitschrift für Psychiatrie* 86 (1927), 1–44.

Hellweg, R., *Stilistische Untersuchungen zu den Krankengeschichten der Epidemien Bücher I und III des Corpus Hippocraticum* (Bonn, 1985).

Hempel, C.G., 'Fundamentals of Taxonomy' (1965), cited from J.Z. Sadler, O.P. Wiggins, and M.A. Schwartz (eds.), *Philosophical Perspectives on Psychiatric Diagnostic Classification* (Baltimore, 1994), 317–331.

Henderson, J., *The Maculate Muse: Obscene Language in Attic Comedy* (Oxford, 1991).

Herman, G., 'Greek Epiphanies and the Sensed Presence', *Historia* 60 (2011), 127–157.

Hershkowitz, D., *The Madness of Epic: Reading Insanity from Homer to Statius* (Oxford, 1998).

Hicks, R.D., *De Anima. Edition and Commentary* (Oxford, 1907).

Hillgruber, M., 'Liebe, Weisheit und Verzicht. Zu Herkunft und Entwicklung der Geschichte von Antiochos und Stratonike', in M. Brüggemann, B. Meissner, C. Mileta, A. Pabst and O. Schmitt (eds.), *Studia hellenistica et historiographica. Festschrift für Andreas Mehl* (Möhrlenbach, 2010), 73–102.

Holmes, B., 'Body, Soul, and Medical Analogy in Plato', in K. Bassi and J.P. Euben (eds.), *When Worlds Elide: Classics, Politics, Culture* (Lanham, MD, 2010), 345–385. (Holmes 2010a).

—— *The Symptom and the Subject. The Emergence of the Physical Body in Ancient Greece* (Princeton, 2010). (Holmes 2010b).

—— 'Sympathy between Hippocrates and Galen: The Case of Galen's Commentary on *Epidemics* II', in Pormann 2012, 49–70.

Holowchak, M.A., 'Aristotle on Dreaming: what Goes on in Sleep when the Big Fire Goes out', *Ancient Philosophy* 16 (1996), 405–423.

Hornblower, S., 'Epic and Epiphanies: Herodotus and the 'New Simonides''', in D. Boedeker and D. Sider (eds.), *The New Simonides: Contexts of Praise and Desire* (Oxford, 2001), 135–147.

Horstmanshoff, H.F.J., and Stol, M. (eds.), *Magic and Rationality in Ancient Near Eastern and Graeco-Roman Medicine* (Amsterdam, 2004),

Horwitz, A.V., and Wakefield, J.C., *The Loss of Sadness: How Psychiatry Transformed Normal Sorrow into Depressive Disorder* (Oxford, 2007).

Hubert, R., 'Veille, sommeil et rêve chez Aristote', *Revue de Philosophie Ancienne* 17 (1999), 75–111.

Hüffmeier, F., 'Phronesis in den Schriften des Corpus Hippocraticum', *Hermes* 89 (1961), 51–84.

Hughes, J.C., *Thinking through Dementia* (Oxford, 2011).

Hutchinson, G.O., *Aeschylus' Septem contra Thebas* (Oxford, 1985).

Ideler, J.L., *Physici et medici Graeci minores* I (Berlin 1841–1842).

Ilberg, J., 'Über die Schrifstellerei des Klaudios Galenos', *Rheinisches Museum* 51 (1896), 165–196.

Ingleby, D., 'The Social Construction of Mental Illness', in P. Wright and A. Treacher (eds.), *The Problem of Medical Knowledge. Examining the Social Construction of Medicine* (Edinburgh, 1982), 123–143.

Ingrosso, P. (ed.), *Menandro. Lo scudo* (Lecce, 2010).

Insel, T., Cuthbert, B., Garvey, M., Heinssen, R., Pine, D., Quinn, K., Sanislow, C., and Wang, P., 'Research Domain Criteria (RDoC): Toward a New Classification Framework for Research on Mental Disorders', *AJPsy* 167 (2010), 748–751.

Inwood, B., *Ethics and Human Action in Early Stoicism* (Oxford, 1985).

—— (ed.), *The Cambridge Companion to the Stoics* (Cambridge, 2003).

—— and Gerson, L.P., *The Stoics Reader. Selected Writings and Testimonia* (Indianapolis, 2008).

al-Issa, I., 'The Illusion of Reality or the Reality of Illusion. Hallucinations and Culture', *British Journal of Psychiatry* 166 (1995), 368–373.

Jackson, S.W., 'Galen—on Mental Disorders', *Journal of the History of the Behavioural Sciences* 5 (1969), 356–384.

—— *Melancholy and Depression: from Hippocratic times to the present day* (New Haven, 1987).

Jacoby, A., 'Stigma, Epilepsy, and Quality of Life', *Epilepsy and Behaviour* 3 (2002), 10–20.

—— and Austin, J.K., 'Social Stigma for Adults and Children with Epilepsy', *Epilepsia* 48 (2007), 6–9.

Jandolo, M., 'Manifestazioni somatiche delle psicosi in Ippocrate', *Rivista di storia della medicina* 11 (1967), 45–48.

Jannaway, C., *Images of Excellence: Plato's Critique of the Arts* (Oxford, 1995).

Jaynes, J., *The Origin of Consciousness and the Breakdown of the Bicameral Mind* (Boston, 1976).

Jeanmaire, H., *Dionysos. Histoire du culte de Bacchus* (Paris, 1951).

Johansen, T.K., 'Body, Soul, and Tripartition in Plato's *Timaeus*', *OSAP* 19 (2000), 87–111.

—— *Plato's Natural Philosophy: a Study of the* Timaeus-Critias (Cambridge, 2004).

Johns, L.C., and Van Os, J., 'The Continuity of Psychotic Experiences in the General Population', *Clinical Psychology Review* 21 (2001), 1125–1141.

Johnston, A., and Smith, P., 'Epilepsy: A General Overview', in V.P. Prasher and M.P. Kerr (eds.), *Epilepsy and Intellectual Disabilities* (Heidelberg, 2008).

Johnston, D., *Roman Law in Context* (Cambridge, 1999).

Jolivet, J. (ed.), *L'Intellect selon Kindi* (Leiden, 1971).

Jones, C., 'Plague and Its Metaphors in Early Modern France', *Representations* 53 (1996), 97–127.

Jones, W.H.S., Withington, E.T., Potter, P., and Smith, W.D. (eds.), *Hippocrates* (Cambridge, MA, and London, 1923–2012), 10 vols.

Joosse, N.P. and Pormann, P.E., 'Commentaries on the Hippocratic *Aphorisms* in the Arabic Tradition: The Example of Melancholy', in Pormann forthcoming 2012, 211–249.

Jouanna, J., 'La théorie de l'intelligence et de l'âme dans le traité hippocratique *Du régime*', *Revue des Etudes Grecques* 79 (1966), 15–18.

—— *Hippocrate et l'école de Cnide* (Paris, 1974).

—— (ed.), *Hippocrate: Des vents, De l'art* (Paris, 1988).

—— *Hippocrate* (Paris, 1992) (trans. M.B. DeBevoise as *Hippocrates*, Baltimore, 1999).

—— 'L'interprétation des rêves et la théorie micro-macrocosmique dans le traité hippocratique du *Régime*: sémiotique et mimésis', in K.-D. Fischer, D. Nickel, and P. Potter (eds.), *Text and Tradition. Studies in Ancient Medicine and its Transmission* (Leiden, 1998), 161–174.

—— *Hippocrate. Épidémies V et VII* (Paris, 2000).

—— 'Alle radici della melancolia: Ippocrate, Aristotele e l'altro Ippocrate', in A. Garzya, A.V. Nazaro and F. Tessitore (eds.), *I Venerdì delle Accademie Napoletane nell'anno accademico 2005–2006* (Naples, 2006), 43–71. (Jouanna 2006a).

—— 'La postérité du traité hippocratique de la *Nature de l'homme*: la théorie des quatre humeurs', in C.W. Müller, C. Brockmann, and C.W. Bunschön (eds.), *Ärzte und ihre Interpreten. Medizinische Fachtexte der Antike als Forschungsgegenstand der klassischen Philologie. Fachkonferenz zu Ehren von Diethard Nickel (14. bis 15. Mai 2004)* (Munich and Leipzig 2006), 117–141. (Jouanna 2006b).

—— 'La théorie de la sensation, de la pensée et de l'âme dans le traité hippocratique du *Régime*: ses rapports avec Empédocle et le *Timée* de Platon', *Aion* 29 (2007), 9–38. (Jouanna 2007a).

—— 'Aux racines de la mélancolie: la médecine grecque est-elle mélancolique?', in J. Clair and R. Kopp (eds.), *De la mélancolie. Les entretiens de la fondation des Treilles* (Paris, 2007), 11–51. (Jouanna 2007b).

—— 'Does Galen Have a Medical Programme for Intellectuals and the Faculties of the Intellect?', in Gill et al. 2009, 190–205.

—— 'La traduction arabe et la traduction latine du *Testament* d'Hippocrate (= *Quel doit être le disciple du médecin*) avec en appendice une nouvelle édition de la traduction latine', in I. Garofalo, S. Fortuna, A. Lami and A. Roselli (eds), *Sulla tradizione indiretta dei testi medici greci: le traduzioni* (Pisa, 2010), 11–31.

—— *Greek Medicine from Hippocrates to Galen: Selected Papers* (trans. N. Allies) (Leiden, 2012).

—— 'The Theory of Sensation, Thought and the Soul in the Hippocratic Treatise Regimen: Its Connections with Empedocles and Plato's *Timaeus*', in J. Jouanna, *Greek Medicine from Hippocrates to Galen. Selected Papers* (Leiden, 2012), 195–228.

—— and Demont, P., 'Le sens d'ἰχώρ chez Homère (Iliade v, v. 340 et 416) et Eschyle (Agamemnon, v. 1480) en relation avec les emplois du mot dans la Collection hippocratique', *Revue des études anciennes* 83 (1981), 197–209.

—— and Grmek, M., *Hippocrates. Épidémies V, VII* (Paris, 2000).

Joubaud, C., *Le corps humain dans la philosophie platonicienne* (Paris, 1991).

Kafka, M.P., 'Hypersexual Disorder: A Proposed Diagnosis for DSM-V', *Archives of Sexual Behavior* 39 (2009), 377–400.

Kahn, C., 'Plato's Theory of Desire', *Review of Metaphysics* 41 (1987), 77–103.

Kany-Turpin, J., and Pellegrin, P., 'Cicero and the Aristotelian Theory of Divination by Dreams', in Fortenbaugh and Steinmetz 1989, 221–245.

Karenberg, A., 'Reconstructing a Doctrine: Galen on Apoplexy', *Journal of the History of Neurosciences* 3 (1994), 85–101.

Kaser, M., *Römisches Privatrecht: Ein Studienbuch* (fifteenth ed., Munich, 1989).

Kass, L. (ed.), *Beyond Therapy: Biotechnology and the Pursuit of Happiness*, (Washington DC, 2003).

Kazantzidis, G., *Melancholy in Hellenistic and Latin poetry. Medical readings in Menander, Apollonius Rhodius, Lucretius and Horace*, (unpublished D.Phil dissertation, Oxford, 2011)

Kelsen, H., *Society and Nature: A Sociological Inquiry* (London, 1946).

Kendler, K., Aggen, H., Knudsen, G.P., Røysamb, E., Neale, M.C., and Reichbron-Kjennerud, T., 'The Structure of Genetic and Environmental Risk Factors for Syndromal and Subsyndromal Common DSM-IV Axis I and All Axis II Disorders', *AJPsy* 168 (2011), 29–39.

Kenny, A.J.P., 'Mental Health in Plato's *Republic*', *Proceedings of the British Academy* 55 (1969), 229–253, repr. in Kenny, *The Anatomy of the Soul. Historical Essays in the Philosophy of Mind* (Oxford, 1973), 1–27.

Kent, G., and Wahass, S., 'The Content and Characteristics of Auditory Hallucinations in Saudi Arabia and the UK: A Cross-cultural Comparison', *Acta Psychiatrica Scandinavica* 94 (1996), 433–437.

Keuls, E., 'The Greek Medical Texts and the Sexual Ethos of Ancient Athens', in van der Eijk et al. 1995, II, 261–274.

King, H., 'Once upon a Text: the Hippocratic Origins of Hysteria', in S. Gilman, H. King, R. Porter, G.S. Rousseau, and E. Showalter (eds), *Hysteria Beyond Freud* (Berkeley, 1993), 3–90.

—— *Hippocrates' Woman. Reading the Female Body in Ancient Greece* (London and New York, 1998).

—— 'Recovering Hysteria from History: Herodotus and 'the First Case of Shell Shock'', in P. Halligan, C. Bass, and J.C. Marshall (eds), *Contemporary Approaches to the Science of Hysteria: Clinical and Theoretical Perspectives* (Oxford, 2001), 36–48.

—— *The Disease of Virgins: Green Sickness, Chlorosis and Problems of Puberty* (London, 2004).

King, P., *The 'Cognitio' into Insanity* (diss. University of North Carolina, 2000).

King, R.A.H. (ed.), *Common to Body and Soul: Philosophical Approaches to Explaining Living Behaviour in Greco-Roman Antiquity* (Berlin, 2006).

Klibansky, R., Panofsky, E., and Saxl, F., *Saturn and Melancholy: Studies in the History of Natural Philosophy, Religion, and Art* (London, 1964). (Also cited from *Saturn und Melancholie*, Frankfurt am Main, 1990).

Knox, B.M.W., *Word and Action: Essays on the Ancient Theater* (Baltimore and London, 1979).

Kollesch, J., *Untersuchungen zu den pseudogalenischen Definitiones Medicae* (Berlin, 1973).

Konstan, D., *Before Forgiveness: The Origins of a Moral Idea* (Cambridge, 2010). (Konstan 2010a).

—— 'The Passions of Achilles: Translating Greece into Rome', *Electronic Antiquity* 14, 1 (2010). (Konstan 2010b).

Korshak, Y., *Frontal Faces in Attic Vase Painting of the Archaic Period* (Chicago, 1987).

Kosak, J.C., *Heroic Measures: Hippocratic Medicine in the Making of Euripidean Tragedy* (Leiden, 2004).

Kouretas, D., *Caractères anormaux dans les drames grecs antiques. Études psychanalytiques et psychopathologiques* (Athens, 1930).

Krause, J.-U., *Gefängnisse im Römischen Reich* (Stuttgart, 1996).

Kraut, R. (ed.), *The Cambridge Companion to Plato* (Cambridge, 1992).

Kraut, R., 'Plato on Love', in G. Fine (ed.), *The Oxford Handbook on Plato* (Oxford, 2008), 286–310.

Kudlien, F., *Der Beginn des medizinischen Denkens in der Antike* (Zurich and Stuttgart, 1967).

Lain Entralgo, P., *The Therapy of the Word in Antiquity* (trans. L.J. Rather and J.M. Sharp, New Haven, 1970) (original ed.: *La Curación por la palabra en la antigüedad clásica*, Madrid, 1958).

Lami, A., 'Lo scritto ippocratico *Sui disturbi virginali*', *Galenos* 1 (2007), 15–59.

Lanata, G., 'Linguaggio scientifico e linguaggio poetico. Note al lessico del De Morbo Sacro', *QUCC* (1968), 22–36.

Landels, J.G., *Music in Ancient Greece and Rome* (London and New York, 1999).

Langer, A., Cangas, A., and Serper, M. 'Analysis of the Multidimensionality of Hallucination-like Experiences in Clinical and Nonclinical Spanish Samples and their Relation to Clinical Symptoms', *International Journal of Psychology* 46 (2011), 46–54.

Langholf, V., 'Die parallelen Texte in *Epidemien* V und VII', in R. Joly (ed.), *Corpus hippocraticum: Actes du Colloque Hippocratique de Mons* (22–26 Septembre 1975) (Mons, 1977), 264–274.

—— *Medical Theories in Hippocrates: Early Texts and the* Epidemics (Berlin and New York, 1990).

—— 'Structure and Genesis of some Hippocratic Treatises', in Horsmanshoff and Stol 2004, 219–275.

Lanza, D., *Lingua e discorso nell' Atene delle professioni* (Naples, 1968).

Lawson-Tangred, H., *Aristotle. De Anima (On the Soul)* (London, 1986).

Le Blay, F., 'Microcosm and Macrocosm: The Dual Direction of Analogy in Hippocratic Thought and the Meteorological Tradition', in van der Eijk 2005b, 251–269.

Leahy, D.M., 'The role of Cassandra in the *Oresteia* of Aeschylus', *Bulletin of the John Rylands Library* 52 (1969), 144–177.

Lear, J., 'Inside and Outside the Republic', in J. Lear, *Open Minded: Working out the Logic of the Soul* (Cambridge, 1998), 219–246.

Lebeck, A., *The Oresteia. A Study in Language and Structure* (Cambridge, MA, 1971).

Leclerc, D., *Histoire de la médecine* (Amsterdam, 1723).

LeDoux, J.E., 'The Neurobiology of Emotion', in J.E. LeDoux and W. Hirst (eds.), *Mind and Brain: Dialogues in Cognitive Neuroscience* (New York and Cambridge, 1986).

Lehane, D., *Shutter Island* (New York, 2003).

Leibbrand, W., and Wettley, A., *Der Wahnsinn: Geschichte der abendländischen Psychopathologie* (Freiburg and Munich, 1961).

Leinieks, V., *The City of Dionysos: a Study of Euripides' Bakchai* (Stuttgart and Leipzig, 1996).

Lent, F., 'The Life of St. Simeon Stylites', *Journal of the American Oriental Society* 35 (1915), 103–198.

Leven, K.H., '"At times these ancient facts seem to lie before me like a patient on a hospital bed"—Retrospective Diagnosis and Ancient Medical History', in Horstmanshoff and Stol 2004, 369–386.

Levy, J.E., *Recherches sur 'Les Académiques' et sur la philosophie cicéronienne*. (Rome, 1992).

—— 'Epilepsy', in K.F. Kiple (ed.), *The Cambridge World History of Human Disease* (Cambridge, 1993), 713–717.

Lewis, A., 'Extract from: Discussion, Various Contributors', in J. Zudin (ed.), *Field Studies in the Mental Disorders* (New York, 1961), 34.

—— 'Foreword', in World Health Organization, *Glossary of Mental Disorders and Guide to their Classification, for use in Conjunction with the International Classification of Diseases, 8th revision* (Geneva, 1974).

Lichtenthaeler, C., *Neuer Kommentar zu den ersten zwölf Krankengeschichten im III Epidemienbuch* (Stuttgart, 1994).

Lightfoot, J.L., *The Sibylline Oracles* (Oxford, 2007).

Linforth, I.M., 'The Corybantic Rites in Plato', *University of California, Publications in Classical Philology* 13 (1946), 121–162.

Lloyd, G.E.R., 'The Empirical Basis of Physiology in the *Parva Naturalia*', in Lloyd and Owen 1978, 215–240.

—— *Magic, Reason and Experience* (Cambridge, 1979).

—— 'Scholarship, Authority and Argument in Galen's *Quod animi mores*', in Manuli and Vegetti 1988, 11–42.

—— *Demystifying Mentalities* (Cambridge, 1990).

—— 'The Definition, Status, and Methods of the Medical τέχνη in the Fifth and Fourth Centuries', in A.C. Bowen (ed.), *Science and Philosophy in Classical Greece* (New York and London, 1991), 249–260.

—— *Aristotelian Explorations* (Cambridge, 1996).

—— *In the Grip of Disease. Studies in the Greek Imagination* (Oxford, 2003).

—— and Owen, G.E.L. (eds.), *Aristotle on Mind and the Senses. Proceedings of the 7th Symposium Aristotelicum* (Cambridge, 1978).

Logan, R.K., *The Extended Mind: The Emergence of Language, the Human Mind, and Culture* (Toronto, Buffalo and London, 2007).

Long, A.A., 'Cicero's Plato and Aristotle', in J.G.F. Powell (ed.), *Cicero the Philosopher: Twelve Papers* (Oxford, 1995).

—— 'Soul and Body in Stoicism', *Phronesis* 27 (1982), 34–57, cited from the reprint in *Stoic Studies* (Cambridge, 1996), 224–249.

—— *Epictetus: A Stoic and Socratic Guide to Life* (Oxford, 2002).

—— 'How does Socrates' Divine Sign Communicate with Him?' in S. Ahbel-Rappe and R. Kamtekar (eds.), *A Companion to Socrates* (Oxford 2005), 63–74.

López Férez, J.A., (ed.), *Tratados Hipocraticos (estudios acerca de su contenido, forma e influencia). Actas del VII Colloque international hippocratique, Madrid, 24–29 de Septiembre de 1990* (Madrid, 1992).

—— 'Algunos datos sobre el léxico de los tratados hipocráticos', in J-A. López Férez (ed.), *La Lengua científica griega: origins, desarrollo e influencia en las lenguas modernas europeas* (Madrid, 2000), I, 31–59.

López-Ibor, J.J., Christodoulou, G., Maj, M., Sartorius, N., and Okasha, A. (eds.), *Disasters and Mental Health* (London, 2005).

López-Morales, D., 'Dos interpretaciones de la anormalidad psíquica: *Vict. 35* et *Morb.Sacr. 15*', in A. Thivel and A. Zucker (eds.), *Le normal et le pathologique dans la Collection hippocratique. Actes du Xe Colloque international hippocratique* II (Nice, 2002), 509–522.

Lo Presti, R., *In forma di senso. L'encefalocentrismo del trattato ippocratico* Sulla malattia sacra *nel suo contesto epistemologico* (Rome, 2008).

—— 'The Matter of Sense, the Sense of Matter. What does the Brain-*hermeneus* Perform according to *On the Sacred Disease?*', *Rhizai* 7 (2011), 147–180.

—— 'Approches hippocratiques du sommeil', in V. Leroux, N. Palmieri and C. Pigné (eds.), *Approches philosophiques et médicales du sommeil de l'Antiquité à la Renaissance*, forthcoming.

Lorenz, H., *The Brute Within: Appetitive Desire in Plato and Aristotle* (Oxford, 2006).

Louis, P. (ed.), *Aristote. Problèmes. Tome III* (Paris, 1994).

Lowe, M., 'Aristotle's *De somno* and his Theory of Causes', *Phronesis* 23 (1978), 279–291.

MacKenzie, M.M., *Plato on Punishment* (Berkeley, 1981).

Magdelaine, C., 'Microcosme et macrocosme dans le *Corpus hippocratique*: Réflexions sur l'homme et la maladie', in J.-L. Cabanès (ed.), *Littérature et médecine: articles* (Talence, 1997), 11–39.

Maire, B., and Bianchi, O., *Caelii Aureliani operum omnium quae exstant concordantiae* (Hildesheim, 2003). 4 vols.

Mannuzza, S., Fyer, A.M., Liebowitz, M.R., and Klein D.F., 'Delineating the Boundaries of Social Phobia: its Relationship to Panic Disorder and Agoraphobia', *Journal of Anxiety Disorders* 4 (1990), 41–59.

Mansfeld, J., 'The Idea of the Will in Chrysippus, Posidonius, and Galen', in *Boston Area Colloquium in Ancient Philosophy* 7 (1991), 107–145.

Manuli, P., 'Galen and Stoicism', in J. Kollesch and D. Nickel (eds), *Galen und das hellenistische Erbe: Verhandlungen des IV. Internationalen Galen-Symposiums* (Stuttgart, 1993), 53–61.

Manuli, P., and Vegetti, M., *Cuore sangue cervello. Biologia e antropologia nel pensiero antico* (Milan, 1977).

—— (eds.), *Le opere psicologiche di Galeno, Atti del terzo colloquio Galenico internazionale (Pavia, 10–12 settembre 1986)* (Naples, 1988).

Marcovich, M., 'Sappho fr. 31: Anxiety Attack or Love Declaration?', *CQ* 22 (1972), 19–32.

Marelli, C., 'Il sonno tra biologia e medicina in Grecia antica', *Bollettino dell'Istituto di filologia greca dell'Università di Padova* 5 (1979–1980), 122–137.

Marenghi, G., *Aristotele. Problemi di medicina* (Milan, 1966).

Marks, I.M., *Fears and Phobias* (London, 1969).

Marzari, M., 'Paradigmi di follia e lussuria virginale in Grecia antica: le Pretidi fra tradizione mitica e medica', *I Quaderni del Ramo d'Oro on-line* n. 3 (2010), 47–74.

Mason, P.G., 'Kassandra', *Journal of Hellenic Studies* 79 (1959), 80–93.

Massimiliano, B., 'Il lessico della 'melancholia' nella tradizione aristotelica', in P. Cuzzolin and M. Napoli (eds.), *Fonologia e tipologia lessicale nella storia della lingua greca* (Milan, 2006), 32–48.

Matentzoglu, S., *Zur Psychopathologie in den hippokratischen Schriften* (Diss. Erlangen-Nürnberg, Berlin, 2011).

Mattes, J., *Der Wahnsinn im griechischen Mythos und in der Dichtung bis zum Drama des fünften Jahrhunderts* (Heidelberg, 1970).

Maturana, H.R., and Varela, F.J., *Autopoiesis and Cognition. The Realization of the Living* (Dordrecht, 1980).

—— and Varela, F.J., *The Tree of Knowledge: The Biological Roots of Human Understanding* (Boston, 1987).

Maudsley, H., *Pathology of the Mind* (third ed., London, 1879).

Mauri, A, 'Funzione e lessico della follia guerriera nei poemi omerici', *Acme* 43 (1990), 51–62.

McCarthy, R.J., 'Al-Kindi's Treatise on the Intellect', *Islamic Studies* 3 (1964), 119–149

McDonald, G.C., *Concepts and Treatments of Phrenitis in Ancient Medicine* (diss. University of Newcastle, 2009).

McPherran, M.L., 'Socratic Religion', in D.R. Morrison, *The Cambridge Companion to Socrates* (Cambridge, 2011), 111–137.

Meagher, R.E., *Herakles Gone Mad: Rethinking Heroism in an Age of Endless War* (Northampton, MA, 2006).

Meehl, P.E., 'Theoretical Risks and Tabular Asterisks: Sir Karl, Sir Ronald, and the Slow Progress of Soft Psychology', *Journal of Consulting and Clinical Psychology* 46 (1978), 806–834.

—— 'Bootstrap Taxometrics: Solving the Classification Problem in Psychopathology', *American Psychologist* 50 (1995), 266–275.

Mellers, J.D.C., 'The Approach to Patients with Non-epileptic Seizures', *Postgraduate Medical Journal* 81 (2005), 498–504.

Menn, S., 'Aristotle's Definition of Soul and the Programme of the *De anima*', *OSAP* 22 (2002), 83–139.

Menninger, K., *The Vital Balance: The Life Process in Mental Health and Illness* (New York, 1963).

Mercuriale, G., *De arte gymnastica* (ed. C. Pennuto, trans. V. Nutton, Florence, 2008) (original ed.: Venice, 1569).

Meyerhof, M., 'Autobiographische Bruchstücke Galens aus arabischen Quellen', *Sudhoffs Archiv* 22 (1929), 72–86.

Miller, H.W., 'A Medical Theory of Cognition', *Transactions of the American Philological Association* 79 (1948), 168–183.

—— 'The Aetiology of Disease in Plato's *Timaeus*', *Transactions of the American Philological Association* 93 (1962), 175–187.

Miller, J.B.F., *Convinced that God Had Called Us: Dreams, Visions and the Perception of God's Will in Luke-Acts* (Leiden, 2007).

Montiglio, S., *Silence in the Land of Logos* (Princeton, 2000).

Morel, P.-M. ''Common to Soul and Body' in the *Parva Naturalia* (Aristotle, *Sens*. 1. 436b1–12)', in R.A.H. King 2006, 121–139.

Moss, G.E., 'Mental Disorder in Antiquity', in D. Brothwell and A.T. Sandison (eds.), *Diseases in Antiquity* (Springfield, IL, 1967), 709–722.

Moss, J., 'Shame, Pleasure, and the Divided Soul', *OSAP* 29 (2005), 137–170.

—— 'Pleasure and Illusion in Plato', *Philosophy and Phenomenological Research* 72 (2006), 503–535.

—— 'Appearances and Calculations: Plato's Division of the Soul', *OSAP* 34 (2008), 35–68.

Most, G.W., *Doubting Thomas* (Cambridge, MA, 2005).

Mudry, P. (ed.), *Le traité des Maladies Aiguës et des Maladies Chroniques de Caelius Aurelianus: Nouvelles Approches* (Nantes, 1999).

—— and Pigeaud, J. (eds.), *Les Écoles médicales à Rome* (Geneva, 1991).

Müri, W., 'Melancholie und schwarze Galle', *Museum Helveticum* 10 (1953), 21–38 (reprinted in H. Flashar (ed.), *Antike Medizin*, Darmstadt, 1971, 165–191).

Murray, O., 'Sympotic History', in Murray 1990, 3–13.

—— (ed.), *Sympotica: a Symposium on the Symposion* (Oxford, 1990).

Nardi, E., *Squilibrio e deficienza mentale in diritto romano* (Milan, 1983).

Nayani, T.H., and David, A.S., 'The Auditory Hallucination: A Phenomenological Survey', *Psychological Medicine* 26 (1996), 177–189.

Neria, Y., Galea, S., and Norris, F.H. (eds.), *Mental Health and Disasters* (Cambridge, 2009).

Nony, S., *Les variations du mouvement. Abû al-Barakât, un physicien à Bagdad (XIIe siècle), Textes arabes et études islamiques* (forthcoming, Cairo, 2013).

Norris, F.H., Friedman, M.J., Watson, P.J., Byrne, C.M., Diaz, E. and Kaniasty, K., '60,000 Disaster Victims Speak: Part 1. An Empirical Review of the Empirical Literature, 1981–2001', *Psychiatry* 65 (2002), 207–239.

Nussbaum, M.C., *The Therapy of Desire: Theory and Practice in Hellenistic Ethics* (Princeton, 1994).

—— *Upheavals of Thought: The Intelligence of Emotions* (Cambridge, 2001).

Nutton, V., 'Hippocrates in the Renaissance', *Sudhoffs Archiv* 27 (1990) 421–439.

—— *Ancient Medicine* (London, 2004).

Oakley, J.H., *Picturing Death in Classical Athens: the Evidence of the White* lekythoi (Cambridge, 2004).

O'Brien-Moore, A., *Madness in Ancient Literature* (Weimar, 1924).

Ogden, D., *Magic, Witchcraft, and Ghosts in the Greek and Roman Worlds: A Sourcebook* (Oxford, 2002).

Oliver, J.R., 'The Psychiatry of Hippocrates. A Plea for the Study of the History of Medicine', *AJPsy* 82 (1925), 107–115.

Onians, R.B., *The Origins of European Thought about the Body, the Mind, the Soul, the World, Time and Fate* (second ed., Cambridge, 1954).

Oser-Grote, C.M., *Aristoteles und das Corpus Hippocraticum: die Anatomie und Physiologie des Menschen* (Stuttgart, 2004).

Padel, R., *In and Out of the Mind. Greek Images of the Tragic Self* (Princeton, 1992).

—— *Whom Gods Destroy: Elements of Greek and Tragic Madness* (Princeton, 1995).

Paduano, G., 'Citazione ed esistenza (Menandro, Aspis 407 sgg.', in *Miscellanea di Studi in memoria di Marino Barchiesi* III = *Rivista di Civiltà Classica e Medievale* 20 (1978), 1055–1065.

Panno, G., *Dionisiaco e alterità nelle «Leggi» di Platone. Ordine del corpo e automovimento dell'anima nella città-tragedia* (Milan, 2007).

Papadopoulou, T., 'Cassandra's Radiant Vigour and the Ironic Optimism of Euripides' Troades', *Mnemosyne* 53 (2000), 513–527.

—— *Heracles and Euripidean Tragedy* (Cambridge, 2005).

Pappas, N., 'Plato's Aesthetics,' *Stanford Encyclopedia of Philosophy* (2008), ⟨http://plato.stanford.edu/entries/plato-aesthetics/⟩

Parlamento, E., '*Servus melancholicus*: I *vitia animi* nella giurisprudenza classica', *Rivista di Diritto Romano* 1 (2001), 1–20.

Passouant, P., 'Historical Views on Sleep and Epilepsy', in M.B. Sterman, M.N. Shouse, and P. Passouant (eds.), *Sleep and Epilepsy* (New York and London, 1982), 1–6.

Patillon, M. (trans.), *Hermogène: L'art rhétorique* (Paris, 1997).

Payne, M.S. (ed.), *Hallucinations: Types, Stages and Treatments* (New York, 2011).

Pellizer, E., 'Outlines of a Morphology of Sympotic Entertainment', in Murray 1990, 177–184.

Pelosi, F., *Plato on Music, Soul and Body* (Cambridge, 2010).

Penfield, W., and Jasper, H.H., *Epilepsy and the Functional Anatomy of the Human Brain* (Boston, 1954).

Perdicoyanni-Paleologou, H., 'The Vocabulary of Madness from Homer to Hippocrates. Part 1: The Verbal Group of *mainomai*', *History of Psychiatry* 20 (3) (2009), 311–339.

—— 'The Vocabulary of Madness from Homer to Hippocrates. Part 2: The Verbal Group of *Bagcheuo* and the Noun *lyssa*', *History of Psychiatry* 20 (4) (2009), 457–467.

Périer, A., *Petits traités apologétiques de Yaḥyâ ben 'Adî* (Paris, 1920).

Perilli, L., Brockmann, C., Fischer, K.-D., and Roselli, A. (eds.), *Officina Hippocratica. Studies in Honour of Anargyros Anastassiou and Dieter Irmer* (Berlin and New York, 2011).

Petsko, G.A., 'The Coming Epidemic of Neurologic Disorders: What Science Is—and Should Be—Doing about it', *Daedalus* 141, 3 (2012), 98–107.

Pfister, F. 'Epiphanie', in *Real-Encyclopädie der classischen Alterthumswissenschaft* Supplementband IV (1924), cols. 277–323.

Pigeaud, J., 'Une physiologie de l'inspiration poétique', *Les Études Classiques* 46 (1978), 23–31.

—— 'Quelques aspects du rapport de l'âme et du corps dans le Corpus hippocratique', in Grmek 1980, 417–433.

—— *La maladie de l'âme: étude sur la relation de l'âme et du corps dans la tradition médico-philosophique antique* (Paris, 1981).

—— *Folie et cures de la folie chez les médecins de l'Antiquité gréco-romaine, La Manie* (Paris, 1987; second ed., Paris, 2010).

—— 'Die Medizin in der Lehrdichtung des Lukrez und des Vergil', in G. Binder (ed.), *Saeculum Augustum II: Religion und Literatur* (Darmstadt, 1988), 216–239. (Pigeaud 1988a).

—— 'La psychopathologie de Galien', in Manuli and Vegetti 1988, 153–183, repr. in Pigeaud 2008a, 561–585 (Pigeaud 1988b).

—— *L'homme de génie et la mélancolie. Aristote, Probléme XXX, 1* (Paris, 1988). (Pigeaud 1988c).

—— 'Les fondements théoriques du méthodisme à Rome', in Mudry and Pigeaud 1991, 7–50.

—— *La follia nell'antichità classica* (Bologna, 1995).

—— 'Les fondements philosophiques de l'éthique médicale: le cas de Rome', in *Entretiens sur l'Antiquité Classique* [de la Fondation Hardt] 43 (1997), 255–296.

—— 'The Triumph of Dualism in Ancient Psychopathology', in L. de Goei and

J. Vijselaar (eds.), *Proceedings of the 1st European Congress on the History of Psychiatry and Mental Health Care* (Rotterdam, 1993), 287–301, repr. in *Poétiques du corps* (Paris, 2008), 599–619.

—— *Aux portes de la psychiatrie: Pinel, l'Ancien et le Moderne* (Paris, 2001).

—— *Poétiques du corps: Aux origines de la médecine* (Paris, 2008). (Pigeaud 2008a).

—— *Melancholia: La malaise de l'individu* (Paris, 2008) (Pigeaud 2008b).

Pigeaud 2010: see Pigeaud 1987.

Pinel, P., *Nosographie philosophique, ou La Méthode d'analyse appliquée à la médecine* (Paris, 1798).

—— *Traité médico-philosophique sur l'aliénation mentale* (Paris, 1801).

Pirovano, L., *Le* Interpretationes vergilianae *di Tiberio Claudio Donato: Problemi di retorica* (Rome, 2006).

Plummer, C., 'Charles Bonnet Syndrome', in Payne 2011, 97–112.

Polansky, R., *Aristotle. De Anima. Commentary* (Cambridge, 2007).

Pollito, R., 'On the Life of Asclepiades of Bithynia', *JRS* 119 (1999), 48–66.

Pormann, P.E., 'The Alexandrian Summary (*Jawāmiʿ*) of Galen's *On the Sects for Beginners*: Commentary or Abridgment?', in P. Adamson, H. Baltussen and M.W.F. Stone (eds.), *Philosophy, Science and Exegesis in Greek, Arabic and Latin Commentaries, Bulletin of the Institute of Classical Studies*, Supplement 83 (London, 2004), II, 11–33.

—— (ed.) *Rufus of Ephesus, On Melancholy* (Tübingen 2008).

—— *Epidemics in Context: Hippocrates, Galen and Hunayn between East and West* (Berlin, 2012).

—— 'Avicenna on Medical Practice, Epistemology, and the Physiology of the Inner Senses', in P. Adamson (ed.), *Interpreting Avicenna* (Cambridge, 2013), 91–108.

—— 'New fragments from Rufus of Ephesus' *On Melancholy*', *CQ* forthcoming.

Porter, R., *A Social History of Madness* (London, 1987).

—— *The Greatest Benefit to Mankind: a Medical History of Humanity* (London, 1997).

—— *Madness. A Brief History* (Oxford, 2002).

Pradeau, J.-F., 'L'âme et la moelle. Les conditions psychiques et physiologiques de l'anthropologie dans le *Timée* de Platon', *Archives de philosophie* 61 (1998), 489–518.

Prandi, L., 'Considerazioni su Bacide e le raccolte oracolari greche', in M. Sordi (ed.), *La profezia nel mondo antico* (Milan, 1993), 51–62.

Preus, A., 'Aristotle on Healthy and Sick Souls', *The Monist* 69 (1986), 416–433.

Pritchett, W.K., *The Greek State at War* III (Berkeley and Los Angeles, 1979).

Psaroudakes, S., 'The *auloi* of Pydna', in A.A. Both, R. Eichmann, E. Hickmann and L. Koch (eds.), *Studien zur Musik-Archäologie 6. Orient-Archäologie 22* (2008), 197–216.

Pulitano, F., *Studi sulla prodigalità nel diritto romano* (Milan, 2002).

Putnam, H., *Words and Life* (Cambridge, MA, 1995).

Radden, J., *The Nature of Melancholy: From Aristotle to Kristeva* (Oxford, 2000).

—— *Moody Minds Distempered: Essays on Melancholy and Depression* (Oxford, 2009).

Rapp, C., 'Interaction of Body and Soul: What the Hellenistic Philosophers Saw and Aristotle Avoided', in R.A.H. King 2006, 187–208.

Rawson, E., 'The Life and Death of Asclepiades of Bithynia', *CQ* 32 (1982), 358–370.

——— *Intellectual Life in the Late Roman Republic* (London, 1985).

Raz, J., rev. of Wolf 2010, *Ethics* (2010), 232–236.

Redfield, J.M., *Nature and Culture in the Iliad: the Tragedy of Hector* (Chicago, 1975).

Reiss, D., Plomin, R., and Hetherington, E.M., 'Genetics and Psychiatry: an Unheralded Window on the Environment', *AJPsy* 148 (1991), 283–291.

Renberg, G. *'Commanded by the Gods'. An Epigraphical Study of Dreams and Visions in Greek and Roman Religious Life* (diss. Duke University, 2003).

——— 'Dream-Narratives and Unnarrated Dreams in Greek and Latin Dedicatory Inscriptions', in E. Scioli and C. Walde (eds.), Sub Imagine Somni: *Nighttime Phenomena in Greco-Roman Culture* (Pisa, 2010), 33–61.

Repici, L., 'Aristotele, gli stoici e il libro dei sogni nel *De divinatione* e nel *De Finibus* di Cicerone', *Metis* 6 (1991), 167–203.

——— *Aristotele. Il sonno e i sogni* (Venice, 2003).

Richards, M., and Brayne, C., 'What do we Mean by Alzheimer's Disease?' *British Medical Journal* 341 (2010) 865–867.

Richardson-Lear, G., 'Permanent Beauty and Becoming Happy in Plato's *Symposium*', in J. Lesher, D. Nails, and F. Sheffield (eds.), *Plato's Symposium: Issues in Interpretation and Reception* (Cambridge, MA, 2007).

Riley, K., *The Reception and Performance of Euripides' Herakles: Reasoning Madness* (Oxford, 2008).

Roberts, J., 'Plato on the Causes of Wrongdoing in the *Laws*', *Ancient Philosophy* 7 (1987), 23–37.

Robinson, D.N., *Wild Beasts and Idle Humours: The Insanity Defense from Antiquity to the Present* (Cambridge, MA, 1996).

Rocca, J., *Galen on the Brain: Anatomical Knowledge and Physiological Speculation in the Second Century AD* (Leiden, 2003)

Rodgers, V.A., 'Σύνεσις and the Expression of Conscience', *Greek, Roman, and Byzantine Studies* 10 (1969), 241–254.

Rodríguez, H., Quarantelli, E.L., and Dynes, R.R. (eds.), *Handbook of Disaster Research* (New York, 2007).

Rose, M., *The Staff of Oedipus: Transforming Disability in Ancient Greece* (Ann Arbor, 2003).

Rosen, G., *Madness in Society: Chapters in the Historical Sociology of Mental Illness* (New York, 1968).

Ross, W.D., *Aristotle. Metaphysics. Edition and Commentary* (Oxford, 1924), 2 v.

Rotondaro, S., 'Il *pathos* della ragione e i sogni: *Timeo* 70D7–72B5', in Calvo and Brisson 1997, 275–280.

Roussel, F., 'Le concept de mélancolie chez Aristote', *Revue d'histoire des sciences et de leurs applications* 41 (1988), 299–330.

Ruffinengo, P.P., 'Al-Kindî, *Trattato sull'intelletto. Trattato sul sogno e la visione*', *Medioevo* 23 (1997), 337–394.

Rütten, T., *Demokrit, lachender Philosoph und sanguinischer Melancholiker. Eine pseudohippokratische Geschichte* (Leiden, 1992).

Sadler, J.Z., *Values and Psychiatric Diagnosis* (Oxford and New York, 2005).

Saïd, S., *La faute tragique* (Paris, 1978).

Sambursky, S., *Physics of the Stoics* (London, 1959).

Sarbin, T.R., and Juhasz, J.B., 'The Historical Background of the Concept of Hallucination', *Journal of the History of the Behavioral Sciences* 3 (1967), 339–358.

Sassi, M.M., *The Science of Man in Ancient Greece* (trans. P. Tucker, Chicago and London, 2001) (original ed.: *La scienza dell'uomo nella Grecia antica*, Turin, 1989).

—— 'The Self, the Soul, and the Individual in the City of the *Laws*', *OSAP* 35 (2008), 125–148.

Saunders, T.J., *Platos' Penal Code. Tradition, Controversy, and Reform in Greek Penology* (Oxford, 1991).

Savage-Smith, E., 'Galen's Lost Ophthalmology and the *Summaria Alexandrinorum*', in V. Nutton (ed.), *The Unknown Galen, Bulletin of the Institute of Classical Studies*, Supplement 77 (London, 2002), 121–138.

Savas, M.Y., *Feminine Madness in the Japanese Noh Theatre* (diss. Ohio State University, 2008).

Scadding, J.G., 'Essentialism and Nominalism in Medicine: Logic of Diagnosis in Disease Terminology', *Lancet* 348 (1996), 594–596.

Schäublin, C., *Marcus Tullius Cicero: Über die Wahrsagung* (De divinatione) (Munich, 1991).

Scharper, E., *Prelude to Aesthetics* (London, 1968).

Schein, S., 'The Cassandra Scene in Aeschylus' 'Agamemnon'', *Greece & Rome* 29 (1982), 11–16.

Schironi, F., 'Technical Languages: Science and Medicine', in Bakker 2010, 338–354.

Schlesier, R., 'Der Stachel der Götter. Zum Problem des Wahnsinns in der Euripideischen Tragödie', *Poetica* 17 (1985), 1–45.

Schofield, M., 'Cicero for and against Divination', *JRS* 76 (1986), 47–64.

Schuhl, P.-M., *La fabulation platonicienne* (Paris, 1968).

Screech, M.A., 'Good Madness in Christendom', in W.F. Bynum, R. Potter and M. Shepherd (eds.), *The Anatomy of Madness: Essays in the History of Psychiatry* (London, 2004), 25–39.

Scurlock, J., and Anderson, B.R., *Diagnoses in Assyrian and Babylonian Medicine: Ancient Sources, Translations, and Modern Medical Analyses* (Urbana and Chicago, 2005).

Seaford, R., *Money and the Early Greek Mind: Homer, Philosophy, Tragedy* (Oxford, 2004).

Seeskin, K., 'Plato and the Origin of Mental Health', *International Journal of Law and Psychiatry* 31 (2008), 487–494.

Seiler, H., 'Homerisch ἀάομαι und ἄτη', in *Sprachgeschichte und Wortbedeutung: Festschrift Albert Debrunner gewidmet von Schülern, Freunden und Kollegen* (Bern, 1954), 409–417.

Sellars, J., *The Art of Living: The Stoics on the Nature and Function of Philosophy* (Aldershot, 2003).

—— 'Stoic Practical Ethics in the Imperial Period', in Sorabji and Sharples 2007, I, 115–140.

Semelaigne, L., *Études historiques sur l'aliénation mentale dans l'antiquité* (Paris, 1869).

Serghidou, A., 'Athena *Salpinx* and the Ethics of Music', in S. Deacy and A. Villing (eds.), *Athena in the Classical World* (Leiden, 2001), 57–74.

Sesto, G.J., *Guardianship of the Mentally Ill in Ecclesiatical Trials: A Canonical Commentary with Historical Notes* (Washington DC, 1956).

Sharples, R., *Theophrastus of Eresus: Sources for his Life, Writings, Thought, and Influence. Commentary 5. Sources on Biology* (Leiden, 1995).

—— 'Common to Body and Soul: Peripatetic Approaches after Aristotle', in R.A.H. King 2006, 165–186.

Sheffield, F., *Plato's Symposium: The Ethics of Desire* (Oxford, 2006).

Shepherd, M., 'ICD, Mental Disorder and British Nosologists. An Assessment of the Uniquely British Contribution to Psychiatric Classification', *British Journal of Psychiatry* 165 (1994), 1–3.

Shibre, T., Teferra, S., Morgan, C., and Alem, A., 'Exploring the Apparent Absence of Psychosis amongst the Borona Pastoralist Community of Southern Ethiopia: a Mixed Method Follow-up Study', *World Psychiatry* 9 (2010), 98–102.

Sideras, A., 'Rufus von Ephesos und sein Werk im Rahmen der antiken Welt', *ANRW* II.37.2 (Berlin, 1994), 1080–1253.

Siegel, R.E., *Galen's System of Physiology and Medicine: An Analysis of His Doctrines and Observations on Bloodflow, Respiration, Tumors, and Internal Diseases* (Basel, 1968).

—— *Galen on Psychology, Psychopathology and Function and Diseases of the Nervous System: an Analysis of his Doctrines, Observations and Experiments* (Basel, 1973).

Simon, B., 'Plato and Freud—The Mind in Conflict and the Mind in Dialogue' *Psychoanalytical Quarterly* 42 (1973), 91–122.

—— *Mind and Madness in Ancient Greece: The Classical Roots of Modern Psychiatry* (Ithaca, NY, 1978).

—— 'Mind and Madness in Classical Antiquity', in E.R. Wallace and J. Gach (eds.), *History of Psychiatry and Medical Psychology* (New York, 2008), 171–197.

Singer, P.N., 'Aspects of Galen's Platonism', in J.A. López Férez (ed.), *Galeno: Obra pensamiento e influencia: Coloquio internacional celebrado en Madrid, 22–25 de Marzo de 1988* (Madrid, 1991), 41–55.

—— 'Some Hippocratic Mind-body Problems', in López Férez 1992, 131–143.

—— (ed.), *Galen: Psychological Writings* (forthcoming, 2013).

Simms, R. (trans.), *Jorge Luis Borges: Other Inquisitions* (Austin, 1993).

Slade, P.D., and Bentall, R.P., *Sensory Deception: A Scientific Analysis of Hallucinations* (Baltimore, 1988).

Slings, S.R., 'Figures of Speech and their Lookalikes. Two Further Exercises in the Pragmatics of the Greek Sentence', in E.J. Bekker (ed.), *Grammar as Interpretation* (Leiden, 1997), 169–214.

—— 'Written and Spoken Language: an Exercise in the Pragmatics of the Greek Sentence', *Classical Philology* 87 (1992), 95–105.

Smith, M., *Jesus the Magician* (New York, 1978).

Smith, M.F. (ed.), *Diogenes of Oinoanda: the Epicurean Inscription* (Naples, 1993).

Smith, W.D., 'Disease in Euripides' Orestes', *Hermes* 95 (1967), 291–307.

—— *The Hippocratic Tradition* (Ithaca; London, 1979).

—— (ed. and trans.), *Hippocrates, Pseudepigraphic Writings* (Leiden, 1990).

Snell, B., *The Discovery of the Mind: The Greek Origins of European Thought* (trans. T.G. Rosenmeyer, Cambridge, MA, 1953) (original ed.: *Die Entdeckung des Geistes*, Hamburg, 1948).

Soardi, M., 'Né uomo né bestia. Riflessioni sulla *theriotes* a partire dal VII libro dell'*Etica Nicomachea*', in V. Andò and N. Cusumano (eds.), *Come bestie? Forme e paradossi della violenza tra mondo antico e disagio contemporaneo* (Caltanissetta and Roma, 2010), 78–88.

Solmsen, F., 'Greek Philosophy and the Discovery of the Nerves', *Museum Helveticum* 18 (1961), 169–197.

Sommerstein, A., *The Comedies of Aristophanes*: Volume 8, *The Thesmophoriazusae* (London, 1994).

Sorabji, R., 'The Mind-Body Relation in the Wake of Plato's *Timaeus*', in G.J. Reydams-Schils (ed.), *Plato's* Timaeus *as Cultural Icon* (Notre Dame, IN, 2003), 152–163.

—— *The Philosophy of the Commentators* (London, 2004), 3 v.

—— *Emotion and Peace of Mind: From Stoic Agitation to Christian Temptation* (Oxford, 2005).

Sorabji, R., and Sharples, R.W. (eds.), *Greek and Roman Philosophy 100 BC–200 AD* (*Bulletin of the Institute of Classical Studies*, Supplement 94) (London, 2007).

Souques, A., 'Connaissances neurologiques d'Hippocrate', *Revue Neurologique* 1 (1934), 1–33 and 177–205.

—— *Étapes de la neurologie dans l'antiquité grecque: d'Homère à Galien* (Paris, 1936).

Sprague, R.K., 'Aristotle and the Metaphysics of Sleep', *Revue of Metaphysics* 31 (1977), 230–241.

Stalley, R.F., 'Punishment and the Physiology of the *Timaeus*', *CQ* 46 (1996), 357–370.

Stallmach, J., Ate. *Zur Frage des Selbst- und Weltverständnisses des frühgriechischen Menschen* (Meisenheim, 1968).

Starobinski, J., *Geschichte der Melancholiebehandlung von den Anfängen bis 1900* (revised ed., Berlin, 2011).

Starr, C.G., 'An Evening with the Flute-girls', *Parola del passato* 33 (1978), 401–410.

Stathakopoulos, D.C., *Famine and Pestilence in the Late Roman and Early Byzantine Empire: a Systematic Survey of Subsistence Crises and Epidemics* (Aldershot, 2004).

Stengel, E., 'Classification of Mental Disorders', *Bulletin of the World Health Organization* 21 (1959), 601–633.

Sterman, M.B., Shouse, M.N., and Passouant, P. (eds.), *Sleep and Epilepsy* (New York and London, 1982).

Stern-Gillet, S., 'On (Mis)interpreting Plato's 'Ion'', *Phronesis* 49 (2004), 169–201.

Stirling, J., *Representing Epilepsy: Myth and Matter* (Liverpool, 2010).

Stobart, H., 'Bodies of Sound and Landscapes of Music: a View from the Bolivian Andes', in P. Gouk (ed.), *Musical Healing in Cultural Contexts* (Aldershot, 2000), 26–45.

Stok, F., 'Follia e malattie mentali nella medicina dell'età romana', *ANRW* II.37.3 (Berlin, 1996), 2282–410.

—— 'Il pazzo e il suo medico', *Medicina nei secoli. Arte e scienza* 9 (1997), 261–276.

—— 'Struttura e modelli dei trattati di Celio Aureliano', in Mudry 1999, 1–26.

Strawson, G., 'The Impossibility of Moral Responsibility', *Philosophical Studies* 75 (1994), 5–24.

Stumfohl, H., 'Zur Psychologie der Sibylle', *Zeitschrift für Religions- und Geistesgeschichte* 23 (1971), 84–103.

Szasz, T.S., 'The Myth of Mental Illness', *American Psychologist* 15 (1960), 113–118.

Taplin, O., *The Stagecraft of Aeschylus. The Dramatic Use of Exits and Entrances in Greek Tragedy* (Oxford, 1977).

Tecusan, M., *The Fragments of the Methodists: Methodism outside Soranus*, I, *Text and Translation* (Leiden, 2004)

Temkin, O., 'Geschichte des Hippokratismus im ausgehenden Altertum', *Kyklos* 4 (1932), 1–80.

—— *The Falling Sickness. A History of Epilepsy from the Greeks to the Beginnings of Modern Neurology* (second ed., 1971; first ed., 1945).

Tetamo, E., 'L'anima e le passioni nel Timeo', *Atti dell'Istituto Veneto di Scienze, Lettere ed Arti* 151 (1993), 915–940.

Thalmann, W.G., *Dramatic Art in Aeschylus' 'Seven against Thebes'*, (New Haven and London, 1978).

Theodorou, Z., 'Exploring Madness in Orestes', *CQ* 43 (1993), 32–46.

Thivel, A., 'La doctrine des περισσώματα et ses parallèles hippocratiques', *Revue de Philologie* 39 (1965) 266–282.

Thorpe, S.J., and Salkovskis, P.M., 'Animal Phobias', in Davey 1997, 81–106.

Thumiger, C., *Hidden Paths. Self and Characterization in Greek Tragedy: Euripides' Bacchae* (*Bulletin of the Institute of Classical Studies*, Supplement 99) (London, 2007).

—— 'Insanity in the Hippocratic Texts: a Pragmatic Perspective', forthcoming.

Tieleman, T., 'Galen on the Seat of the Intellect: Anatomical Experiment and Philosophical Tradition', in T. Rihll and C. Tuplin (eds.), *Science and Mathematics in Ancient Greek Culture* (Oxford, 2002), 256–273.

—— *Chrysippus' On Affections: Reconstruction and Interpretation* (Leiden, 2003). (Tieleman 2003a).

—— 'Galen's Psychology', in J. Barnes and J. Jouanna (eds.), *Galien et la philosophie* (Geneva, 2003), 131–161 (Tieleman 2003b).

—— 'Galen and the Stoics; Or, the Art of Not Naming', in Gill et al. 2009, 282–299.

Todd, R.B., *Alexander of Aphrodisias on Stoic Physics* (Leiden, 1976).

Toner, J., *Popular Culture in Ancient Rome* (Cambridge, 2009).

Toohey, P., *Melancholy, Love, and Time: Boundaries of the Self in Ancient Literature* (Ann Arbor, 2004).

—— 'Rufus of Ephesus and the Tradition of the Melancholy Thinker', in P.E. Pormann (ed.), *Rufus of Ephesus, On Melancholy* (Tübingen, 2008), 221–243.

Tracy, T.J., *Physiological Theory and the Doctrine of the Mean in Plato and Aristotle* (The Hague and Paris, 1969).

Trede, K., Salvatore, P., Baethge, C., Gerhard, A., Maggini, C., and Baldessarini, R.J., 'Manic-Depressive Illness: Evolution in Kraepelin's Textbook 1883–1926', *Harvard Review of Psychiatry* 13 (2005), 155–178.

Trenchard-Smith, M., 'Insanity, Exculpation and Disempowerment in Byzantine Law', in W.J. Turner (ed.), *Madness in Medieval Law and Custom* (Leiden and Boston, 2010), 39–56.

Tristán, P.D., *El 'prodigus' y su condición jurídica en derecho romano clásico* (Barcelona, 2000).

Tsouna, V., 'Epicurean Therapeutic Strategies', in J. Warren (ed.), *The Cambridge Companion to Epicureanism* (Cambridge, 2009), 249–265.

Tucker, W. (ed.), *Ptolemaic Astrology* (Sidcup, 1961).

Tuominen, M., 'Receptive Reason: Alexander of Aphrodisias on Material Intellect', *Phronesis* 55 (2010), 170–190.

Ullmann, M. (ed.), *Rufus von Ephesus. Krankenjournale* (Wiesbaden, 1978).

——, 'Die arabische Überlieferung der Schriften des Rufus von Ephesos', *ANRW* II.37.2 (Berlin, 1994), 1293–1349.

——, *Wörterbuch der griechisch-arabischen Übersetzungen*. Supplement (Wiesbaden, 2006–2007), 2 v.

Urso, A.M., *Dall' autore al traduttore: Studi sulle Passiones celeres e tardae di Celio Aureliano* (Messina, 1997).

Vallance, J.T., *The Lost Theory of Asclepiades of Bithynia* (Oxford, 1990).

—— 'The Medical System of Asclepiades of Bithynia', *ANRW* II.37.1 (Berlin, 1993), 693–727.

Valles, Francisco, *Commentaria in septem libros de Hippocrates. De morbis popularibus* (Orleans, 1554).

van der Eijk, P.J., 'Divine Movement and Human Nature in Eudemian Ethics 8,2', *Hermes* 117 (1989), 24–42.

—— 'Aristoteles über die Melancholie', *Mnemosyne* 43 (1990), 33–72.

—— 'Aristotelian Elements in Cicero's *De Divinatione*', *Philologus* 137 (1993), 223–231.

—— (trans. and ed.), *Aristoteles: De insomniis. De divinatione per somnum* (Berlin, 1994).

—— 'Towards a Rhetoric of Ancient Scientific Discourse: Some Formal Characteristics of Greek Medical and Philosophical Texts', in E.J. Bakker (ed.), *Grammar as Interpretation. Greek Literature in its Linguististic Context* (Leiden, New York and Köln, 1997), 77–129.

—— 'The Matter of Mind: Aristotle on the Biology of "Psychic" Processes', in W. Kullmann and S. Föllinger (eds.), *Aristotelische Biologie. Intentionen, Methoden, Ergebnisse* (Stuttgart, 1997), 231–259, repr. in van der Eijk 2005a, 206–237.

—— 'The Anonymus Parisinus and the Doctrines of "The Ancients"', in P.J. van der Eijk (ed.), *Ancient Histories of Medicine: Essays in Medical Doxography and Historiography in Classical Antiquity* (Leiden, 1999), 295–331. (van der Eijk 1999a).

—— 'The Methodism of Caelius Aurelianus: some Epistemological Issues', in Mudry 1999, 47–83. (van der Eijk 1999b).

—— 'Aristotle's Psycho-Physical Account of the Soul-Body Relationship', in Wright and Potter 2000, 57–77. (van der Eijk 2000a).

—— (ed.), *Diocles of Carystus* (Leiden, 2000–2001). (van der Eijk 2000b).

—— 'Divination, Prognosis, Prophylaxis: the Hippocratic work 'On Dreams' (*De victu* 4) and its Near Eastern Background', in Horstmanshoff and Stol 2004, 187–218.

—— *Medicine and Philosophy in Classical Antiquity: Doctors and Philosophers on Nature, Soul, Health and Disease* (Cambridge, 2005). (van der Eijk 2005a).

—— (ed.), *Hippocrates in Context: Papers Read at the XIth International Hippocratic Colloquium, University of Newcastle upon Tyne, 27–31 August 2000* (Leiden, 2005). (van der Eijk 2005b).

—— 'On Galen's Therapeutics', in Hankinson 2008, 283–303. (van der Eijk 2008a).

—— 'Rufus' *On Melancholy* and its Philosophical Background', in P.E. Pormann

(ed.), *Rufus of Ephesus: On Melancholy* (Tübingen, 2008), 159–178. (van der Eijk 2008b).
—— 'The Role of Medicine in the Formation of Early Greek Philosophical Thought', in P. Curd and D. Graham (eds.), *Oxford Guide to Pre-Socratic Philosophy* (Oxford, 2008), 385–412. (van de Eijk 2008c).
—— 'Modes and Degrees of Soul-body Relationship in *On Regimen*', in Perilli et al. 2011, 255–270.
—— 'Galen and the Scientific Treatise: a Case Study of *Mixtures*', in M. Asper (ed.), *Writing Science* (Berlin, 2013), 145–175. (van der Eijk 2013a).
—— 'Galen on the Nature of Human Beings', in P. Adamson and J. Wilberding (eds.), *Galen and Philosophy* (forthcoming, London, 2013). (van der Eijk 2013b).
——, Horstmanshoff, H.F.J., and Schrijvers, P.H. (eds.), *Ancient Medicine in its Social-Cultural Context* (Amsterdam and Atlanta, 1995), 2 v.
—— and Pormann, P.E., 'Galen, *On Affected Places* III.9–10: Greek Text and English and Arabic Translations', in P. Pormann (ed.), *Rufus on Melancholy* (Tübingen, 2008), 265–287.
—— and Singer, P.N. (trans.), *Galen: Works on Human Nature* (forthcoming, Cambridge, 2014).
Van Hoof, L., *Plutarch's Practical Ethics: The Social Dynamics of Philosophy* (Oxford, 2010).
Varela, F.J., Thompson, E., and Rosch, E., *The Embodied Mind: Cognitive Science and Human Experience* (Cambridge, MA, 1991).
Vázquez-Buján, M.E., 'La nature textuelle de l'oeuvre de Caelius Aurelianus', in Mudry 1999, 121–140.
Vegetti, M., 'Il *De locis in homine* fra Anassagora ed Ippocrate', *Rendiconti dell'Istituto lombardo di scienze e lettere, Classe di lettere e scienze morali e storiche* 99 (1965), 193–213.
—— 'La terapia dell'anima. Patologia e disciplina del soggetto in Galeno', in M. Menghi and M. Vegetti (eds.), *Le passioni e gli errori dell'anima* (Venice, 1984), 131–155.
Versnel, H.S., 'What Did Ancient Man See When He Saw a God? Some Reflections on Greco-Roman Epiphany', in D. van der Plas (ed.), *Effigies Dei. Essays on the History of Religions* (Leiden, 1987), 42–55.
Vickers, M., 'Attic *symposia* after the Persian Wars', in Murray 1990, 105–121.
von Staden, H., *Herophilus: The Art of Medicine in Early Alexandria* (Cambridge, 1989).
—— 'Incurability and Hopelessness: The Hippocratic Corpus', in P. Potter, G. Maloney, and J. Desautels (eds.), *La maladie et les maladies dans la Collection Hippocratique* (Quebec, 1990), 75–112.
—— 'The Discovery of the Body: Human Dissection and Its Cultural Contexts in Ancient Greece', *Yale Journal of Biology and Medicine* 65 (1992), 223–241. (von Staden 1992a).
—— 'The Mind and the Skin of Heracles: Heroic Diseases', in D. Gourevitch (ed.), *Maladie et maladies. Histoire et conceptualisation* (Geneva, 1992), 131–150. (von Staden 1992b).
—— 'Anatomy as Rhetoric: Galen on Dissection and Persuasion', *Journal of the History of Medicine and Allied Sciences* 50 (1995), 47–66.

―――― 'Body, Soul, and Nerves: Epicurus, Herophilus, Erasistratus', in Wright and Potter 2000, 79–116.

―――― ''A Woman Does Not Become Ambidextrous': Galen and the Culture of Scientific Commentary', in R. Gibson and C.S. Kraus (eds.), *The Classical Commentary. Histories, Practices, Theory* (Leiden, 2002), 109–139.

Wallace, R.W., 'An Early Fifth-Century Athenian Revolution in Aulos Music', *Harvard Studies in Classical Philology* 101 (2003), 73–92.

―――― 'Damon of Oa: a Music Theorist Ostracized?', in Murray and Wilson 2004, 249–268.

Waller, N.G., 'Carving Nature at its Joints: Paul Meehl's Development of Taxometrics', *Journal of Abnormal Psychology* 115 (2006), 210–215.

Walsham, A., 'Invisible Helpers: Angelic Intervention in Post-Reformation England', *Past and Present* 208 (2010), 77–130.

Wardle, D., *Cicero on Divination:* De divinatione I (Oxford, 2006).

Warren, J., *Facing Death: Epicurus and his Critics* (Oxford, 2004).

Wedgwood, R., 'Diotima's Eudaimonism: Intrinsic Value and Rational Motivation in Plato's *Symposium*,' *Phronesis* 54 (2009), 297–325.

West, M.L. (ed. and trans.), *Euripides' Orestes* (Warminster, 1989).

―――― *Ancient Greek Music* (Oxford, 1992).

Westphal, C., 'Die Agoraphobie: eine neuropatische Erscheinung', *Archiv für Psychiatrie und Nervenkrankheiten* 3 (1872), 138–161.

White, M.J., 'Stoic Natural Philosophy (Physics and Cosmology)', in Inwood 2003, 124–152.

Whitteridge, G., *Disputations Touching the Generation of Animals by William Harvey* (Oxford, 1981).

Whitwell, J.R., *Historical Notes on Psychiatry* (Philadelphia, 1937).

Wiesner, J., 'The Unity of the Treatise *De somno* and the Physiological Explanation of Sleep in Aristotle', in Lloyd and Owen 1978, 241–280.

Wijsenbeek-Wijler, H., *Aristotle's Concept of Soul, Sleep and Dreams* (Amsterdam, 1976).

Willink C.W., *Euripides, Orestes, with Introduction and Commentary* (Oxford, 1986).

Wilson, E.A., *Psychosomatic: Feminism and the Neurological Body* (Durham, 2004).

Wilson, M., 'Six Views of Embodied Cognition', *Psychonomic Bulletin & Review* 9 (2002), 625–636.

Wilson, P., 'The *aulos* in Athens', in S. Goldhill and R. Osborne (eds.), *Performance Culture and Athenian Democracy* (Cambridge, 1999), 58–91.

Witt, C., 'Dialectic, Motion, and Perception: *De Anima* Book 1', in M.C. Nussbaum and A.O. Rorty (eds.), *Essays on Aristotle's De Anima* (Oxford, 1992), 169–183.

Wittern, R., 'Die psychische Erkrankung in der klassischen Antike', *Sitzungsberichte der Physikalisch-Medizinischen Sozietät zu Erlangen*, N.F. Bd. 3, Heft 1 (1991).

Wittgenstein, L., *Culture and Value: a Selection from the Posthumous Remains* (trans. P. Winch, Oxford, 1980).

Wöhrle G., *Studien zur Theorie der antiken Gesundheitslehre* (*Hermes Einzelschriften* 56) (Stuttgart, 1990).

Wolf, S., *Meaning in Life and Why it Matters* (Princeton, 2010).

World Health Organization, *The ICD-10 Classification of Mental and Behavioural Disorders: Clinical Descriptions and Diagnostic Guidelines* (Geneva, 1992).

Wright, J.P., and Potter, P. (eds.), *Psyche and Soma: Physicians and Metaphysicians on the Mind-body Problem from Antiquity to Enlightenment* (Oxford, 2000).

Wright, M.R. (ed.), *Reason and Necessity. Essays on Plato's* Timaeus (London, 2000).

Wyatt, W.F., 'Homeric ἄτη', *American Journal of Philology* 103 (1982), 247–276.

Yonge, C.D., *Cicero: The Academic Questions, Treatise* De finibus *and Tusculan Disputations* (London, 1880).

INDEX

For the terms that are used for mental disorders in the Hippocratic corpus see 83–93.